This
a.

1

2

HARD CAPSULES

DEVELOPMENT AND TECHNOLOGY

HARD CAPSULES

DEVELOPMENT AND TECHNOLOGY

Edited by

K. Ridgway

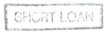
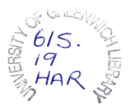
London
THE PHARMACEUTICAL PRESS
1987

Copies of this book may be obtained through any good bookseller, or in any case of difficulty, direct from the publisher or the publisher's agents:

The Pharmaceutical Press
(publications division of The Pharmaceutical Society of Great Britain)
1 Lambeth High Street, London SE1 7JN, England

Australia
The Australian Pharmaceutical Publishing Co. Ltd
35 Walsh Street, West Melbourne 3003

Canada
McAinsh & Co. Ltd
2760 Old Leslie Street, Willowdale, Ontario M2K 2X5

Japan
Maruzen Co. Ltd
3–10 Nihonbashi 2-chome, Chuo-ku, Tokyo 103

New Zealand
The Pharmaceutical Society of New Zealand
124 Dixon Street, PO Box 11–640, Wellington

U.S.A.
Rittenhouse Book Distributors, Inc.,
511 Feheley Drive, King of Prussia, Pennsylvania 19406

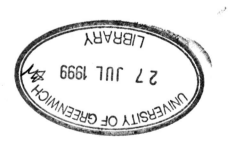

International Standard Book Number (ISBN): 0 85369 159 2. All rights reserved. No part of this publication may be reproduced, stored in a retrieval system, or transmitted in any form or by any means—electronic, mechanical, photocopying or otherwise—without the prior written permission of the copyright holder. Typeset, printed and bound in Great Britain by The Bath Press, Bath BA2 3BL, Avon.

Editor

K. Ridgway, BA, BSc, PhD, Dip Chem Eng, C Chem, FRSC, C Eng, FIChemE
Formerly Senior Lecturer, School of Pharmacy, University of London

Contributors

G. C. Cole, BA, CEng, MIChemE
Staff Specialist—Pharmaceuticals, Davy McKee, London

B. E. Jones, MPharm, MPS
Advisor, Customer Technical Services, Elanco Qualicaps, Lilly Industries Ltd, Basingstoke, Hampshire

R. T. Jones, BSc
Director of Research and Development, Croda Colloids Ltd, Widnes, Cheshire

J. M. Newton, BPharm, PhD, FPS
Professor of Pharmaceutics, School of Pharmacy, University of London

Contents

Preface

The gelatin capsule was originally devised about 150 years ago as a means of masking the unpleasant taste of certain liquid medicaments. These capsules were crudely hand-made. In the intervening years, a sophisticated technology for the mass production of high quality capsules has been developed, and the capsule has become a popular alternative to tablets as a dosage form.

Information on the techniques used in the production of capsules has not been readily available because much of it has been confined to research papers published in a variety of technical journals. This book has been designed to fill the need for a concise description of the history, manufacture, and filling of hard gelatin capsules. The text is supported by nearly 150 illustrations.

The book traces the history of capsule making and filling. The original method of forming capsules by dipping moulds into gelatin solution has not changed, but the mass production of high quality capsules has required the development of complex machinery. After manufacture, capsules must be printed with a name and code number for identification purposes, and then filled. Numerous automated systems have been devised for filling capsules with powders, although manual methods may still be used for small batches for experimental purposes. In addition, pellets, pastes, and liquids can now be filled into hard capsules. Capsules which have been filled must then be check-weighed, cleaned and inspected for faults. The methods and equipment used in all these processes are described.

Gelatin is almost the perfect substance for making capsules and two chapters cover the essential details of the structure, manufacture, and physical and chemical properties of gelatin. However, although gelatin is ideal for the purpose, other materials which might be used as substitutes or extenders have been investigated. There are also various additives which may be used to modify the properties of gelatin.

Capsules must be manufactured to a high quality because of the legislative requirements consequent upon the need for therapeutic effectiveness and patient acceptability. In addition, the manufacturing process requires high standards of inspection and control in order to avoid stoppages and breakdowns due to defective capsules. Guidance is given on pharmacopoeial, manufacturing, and other standards.

Powders which are to be filled into hard capsule shells must have flow properties which allow accurate dosing at high speed. Moreover, the formulation of the powder must take into account the release of the drug (the bioavailability) after ingestion of the capsule. The parameters which must be considered in the formulation of powders for filling into capsules are described and discussed.

The text contains many literature references relevant to the subject matter: these are listed at the end of each chapter. In addition, an extensive structured Bibliography at the end of the book contains over 1300 references on all aspects of capsule technology.

It has not proved possible to include an up-to-date account of the development and manufacture of soft gelatin capsules, but appropriate comparison with hard capsules will be found in several chapters, and relevant references are included in the Bibliography.

Acknowledgments

The expenses of writing and editing this volume were underwritten by Merck Sharp and Dohme Ltd, Hoddesdon, Hertfordshire and their support is gratefully acknowledged.

The assistance of manufacturers in allowing publication of illustrations and details of their machinery and capsules is duly acknowledged. The general editorial staff of the Department of Pharmaceutical Sciences of The Pharmaceutical Society of Great Britain, who assisted in checking and preparing the manuscript for press, are acknowledged with thanks.

Chapter 1

The History of the Gelatin Capsule

B. E. Jones

The word 'capsule' in the English language is derived from the Latin word 'capsula', which means a small box or container. The word occurs in many scientific disciplines, ranging from anatomy, as an enclosing membrane, and botany, as a descriptive word for fruit, to astrophysics, as a space vehicle. In pharmacy, 'capsule' has been used to describe a glass ampoule (e.g. amyl nitrite capsules) and also as a name for a protective cap over the stopper of a bottle of medicine. In more recent times, 'capsule' has been used primarily to describe a solid oral dosage form which consists of a container, usually made of gelatin, filled with a medicinal substance. The word can be used to refer either to the gelatin container itself or to the whole object, container plus drug. In this book it will be used chiefly to mean a single-dose medicine container.

There are many forms of capsule and they can be divided into two main categories which in current usage are described by the adjectives 'hard' and 'soft'. The *hard gelatin capsule* consists of two separate parts, each a semi-closed cylinder in shape, one part being called the 'cap', having a slightly larger diameter than the other, which is called the 'body' and which is longer. The cap fits closely over the body to form a sealed unit. The *soft gelatin capsule* is a one-piece container which has a variable shape, and, due to its method of manufacture, may be either seamed, along its axis, or seamless. The adjectives hard and soft are sometimes applied to soft gelatin capsules, and in this context the terms refer to whether the capsule wall contains glycerol or other plasticiser which makes it soft and elastic, if included, or hard and rigid, if omitted. In current manufacturing practice all one-piece gelatin capsules are soft and elastic.

The Invention of the Gelatin Capsule

The gelatin capsule was invented in the early nineteenth century as a result of the need to mask the obnoxious taste of many of the medicinal substances which were in vogue at that time. One important such drug was the oleoresin of copaiba, which is extremely nauseating when taken by mouth. It was used in the treatment of venereal disease, the incidence of which appears to have been high as a result of the Napoleonic wars and the associated social unrest in Europe. Many unsuccessful attempts were made to overcome this taste problem. Mixtures with the standard pharmaceutical vehicles, aromatic waters, essential oils, honey, and syrups were made, but to no avail. All the culinary arts were employed, even going so far as the making of a 'copaiba custard'. The first successful solution to the problem was the invention of the capsule, which covered the individual dose in a bland tasteless film of gelatin, enabling it to be swallowed easily and without interfering with its activity.

The first recorded patent for a gelatin capsule was French Patent 5648, granted in Paris on 25th March 1834 to Dublanc and Mothes. The idea was quickly acclaimed and its use spread rapidly both inside and outside France. This rapid spread might have been caused either by simultaneous discovery by other workers, or, what is more probable, by the fact that it filled an undoubted need and was a good commercial proposition. In 1835, the year following the first patent, capsules were being manufactured in places as far apart as Berlin and New York (Anon., *Pharm. Era*, 1896a; Schlenz-Casel, 1897).

The actual inventor of the gelatin capsule appears to have been Mothes. In the preamble to the first addition to the patent of Mothes and Dublanc, granted in December 1834, it was stated that Mothes was a pharmacy student, and so was under the legal age to obtain his pharmacy diploma; in order to present the patent he became associated with Dublanc, who was already an established pharmacist. The addition to the patent is further described as being made by Mothes 'in

1

his personal name and in his own private interest'. In 1837 Mothes applied for an extension to the period of validity of the original patent. The French Academy in reviewing his case noted that he had broken off his association with Dublanc (Planche and Gueneau de Mussy, 1837), and granted to him a ten-year extension as the sole proprietor of the invention. Dublanc's name was soon omitted in the many references to capsules made in the contemporary literature.

No copy of the original patent seems to be available. However, the first addition to the patent described the method of manufacture in full, said that 'It was not without its own inconveniences' and went on to describe improvements. The capsules were formed on moulds which were small round pouches made of soft leather tied to a small long-necked metal funnel by a waxed string. The moulds were filled with mercury to make them firm, then dipped into a solution of gelatin, removed and placed in a heated box at 40° to dry. To remove the capsules from the moulds the mercury was emptied out and the gelatin shape was then carefully taken off the mould. To prevent the gelatin adhering to the moulds they were covered in 'baudruche', gold-beater's skin. As a result the capsules had walls consisting of two layers. Mothes considered that this method was expensive and not capable of producing capsules of a large enough size. The improved method of the first addition was to use solid moulds, in the shape of an elongated sphere, and made of burnished brass to prevent oxidation. They were dipped into concentrated solutions of flavoured and sweetened gelatin, then placed upright on a special board and allowed to cool. The capsules were removed before they were completely dry and finished off by being placed on a sieve in a slightly heated room. They were carefully filled with the balsam and then sealed with a drop of gelatin solution.

In France, capsules acquired an immediate popularity. An idea of the extent of this can be gained from the quantities of materials which Mothes was reported as having used in his process: in 1835, 3500 kg of gelatin and in 1836, 1500 kg of copaiba balsam (equivalent to 750 000 doses) (Herpin, 1837). To purchase this large quantity of copaiba he had to travel to London because Paris was unable to supply his needs. His business was extended by increasing the number of types of oil filled into capsules and also by supplying empty capsules to pharmacists.

Capsules rapidly achieved official recognition. When Mothes presented his invention to the Académie Royale de Médecine they paid him a high compliment, saying that he had rendered an immense service to science and humanity (Anon., *Chemist Drugg.*, 1889). In 1837 Dr Ratier made an entry in the '*Dictionnaire de Médecine et de Chirurgie pratiques*' to the effect that capsules were a means of directly administering copaiba without in any way altering its virtues.

In 1838 Mothes ceased to supply empty capsules to the pharmaceutical trade and, as a result, several attempts were made to overcome his patent, which he was rigorously enforcing. In the previous year, when the Economic Committee of the French Academy investigated his application for a patent extension, they found he was employing twenty workmen in his business (Herpin, 1837). They surmised that if the patent was not renewed there would be a rush of other companies into the field. They held the capsule in such high regard that it was proposed that it should be brought to the attention of other industries, and Herpin suggested to the Academy that because of the importance of capsules they should be filled with native resinous medicines that were similar to copaiba, such as turpentine oil. This would have a favourable economic effect and would also be of strategic importance. He obviously suggested this because of the very successful English naval blockade during the Napoleonic wars, which were then still fresh in people's memories. In this year a method was published for masking the flavour of cubeb, copaiba, and other nauseous materials using gelatin, but not as a capsule as defined in the patent (Garot, 1838). The drugs were first formed into standard pill masses, each of which was mounted on a pin and then dipped into a gelatin solution. After drying, the pins were removed and the resulting holes sealed with a drop of gelatin. Garot stated that he had devised this method only because of Mothes's refusal to sell empty capsules.

For some reason, the method mainly quoted in the literature as being used by Mothes was the cumbersome one described in the first patent. This may have been deliberately brought about for commercial reasons, or may have been due to the fact that French patents at that time were handwritten documents and it would have been necessary to attend the patent office in person to read them. The standard source for information was a report on the original patent by Cottereau published in the journal *Traité de Pharmacologie*. As a result, several workers published 'new methods' for making capsules using metal moulds.

In 1846 in the *Journal de Pharmacie et de Chimie*, Giraud claimed a method using iron moulds (Giraud, 1846). The editor in a footnote to the article pointed out that this infringed Mothes's patent. In 1850, in the same journal, there was a report on Mothes's improved method of making capsules using metal moulds which, rather strangely, described the method used by him in his first patent addition fifteen years previously. Alpers, in a history of capsules published in 1896, upbraided Mothes for taking Giraud's idea and claiming it as his own (Alpers, 1896a).

In the United States of America the first mention of capsules in the pharmaceutical literature was in 1835 in the *American Journal of Pharmacy*, which published an abstract of the paper by Cottereau describing their method of manufacture (Cottereau, 1835–6). In the same journal two years later, Alfred Guillou of Philadelphia reported the results of a series of experiments on capsules (Guillou, 1837). These enabled him to make capsules which looked identical to those made in France, so much so that they could not be distinguished from them. In fact he sold them as being of French origin. He used metallic ovoid moulds, mounted on tin dishes, a method exactly as described in Mothes's addition to his patent. Alpers credited Guillou with being the first to suggest this method of manufacture. No practical use appears to have been made of this invention and there is no further record of Guillou's association with capsules.

The first American capsule business was started in New York in 1836 by H. Planten, a Dutchman who had emigrated there in 1835 (Alpers, 1896a). He was described as using French manufacturing methods, selling his capsules as 'Mothes's capsules' and packing them with directions for use in both English and French. The medical profession in America had very rapidly accepted that capsules were an excellent method of administration for copaiba and that France was the source of high quality material. It was many years before capsules of American origin were sold openly and made with American-manufactured gelatin.

In the German-speaking states the invention appears to have been first reported by Buchner (1837). He described Mothes's capsules as copaiba balsam covered in a bubble of glue, and said that the method of making them was unknown. Later

the same year, a Munich physician, Dr Feder, disclosed the secret of their manufacture to those interested (Schlenz-Casel, 1897). He described a method similar to that of Mothes, using solid moulds of hard wood or, later, iron, which were lubricated by dipping in soap spirit. Feldhaus (1912), commenting on the spread of capsule usage in Germany, referred to the fact that there was no uniform patent law at that time and it was only in Prussia, where patents were examined carefully, that the patent of Mothes and Dublanc was upheld. The first large-scale manufacture in Germany is credited to a Berlin pharmacist, J. E. Simon, also in 1837. Schlenz-Casel remarked in 1897 that the rapid spread of capsules in Germany was due to the high profit margin in their manufacture; in that year there were 13 capsule factories listed in the Pharmaceutical Calendar.

In Britain, although capsules appear to have been widely used from an early date, the only references to their manufacture were reports from other countries. The first was an abstract in the *Lancet* in 1840 of a paper by Desfontenelles from the *Journal de Chimie*. This described a method of making 'gelatinous capsules' by an adaptation of the original Mothes and Dublanc patent but using a rather strange mould, the swimming bladder of a tench or other fish from 5 to 7 inches long. This was tied by a ligature to a copper tube, inflated, greased with lard, then dipped in a hot solution of gelatin made to the formula of Garot. When set, the capsule was removed by deflating the bladder.

The first mention in the *Pharmaceutical Journal* came in 1843 with the translation of an article by Adolph Steege, Court Apothecary at Bucharest, called 'On the formation of the gelatinous capsules of Balsam of Copaiba'. The moulds were made of iron, mounted on a wooden plate, and after lubrication with almond oil were dipped in gelatin solution. When the gelatin had set, the capsules were trimmed to the right length, carefully pulled off the moulds and dried on a loose hair sieve. The balsam was filled into them using a glass dropper tube and they were sealed by carefully dipping them into gelatin solution. Steege claimed that capsules could be made elastic by adding sugar to the gelatin solution, and transparent by using isinglass instead of gelatin.

In France, the commercial success of the gelatin capsule stimulated many workers to try to devise ways of overcoming Mothes's patent, which he was enforcing with litigation. Mothes's precise methods were apparently only known to a few people, which led to his improved process, using metallic moulds, being reinvented several times. Sinninoir from Nancy in 1841 suggested the use of wax moulds mounted on metallic pins (Schlenz-Casel, 1897). The moulds were removed from the capsule by heating them and melting the wax, a tedious process which did not prove viable. Moulds for dipping were best made from metal, and there was no success in the search for alternative materials.

Improved Methods of Manufacture of One-piece Gelatin Capsules

Many inventors applied themselves to devising improved mechanical systems. In 1844, Viel obtained a French patent for a method of making and filling the capsule on the same piece of apparatus. He formed a tube of gelatin by dipping hollow cylindrical moulds. The gelatin tubes could be pulled off the moulds and at the same time could have liquid medicaments pumped into them through the centre of the moulds. The filled tubes were cut up into capsules using a special pair of pincers developed from the castration scissors used by farmers (Schlenz-Casel, 1897). Mothes and his new partner Lamouroux claimed infringement, and a panel of three experts considered the case. Two of them considered that Viel's process was an infringement of Mothes's patent, but the third, Professor Chevallier of the School of Pharmacy, Paris, thought Viel's method was significantly different from Mothes's because of the use of a single mould for both making and filling the capsules. He complained also of Mothes's restrictive practices in refusing to sell empty capsules and trying to obtain a monopoly in the supply of copaiba capsules. The Chambre du Conseil accepted the minority opinion, and gave judgement in favour of Viel. Mothes and Lamouroux appealed against the decision, but at the same time purchased Viel's process from him for 37 000 francs. Their appeal was subsequently rejected.

In Italy, also in 1844, Pegna made capsules by casting in moulds instead of by dipping. He used moulds which consisted of a closely-fitting pair of brass plates with the forms of the capsules on their inside surfaces. A gelatin solution was poured into the moulds to form the capsule. A similar process was patented in France in 1846 by Lavalle, a doctor, and Thévenot, a pharmacist, from Dijon (French Patent 3906). Their capsule moulds were a pair of hexagonal copper or iron plates in which suitable cavities had been formed and a plate which acted as a guide to locate the moulds accurately together. Their capsule mass was a solution of gum, sugar, gelatin, and a little honey which they claimed was more soluble than the mixture used by Mothes. It was cast into thin sheets, and a sheet was laid on top of one of the plates, so that it took up the shape of the cavities. The medicament was placed in the hollows. A second sheet was placed on the first and the second plate was put into position by means of the guide plate. The whole assembly was placed in a press and the capsules stamped out. These capsules were much more regular in shape than Mothes's, and they later became known as 'perles'. The inventors made capsules containing liquids, such as copaiba, cod-liver oil, and turpentine oil, and powders such as quinine sulphate and rhubarb. In an addition to this patent in 1850 in the names of Clertan and Lavalle, the capsules were coated with syrup and presented as a bonbon.

Mothes and Lamouroux, using some of Viel's ideas, obtained a patent in December 1846 for a 'machine to prepare and manufacture a large number of Mothes capsules' (French Patent 4780). Their machine was a rotary die type apparatus, a forerunner to the main process in use today. Gelatin ribbons were passed between two sets of rollers. The first set positioned the ribbons. The second set had capsule-shaped cavities in their surfaces so that as the rollers came together capsules were cut out of the ribbons. They called this machine a 'Capsulateur Mécanique', but do not appear to have used it because Mothes obtained another patent for making capsules by dipping in 1850 (Anon., *J. Pharm. Chim.*, *Paris*, 1850). Their problem was probably the difficulty in filling the capsules during manufacture. However, Viel, who had obviously not relinquished his interest in capsules, obtained a patent in 1859 for a 'Capsulateur Viel' (French Patent 43 022). He used large ribbons of gelatin which were passed between rollers turned by hand in a device similar to a clothes mangle. The liquid to be filled was held in a pear-shaped flask and was delivered into the nip of the rollers just where the capsules were formed.

Berthiot, a Parisian pharmacist, patented another method in 1860 (French Patent 43 963). Gelatin solution was forced through an annular orifice to form a tube which was continuously filled with liquid from a concentric tube in the centre. The gelatin tube was chilled to set it and then formed into capsules by passing it between two engraved rollers. This process is the forerunner of that used to make seamless soft gelatin capsules today. Many other patents were granted about this time for improvements to the system for making capsules (Thuret, 1943) which is indicative of the commercial success of the capsule as a dosage form.

Other workers explored the use of alternative materials from which to prepare capsules to defeat Mothes's limitations on trade. Substances were chosen on the basis of alleged improvements in performance *in vivo* over gelatin, perhaps anticipating the present-day interest in drug release. In 1843, Savaresse, father and son, and Douillet obtained a patent for the manufacture of organic capsules called 'Savaresse' (French Patent 15 212). The elder Savaresse was a manufacturer of musical strings and they used the catgut process to prepare thin membranes from the small intestines of sheep. These were cut into small lengths, dipped into sulphurous acid solution as a preservative, and then placed over capsule-shaped moulds. When dry they were removed and filled, the open end being closed with a knot of fine thread and sealed with a drop of gelatin. The inventors argued that a gelatin capsule dissolved too quickly, perhaps even in the mouth, and as a result patients could experience 'nauseous eructations'. They claimed that the membrane passed through the stomach unaffected and disintegrated only in the intestines. This description of an enteric product was made 40 years before the generally-acknowledged inventor of this idea, Unna, published it (Dumez, 1921).

In 1845 a patent for the same membrane capsule was granted in Britain to Evans and Lescher (Anon., *Pharm. J.*, 1845–6). Alpers refers to them as French pharmacists. The same journal also published a letter from a Dr Garrod reporting that a trial of membrane capsules showed that they protected his patients from the taste of copaiba without detracting from its efficacy. A few months later, in the same journal, Dr William Acton wrote a paper entitled 'On the best means of disguising the taste of nauseous medicines', in which he stated that capsules were the best modern method of giving nauseous liquids and that membrane capsules were an improvement over gelatin ones because the latter were often too thin and burst on swallowing. A contemporary advertisement for gelatin capsules made the counter-claim 'They are very easily dissolved in the most delicate stomachs without any effort (the envelope being gum, sugar, and gelatin); they are superior to those made of gluten or membrane, which frequently pass through the stomach without dissolving or are thrown up after uselessly fatiguing the stomach' (Anon., *Chemist Drugg.*, 1868). The relationship between Savaresse, Evans, and Lescher is unknown, but in a letter in the *American Journal of Pharmacy* in 1896 the firm of Evans and Sons of Boston are reported to have been manufacturers of Savaresse capsules (Alpers, 1896b).

Developments in the Use of One-piece Gelatin Capsules

Following on from the numerous patents granted in the 1850s and 1860s the one-piece gelatin capsule became a well-established pharmaceutical item. The extent of the spread of usage can be gauged from the numerous advertisements which appeared in the pharmaceutical press, and from the increasing mention of capsules in books of reference. The first pharmacopoeia to include a monograph on capsules was the French Codex of 1884, which was closely followed by the Dutch Pharmacopoeia of 1889 and the German Pharmacopoeia of 1896 (Jones and Törnblom, 1975).

At the end of the last century the only other significant development was the production of an elastic soft gelatin capsule which is the form that we know today. This was achieved by the addition of glycerol to the mass. Several authors have credited Detenhoff with being the originator of this idea (Alpers, 1896a; Wilkie, 1913). His work was published in the *Pharmazeutische Zeitung für Russland* in 1876. He suggested using a capsule mix consisting of 1 part of gelatin, 2 parts of water, and 2 parts of glycerol, and prepared capsules from this by the standard dipping technique. However, in the previous year, Taetz had been granted a patent for 'an elastic capsule to make it easier to swallow medicines' (French Patent 106 325). His formula was 1 part of gelatin, $1\frac{1}{2}$ parts of glycerol, and $2\frac{1}{2}$ parts of water. The glycerol in these formulations acted as a plasticiser. Since his time other substances have been used to obtain the same effect.

In France, capsules were well established by the end of the nineteenth century. In Britain, the spread was similar but slower. In the pharmaceutical press several attempts were made to popularise their use, particularly for extemporaneous dispensing. The *Chemist and Druggist* in 1888 published an article on capsule manufacture. It explained that if it were known that a dozen capsules could be made in the same time as a dozen suppositories then every pharmacist would adopt this art. It gave a detailed description of how to make moulds, and contained recipes for making both hard and soft capsules. It referred to the perle or globule, which was only popular in France, and included a diagram of how it was made. In 1889 there was an article in the same journal on the Paris Exhibition, which described the part concerning capsules. It posed the question 'Why should English pharmacists have lived for so long with the idea that the industry is a secret one?'. It described the small-scale equipment available. Amongst the exhibitors was a company, Capgrand-Mothes and Company, Paris, which was apparently the successor to Mothes's previous business ventures. Mothes was offering for sale an 'encapsuleur' for filling powders into capsules and also pepsinised capsules, with pepsin in their walls. This article was followed in 1890 by another, by Forret, on the extemporaneous manufacture of flexible gelatin capsules. Ten years later, in the same journal, there was another article on flexible gelatin capsules by a manufacturer who commented that 'it is no unusual thing nowadays to see a prescription for gelatin capsules in place of pills' (Anon., *Chemist Drugg*, 1900).

The rate of increase of capsule usage in Britain can be clearly seen from an examination of *The Extra Pharmacopoeia* started by Martindale and Westcott. The 1st edition was published in 1883 and listed only one capsule product, Oil of Santal. The 5th edition of 1888 listed nine products and also included the first references to a hard two-piece gelatin capsule. This rate of increase gradually accelerated in succeeding years: in the 7th edition of 1892, there were 14 products listed: in the 9th edition of 1898, 24; in the 10th edition of 1901, 31; and in the 11th edition of 1904, 95.

There was a gradual decline in the extemporaneous manufacture of capsules as more and more manufacturers offered for sale an extensive list, covering nearly all the possible requirements. In 1906, A. M. Hance presented a paper to the American Pharmaceutical Association on 'Machine-made vs hand-made soluble elastic capsules'. He said that the improvements in manufacturing technique had almost rendered the hand-made capsule obsolete. He listed nine points of superiority of the machine-made variety which included uniformity, appearance, solubility, stability, and profit (Anon., *Pharm. J.*, 1907).

An account of how the industrial manufacturers of soft gelatin capsules had revolutionised their output was given several years earlier, (Anon., *Chemist Drugg.*, 1890). An American firm of capsule makers had got a new machine for making these useful aids to medication. It had four iron plates, each of which, bearing from 200–250 olives, was dipped automatically into gelatin and sent rolling down a track to the cutter which automatically cut off the waste. Without manual help, these plates rolled on to an elevator and were hoisted on to another track, which rolled them back to the place they started off from, after the capsules had been cleaned. There they were pulled off and tipped into bins. The whole process required but a short time, the greater part of which was the drying step. The machine did the work of about 175 people.

The invention which led to the present large-scale industrial manufacture of capsules was the perfection of the rotary die technique in 1933 by R. P. Scherer, an American citizen of German birth. This process produced capsules of high quality and significantly reduced manufacturing costs. Scherer established a large business, both in making generic preparations and in filling other companies' specialities. After 1945 he established companies in Europe to extend the availability of his service, and since then other companies have entered the field.

The Invention of the Hard Gelatin Capsule

One successful way of overcoming Mothes's patent resulted in the production of a new type of capsule, the hard two-piece, which was the forerunner to the modern hard gelatin capsule. This was invented by another Parisian pharmacist, J. C. Lehuby, who was granted a patent on 20th October, 1846, for 'Mes enveloppes médicamenteuses' (French Patent 4435). The name medicinal envelopes was probably chosen to avoid any patent problems with capsules. Lehuby described them as cylindrical in shape, like silk-worm cocoons, composed of two compartments or cups which fitted one inside the other to form a box. The moulds used were silver-plated metal cylinders about 4 to 5 centimetres long, varying in diameter from several millimetres to several centimetres. The diameters of the two half-moulds were different, so that the cast halves fitted together snugly. Capsules were made by dipping the moulds into a decoction of starch or tapioca, the consistency of a bouillie, which was sweetened with a little sugar, and coloured with 'fish silver'.

The patent was quickly followed by three additions. The first was granted on 20th January 1847, extending the range of materials to be used for making the envelopes, and referring to them for the first time as capsules. The prime material recommended was carragheen, to which could be added, if necessary, various gelatins, gums, and glues. On the same day he was granted a completely separate patent for a new gelatin derived from carragheen moss, *Fucus crispus*. This he described as having superior properties to animal gelatins, which were too brittle. His second addition was made in November 1847, and here he called his envelopes 'capsules-boîtes', capsule boxes. He described improvements in his equipment for making capsules, using several moulds mounted on a disc, and an improved method for making his new gelatin from carragheen. The third addition, granted in 1850, was in the name of Lehuby, Silbermann and Garnier. This commented that earlier capsules were either brittle or had an unpleasant smell, and a further-improved process was given for extracting gelatin from carragheen moss. This was still the preferred material for the manufacture of capsules which they called 'capsules en lichen'. The formulation for the solution for making capsules was: 10 litres of water, 1.8 kg of dried carragheen extract, 0.9 kg of animal gelatin to reduce the hygroscopicity of the capsules, and 2 or 3 litres of a decoction of marshmallow root to overcome the brittleness caused by the gelatin.

Although Lehuby was the undoubted inventor of the two-piece gelatin capsule, many authors have credited it to J. Murdoch, who was granted British Patent 11 937 in London on 2nd May 1848 for 'An improved capsule or small case for protecting matters enclosed therein from the action of air; and an improved material to be used in their manufacture'. The patent described, in the same wording as used in Lehuby's patent, two-piece capsules, a method for their manufacture, and how to make a vegetable gelatin from carragheen moss. It was also the first patent which admitted the sole use of animal gelatin for making capsules.

Murdoch was a patent agent by profession, a fact stated in the patent. Thuret (1943) was the first to point out the similarities between the patents of Lehuby and Murdoch, particularly in the use of vegetable gelatin. Murdoch's patent preamble states that 'it was communicated to me from abroad,' and all the evidence points to Lehuby's being the original inventor. The probable reason for Murdoch's being credited with the invention was the commercial and communication problems of that time. The use of Mothes's capsules spread quickly into many countries, which resulted in many references to them in the literature and caused them to be sold under a French guise, acknowledging their origin. Lehuby's capsules, on the other hand, were not so quickly taken up by the pharmaceutical trade. There was a 30-year gap between the patents and the proper commercial use of hard gelatin capsules, and very few references to them appeared in the literature. In fact two authoritative papers on the history of capsules by Alpers (1896a) and Wilkie (1913), failed to mention either Lehuby's or Murdoch's part in the development of capsules.

In both Britain and Germany at the beginning of this century, hard gelatin capsules were referred to as being of American origin. The first published reference to them outside Britain and France was in 1848 in *Dingler's Polytechnischen Journal* which had an abstract taken from the *London Journal of the Arts* recording Murdoch's patent. Feldhaus (1912) in Germany, in a history of capsules, dismissed the claims of a Viennese pharmacist, Gross von Figely, to have invented them, and recorded Murdoch as the inventor. He used *Dingler's Polytechnischen Journal* as his information source. Two years later, Urdang (1914) in the U.S.A. also gave credit to this belief. These works have become the standard historical reference sources for others and as a result the original error has been perpetuated.

Mothes appears to have been unsuccessful in maintaining the exclusive use of his patent for making soft gelatin capsules, despite resorting to litigation. In countries outside France, capsules were sold openly under the guise of being made in France, or of French origin, even when manufactured locally. His efforts are illustrated by an amusing story from the *Pharmaceutical Journal* of 1857 called 'Mothes' Capsules—extraordinary proceedings'. A London pharmacist was taken to court by Mothes's agents for selling counterfeit capsules. These had been purchased from a recognised wholesaler, and there was an out-of-court settlement for £19. 3s. 4d. It was found that a London company had been making and selling capsules as 'genuine Mothes' for at least 10 years previously, packing them as Mothes's with a green label, seal, and signature. A solicitor's letter warned all pharmacists that they should not be fooled by such crude imitations and that they would be prosecuted if they sold counterfeit capsules. The editor noted that during his enquiries he had purchased two genuine boxes of Mothes's capsules which were dissimilar, and that the London 'imitation' capsules were closer in appearance to one of the genuine specimens than the genuine ones were to each other.

The Development of Hard Gelatin Capsules

After the first patents, the spread in the use of hard gelatin capsules appears to have been delayed for two reasons. Firstly, the most popular medicinal substances in use were galenicals, which were frequently liquid or semi-solid and thus were more suited to being filled into soft gelatin capsules. Secondly, to make a two-piece capsule which fitted together properly required numbers of accurately-made moulds, which were an expensive item.

The first recorded large-scale manufacture of hard two-piece capsules was by an American company, H. Planten of New York. They were an old-established capsule house, having started making soft gelatin capsules as early as 1836. In the early 1860's they produced two-piece capsules made from jujube paste, a material used in the confectionery trade. This was similar to the material described by Lehuby in the first patent. Problems arose because of their poor fit and they were discontinued.

The first successful manufacturer of hard gelatin capsules on a commercial scale was a Detroit pharmacist, F. A. Hubel (Wilkie, 1913). He overcame the problem of making low-cost but accurate moulds by using pieces of gauge iron rod or wire set in wooden blocks. It is recorded by Wilkie that Hubel became interested in such capsules after being told of them by one of his friends who had watched them being made in Italy. Crude lead moulds had been used, and the two parts of the capsules, which had the same diameter, had to be dampened afer filling to allow them to be forced together. In 1874, Hubel started manufacturing capsules. For each size he used two sets of mould pins, one for the cap and one for the body, with different diameters, so that a good telescopic fit of the two halves was obtained. The mould pins were set in wooden blocks. They were dipped into gelatin solution and withdrawn to produce a film that, whilst still wet, was cut to the required length using a pen-knife. The coated moulds were left to stand for the films to air-dry; when ready, the capsule pieces were removed from the moulds with brass tongs and joined together.

The capsule quickly achieved popularity, particularly after 1875, when the whole of Hubel's output was sold for him by another Detroit company, Parke, Davis, who applied aggressive sales and promotional methods (Stadler, 1959). Hubel continually improved his methods and in February 1877 was granted the first of several patents for his equipment. In the period 1877 to 1883 a large number of patents were granted for capsule-making machines (Alpers, 1896a). Disputes arose over priority but in the lawsuits which followed Hubel was successful in establishing his claims. When he retired in 1900 his plant had a production capacity of one million capsules per day.

The commercial success of hard gelatin capsules soon brought other companies into the field. Several of these were in Detroit, and one of them was the Merz Capsule Co. This company, which was founded in 1887, started manufacture in a 1200-square foot loft, and was one of several companies that, in 1894, successfully opposed the 'Capsule Trust', a group of companies that tried to force up the price of capsules (Anon., *Pharm. Era*, 1896b). The Trust was defeated after extensive litigation, which had an unsettling effect on the market. By 1896, however, Merz's output had expanded and the plant occupied a three-storey factory with a floor space of 25 200 square feet. Its capacity was then 750 000 capsules per day, and it was exporting to Canada, the West Indies, Central and South America, and the Hawaiian Islands.

The local concentration of small manufacturers led to an amalgamation of a number of competing firms who, under the aegis of W. Wilkie, a pioneer of capsule engineering, formed the U.S. Capsule Company, which supplied most of its products to Parke, Davis. In 1901 this company, together with its subsidiary the M.L. Capsule Company, were purchased by Parke, Davis, who now acquired their own manufacturing capacity for the first time, despite the fact that they had been active in capsule selling since 1875. In 1897 Eli Lilly & Co., Indianapolis, included capsules of their own manufacture in their price list. Their first capsule-plant manager was R. P. Hobbs, who in 1894 was granted two patents for self-locking capsules (U.S. Patents 525 844 and 525 845). This invention antedated by some 70 years the modern use of this idea.

The manufacture of capsules was largely, but not wholly, restricted to the U.S.A. In 1910 the estimated world production was over one thousand million capsules per year, of which 90% were made in the U.S.A. The only other country in which there appears to have been production activity was Germany. In the 1890s, 13 companies were listed in the German pharmaceutical calendar as manufacturers of capsules, the bulk of their output being the various forms of soft gelatin capsule, but at least one manufacturer, G. G. Pohl of Schönbaum near Danzig, made hard gelatin capsules. These were recommended for oils though, surprisingly, not powders, and appear to have been widely used. A stand for holding capsules whilst filling them with oil, devised by Tschanter, was shown in several journals (Anon., *Pharm. J.*, 1896).

The large demand for capsules gave a stimulus to continued engineering development to improve both the product and the efficiency of the process. Capsules made on the original iron moulds became discoloured, but Wilkie introduced first phosphor-bronze, then stainless steel, mould pins. Initially the capsules were cut to the correct length immediately after dipping, but eventually they were cut at a later stage, when the film had dried, in order to improve the quality of the cut edge; this facet of capsule quality was frequently mentioned in sales literature at the turn of the century (Eli Lilly & Co.).

The two factors which have contributed most to the vast increase in capsule output are air-conditioning and machinery design. Most of the production cycle is taken up by the drying process, and it was not until manufacturing machines were installed in air-conditioned areas that it was possible to produce capsules efficiently all the year round, without halting production during the hot humid summer months. The first recorded all-the-year-round manufacture was in 1912 (Eli Lilly & Co.).

There has been a continuous improvement in machine design. In 1896 each capsule machine, operated by one man, could produce 10 000 to 12 000 per day. Each capsule had to be manually trimmed and individually joined, but this last manual step was eliminated in 1913 by the first fully-automatic machine for making hard gelatin capsules, designed by B. W. Scott, of the Arthur Colton Co. of Detroit, for Eli Lilly & Co. (U.S. Patent 1 076 459). This machine was called the 'Stacker machine' because it took the pin bars, with dried capsule films on them, and stacked them in an upright position before feeding them through the section where the capsule parts were stripped, cut to length, and the the two halves joined. The capsule moulds were mounted 30 to each bar and

there were 175 pairs of bars on the machine. The whole cycle was now automatic and the output was about 8000 capsules per hour. Originally there was only one gelatin container and as a result only single-coloured capsules could be produced. Several years later, the machine was modified to enable two-coloured capsules to be made. A second gelatin container was added and a device incorporated to separate the body and cap mould bars for the dipping operation. Another feature of the machine was that the pin bars were held stationary in an inverted position and the gelatin solution container was raised up to them.

The design on which nearly all modern large-scale machines are based was patented by Arthur Colton in 1931 and assigned to Parke, Davis & Co. (U.S. Patent 1 787 777, and British Patent 360 427). This differed from previous machines in that the machine was divided into two parts through which the cap and body pins passed separately but synchronously. The machine was much larger, holding over 700 pairs of pin bars, and had an output of 30 000 capsules per hour. It was able to produce two-coloured capsules because there were separate gelatin containers. The capsules produced were of a more uniform thickness, due to the procedure of lowering the moulds into the gelatin solution and then removing them to spread the gelatin film more evenly over the pins.

Modern machines, as well as running faster, have been improved so that they can run on a 24-hour day, all-year-round basis with only short periodic stops for maintenance and holidays (Martyn, 1974). The machines are constructed either by the manufacturers themselves or by specialist machinery manufacturers such as Cherry Burrell of Detroit.

The Use of Capsules as a Dosage Form

Capsules, because of their elongated shape, are easy to swallow, which is one reason for the number of capsule-shaped tablets manufactured today. Patients are sometimes timid about their ability to swallow a capsule because they look at its largest dimension, its length, and imagine that it will never go down their throats. They do not realise that the tongue reflexively lines up a capsule end-on for swallowing. Advice on how to take capsules has been given since earliest times. Dr William Acton (1845–6) said to 'recommend such sceptics (people unable to swallow) to take about a dessert spoonful of water in their mouth, and then place the capsule on the tongue, when the whole will be swallowed without difficulty, whereas, if the capsule be placed on the tongue and water be drunk, the patient will often swallow the water, but the capsule will remain and produce convulsive action of the pharynx'.

The consumers of hard gelatin capsules are still not too familiar with them despite their long history. Many patients are under the misapprehension that they are made of plastic. This, in the loosest chemical terms, could be said to be true in that gelatin is a polymer prepared from an organic starting material. The apocryphal story about the use of capsules is of the patient who thinks the shells are inedible and empties out the contents to take them. Like all tales of this nature its origins go back many years. Taylor (1915) quoted an item from the Louisville Medical News of 1877: 'physician states that an intelligent gentleman has been given capsules to take without specific directions and later informed the physician that he did not like them at all, his idea of taking them being to peel off the hulls and put the stuff in water'.

Soft gelatin capsules come in a wide range of shapes and sizes, governed solely by the dose required and the method of manufacture. However, because hard gelatin capsules are manufactured empty by one supplier and filled by another there has been the need to produce standard sizes, particularly when machine-filling is involved. Hubel in 1875 was already making capsules in three standard sizes known as numbers 1, 2, and 3 (Stadler, 1959). No reference appears in the literature as to how the standard sizes 000, 00, 0, 1, 2, 3, 4, and 5 were arrived at. It has been suggested that they were simply based on standard engineering dimensions for iron rods (Jones and Turner, 1974). Wilkie, one of the early capsule experts, is reported to have entered capsule manufacturing because he had been a salesman supplying capsule makers with accurately-gauged iron for their moulds.

Lehuby described capsules as being preferably cylindrical in shape with hemispherical ends. Over the years several variations on that theme have been patented. In 1865 an American, D. Dick, was granted a patent for a cone-shaped capsule (Alpers, 1896a). Parke, Davis in 1896 offered for sale in Britain a rectal capsule which differed from the normal one in that it had a pointed cap-half to facilitate insertion (Chemist Drugg., 1896). In 1914 R. J. Estes of Oklahoma was granted a patent

for a capsule which had its body-end edge cut away at an oblique angle to facilitate the closing of the two halves together (U.S. Patent 1 122 089). Non-standard shapes of capsules are produced by several large pharmaceutical companies in the U.S.A. in order to prevent counterfeiting of their products. For example, Smith Kline & French use capsules with flat ends and bevelled shoulders, and Eli Lilly & Co. use capsules with paraboloidal ends to the bodies (Physicians' Desk Reference, 1985).

Probably the only significant change in basic design since the time of Lehuby has been the development of the self-locking capsule. One of the drawbacks in the industrial use of hard gelatin capsules was that when filled they could be vibrated apart, with consequent powder spillage, especially when handled on automatic packaging machines. To overcome this, two methods of sealing capsules were used, banding and dot-sealing, but both have the disadvantages of being time-consuming, costly, and spoiling the appearance of the capsule (Jones, 1969). It was pointed out in the Pharmaceutical Journal, in 1912, that capsules which were trimmed before they were dry had a rough body edge, which acted as a sort of spring lock to hold the capsules together (Anon., Pharm. J., 1912).

The best solution to the problem was the development of the self-locking capsule which enabled the two halves to stay closed during rough handling without the need for a post-filling operation. The first recorded patent, as mentioned earlier, for a self-locking capsule was granted in 1894, to R. P. Hobbs of Indianapolis (U.S. Patent 525 844). His capsules had a circular constriction ring around the cap and a slightly bell-shaped body. The patent stated 'This tight fit or lock fit will prevent separation during joining or handling'.

In 1913, M. Pollock of New York obtained a patent for a cylindrical flat-ended capsule which had engaging notches in the cap and body to prevent the capsule's coming apart (U.S. Patent 1079 438). However, either these ideas presented production problems or they were not required by the users, because they were not commercially exploited. The first modern patent for such a system was granted to Eli Lilly & Co. in 1963, for capsules called 'Lok-Caps' (French Patent 1 343 698). A series of indentations inside the capsule cap forms a friction seal when the capsule is closed after filling. Since then two other companies, Parke, Davis and R. P. Scherer, have patented similar systems to perform this function; these capsules are described in Chapter 11.

Enteric Capsules

Capsules are usually required to dissolve in the stomach as rapidly as possible, releasing their contents, but for certain purposes they are designed to pass through the stomach and into the intestine before dissolving. Such products are described by a variety of terms, including gastric-resistant, entero-soluble, and enteric. Their production was first suggested in the 1880s as a means of administering medicines which were very irritant to the gastric mucosa. The first true enteric coating of products is credited to the German, Dr Unna (Dumez, 1921). Prior to this time people had used fats and waxes to coat the products to try to prevent disintegration in the stomach. Unna suggested the use of a keratin coating on pills so that they were insoluble in the acid secretion of the stomach but soluble in the alkaline secretions of the intestine. Unna's pills were first sold in Germany in 1884. Subsequently the firm of Pohl, in Schönbaum, offered for sale keratinised capsules 'kapsulae keratinosae', prepared not from gelatin but from a mixture of keratin, shellac, borax, and colophony. They did not perform well *in vivo* because the contents tended to absorb water and swell, bursting the capsule shell (Pohl, 1892).

In 1895 a Swiss pharmacist, Dr Weyland, offered a different solution to the problem by suggesting the use of formaldehyde to 'harden' the capsules so that the consequent increase in their solution time would carry them through the stomach before they dissolved (Dumez, 1921). The capsules were treated by soaking them in an aqueous solution of formaldehyde for a short period then drying them in a warm place. This process was patented in Germany by Hausmann, Weyland's employer, in 1895. Hausmann obtained a second patent in the same year for a similar process which used another aldehyde, acrolein.

In 1904, Rumpel suggested a means whereby empty capsules could be treated with formaldehyde. However, his method lacked some logic because he recommended that after filling, the capsule should be sealed by painting the joint with collodion or gelatin solution and re-treating; the latter process, it would seem, obviated the need for the initial treatment. Capsules produced by Rumpel's method were called 'kapsulae geloderatae' and were sold in Germany by the firm of Pohl of Schönbaum. They were also sold in America where they were known as 'Pohl's enteric capsules'.

In 1907 the firm of Evans Sons Lescher and Webb obtained a patent for 'Improvements relating to gelatine capsules containing medicines for internal use' (British Patent 23 337). They described the manufacture of a two-layered capsule from prepared animal intestinal membranes, which were rendered enteric by coating them with cocoa butter, paraffin wax, or other suitable vegetable, animal, or mineral fat.

Enteric products fell into disrepute for two reasons, both of which led to poor *in vivo* results. The first was that the formaldehyde treatment, despite being a simple process, had its limitations. The reaction between gelatin and formaldehyde proceeds by a cross-linking mechanism which, once started, continues even when the capsules are removed from the aldehyde. In *The Extra Pharmacopoeia* in 1910, there is an entry for formagules, formolised gelatin capsules, which states that 'they cannot be relied upon if stored for too long' (Martindale and Westcott, 1910). Dumez, in 1921, in his history of the development of enteric-coated capsules, pointed out that despite what certain workers had said there was evidence pointing to the instability of formaldehyde-treated capsules and concluded that 'only time would tell'.

The second reason was that the coating materials, whose function relied upon the changes in solubility with pH, were chosen on the basis of an incorrect physiological assumption. They were intended to be insoluble at the acid pH of the stomach but to be soluble at an alkaline pH, which was assumed to be the condition in the duodenum. It has more recently been shown that the pH of the duodenum is seldom, if ever, alkaline (Kanig, 1954). During the first half of this century many workers searched for suitable materials and amongst others, shellac, tolu, mastic, resin, carnauba wax, and salol were tried.

It was not until the development of modified cellulose derivatives such as cellacephate, which had the correct solubility properties, i.e. insoluble in strongly acid solution but soluble at slightly acid pH values, that satisfactory products were produced (Jones, 1970).

References

Acton, W., *Pharm. J.*, 1845–6, *5*, 502–505.
Alpers, W. C., *Am. J. Pharm.*, 1896a, *68*, 481–494.
Alpers, W. C., *Am. J. Pharm.*, 1896b, *68*, 575.
Anon., *Chemist Drugg.*, 1868, *9*, 835.
Anon., *Chemist Drugg.*, 1888, *32*, 496.

Anon., *Chemist Drugg.*, 1889, *35*, 214.
Anon., *Chemist Drugg.*, 1890, *36*, 64.
Anon., *Chemist Drugg.*, 1896, *48*, 584–585.
Anon., *Chemist Drugg.*, 1900, *56*, 131–133.
Anon., *Dingler's Polytech. J.*, 1848, *109*, 397–399.
Anon., *J. Pharm. Chim.*, *Paris*, 1850, *17*, 204–205.
Anon., *London Journal of the Arts*, 1848, *2*(5), 42–44.
Anon., *Pharm. Era*, 1896a, *29*, 992–993.
Anon., *Pharm. Era*, 1896b, *29*, 994.
Anon., *Pharm. J.*, 1845–6, *5*, 361–363.
Anon., *Pharm. J.*, 1857–8, *17*, 43–44.
Anon., *Pharm. J.*, 1896, *56*, 307.
Anon., *Pharm. J.*, 1912, *88*, 778–779.
Buchner, A., *Repertorium für die Pharmazie*, 1837, *61*, per Schlenz-Casel, *Apothekerzeitung, Berl.*, 1897, *34*, 275–276.
Cottereau, *Traité de Pharmacologie*, per *Am. J. Pharm.*, 1835–6, *1*, 351–352.
Desfontenelles, *J. Chim.*, per *Lancet*, 1839–40, *1*, 901.
Detenhoff, *Pharmazeutische Zeitung für Russland*, 1876, per *Am. J. Pharm.*, 1878, *50*, 295, and *J. Pharm. Chim.*, *Paris*, 1878, *28*, 73–74.
Dumez, A. G., *J. Am. pharm. Ass.*, 1921, *10*, 372–376.
Eli Lilly & Co., Indianapolis, U.S.A., company archives.
Feldhaus, F. M., *Chemikerzeitung*, 1912, *35*, 697.
Forret, J. A., *Chemist Drugg.*, 1890, *37*, 291–292.
Garot, M., *J. Pharm.*, *Paris*, 1838, *24*, 78-80.
Giraud, A., *J. Pharm. Chim.*, *Paris*, 1846, *9*, 354–355.
Guillou, A., *Am. J. Pharm.*, 1837, *3*, 20–22.
Gueneau de Mussy and Guibourt, *J. Pharm. Chim.*, *Paris*, 1848, *14*, 350–352.
Hance, A., *Pharm. J.*, 1907, *78*, 205–206.

Herpin, *Bulletin de la Société d'Encouragement pour l'Industrie Nationale*, 1837, *36*, 219–221.
Jones, B. E., *Mfg Chem.*, 1969, *40*(2), 25–28.
Jones, B. E., *Mfg Chem.*, 1970, *41*(5), 53–54 and 57.
Jones, B. E., and Turner, T. D., *Pharm. J.*, 1974, *213*, 614–617.
Jones, B. E., and Törnblom, J.-F. V., *Pharm. Acta Helv.*, 1975, *50*, 33–45.
Kanig, J. L., *Drug Stand.*, 1954, *22*, 113–121.
Martindale, W. H. and Westcott, W. W., *The Extra Pharmacopoeia*, 14th Edn, London, H. K. Lewis, 1910, pp. 542–545.
Martyn, G. W., *Drug Devel. Comm.*, 1974–5, *1*, 39–49.
Physicians Desk Reference, 39th Edn, Oradell, New Jersey, Medical Economics Co. Inc., 1985.
Planche and Gueneau de Mussy, *Bulletin de l'Académie Royale de Médecine*, 1837, 442–443.
Pohl, G., per *Pharmazeutische Centralhalle für Deutschland*, 1892, *33*, 512–514.
Ratier, M. F., *Dictionnaire de Médecine et de Chirurgie pratiques*, Vol. XV, p. 285–8, per Alpers, W. C., *Am. J. Pharm.*, 1896a, *68*, 481–494.
Schlenz-Casel, *Apothekerzeitung, Berl.*, 1897, *34*, 275–276.
Stadler, L. B., *J. Am. Pharm. Ass.*, pract. Pharm. Edn, 1959, *20*, 723–724.
Steege, A., *Repertorium für die Pharmazie*, per *Pharm. J.*, 1842–3, *2*, 769–770.
Taylor, F. O., *J. Am. pharm. Ass.*, 1915, *4*, 468–481.
Thuret, A., *Travaux des Laboratoires de Matière Médicale et de Pharmacie Galénique de la Faculté de Pharmacie de Paris*, 1943 to 1945, *32*(76), Pt 1, 7–257.
Urdang, G., *Pharm. Archs*, 1914, *14*, 58–59.
Wilkie, W., *Bull. Pharm.*, Detroit, 1913, *27*, 382–384.

Chapter 2

Gelatin: Structure and Manufacture

R. T. Jones

Gelatin has all the properties required to meet the needs of the pharmaceutical capsule industry. These include solubility, solution viscosity, and thermally reversible gelation properties in aqueous solution. It produces strong, clear, flexible, high-gloss films which dissolve readily under the conditions existing in the stomach. However, other industries could also claim gelatin as their own. The solution viscosity, gelation, melting point, clarity, and texture characteristics which are peculiar to gelatin go to make the edible table jelly; it has so far remained unmatched by other hydrocolloids for this purpose. The photographic film industry is based upon the unique ability of gelatin to suspend silver halide crystals and to control their growth during the digestion and ripening stages, coupled with its solution, gel, and film properties. In fact, the origins of gelatin manufacture can be traced back as far as 4000 B.C.

Crude gelatin was extracted by cooking hide pieces in water, and its interest lay in the adhesive properties of this animal glue. The history of gelatin manufacture has been traced by Bogue (1922), by Smith (1929) and by Koepff (1985). It shows that the earliest practical manufacture of animal glue which can be related to the present day gelatin industry was established in Holland in the seventeenth century and was introduced into England during the early part of the eighteenth century. In the United States, the earliest records show that glue manufacture dates back to 1808.

The first reference to glue in the patent literature was in 1754 when a patent assigned to Zomer (British Patent 691) described glue preparation from fish waste.

Bone glue extraction was apparently covered in an 1814 patent (Bogue, 1922) and over the following forty years or so patents covering various aspects of glue manufacture were granted, including the demineralisation of bone, the use of sulphurous acid, the vacuum evaporation of liquors, and the use of dehumidified air in drying. The basis of modern gelatin manufacturing practice had been established by about 1850.

The first mention of the use of gelatin for edible purposes is found in a patent assigned to Cooper in 1845, which described the preparation of jellies by mixing gelatin with 'sugar, lemon or lime juice, eggs and sundry spices'. About the same time, hard and soft gelatin capsules were developed. In 1878, gelatin was first used in photographic emulsions. Today, it finds application in industries as diverse as pharmaceuticals, photography, food, wine, cosmetics, paper, printing, and abrasives. Koepff (1985) gives a very detailed summary of industrial gelatin production in Western Europe from the mid 19th century to 1983.

There are no official published figures for the total world-wide consumption of gelatin but it was estimated by Flausch (1978) to be of the order of 120 000 tons per annum in 1976, and by Koepff (1985) to be approximately 140 000 tons in 1982.

The major outlet for gelatin is still the food industry, which takes about 70% of the gelatin produced. Approximately 15% is consumed by the pharmaceutical industry, 10% by the photographic industry, and the remaining 5% or so finds its way into other markets.

Within the pharmaceutical industry, hard and soft capsules constitute the major use for gelatin but other applications exist, such as micro-encapsulation, tablet binding, tablet coating, emulsion stabilisation, and the manufacture of pastes and suppositories. The pharmaceutical and medical applications of gelatin have been reviewed (Jones, 1971).

THE STRUCTURE OF GELATIN

Gelatin is not a naturally-occurring protein, but is derived from the fibrous protein collagen, which is the principal constituent of animal skin, bone, sinew, and connective tissue. Any discussion of the structure of gelatin requires, therefore, an

13

understanding of the nature and structure of collagen and of its conversion to gelatin.

The Structure of Collagen

The primary structure of collagen arises from the linkage of α-amino and imino acids by peptide bonds to form a polymer. The amino acid compositions of a variety of mammalian collagens have been compared by Eastoe and Leach (1958), Eastoe (1967), and Eastoe and Leach (1977), and although some differences are apparent between collagens from different sources, there are certain features which are common to, and uniquely characteristic of, collagen. Collagen is the only mammalian protein containing large amounts of hydroxyproline and hydroxylysine and the total imino acid (proline and hydroxyproline) content is high; approximately one-third of the residues consist of glycine, and methionine is the only sulphur-containing amino acid present: cysteine and cystine are absent, as is tryptophan.

It is now known that the similarities between mammalian collagens of different sources, as noted by Eastoe and others, belie the existence of several different types of collagen existing in various tissues and organs. Although they show the general characteristics of collagen, the various collagen forms differ in amino acid composition and molecular weight species. This was first noted by Miller and Matukas (1969), and by 1982 (Miller and Gay, 1982), the existence of nine collagen types had been demonstrated. By 1986, the number stood at eleven. Fortunately for the consideration of commercial gelatin production, a single collagen type, 'Type I', constitutes practically all the collagen present in bone and tendon and predominates (80% or more) in hide.

Wide-angle X-ray diffraction studies show that collagen has a pattern indicative of long intertwined filaments (Ramachandran and Kartha, 1954; Cowan et al., 1955; Rich and Crick, 1961), and narrow-angle X-ray diffraction shows that there exists a characteristic spacing of approximately 64 nm for dry collagen. This pattern can also be seen under the electron microscope, indicating that the microscopic fibrils are composed of much thinner filaments, or protofibrils, which possess specifically ordered chemical and structural variations along their main axes (Wolpers, 1941, 1950; Hall et al., 1942; Schmitt et al., 1945; Schmitt and Gross, 1948).

The structure of collagen has been studied intensively, and several useful reviews have been published (Gustavson, 1956; Harrington and von Hippel, 1961; Ward, 1964; Harding, 1965; Bailey, 1968; Piez, 1968; Balian and Bowes, 1977; Fraser et al., 1979; Glanville and Kühn, 1979; Miller and Gay, 1982; Privalov, 1982).

There is now a generally accepted model of the collagen molecular structure, although certain details remain vague. The collagen unit, or monomer (tropocollagen), consists of a triple helix of three polypeptide chains, each of which has a helically coiled configuration. This is a threefold left-handed screw, in which each amino acid extends 120 degrees around the coil axis and 0.312 nm along the direction of the axis. Thus each chain is built up of triplets of amino acids, with every third residue being in a similar environment, and glycine appearing as every third residue. The three coiled chains are coiled around each other to give a right-handed coil of about 1.4 nm diameter, forming a tropocollagen molecule, which behaves as a rigid rod with a length of 300 nm and a molecular weight of approximately 300 000.

The triple helical structure arises from two factors. Firstly, the glycine residues permit triple chain packing by allowing the chains to come close enough for hydrogen bonding to occur and, secondly, the high content of imino acids directs the individual chains into a poly-L-proline II-type helix (Cowan and McGavin, 1955), through steric hindrance to rotation.

The tropocollagen molecules are joined together in an end-to-end fashion to form protofibrils and these, in turn, form fibrils by aggregation. Freely dangling, single peptide chains (telopeptides) at one or both ends of the tropocollagen molecule are believed to be responsible for 'cementing' together the basic units. A periodicity of 64 nm in the axial direction of the collagen fibril is apparent when the fibril has been negatively stained with phosphotungstic acid and observed under the electron microscope. Hodge and Petruska (1962) have explained this banded structure as being due to a regular staggered arrangement of molecules in which the dark bands represent gaps between adjacent molecules. This is most easily understood by reference to the schematic model shown in Fig. 2.1A, and the molecular geometry diagram in Fig. 2.1B.

The explanation for the ordered arrangement of molecules in the fibrils appears to lie in the side-chain groups of the amino acid residues (Hulmes et al., 1973). These can interact with

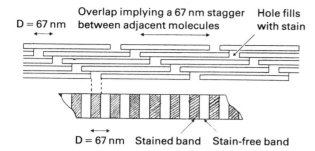

Fig. 2.1A. Schematic diagram of the packing arrangement of tropocollagen molecules in the native fibril, according to the model of Hodge and Petruska (1962).

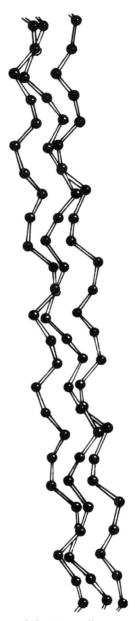

Fig. 2.1B. Diagram of the tropocollagen molecule, showing only the α-carbon atoms in the chains.

side-chain groups on an adjacent molecule, and that spatial arrangement which allows the maximum number of favourable interactions will be the most stable thermodynamically. These pairs of interacting amino acids apparently occur 64 nm apart in the sequence, and this is true not only for ionic interaction, between, for example, the positively charged side chain of arginine and the negatively charged aspartic acid residue, but also for the hydrophobic bonds formed by eliminating water from between two amino acids.

In addition to these bonds there are a smaller number of stronger covalent cross-links between chains in adjacent molecules (intermolecular cross-links) and also between chains within the same tropocollagen molecule (intramolecular cross-links). Evidence for the existence of various types of covalent bonds in native collagen has been reviewed by Harding (1965). Bonds involving ester, carbohydrate, aldehyde, ε-amino, and γ-glutamyl groups were considered. Subsequently, the principal intermolecular and intramolecular cross-links have been shown to be those involving aldehyde groups formed from lysine residues (Bailey *et al.*, 1974; Light and Bailey, 1979). The initial stage in the formation of intermolecular bonds is the oxidative deamination of lysine residues (in the case of skin collagen) or hydroxylysine residues (in the case of bone collagen) located in the non-helical, end-chain regions of the molecules by the enzyme lysyloxidase. The aldehydes produced then condense with side-chain amino groups of hydroxylysine residues situated in the helical regions of neighbouring molecules. Intramolecular cross-links are established by the aldol condensation of lysine aldehyde groups on adjacent chains. These bonds are important in conferring

high tensile strength and resistance to chemical attack on the collagen fibres.

SOLUBLE COLLAGEN
Certain solutions, such as dilute alkali buffers (Harkness *et al.*, 1954), salt solutions (Gross *et al.*, 1955; Jackson and Fessler, 1955; Gallop *et al.*,

1957), and acid buffers (Orekhovich *et al.*, 1948) are able to extract a small proportion of collagen in a soluble form. The existence of a biological precursor of tropocollagen, 'procollagen', has been identified (Layman *et al.*, 1971; Bellamy and Bornstein, 1971). However, the situation is simplified for Type I collagen for which procollagen exists fleetingly, if at all, outside the fibroblast cells. The extent to which collagen can be solubilised in this way depends upon the collagen source and its age (Johns, 1977). Present knowledge of the structure of collagen owes much to studies on this soluble form and particularly to the discovery that it can be precipitated in various forms, some of which exhibit the characteristic banding pattern of insoluble collagen under the electron microscope (Highberger *et al.*, 1951; Gross *et al.*, 1954). The explanation is that the monomer unit, tropocollagen, is a rigid rod about 300 nm long and 1.5 nm wide. Subsequent studies, using such techniques as viscometry, light-scattering, ultra-centrifugation and osmometry, have confirmed this view (Boedtker and Doty, 1956; Harrington and von Hippel, 1961; Veis, 1964; von Hippel, 1967).

Optical rotation studies have shown soluble collagen to exhibit a high negative value ($-350°$ to $-400°$) of specific optical rotation, α_D, which is explained by the helical conformation of the chains (Harrington and von Hippel, 1961). The evidence for the existence of non-helical peptide chains (telopeptides) at the ends of the tropocollagen molecules, and their role in building up the collagen fibre structure, is that peptides are released on enzymatic hydrolysis, whilst the helical region remains unaffected. The tropocollagen is then less able to reform into native-type fibrils (Bornstein *et al.*, 1966a and b).

Conversion of Collagen to Gelatin

The triple helix structure of tropocollagen can be destroyed (denaturation) by the application of heat (Flory and Weaver, 1960) or by the use of compounds which destroy hydrogen bonds (Steven and Tristram, 1962), with resultant conversion to gelatin. The tropocollagen–gelatin transformation has been extensively studied and reviewed (Harding, 1964; Veis, 1964; Ward, 1964; Johns and Courts, 1977). Denaturation involves breaking only the hydrogen bonds and those hydrophobic bonds that help to stabilise the collagen helix. This is followed by the disentanglement of the chains and dissociation into smaller components with a random coil configuration. Loss of helical

structure results in a marked fall in intrinsic viscosity (Doty and Nishihara, 1958), an alteration in specific optical rotation (from about $-400°$ to $140°$) (Burge and Hynes, 1959), a reduction in the angular dependence of light scattering (Engel, 1962), and an increase in partial specific volume (Christiensen and Cassel, 1967).

Thermal denaturation normally occurs at about 40°C, at pH 7, but this temperature varies with the collagen source (Crosby and Stainsby, 1962), the pH (Dick *et al.*, 1965), and the ionic strength (Woodlock and Harrap, 1968). It is convenient to define the transition in terms of a denaturation temperature, T_D, which is the temperature at which the viscosity, or optical rotation, falls by 50% of its original (stable) value in 30 minutes (von Hippel, 1967).

The presence of interchain cross-links within the tropocollagen molecule appears to have little influence on T_D, since the introduction of 10 intramolecular bonds into ichthyocol tropocollagen by reaction with formaldehyde increases T_D by only 1.4°C (Veis and Drake, 1963). The value of T_D for different collagens correlates with the total imino acid (proline + hydroxyproline) content. For example, fish collagens with relatively low imino acid contents exhibit T_Ds in the range 10–30°C compared with values of 36–40°C for mammalian collagens (Piez, 1960; von Hippel and Wong, 1963; Rigby, 1967). Denaturation occurs more readily as the pH is reduced but the effect is somewhat influenced by the acid used (Burge and Hynes, 1959; Dick *et al.*, 1965). Lower values result from the addition of neutral salts at constant pH (Woodlock and Harrap, 1968). Not surprisingly, compounds which destroy hydrogen bonds, such as urea, guanidine, and potassium thiocyanate, can bring about denaturation in the cold (Steven and Tristram, 1962).

The products of the denaturation of tropocollagen depend upon whether cross-links remain between the three component protein chains, and the situation is further complicated by the fact that the three chains are not identical. Single-chain species (α-type) of approximately 100 000 molecular weight (Kang *et al.*, 1966, 1969; Piez *et al.*, 1968) and two-chain species (β-type) of approximately 200 000 are the main components, although a disordered form of tropocollagen itself (γ-type), having a molecular weight of approximately 300 000 has been found (Piez *et al.*, 1961; Piez, 1967). Its link can be broken by alkali to give the α-species. Chromatographic separations on carmellose have shown that two α and two β components exist. The two α components, designated α_1 and α_2, differ in amino acid composition. The α_1 form contains smaller amounts of histidine, hydroxylysine, tyrosine, and those amino acids possessing large hydrophobic side-chains, but is richer in hydroxyproline.

The β components consist of dimers formed from two α_1 chains (β_{11}) or an α_1 and an α_2 chain (β_{12}), whilst the γ component is made up of two α_1 chains and one α_2 chain and is designated γ_{112}. The proportion of α to β components varies with the collagen source and the method of solubilisation.

The amino acid sequence of the α chain has been pieced together from various studies on specific cleavage of tropocollagen using enzymes or cyanogen bromide (Hulmes et al., 1973). Most of the chain is composed of triplets of the form Gly-X-Y, with Gly-Pro-Y occurring frequently and in particular Gly-Pro-Hypro. The terminal regions of the α chain do no show this triplet sequence and cannot therefore possess a helical structure.

The thermal denaturation of tropocollagen represents the simplest situation in the conversion of collagen to gelatin but, since the proportion of mature collagen which is soluble in cold buffer solutions is small, it does not present a commercially viable route to gelatin production. However, increased proportions of collagen can be solubilised by more drastic treatments.

Pretreatment of collagen with cold alkali can result in subsequent increased solubility in weak acid buffers (Courts and Stainsby, 1959), but this more drastic treatment breaks some peptide bonds (mainly at glycine residues) in addition to cross-links. This type of solubilised collagen has been termed 'eucollagen' (Courts, 1960); it closely resembles tropocollagen in its physicochemical properties (Crosby et al., 1962; Reed and Stainsby, 1962; Higgs and Reed, 1963), except for its lower isoelectric pH, a reduced tendency to show the characteristic banded pattern of collagen fibrils under the electron microscope, and a slightly reduced denaturation temperature.

British Patent 1 239 861 (1971) describes a more intensive alkali treatment which makes it possible to dissolve the collagen in the alkali itself, and gives a product similar to eucollagen. Other variations on the alkali pretreatment method have been described (Hey and Stainsby, 1965; Fujii, 1969). An acid treatment, which involves shaking minced collagen with hydrochloric acid and homogenising at high speed for a short time, is effective in partly solubilising it (U.S. Patent 3 293 237, 1966; Yates, 1968).

A number of patents exist which claim methods for solubilising collagen using proteolytic enzymes (U.S. Patent 2 979 438, 1961; Japanese Patent 9295, 1963; French Patent 1 450 430, 1966; British Patent 1 062 083, 1967; U.S. Patent 3 314 861, 1967; British Patent 1 119 342, 1968). The enzymes are believed to attack the terminal peptides, leading to breakage of intra- and intermolecular cross-links, whilst the helical region remains intact. Certainly, this is the mode of action demonstrated for soluble collagen treated with trypsin or chymotrypsin (Kühn et al., 1966; Martin et al., 1966), pronase (Drake et al., 1966), and pepsin (Hodge et al., 1960).

Conventional processes for converting collagen to gelatin do not involve the intermediate stage of conversion to soluble collagen but instead involve the direct conversion of purified collagen to gelatin. Insoluble collagen can be thermally denatured in a similar manner to soluble collagen, but the change occurs approximately 20°C higher than the denaturation temperature for the same tissues, and instead of being solubilised the collagen fibres shrink to one third of their original length (Rigby, 1967). The shrinkage temperature, T_S, in common with the denaturation temperature, T_D, is affected by the imino acid content, by pH, and by salt concentration. Alkaline pretreatment reduces T_S (Blazej and Galatik, 1966) whilst intermolecular cross-linking increases it, a fact which is utilised to advantage in leather tanning.

Apart from denaturation of the helical structure, it is necessary to break a sufficient number of intermolecular bonds to solubilise the protein and, in practice, intramolecular cross-links and certain labile main-chain peptide bonds may also be broken during the pretreatment and extraction processes. Residual intermolecular links can give rise to the appearance of components with molecular weights in excess of that of the γ-component (Flory and Weaver, 1960).

Molecular Weight of Gelatin

Because gelatins are obtained by denaturation and degradation of collagen, a heterogeneous product normally results, with a range of molecular weight species. In such a polydisperse system the average molecular weight attributed to a gelatin will depend upon the method of determination. Molecular weight studies on gelatins, as with tropocollagens, have been made using the techniques of osmometry (Pouradier *et al.*, 1950; Pouradier and Venet, 1950, 1952; Boedtker and Doty, 1956), light scattering (Boedtker and Doty, 1954; Gouinlock *et al.*, 1955; Veis *et al.*, 1955, 1958, 1960; Veis and Cohen, 1956, 1957; Courts and Stainsby, 1958), viscometry (Pouradier and Venet, 1950, 1952; Gouinlock *et al.*, 1955; Bourgoin and Joly, 1958; Veis *et al.*, 1960), ultracentrifugation (Scatchard *et al.*, 1944; Williams, 1954; Williams and Saunders, 1954; Williams *et al.*, 1954, 1958), end-group analysis (Courts and Stainsby, 1958), gel filtration or gel permeation chromatography (Cheve, 1966; Robinson, 1975; Tomka, 1976; Itoh and Okamoto, 1985), high pressure size-exclusion chromatography (HPSEC) (Lorry and Vedrines, 1985; Xiong-fong and Bi-xion, 1985; Beutel, 1985), and gel electrophoresis (Bartley, 1973; Bartley and Marrs, 1974; Tomka *et al.*, 1975; Tomka, 1976, 1979; Koepff, 1979; Aoyagi, 1985). Gel electrophoresis and HPSEC are proving to be the most useful techniques since they give good resolution of molecular species and also allow calculation of values of weight average molecular weight (M_w) and number average molecular weight (M_n).

The weight average molecular weight of commercial gelatins may vary from about 20 000 to 200 000, but very much higher molecular weights (in excess of 10^6) have been reported for gelatin fractions separated by alcohol coacervation (Veis, 1964) or gel electrophoresis (Tomka *et al.*, 1975; Tomka, 1979). These high molecular weight species have been shown not to be due to aggregation in solution (Veis, 1964). Number average chain weights in the range 40 000 to 80 000 have been reported (Courts, 1954) for high-grade commercial gelatins but other reports (Courts and Stainsby, 1958; Stainsby, 1977) suggest that these estimates may be on the high side (see later). Values of number average molecular weights also falling within this range have been reported for hard capsule gelatins (Robinson *et al.*, 1975).

Comparative molecular weight data obtained by light scattering (weight average molecular weight) and end-group analysis (number average chain molecular weight) demonstrated that high molecular weight fractions from both acid and limed gelatins are branched structures (Courts and Stainsby, 1958). More recent work suggests that the degree of branching may be even greater than was originally thought, due to limitations of the technique and the presence of chains possessing no terminal amino groups (Stainsby, 1977).

The lower intrinsic viscosities exhibited by acid-processed gelatins compared with lime-processed gelatins of comparable molecular weights have been interpreted as indicating a more compact, more highly cross-linked structure for these so-called acid gelatins (Robinson *et al.*, 1975).

The average molecular weight and the molecular weight distribution are functions of the collagen-to-gelatin conversion process and they have an important effect on the physical properties of the gelatin. A typical molecular weight distribution for hard capsule grade limed ossein gelatin determined by gel electrophoresis is illustrated in Fig. 2.2, and the molecular weight fractions are detailed in Table 2.1. This shows the prominent α-peak characteristic of limed gelatins which is a consequence of the selective breaking of cross-links.

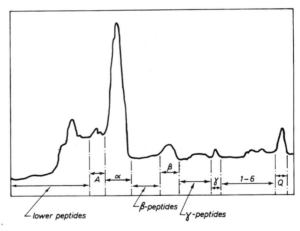

Fig. 2.2. The molecular weight distribution of a hard capsule grade, limed ossein gelatin (Bloom strength, 250 g), determined by polyacrylamide gel electrophoresis (2.5% gel).

The amino acid compositions of gelatins are quite similar to those of the parent collagens, except for the amide group and the organic residue. Amino acid analyses of several diverse animal gelatins are illustrated in Table 2.2 (Eastoe and Leach, 1977).

COMMERCIAL MANUFACTURE OF GELATIN

Boiling animal bones or skins in water results in a low yield of impure gelatin with poor physical and organoleptic properties. Commercial processes for converting collagen stock into gelatin

Table 2.1. Molecular weights and relative proportions of molecular species separated by gel electrophoresis of limed ossein gelatin.

Molecular species	Molecular weight	Fraction %
<A	<86 000	39.8
A	86 000	8.3
α	95 000	14.4
β-peptides	145 000	6.8
β	190 000	5.2
γ-peptides	237 000	9.3
γ	285 000	1.3
1–6	380 000–855 000	11.7
Q (microgel)	1.5×10^6–1.5×10^7	3.2

NOTES
1. The molecular species α, β, and γ are as defined in the text.
2. A and <A are molecules of progressively lower weight than α molecules.
3. β-Peptides are molecules intermediate in size between α and β molecules.
4. γ-Peptides are partially hydrolysed γ molecules.
5. Molecules designated 1–6 are species identifiable as greater in molecular weight than γ molecules, and are oligomers of the α chain.
6. Molecules designated Q (known as microgel) are polymerised species of extremely high molecular weight.

Table 2.2. Composition of mammalian gelatins (values are given as numbers of residues per 1000 total residues)

	Rabbit skin	Whale skin	Pig skin	Ox skin	Ox bone
Alanine	105.0	110.5	111.7	112.0	116.6
Glycine	325	326	330	333	335
Valine	20.7	20.6	25.9	20.1	21.9
Leucine	22.2	24.8	24.0	23.1	24.3
Isoleucine	13.0	11.0	9.5	12.0	10.8
Proline	132.0	128.2	131.9	129.0	124.2
Phenylalanine	14.0	13.0	13.6	12.3	14.0
Tyrosine	3.0	3.6	2.6	1.5	1.2
Serine	34.7	41.0	34.7	36.5	32.8
Threonine	20.0	24.0	17.9	16.9	18.3
Cystine	0.5				
Methionine	5.4	4.7	3.6	5.5	3.9
Arginine	47.3	50.1	49.0	46.2	48.0
Histidine	5.5	5.7	4.0	4.5	4.2
Lysine	27.4	25.9	26.6	27.8	27.6
Aspartic acid	47.5	46.3	45.8	46.0	46.7
Glutamic acid	67.5	69.6	72.1	70.7	72.6
Hydroxyproline	105.1	89.1	90.7	97.6	93.3
Hydroxylysine	4.4	5.8	6.4	5.5	4.3
Amide*	38.4	25.6	41.5	7.5	15.7
Recovery by wt. (%)	96.9	99.7	97.2	99.8	
Total N (%)	18.1	18.6	18.3	18.1	
Recovery of N (%)	99.6	100.5	101.5	100.9	
Process	alkali	?	acid	alkali	alkali

*No. of molecules of NH_3 released during hydrolysis per 1000 total residues.

are designed with the object of achieving the maximum yield of gelatin consistent with commercially acceptable values of properties such as gel strength, viscosity, colour, clarity and taste. Manufacture basically involves the removal of non-collagenous material, conversion of collagen to gelatin, purification, then recovery of gelatin in a dry form. The details of the process vary depending upon the nature of the raw material used; the exact operating conditions adopted by manufacturers are, in many instances, commercial secrets. The basic operations involved in pharmaceutical gelatin manufacture are illustrated in Fig. 2.3.

Collagenous Raw Materials

It is possible to utilise a fairly wide range of collagenous raw materials for conversion into gelatin. Bogue (1922) has reported typical values for glue yields and moisture contents for a wide range of skin and bone materials. In practice, the choice is largely restricted, for economic, processing and quality reasons, to cattle bone, cattle skin (hide), and pigskin. Typical compositions for these materials, in terms of water, grease content, and gelatin yield, have been reported (Hinterwaldner, 1977).

In the U.S.A., pigskin is the principal raw material for gelatin production because of its availability in a fresh, frozen condition from the large meat packers. It has been used to a much smaller extent in Europe because of such factors as consumer taste for 'crackling' on pork joints and its use for, amongst other things, a meat extender in sausages, but its use is increasing.

An important raw material is hide scrap arising from tanneries. Apart from trimmings from the hides themselves, the inner, non-grain layer, or corium (known commercially as 'splits') is utilised. Hide may be received in either a wet or dry state, limed or unlimed, and dehaired or not, depending upon the stage in leather manufacture at which the scrap arises. It can also vary in type and age from thin calfskin splits to thick, mature buffalo hide, which behave quite differently in terms of the processing required for their conversion to gelatin.

Bone for gelatin manufacture may be either fresh bone, from slaughtered animals, which has a high moisture and fat content and probably some adhering sinew and meat, or the sun-dried material obtained primarily from India. The latter type of bone has been naturally cleaned and generally

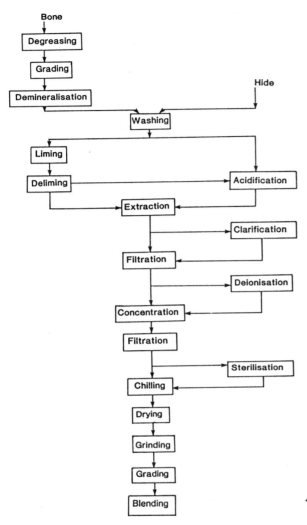

Fig. 2.3. A flowsheet of the commercial process for the conversion of collagen to gelatin.

Other raw materials, which may be locally in good supply, such as sheepskin or sheep's trotters, may be used, and will have their own particular processing requirements. It is also possible to extract gelatin from chrome-tanned leather scrap, provided either that chromium is first removed or the process is designed to prevent its passing into solution.

The pretreatment of raw materials is necessary. This refers to those procedures necessary to clean up the material and to remove inorganic and organic matter which would otherwise have an adverse effect on the subsequent 'chemical conditioning' of the collagen and on gelatin extraction.

Bone requires a very different pretreatment from hide and skin, principally because of its high inorganic content. In all pretreatment processes the aim is to maintain the collagen in an 'undamaged' form to prevent loss of potential gelatin yield or quality.

BONE

Crushing. Indian bone is crushed before shipment and can vary in size from about 6 to 18 mm pieces. Fresh bones have to be sorted to remove inferior raw material and foreign matter; this is still done by hand, with the assistance of electromagnets for the removal of tramp iron as the bone is fed on a conveyor belt to the bone cutter. Various types of bone cutter can be used; the design may involve either a true knife-cutting action or a hammer blow. The important parameters are, firstly, that the bone pieces should be sufficiently small to minimise the time spent in the degreasing and demineralisation stages, and, secondly, that they should not be so small that they create problems in subsequent wet processing, for example poor drainage rate or loss due to fines passing solids-retaining screens. Generally the upper size limit will be about 12 mm and the lower about 3 mm. Apart from the size of the bone pieces, their shape can also be important in influencing fat removal, and again this is a function of the design of the cutter.

Degreasing. Indian bone generally has a grease content of 1–2%, which means that no further degreasing is needed. In contrast, fresh bone will contain, typically, about 35% moisture and 15% fat. This fat must be removed or it will cause processing problems. For example, during the liming stage, fat, or calcium soaps formed from it, can clog the capillary spaces in the demineralised bone (ossein) and impede the penetration of alkali. Fat

shows a much lower level of attached tissue, but still contains a considerable quantity of impurity in the form of dried blood.

The composition of bone varies with the species and age of the animal from which it is obtained, and also from one part of the skeleton to another (Johns, 1977). The outer and inner portions of the bones give rise to 'hard' (or compact) and 'soft' (or spongy) pieces respectively. Figures indicating the possible variation in overall composition of fresh, whole bone have been reported, but despite the difference in physical structure the chemical composition of bovine compact and spongy bone is very similar.

which appears in the gelatin liquor during extraction may become partially emulsified, producing poor-clarity liquors which are difficult to filter. More important still is the fact that gelatins with a high grease or fatty acid content may show localised non-wettability, resulting in 'fish eyes' in photographic films or 'windows' in hard gelatin capsules.

It is important to protect the collagen from thermal denaturation during degreasing. Sinew, attached to the bone, but unprotected by an inorganic phase, is particularly susceptible to thermal damage and will denature at a temperature in the region of its shrinkage temperature (about 65°C).

Also of importance is the quality of the removed fat, which is a valuable by-product. For these reasons, many of the degreasing processes which have been used are unsatisfactory. The simplest method, treatment of the bones with boiling water for several hours, still leaves 3–8% fat (Virnik and Zharkova, 1937) in the bone, and at the same time damages the collagen structure (Chayen and Ashworth, 1953). The use of hot organic solvents or their vapours is much more effective in removing fat but, again, is liable to denature the collagen and also suffers the disadvantage of being an expensive process in time (up to 24 hours) and fuel for steam-raising plant. Such processes have recently been reviewed (Hinterwaldner, 1977). Modern degreasing processes favour rapid water-extraction of fat on a continuous basis.

The 'Chayen Cold Degreasing Process' defined in British Patent 714 671, 1954 established that fat could be extracted in the cold by 'impulse rendering'. This is a process in which the bone is exposed to a series of high speed impulses transmitted through water by a high speed hammer mill, which causes mechanical rupture of the cell membranes so that the fat is liberated and can be removed by the water. After separation from the cold water and solid fat, the bone is given a hot water wash to remove surface fat. The whole process takes only a matter of minutes. A simplified process flowsheet is shown in Fig. 2.4. The residual fat content of the bone is generally less than 2%. Other wet degreasing processes which depend upon the hot water washing of bone have been described (Leiner and Gash, 1972), and the compression of heated bone in a press has been advocated as an alternative procedure for separation of grease (Flausch, 1978).

Grading of Bone. The sinew component of degreased bone has a very different physical form

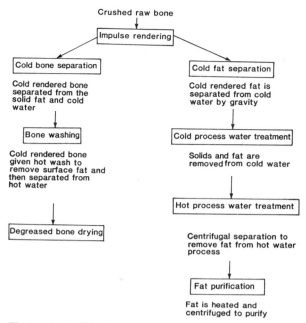

Fig. 2.4. A simplified flowsheet of the degreasing process.

from the hard and soft bone components; it is important to separate it, in order that it may be treated differently in subsequent processing to avoid losses in the yield and quality. Complete separation and processing of sinew from bone is not really a practical proposition. It is usual to separate the degreased bone into hard, soft, and sinew fractions in which:

(1) the hard bone fraction is virtually free from sinew but will contain a proportion of soft bone
(2) the soft bone fraction contains a proportion of hard bone and sinew
(3) the sinew fraction contains a proportion of soft bone but a negligible amount of hard bone.

Separation into these three fractions can be effected in the wet state but is most easily effected after the degreased bone has been dried. Differences in specific gravity of the three components are utilised in their separation on a vibrating screen. Improved separation can be achieved by a second screening.

Demineralisation. The inorganic phase of bone is composed principally of calcium phosphate together with carbonate ions, although it is still not clear whether the major component is hydroxyapatite, tricalcium phosphate hydrate, or octacalcium phosphate. Minor constituents, totalling about 2% of the inorganic matter, include magnesium, sodium, and potassium chlorides and fluorides, together with trace elements at levels below 100 ppm.

Demineralisation of degreased bone is necessary to free the collagen before it can be conditioned and extracted as gelatin. This is achieved by treatment with dilute hydrochloric acid in counter-current flow, so that the fresh bone will meet almost-spent acid, while fresh acid is reacted with the bone which is about to leave the process. The main reaction taking place can be considered to be dissolution of tricalcium phosphate to the monocalcium salt:

$$Ca_3(PO_4)_2 + 4HCl \rightarrow Ca(H_2PO_4)_2 + 2CaCl_2$$

The concentration of acid and the time of treatment are varied according to the type of bone being handled and its grist size. Excessive acid concentrations or over-long treatment times can result in loss of yield and eventual gelatin quality through hydrolysis of the collagen and therefore, in practice, complete demineralisation is not attempted.

Temperature control is also important, since heat is generated in the reaction and increased temperature accelerates the rate of collagen hydrolysis. It is usual to employ refrigeration plant during the summer months, in warm climates, to maintain a demineralisation temperature of 10–15°C. In general, 4–5% v/v hydrochloric acid is used, with treatment times varying from about 4–6 days for the hard bone fraction to 1–2 days for the sinew fraction. The demineralised bone (ossein) normally shows a residual ash content of 1–2%.

The sinew fraction is particularly vulnerable to losses in yield during demineralisation because of its more friable nature, its greater tendency to swell, and the greater risk of thermal denaturation during the previous stages of degreasing and drying. Losses of collagen into the acid liquor can best be assessed by hydroxyproline determination rather than by nitrogen testing, since small amounts of other proteins and mucoproteins present in the bone will also pass into solution.

An important by-product from the demineralisation process is dicalcium phosphate, which is obtained by treating the spent acid leach liquor with lime to precipitate dicalcium phosphate at pH 4.2–4.5. After concentration, the slurry is filtered, washed, and dried to give a white free-flowing powder which is used in animal feeds and fertilisers.

Other acids, such as phosphoric, can be used instead of hydrochloric acid, but, apart from comparative cost considerations and the question of the solubility of the reaction product, which influences diffusion rate, the most important consideration is the economic necessity to recover phosphate in a saleable form.

HIDE

Splits and hide pieces are normally first given a superficial wash to remove any surface contamination and then fed to a cutter in order to reduce the material to a convenient size. Generally the cut pieces will be about 5–20 cm^2 in area, which allows the material to be pumped or 'flumed' with water. Dry hide, which is an extremely tough material, is sometimes given a weak caustic presoak to soften it before cutting, whilst hide which still has hair attached must be dehaired by treatment in a lime slurry containing sodium sulphide for several days.

If the hide is to be acid-extracted without conventional liming treatment it must be given a more thorough washing, and it is sometimes given a short 'clean-up' treatment in dilute caustic solution containing hydrogen peroxide prior to neutralisation and water-washing. These operations are generally performed in paddle washers which ensure effective relative movement between the hide pieces and the solution.

PIGSKIN

Where pigskin is received in a frozen state, which is the case in the U.S.A., the only pretreatment necessary is to thaw the material, and cut and wash it. Despite its high fat content, no attempt is made to remove the fat at this stage, because it is most convenient to separate it during the subsequent acid extraction of gelatin. Any alkaline pretreatment must be avoided to prevent the possible formation of soaps.

Conditioning of Collagen

LIMING PROCESS

The function of the liming process is to 'condition' the collagen so that gelatin with the desired physical properties is obtained in good yield on subsequent extraction at low temperature and near-neutral pH. Liming brings about both physical and chemical changes in the collagen. The amide groups of the glutamine and asparagine residues are converted into carboxyl groups with liberation of ammonia, resulting in a shift in the isoelectric point of the collagen (Ames, 1944). However, the deamidation reaction is incidental to the collagen-to-gelatin conversion (Ames, 1952), the change in isoelectric point being practically complete after 10–20 days, whilst conditioning reactions leading to increased yield of gelatin continue for a very much longer time. The gelatin derived from limed collagen normally has an isoelectric point of pH 4.8–5.2.

Arginine residues may be deguanidated to form ornithine residues and urea (Highberger and Stecker, 1941), but the reaction is slow and becomes important only in the later stages of liming. A 34% conversion of arginine to ornithine has been reported (Hamilton and Anderson, 1954) for extensively limed calfskin, whereas 3% conversion is a more normal figure for conventionally limed collagen (Eastoe, 1955). Ornithine has a side-chain amino group, so that the formation of arginine is accompanied by an apparent decrease in chain average molecular weight where generation of free amino groups is attributed to peptide bond hydrolysis. Some peptide bond hydrolysis undoubtedly does occur but it has been estimated (Courts, 1960; Grassmann et al., 1962) that this represents less than one bond per chain. The peptide bonds most susceptible to hydrolysis during alkaline processing are those involving glycine, serine, threonine, aspartic acid, and glutamic acid at the amino group terminus, and also these same amino acid residues, plus alanine and phenylalanine, at the carboxyl group end. The bonds most stable to hydrolysis involve proline and hydroxyproline (Grassmann and Hörmann, 1953; Courts, 1954; Heyns and Legler, 1958).

Perhaps the most important function of liming is the destruction of cross-links. Alkali-labile bonds almost certainly exist in the non-helical, telopeptide regions where cross-links occur, but not all cross-links are generally destroyed, as evidenced by the existence of very high molecular weight branched gelatin molecules. Indeed, complete removal of cross-links may not necessarily be desirable since these very high molecular weight molecules may be important in determining gel setting rate (Bartley and Marrs, 1974; Tomka et al., 1975).

Soaking collagen in acid (e.g. 9% HCl) prior to liming significantly reduces the liming period (Ames, 1957; Courts, 1960). However, if this 'dual soak' process is reversed and the acid treatment is given after liming the same increase in yield is not observed. This has been interpreted as indicating that two types of insolubilising bonds are present in the collagen, one type being labile in acid (or in a very strong alkali such as 5% NaOH) and the other being labile only in lime (Hodge and Petruska, 1962). When intact, the acid-labile bonds apparently protect some of the alkali-labile bonds from hydrolysis during liming. Another important role of the liming process is the removal of foreign proteins and mucoproteins, which exist as impurities in the collagen, and are soluble at alkaline pH.

Collagen fibres, after liming, are indistinguishable from the native fibres under the electron microscope, except that they are swollen and the internal adhesion of each fibril is reduced by rupture of certain intermolecular links (de La Burde, 1962). Swelling of collagen during liming proceeds in two stages: the initial rapid equilibrium swelling is complete within about three days, and slower swelling, indicative of structural breakdown, proceeds during the entire liming period (Bowes and Kenten, 1950).

The collagenous raw material may be ossein or cattle skin. The sinew fraction of ossein is not used because of its susceptibility to physical and chemical breakdown during liming. Normally, Indian bone or the 'hard fraction' of ossein from fresh bone is used, although the soft fraction can also be utilised provided it has been sufficiently well segregated from sinew to avoid losses in yield.

Liming is carried out in tanks or pits, or occasionally churns, where the collagen stock is soaked in slaked lime slurry (2–5% concentration) for periods of 60–120 days.

The length of time in lime depends upon such factors as the nature of the raw material, temperature, availability of pits, and the properties of the gelatin required. Ideally, the liming pits should be sited indoors where some control of temperature and humidity can be exercised to prevent marked fluctuations. Typically, liming temperatures of 14–18°C are used. At regular intervals the contents of the pits should be aerated to ensure distribution of lime slurry throughout the pits and to discourage the growth of anaerobic bacteria. The lime slurry may be replaced by fresh slurry several times during the conditioning period, to assist in the removal of impurities.

Apart from its low cost, the use of lime has the advantage that, provided undissolved lime is always present, its solubility acts as a built-in regulator of the alkalinity. It also tends to swell collagen to a lesser degree than sodium hydroxide at the same pH.

It is possible to accelerate the conditioning process by 'sharpening' the lime liquor by the addition of sodium hydroxide, sodium carbonate, sodium sulphide, hydroxylamine, or calcium chloride and methylamine. By increasing the concentration of sodium hydroxide to about 2%, it is possible to condition the material in 2–6 weeks without using any lime. However, this shorter and consequently more drastic pretreatment is more difficult to control to give a uniform degree of conditioning and usually leads to a greater loss of yield into solution. Part of the 'over-conditioning' is associated with the higher degree of swelling in caustic solution compared with lime slurry, although this can be minimised by the use of a swelling restrainer such as sodium sulphate. This formed the basis of the so-called Sulphate Process (Ward, 1953) by which it was found possible to alkali-condition collagen in 5 days using 5–10% sodium hydroxide solution containing 20% sodium sulphate as a swelling restrictor.

De-liming

De-liming is effected by washing with water in a log-washer or paddle-washer for about 24 hours, preferably after solid surface lime has been mechanically removed with water. It is then necessary to neutralise the raw material, which at this stage is generally at pH 9–10, with acid. In practice it may be advantageous to over-acidify the material slightly and wash back to the desired pH. However, where the collagen has been extensively limed or caustic-treated, care must be taken not to acidify to the point where the collagen becomes excessively swollen and fragile. During the final stages, when the pH of the material is closer to neutrality and therefore susceptible to bacterial action, the use of sulphurous acid has certain advantages because of its preservative action. The final pH of the collagen stock is normally required to be in the pH range 5.0–6.5, although more acid values are sometimes used.

ACID CONDITIONING

An alternative to the liming process is to acidify the collagen for subsequent extraction at low pH. It is sufficient simply to bring the collagen to the required equilibrium pH and, since this is normally achieved within 24 hours, acid conditioning offers the advantage of very much shorter processing time compared with the liming process. However, if reasonable gelatin yields and qualities are to be achieved, acid processing is generally restricted to

soft bone ossein, sinew, pigskin, and calfskin. It has also been applied to sheepskin and mature cattle skin, but the age of the animal is a significant factor and a maximum age of 2–3 years for cattle skin has been suggested as being suitable for acid processing (Reich *et al.*, 1962). Skins from pigs up to 18 months old give higher gelatin yields and qualities than skins taken from 30-month-old pigs.

The young pigskin widely available in the U.S.A. is particularly amenable to acid processing, which also avoids the problem of saponification of the fat which would occur in alkaline processing. The pigskin is treated with 5% mineral acid solution (hydrochloric acid, sulphuric acid, or phosphoric acid) for 10–30 hours before washing with water to remove excess acid and to provide a suitable extraction pH of about 4. Cattle skin, soft bone ossein and sinew are less easily extracted than young pigskin and it is usual to adjust these materials to a lower pH within the range 2–3.5.

Acid conditioning and extraction yields a gelatin with an isoelectric point well above pH 5. This is because a proportion of the glutamine and asparagine residues remain in the amide form, giving rise to isoelectric points in the region of pH 7.0–9.5 for acid pigskin gelatin and pH 6.0–8.0 for acid ossein gelatins. In contrast to the liming process the 'conditioning effect', in terms of breakage of cross-links and peptide bonds prior to extraction, is minimal. Studies on the titration curves of acid precursor pigskin gelatin and native collagen have shown that peptide bond hydrolysis is the more important reaction in the acid extraction of gelatin (Bowes and Kenten, 1948; Ames, 1952; Loeven, 1954).

Extraction and Purification of Gelatin

The conditions of pH and temperature for extraction are, to a large extent, dictated by the nature of the raw material and the pretreatment it has received, but extraction normally takes place under either acid or neutral conditions and at the minimum temperature needed to give a reasonable extraction rate and a high yield of gelatin. For a given raw material, the extraction rate is greater under acid conditions, but at the same time thermal degradation of gelatin is considerably more rapid than at neutral pH.

ACID EXTRACTION

For materials which have received no alkaline pretreatment but simply acid conditioning, such as soft bone ossein, sinew, and pigskin, it is necessary to extract at acid pH to obtain reasonable extraction rates and good yields without resorting to very high temperatures.

Pigskin is generally extracted at pH 4 or thereabouts, in a traditional batch-by-batch fashion. The material is loaded into extraction pans, constructed from acid-resistant stainless steel, which have false bottoms covered with stainless steel mesh through which liquor can drain. Preferably the pans are fitted with lids and are lagged to reduce heat loss. The general procedure is to load the material, allow it to drain, cover it with hot water, and then heat the liquor by circulation through an external heat exchanger until the required temperature is achieved. When the gelatin concentration reaches 4–10% the liquor is drained and further 'runs' are made in a similar manner, using progressively higher temperatures.

Ossein and sinew are less readily extracted than pigskin. The extraction is normally carried out at pH 3.0–3.5, although a pH as low as 2.0 may be used. The secret of successful acid extraction is the rapid removal of the gelatin from the ossein after it has passed into solution to reduce thermal hydrolysis and consequent deterioration in physical properties. The batch process has largely been replaced by a semi-continuous extraction process in which hot water at a controlled temperature and flow rate is continuously run on to the ossein at the top of the pan, while gelatin liquor at a concentration of 3–6% is continuously run off from the bottom, and is neutralised as soon as possible. The extraction temperature is raised during the process, to maintain the extraction rate, from about 50° at the start to about 75° at the end. It is generally recognised that acid extraction results in a gelatin with a high gel strength/viscosity ratio compared with neutrally extracted limed gelatin. Some control over this ratio can be exercised, however, by selection of the extraction pH within the acid range. In general, high gel strength is favoured by a low pH, whilst higher viscosities are more easily achieved at a higher pH. As extraction progresses the gelatin viscosity generally increases (except for the final extracts, when it may fall again) whereas the gel strength tends to decrease. This is due, in part, to the fact that the pH tends to increase as the extraction progresses.

Limed hide or ossein can be extracted at low pH, and such commercially produced gelatins generally have lower viscosities than neutrally extracted material. However, this lower viscosity arises largely through secondary hydrolysis of the gelatin in solution rather than from breakage of specific bonds in the collagen. High viscosities can in fact be obtained by extraction at a pH as low as 2.0 using continuous extraction under carefully controlled conditions.

The water used for extraction may need to be deionised if it has too high a content of dissolved solids and, more particularly, if it contains a high level of nitrate ions which can affect the performance of the gelatin in particular applications. (Further consideration of the importance of nitrate ions is given in Chapter 3.)

NEUTRAL EXTRACTION

Limed collagen stock is normally extracted at a neutral or weakly acid pH in batches. The extraction pH may vary from 5.0 to 8.0 but is most commonly between 5.0 and 6.5. The gelatin is obtained as a series of extracts with an initial temperature of 50–60°, increasing to boiling point for the final extract. Liquor concentrations of 4–10% are achieved, the rate of extraction being a function not only of temperature but also of the nature of the raw material and the extent of alkaline conditioning.

The first fraction of the total gelatin is obtained simply by the thermal breakdown of the hydrogen bonds which stabilise the helical structure of well-conditioned regions of the collagen. This gelatin fraction is simply 'melted out', with no further rupture of covalent linkages. Later extracts may be obtained as a consequence of further breakdown of collagen resulting from the conditioning action of the prevailing pH and temperature conditions. Neutral extraction tends to give gelatins with lower gel strength/viscosity ratios than acid extraction. High viscosities are favoured by neutral extraction of collagen which has been limed for a long period.

As extraction progresses, the gelatin gel strength generally decreases (the first extract is, anomalously, often lower in gel strength than the second extract) whilst the viscosity tends to increase for successive runs until the final one at near boiling temperature. The 'last run' gelatins generally have poorer physical properties, and are darker in colour and stronger in odour, reflecting the more extensive heat treatment received during extraction.

FILTRATION AND CLARIFICATION

The dilute gelatin liquor from the extraction pans contains suspended collagen particles, fat globules, and foreign proteins (if these have not been removed during the conditioning stage). Preliminary coarse separation can be effected by centrifugation, filtration through muslin, or passage through sludge separators.

The traditional method of filtering gelatin liquors, which is probably still the most effective, is to pressure-filter through compressed pads of cellulose pulp which have previously been sterilised with steam. At the end of filtration the pulp pads are broken up, washed with boiling water to remove gelatin and insoluble matter, and then reformed in a press for re-use.

Self-cleaning centrifugal types of filter are also in use, based on the principle of filtration through diatomaceous earth coated on twilled stainless steel support screens. These round support elements are normally mounted horizontally on a central hollow axial shaft in a closed vertical pressure vessel.

Certain gelatin processes produce liquors which, after filtration, still have poor clarity due to non-collagenous proteins which have been extracted from the raw material, particularly in the last extraction runs. In such cases it is usually possible to improve the clarity by 'chemical clarification' in which a flocculent precipitate is formed, in situ, to adsorb finely divided suspended solids and turbidity-producing colloids. Suitable precipitates should not only be good adsorbents but also separate rapidly under gravity or on centrifugation. In the past, heat-coagulable protein such as egg albumen has been used but, apart from being expensive, the necessity of using temperatures close to boiling point results in thermal degradation. A more acceptable alternative is to produce a flocculent precipitate of an inorganic salt in the liquor.

Various systems have been used (U.S. Patent 3 184 445, 1965), which include dicalcium phosphate, calcium carbonate, and aluminium hydroxide flocs. Such methods can be particularly useful for acid-extracted gelatin liquor since they provide the possibility of neutralising the acid without significantly raising the ash content of the gelatin.

For example, if phosphoric acid is used to condition the collagen for extraction, then by adding lime slurry to gelatin liquor the pH of the liquor can be raised to 5.0–6.5 (depending upon the concentration of phosphate ions), thereby precipitating dicalcium phosphate. The addition of a small amount of aluminium sulphate during precipitation can also assist in producing a more rapidly-separating precipitate.

In general, chemical clarification is more easily and reproducibly applied to acid-processed gelatin liquors, because alkali-processed liquors contain soaps which may interfere. It is common practice to give a 'polishing filtration' to the concentrated gelatin liquor, particularly where there is a risk of salts precipitating from the solution during evaporation.

DEIONISATION

In general, the ash content of even a poor alkali-processed gelatin will be below the 2% maximum limit permitted by the most stringent of the various Pharmacopoeias. However, ash levels below 1% are frequently specified by individual pharmaceutical gelatin users: in such cases it may be necessary to deionise the gelatin. Concern about specific ions such as iron, phosphate, sulphite, nitrate, or nitrite may also be a reason for resorting to ion exchange.

In the case of acid-extracted gelatins, it is generally necessary to raise the pH of the liquor after extraction from around 3.5 to around 6.0 before further processing. This would bring about an increase in ash content, unless an insoluble, filterable precipitate is formed, or ammonium hydroxide is used as the alkali.

Acid pigskin gelatin is frequently offered at pH 4.0–4.5 to avoid this problem, whilst certain acid processes use sulphur dioxide as the conditioning acid, relying on its volatility to increase the pH during evaporation. In most cases, however, acid-extracted gelatins for pharmaceutical applications are treated by ion-exchange to raise the pH without increasing the ash content, yielding products with ash contents as low as 0.1%.

Gelatin liquor can be deionised before or after evaporation, but because of the problems of handling the viscous concentrated solution it is usual to work with the weak liquor. Mixed-bed ion-exchange resin columns are theoretically more effective than separate anion and cation resin columns and also offer the advantage that the pH of the liquor is not greatly altered, thus reducing the risk of hydrolysis. However, separate anion and cation columns are widely used because of their simplicity of operation, and particularly their regeneration. Whether anion exchange should precede or follow cation exchange will depend upon the gelatin liquor. For example, gelatin liquors which have been chemically clarified with dicalcium phosphate should be cation-exchanged first, otherwise precipitation of tricalcium phosphate can occur in the anion resin column as the pH increases above about 7.5. Acid-extracted gelatin liquors, on the other hand, are better anion-exchanged initially since cation exchange is, firstly, less effective at acid pH and, secondly, would make the liquor even more acid, with greater risk of degradation. Since extremes of pH are generally experienced at some stage of ion-exchange it is important to avoid high liquor temperatures and to pass the liquor through the columns are rapidly as possible.

CONCENTRATION

Because gelatin is susceptible to thermal hydrolysis it is necessary to keep the evaporation time and temperature to a minimum and therefore vacuum is applied. Various types of evaporator are used including tubular, plate, thin film, centrifugal, and 'flash' evaporators (Hinterwaldner, 1977). The plate and tubular types are normally operated in a double- or triple-effect arrangement for reasons of heat economy. It should be possible to concentrate the gelatin solution to a final level of 20–25% with a liquor temperature below 55° in the final effect. Higher concentrations, in particular for high-viscosity gelatins, can lead to the risk of localised overheating due to reduced circulation rate, but, because evaporation is a cheaper operation than drying, there is an incentive to reduce the water content as far as possible by evaporation. Thin film, centrifugal, and flash evaporators are frequently used to increase the concentration further. Flash evaporation involves rapidly increasing the temperature of the gelatin solution up to 120–145° in a plate heat exchanger, followed by expansion into a vacuum separator, resulting in rapid evaporation of water and simultaneous cooling of the liquor. The liquor can be recycled through the system until the required concentration is achieved.

STERILISATION

Since the addition of preservatives to gelatin for edible or pharmaceutical use is not permissible (with the possible exception of limited amounts of sulphur dioxide) and yet gelatin will support bacterial growth, it is necessary to operate a regular and rigid programme of plant sterilisation. Monitoring of micro-organisms at various stages of gelatin manufacture from extraction through to the dry gelatin is common practice. Flash evaporators are useful in the sterilisation of gelatin since the short-time, high-temperature sequence is effective against bacteria, whilst gelatin degradation is minimal.

Where heat sterilisation is required without the necessity for concentrating the gelatin, the liquor can be flashed to high temperature (140°) for a few seconds using live steam followed by expansion into vacuum and cooling. The steriliser is suitably placed immediately prior to the chilling and drying operation. The drying process itself, which in its final stages involves air temperatures of around 75°, also contributes to the sterility of the gelatin.

CHILLING AND DRYING

Commercially, dry gelatin is obtained by chilling the concentrated liquor to form a gel which is then air-dried. The rate-determining stage in the removal of moisture from the gel is the diffusion of water from the interior of the gel to the surface where it is evaporated. If evaporation is too rapid then surface skinning, or 'case-hardening' can occur. To reduce the risk of this, the air temperature is kept low to begin with and is slowly increased during the drying cycle. The final moisture content of the gelatin should be in the range of 8–13%. Lower moisture contents than this can cause poor dissolution or even partial insolubility of the gelatin.

Gelation may be achieved using either a slowly rotating, brine-cooled, stainless steel drum, or an endless stainless steel chilled band, or a scraped-tube, brine-cooled heat exchanger in which the gelatin solution is simultaneously chilled and extruded through a noodling or dicing head.

The continuous gel sheet which is taken off the drum or band chiller is fed to a cutter or mincer where it is reduced to 'cubes' or 'crumbs'.

The drying stage may be performed either as a continuous or a batch operation. The continuous drier consists of a stainless steel band moving through a series of controlled temperature and humidity zones in the drying tunnel. The drying air is filtered to remove airborne particles, and may be scrubbed to remove gaseous impurities such as sulphur dioxide. Such a band drier is most conveniently fed with noodled gelatin from a scraped-surface heat exchanger. The total drying time is less than 4 hours.

In a typical batch-drying process the gel pieces are supported on a stainless steel screen and exposed to an upward draught of air of controlled temperature and humidity. Movement of the gelatin gel particles may be effected by rotating 'rakes'.

Rotating drum driers in which the cylindrical wall is permeable to the drying air are also in use.

Maximum drying temperatures of about 75° are employed and the total drying time is normally 6–12 hours. A typical capacity for a batch drier would be 750–1000 kg dry gelatin.

Other drying processes such as the fluidised-bed method have been tried but have generally found little favour. Spray drying is costly because it is necessary to dry comparatively dilute solutions and because it produces a low bulk density, fluffy powder. Drum drying can result in significant thermal degradation of gelatin and produces a very fine powder on milling. Both spray drying and drum drying do offer, however, advantages in the production of cold-water dispersible gelatins by virtue of drying occurring directly from the sol to dry state, without intermediate gel formation.

GRINDING, SIEVING, AND BLENDING

The gelatin from the drier may be in the form of broken sheet, cube, crumb, or noodle, depending upon the particular method of drying used. It may be supplied to the customer in these forms, but usually it is milled and then classified into specific particle size ranges by sieving. The particle size achieved by milling will depend partly on the hardness of the gelatin, which is a function of the grade and moisture content, and partly on the design of the mill. A coarse grade is given by a 'knife-type' mill, whilst finer powder results from the use of a hammer mill.

Commercially, standard gelatin grades are achieved by the blending of individual gelatin batches which have previously been tested for their attainment of physical, chemical, and microbiological standards.

References

Ames, W. M., *J. Soc. chem. Ind., Lond.*, 1944, *63*, 200–204, 234–241, 277–280, 303–306.
Ames, W. M., *J. Sci. Fd Agric.*, 1952, *3*, 454–463.
Ames, W. M., *J. Sci. Fd Agric.*, 1957, *8*, 169–173.
Aoyagi, S., in *Photographic Gelatin*, Proceedings of the Fourth IAG Conference, Fribourg, 1983, H. Amman-Brass and J. Pouradier, (Ed.), 1985, pp. 36–54.
Bailey, A. J., in *Comprehensive Biochemistry*, Vol. 26, Part B, M. Florkin and E. H. Stotz (Ed.), London, Elsevier Publishing Co., 1968, p. 297.
Bailey, A. J. *et al.*, *Nature*, 1974, *251*, 105–109.
Balian, G. and Bowes, J. H., in *The Science and Technology of Gelatin*, A. G. Ward and A. Courts (Ed.), London, Academic Press, 1977, pp. 1–30.
Bartley, J. P., Leatherhead Food R.A., *Technical Circular No. 531*, 1973.
Bartley, J. P. and Marrs, W. M., Leatherhead Food R. A., *Technical Circular No. 582*, 1974.
Bellamy, G. and Bornstein, P., *Proc. natn. Acad. Sci. U.S.A.*, 1971, *68*, 1138.

Beutel, J., in *Photographic Gelatin*, Proceedings of the Fourth IAG Conference, Fribourg, 1983, H. Amman-Brass, and J. Pouradier, (Ed.), 1985, pp. 65–78.
Blazej, A. and Galatik, A., *Kozarstvi*, 1966, *16*, 359–363.
Boedtker, H. and Doty, P., *J. phys. Chem., Ithaca*, 1954, *58*, 968–983.
Boedtker, H. and Doty, P., *J. Am. chem. Soc.*, 1956, *78*, 4267–4280.
Bogue, R. H., *The Chemistry and Technology of Gelatine and Glue*, New York, McGraw-Hill Book Co., 1922.
Bornstein, P. *et al.*, *Biochemistry, N.Y.*, 1966a, *5*, 3803–3812.
Bornstein, P. *et al.*, *Proc. natn. Acad. Sci. U.S.A.*, 1966b, *55*, 417–424.
Bourgoin, D. and Joly, M., in *Recent Advances in Gelatin and Glue Research*, G. Stainsby (Ed.), London, Pergamon Press, 1958, pp. 204–208.
Bowes, J. H. and Kenten, R. H., *Biochem. J.*, 1948, *43*, 358–365.
Bowes, J. H. and Kenten, R. H., *Biochem. J.*, 1950, *46*, 1–8.
Burde, R., de La, *Dissertation Technische Hochschule Aachen*, 1962.
Burge, R. E. and Hynes, R. D., *J. molec. Biol.*, 1959, *1*, 155–164.
Chayen, I. H. and Ashworth, D. R., *J. appl. Chem., Lond.*, 1953, *3*, 529–537.
Cheve, J. L., *Comptes rendus de l'Académie des Sciences, Paris*, 1966, C267.
Christiensen, R. G. and Cassel, J. M., *Biopolymers*, 1967, *5*, 685-689.
Courts, A., *Biochem. J.*, 1954, *58*, 70–74, 74–79.
Courts, A., *Biochem. J.*, 1960, *74*, 238–247.
Courts, A. and Stainsby, G., in *Recent Advances in Gelatin and Glue Research*, G. Stainsby (Ed.), London, Pergamon Press, 1958, pp. 100–105.
Courts, A. and Stainsby, G., per *Nature*, 1959, *183*, 440–441.
Cowan, P. M. and McGavin, S., *Nature*, 1955, *176*, 501–503.
Cowan, P. M. *et al.*, *Nature*, 1955, *176*, 1062–1064.
Crosby, N. T. and Stainsby, G., *Research, Lond.*, 1962, *15*, 427–435.
Crosby, N. T. *et al.*, *J. Soc. Leath. Trades Chem.*, 1962, *46*, 152–161.
Dick, Y. P. *et al.*, *Abs. Fed. Eur. Biochem. Soc., Vienna*, 1965, *2*, 215.
Doty, P. and Nishihara, T. in *Recent Advances in Gelatin and Glue Research*, G. Stainsby (Ed.), London, Pergamon Press, 1958, pp. 92–99.
Drake, M. P. *et al.*, *Biochemistry, N.Y.*, 1966, *5*, 301–312.
Eastoe, J. E., *Biochem. J.*, 1955, *61*, 589–602.
Eastoe, J. E., in *Treatise on Collagen*, Vol. 1, G. N. Ramachandran (Ed.), London, Academic Press, 1967, pp. 1–72.
Eastoe, J. E. and Leach, A. A., in *Recent Advances in Gelatin and Glue Research*, G. Stainsby (Ed.), London, Pergamon Press, 1958, pp. 173–178.
Eastoe, J. E. and Leach, A. A., in *The Science and Technology of Gelatin*, A. G. Ward and A. Courts (Ed.), London, Academic Press, 1977, pp. 77–85.
Engel, J., *Arch. Biochem.*, 1962, *97*, 150–158.
Flausch, A., *L'actualité chimique*, 1978, *2*, 40–45.
Flory, P. J. and Weaver, E. S., *J. Am. chem. Soc.*, 1960, *82*, 4518–4525.
Fraser, R. D. B. *et al.*, in *Fibrous Proteins: Scientific, Industrial and Medical Aspects*, Vol. 1, D. A. D. Parry and L. K. Creamer (Ed.), London, Academic Press, 1979, p. 179–206.

Fujii, T., *Hoppe-Seylers Zeitschrift für physiologische Chemie*, 1969, *350*, 1257–1265.

Gallop, P. M. *et al.*, *J. biophys. biochem. Cytol.*, 1957, *3*, 545–557.

Glanville, R. W. and Kühn, K., in *Fibrous Proteins: Scientific, Industrial and Medical Aspects*, Vol. 1, D. A. D. Parry and L. K. Creamer (Ed.), London, Academic Press, 1979, pp. 133–150.

Gouinlock, E. V. *et al.*, *J. Polym. Sci.*, 1955, *16*, 383–395.

Grassmann, W. and Hörmann, H., *Hoppe-Seylers Zeitschrift für physiologische Chemie*, 1953, *292*, 24–32.

Grassmann, W. *et al.*, *Kolloidzeitschrift*, 1962, *186*, 50–57.

Gross, J. *et al.*, *Proc. natn. Acad. Sci. U.S.A.*, 1954, *40*, 679–688.

Gross, J. *et al.*, *Proc. natn Acad. Sci. U.S.A.*, 1955, *41*, 1–7.

Gustavson, G. H., in *Chemistry and Reactivity of Collagen*, G. H. Gustavson (Ed.), New York, Academic Press, 1956, p. 155.

Hall, C. E. *et al.*, *J. Am. chem. Soc.*, 1942, *64*, 1234.

Hamilton, P. B. and Anderson, R. A., *J. biol. Chem.*, 1954, *211*, 95–102.

Harding, J. J., *J. Soc. Leath. Trades Chem.*, 1964, *48*, 160–173.

Harding, J. J., *Adv. Protein Chem.*, 1965, *20*, 109–190.

Harkness, R. D. *et al.*, *Biochem. J.*, 1954, *56*, 558–569.

Harrington, W. F. and von Hippel, P. H., *Adv. Protein Chem.*, 1961, *16*, 1–138.

Hey, C. D. and Stainsby, G., *Biochim. Biophys. Acta*, 1965, *97*, 364–366.

Heyns, K. and Legler, G., in *Recent Advances in Gelatin and Glue Research*, G. Stainsby (Ed.), London, Pergamon Press, 1958, pp. 186–190.

Higgs, D. G. and Reed, R., *Biochim. Biophys. Acta*, 1963, *78*, 265–277.

Highberger, J. H. and Stecker, H. C., *J. Am. Leath. Chem. Ass.*, 1941, *36*, 368–374.

Highberger, J. H. *et al.*, *Proc. natn. Acad. Sci. U.S.A.*, 1951, *37*, 286—291.

Hinterwaldner, R., in *The Science and Technology of Gelatin*, A. G. Ward and A. Courts (Ed.), London, Academic Press, 1977, pp. 295–314.

Hodge, A. J. and Petruska, J. A., in *Aspects of Protein Structure*, G. N. Ramachandran (Ed.), New York, Academic Press, 1962, pp. 289–300.

Hodge, A. J. *et al.*, *Proc. natn. Acad. Sci. U.S.A.*, 1960, *46*, 197.

Hulmes, D. J. S. *et al.*, *J. molec. Biol.*, 1973, *79*, 137–148.

Itoh, M. and Okamoto, Y., in *Photographic Gelatin*, Proceedings of the Fourth IAG Conference, Fribourg, 1983, H. Amman-Brass and J. Pouradier (Ed.), 1985, p. 125.

Jackson, D. S. and Fessler, J. H., *Nature*, 1955, *176*, 69–70.

Johns, P., in *The Science and Technology of Gelatin*, A. G. Ward and A. Courts (Ed.), London, Academic Press, 1977, pp. 31–72.

Johns, P. and Courts, A., in *The Science and Technology of Gelatin*, A. G. Ward and A. Courts (Ed.), London, Academic Press, 1977, pp. 140–142.

Jones, R. T., *Process Biochem.*, 1971, *6*(7), 19–22.

Kang, A. H. *et al.*, *Biochemistry, N.Y.*, 1966, *5*, 509–515.

Kang, A. H. *et al.*, *Biochem. biophys. Res. Commun.*, 1969, *36*, 345–349.

Koepff, P., *The Use of Electrophoresis in Gelatin Manufacture* at the Royal Photographic Society Symposium on Photographic Gelatin, Oxford, 1979.

Koepff, P., in *Photographic Gelatin*, Proceedings of the Fourth IAG Conference, Fribourg, 1983, H. Amman-Brass and J. Pouradier (Ed.), 1985, pp. 3–35.

Kuhn, K. *et al.*, *Biochemische Zeitschrift*, 1966, *344*, 418–434.

Layman, D. L. *et al.*, *Proc. natn. Acad. Sci. U.S.A.*, 1971, *68*, 454.

Leiner, M. and Gash, P., Symposium on By-products of the Food Industry, Leatherhead Food R.A., *Symposium Proceedings No. 16*, 1972.

Light, N. D. and Bailey, A. J., *Fibrous Proteins: Scientific, Industrial and Medical Aspects*, Vol. 1, D. A. D. Parry and L. K. Creamer (Ed.), London, Academic Press, 1979, pp. 151–177.

Loeven, W. A., *J. Soc. Leath. Trades Chem.*, 1954, *38*, 117–126.

Lorry, D. and Vedrines, M., in *Photographic Gelatin*, Proceedings of the Fourth IAG Conference, Fribourg, 1983, H. Amman-Brass and J. Pouradier (Ed.), 1985, pp. 36–54.

Martin, G. R. *et al.*, in *Environmental Variables in Oral Diseases*, C. J. Kreshover and F. J. McClure (Ed.), Washington, D. C., American Association for Advancement in Science, 1966, p. 155.

Miller, E. J. and Gay, S., Structural and Contractile Proteins, Part A, in *Methods in Enzymology*, Vol. 82, L. W. Cunningham (Ed.), London, Academic Press, 1982, p. 3.

Miller, E. J. and Matukas, V. J., *Proc. natn. Acad. Sci. U.S.A.*, 1969, *64*, 1264.

Orekhovich, V. N. *et al.*, *Biokhimiya*, 1948, *13*, 55–60.

Piez, K. A., *J. Am. chem. Soc.*, 1960, *82*, 247.

Piez, K. A., in *Treatise on Collagen*, Vol. 1, G. N. Ramachandran (Ed.), London, Academic Press, 1967, pp 207–252.

Piez, K. A., *Ann. Rev. Biochem.*, 1968, *37*, 678.

Piez, K. A. *et al.*, *Biochim. Biophys. Acta*, 1961, *53*, 596–598.

Piez, K. A. *et al.*, *Brookhaven Symp. Biol.*, 1968, *21*, 345–357.

Pouradier, J. and Venet, A. M., *J. Chim. phys.*, 1950, *47*, 11–20, 391–398.

Pouradier, J. and Venet, A. M., *J. Chim. phys.*, 1952, *49*, 85–92, 239–244.

Pouradier, J. *et al.*, *J. Chim. phys.*, 1950, *47*, 887–891.

Privalov, P. L., *Adv. Prot. Chem.*, 1982, *35*, 1–104.

Ramachandran, G. N. and Kartha, G., *Nature*, 1954, *174*, 269–270.

Reed, R. and Stainsby, G., *Collagen Symposium*, New York, Madras Interscience, 1962, p. 513.

Reich, G. *et al.*, *Gesammelte Abhandlungen (Deutsches) Lederinstitut*, 1962, *18*, 15–23.

Rich, A. and Crick, F.H. C., *J. molec. Biol.*, 1961, *3*, 483–506.

Rigby, B. J., *Biochim. Biophys. Acta*, 1967, *133*, 272–277.

Robinson, J. A. J., *A Study of Some Physical Properties of Gelatin*, Ph.D. Thesis, University of Nottingham, 1975.

Robinson, J. A. J. *et al.*, *J. Pharm. Pharmac.*, 1975, *27*, 653–658.

Scatchard, G. *et al.*, *J. Am. chem. Soc.*, 1944, *66*, 1980–1981.

Schmitt, F. O. and Gross, J., *J. Am. Leath. Chem. Ass.*, 1948, *43*, 658–675.

Schmitt, F. O. *et al.*, *J. appl. Phys.*, 1945, *16*, 263.

Smith, P. I., *Glue and Gelatine*, London, Pitman Press, 1929.

Stainsby, G., in *The Science and Technology of Gelatin*, A. G. Ward and A. Courts (Ed.), London, Academic Press, 1977, pp. 109–136.

Steven, F. S. and Tristram, G. R., *Biochem. J.*, 1962, *85*, 207–210.

Tomka, I., *Chimia*, 1976, *30*(12), 534–540.

Tomka, I., at the Royal Photographic Society Symposium on Photographic Gelatin, Oxford, 1979.

Tomka, I. *et al.*, *J. photogr. Sci.*, 1975, *23*, 97–103.

Veis, A., *The Macromolecular Chemistry of Gelatin*, London, Academic Press, 1964.

Veis, A. and Cohen, J., *J. Am. chem. Soc.*, 1956, *78*, 6238–6244.

Veis, A. and Cohen, J., *J. Polym. Sci.*, 1957, *26*, 113–116.

Veis, A. and Drake, M. P., *J. biol. Chem.*, 1963, *238*, 2003–2011.

Veis, A. *et al.*, *J. Am. chem. Soc.*, 1955, *77*, 2368–2374.

Veis, A. *et al.*, in *Recent Advances in Gelatin and Glue Research*, G. Stainsby (Ed.), London, Pergamon Press, 1958, pp. 155–163.

Veis, A. *et al.*, *J. Am. Leath. Chem. Ass.*, 1960, *55*, 548–563.

Virnik, D. I. and Zharkova, A. V., *Kino-foto-khimicheskaya promȳshlennost*, 1937, *5*, 51–61.

von Hippel, P. H., in *Treatise on Collagen*, Vol. 1, G. N. Ramachandran (Ed.), London, Academic Press, 1967, pp. 253–338.

von Hippel, P. H. and Wong, K.–Y., *Biochemistry, N.Y.*, 1963, *2*, 1387–1398.

Ward, A. G., *Nature*, 1953, *171*, 1099–1101.

Ward, A. G., *J. roy. Inst. Chem.*, 1964, *88*, 406–413.

Williams, J. W., *J. Polym. Sci.*, 1954, *12*, 351–378.

Williams, J. W., in *Recent Advances in Gelatin and Glue Research*, G. Stainsby (Ed.), London, Pergamon Press, 1958, pp. 106–113.

Williams, J. W. and Saunders, W. M., *J. phys. Chem.*, Ithaca, 1954, *58*, 854–859.

Williams, J. W. *et al.*, *J. phys. Chem.*, Ithaca, 1954, *58*, 774–782.

Williams, J. W. *et al.*, *Chem. Rev.*, 1958, *58*, 715–718.

Wolpers, C., *Naturwissenschaften*, 1941, *28*, 461.

Wolpers, C., *Leder*, 1950, *1*, 3–12.

Woodlock, A. F. and Harrap, B. S., *Aust. J. biol. Sci.*, 1968, *21*, 821–826.

Xiong-fong, C. and Bi-xion, P., in *Photographic Gelatin*, Proceedings of the Fourth IAG Conference, Fribourg, 1983, H. Amman-Brass and J. Pouradier (Ed.), 1985, pp. 55–64.

Yates, J. R., *J. Soc. Leath. Trades Chem.*, 1968, *52*, 425–435.

Chapter 3

Gelatin: Physical and Chemical Properties

R. T. Jones

Acidic and Basic Properties

Several of the amino acid residues of gelatin possess ionisable groups (carboxyl, phenolic, amino, guanidino, and imidazole), which are distributed along the length of the molecule. Together with the terminal amino and carboxyl groups, the acidic and basic side-chain groups enable gelatin to adopt a different net charge, which may be either negative or positive, depending upon the pH of the solution. The numbers of these groups can be determined from titration curves; data for both acid- and lime-processed gelatin are summarised in Table 3.1.

Table 3.1. Content of acidic and basic groups in gelatin*

| Group | pH Titration range (40°) | Concentration mmol/g protein | |
		Acid-processed	Lime-processed
carboxyl	1.5–6.5	0.85	1.23
amide	—	0.35	0.03
α-amino + imidazole	6.5–8.0	0.06	0.07
ε-amino	8.0–11.5	0.42	0.42
guanidino	—	0.49	0.48

* Kenchington and Ward, 1954

The difference in the number of free carboxyl groups present in acid and limed gelatins is due to the differing degrees of deamidation of glutamine and asparagine residues.

The iso-ionic point is the pH of a solution of a protein that contains no non-colloidal ions other than hydrogen or hydroxyl. In the absence of other ions, this pH corresponds to there being zero average net charge on the molecule and coincides with the isoelectric point for gelatin. The isoelectric point is the pH of a gelatin solution in which no net migration of the protein is produced by application of an electric field; it is affected by the ionic strength of the solution. The iso-ionic point is most conveniently determined by deionising a dilute (2–5%) gelatin solution using a mixed-bed ion-exchange column, whilst the isoelectric point can be determined by observing the pH for which there is zero electrophoretic mobility.

The changes in ionisation with pH affect the shape of the gelatin molecules in solution and the interactions between them, and account to some extent for the pH-dependence of the physical properties. The iso-ionic pH is of practical importance since it coincides with extreme values for many of the solution and gel properties of gelatin.

It is generally accepted that the iso-ionic point of lime-processed gelatin falls within the range 4.8–5.2 whilst acid-processed gelatins exhibit values of 6.0–9.4, although it should be noted that the value does not unequivocally differentiate between acid-extracted and neutral-extracted gelatins.

Isoelectric focusing techniques applied to gelatins have shown that a distribution of isoelectric point values occurs, not only in acid-processed gelatins but also in limed gelatins (Maxey and Palmer, 1976; Li-juan et al., 1985; Toda, 1985). For limed gelatins, the range was 0.5–0.7 pH units. A gelatin exhibiting an average isoelectric point of 4.85 showed components ranging from approximately 4.6 to 5.1. Acid-processed gelatins showed a wider distribution (about 2 pH units), as might be expected, due to more widely differing degrees of deamidation of the molecules. The distribution is not merely a characteristic of commercial, blended gelatins since a pure α-component of gelatin gave a similar distribution to that of limed gelatin.

Hydrolysis of limed gelatin by enzymes or alkali results in a reduction of the average isoelectric point, to as low as pH 4.6 in the case of alkaline hydrolysis. This is due to the basicity of the α-amino groups liberated on hydrolysis differing from that of the ε-amino groups, and the acidity of the α-carboxyl groups differing from that of the side-chain carboxyls. In addition, conversion of arginine residues to less basic ornithine residues will contribute to the reduction of the isoelectric point value.

Gel Strength

As a protein, gelatin has the unique ability to form a thermally reversible gel. The sol/gel and gel/sol transformations occur very readily when the temperature is changed over a comparatively small range. Gel strength depends upon the gelatin concentration, pH, temperature, and maturing time.

METHODS OF MEASURING GEL STRENGTH

Commercially, gelatin gel strengths are determined by a standard, but arbitrary, test (BS 757: 1975) which measures the force required to depress the surface of a 6.67% w/w gel, matured at 10° for 16–18 hours, by a distance of 4 mm using a flat-bottomed plunger 12.7 mm in diameter. The force is applied in the form of a stream of lead shot and the weight, in grams, is termed the 'Bloom' strength. A semi-automated version of the Bloom gelometer, the 'Boucher Electronic Jelly Tester' is now also in use and is recognised by the BSI. In this instrument the plunger is suspended from one end of a beam mounted on a torsion wire. Force is applied to the plunger by torque on the wire. The instrument is calibrated to give 'Bloom' values. Another, known as the 'Texture Analyser', is also available.

The procedure used in the U.S.A. for Bloom testing (AOAC 1984) differs from the BSI method in the shape of the plunger. The BS plunger has its bottom edge rounded to a radius of curvature of 0.44 mm whilst the AOAC plunger has a sharp edge. This affects the Bloom result to the extent that the AOAC Bloom will be approximately 3% higher than the BS Bloom.

Whilst Bloom gel strength is widely accepted as a measure of quality, gelatins are rarely used under conditions which even approximate to those of the test procedure. In hard capsule manufacture, for example, the gelatin gel coating the stainless steel pins is formed in a matter of seconds from an approximately 30% w/w solution on cooling from about 50° to 25°. In the manufacture of soft capsules, a concentrated gelatin solution is again rapidly gelled on a chilled drum, but in this case the situation is complicated by the inclusion of a plasticiser, normally glycerol.

Absolute values of rigidity can be obtained by a method involving measurement of the distortion of a gel surface under pressure (Saunders and Ward, 1954). The method is applicable to gels with a wide range of rigidities, but it is not suitable for routine work. Other methods of gel strength measurement applied to gelatin have been reviewed (Finch and Jobling, 1977).

THE NATURE OF THE GELATIN GEL

When an aqueous solution of gelatin above a certain minimum critical concentration is cooled below 40°, a three-dimensional gel network is formed. Gelation is accompanied by changes in optical rotation (Smith, 1919; Kraemer and Fanselow, 1925), X-ray diffraction pattern (Gerngross et al., 1932; Katz, 1932), viscosity (Richardson, 1933; Ferry and Eldridge, 1949; Bohonek et al., 1976), light scattering (French et al., 1971; Moritani et al., 1971; Pines and Prins, 1973; Bohonek et al., 1976), electron microscopic structure (Titova et al., 1973; Bohonek, 1974; Bohonek et al., 1976; Heathcock and Jewell, 1976), and enthalpy (Borchard et al., 1976). These changes have been interpreted as indicating the partial reordering of gelatin molecules into the collagen helical structure.

The transformation can be considered as a three-stage process, the first stage being the intramolecular rearrangement of imino acid-rich chain segments of single-chain gelatin molecules, so that their configurations are similar to those of the same segments in the collagen structure. This is known as the 'collagen fold' and is responsible for the observed increase in optical rotation (von Hippel and Harrington, 1959, 1960; Flory and Weaver, 1960; Engel, 1962). The second stage requires the association of separate chains in 'collagen-fold form' at these regions to form a three-dimensional network. These network junction points formed by association of two or three ordered segments (from two or more individual chains, respectively) create the 'crystallites' indicated by X-ray diffraction studies on gelatin gels, and are linked by the non-helical regions of the gelatin chains (Boedtker and Doty, 1954; Flory and Weaver, 1960; Veis, 1964). The third stage involves the stabilisation of this structure by lateral interchain hydrogen bonding within the helical regions.

The formation of the gelatin gel can therefore be considered as the production of a three-dimensional network of gelatin molecules with water entrapped in the meshes. Development of the equilibrium gel rigidity occurs through the propagation of collagen folding in the junction regions, and by the formation of new, but less stable, links, resulting in a fine network within the coarse network. This gel structure for gelatin has been dramatically demonstrated by freeze-etching electron microscopy studies (Bohonek *et al.*, 1976; Heathcock and Jewell, 1976).

A schematic view of gel formation is shown in Fig. 3.1. Not all gelatin molecules contribute to

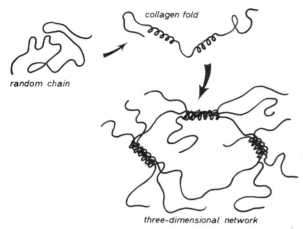

Fig. 3.1. Schematic representation of the formation of a three-dimensional network in gelatin gels.

the gel network. Ultracentrifugation studies (Johnson and Metcalfe, 1967; Bohonek *et al.*, 1976; Gross and Rose, 1976) on gelatin gels have demonstrated the existence of a non-gelling or weakly-gelling 'sol' component. This sol component can also be extracted by dialysis of the gel; the proportion of the total gelatin existing as sol decreases with maturing time and decreasing temperature (Johnson and Metcalfe, 1967). The sol component (which can represent as much as 40% of the gelatin in a 2% gel at 20°, depending on the gelatin used) is more polydisperse and has a lower average molecular weight than the gel component. It also exhibits reduced ability for collagen folding. Moreover, differences in amino acid composition and N-terminal amino acids for the sol and gel fractions have been detected. The evidence is that the sol fraction (at temperatures below about 21°) consists mainly of α_2 chains or their degraded fragments. It has also been observed that the α_2 chains are not found in the sol phase in gelatin containing no molecules smaller than α chains (Bohonek *et al.*, 1976).

EFFECT OF MOLECULAR WEIGHT
It was established 40 years ago (Ferry, 1948b; Ferry and Eldridge, 1949) that there was a linear relationship between the square root of the rigidity modulus G and the weight average molecular weight (M_w) for a series of low molecular weight (33 000–72 000) gelatins prepared from a high molecular weight lime-processed gelatin by progressive thermal hydrolysis. Other workers (Pouradier *et al.*, 1954; Saunders and Ward, 1954; Courts, 1959) showed that above a certain critical average molecular weight the rigidity modulus was practically independent of molecular weight, provided the temperature of the gel was sufficiently below the melting point. The rigidity plateau differed for gelatins of different origins, but this structural feature (called the 'rigidity factor') could not be related to intrinsic viscosity or to the chain average molecular weight (Courts, 1959).

Another factor which influences the position of the plateau is the degree of racemisation of the amino-acid residues in the protein chain. It is known that racemisation can occur at alkaline pH and this can impair the ability to form the collagen fold.

The very high molecular weight components (i.e. greater than that of the α-chain), which of necessity must be multi-chain molecules, exhibit a reduced tendency to form useful gel network links despite their greater tendency to form the collagen fold (Bohonek *et al.*, 1976). It has been suggested that this reflects a tendency for intramolecular aggregation to occur, which would effectively reduce the number of collagen folds available for network formation (Veis, 1964). As the temperature approaches the melting point of the gel the 'critical molecular weight' increases and the rigidity becomes more dependent upon molecular weight (Saunders and Ward, 1958). The rigidity of commercial gelatins possessing a broad distribution of molecular weights depends upon the proportion of molecules with molecular weights below the critical value.

EFFECT OF TEMPERATURE AND TIME
The strength of a gelatin gel increases rapidly during the first few hours and thereafter more slowly, at any given temperature (Saunders and Ward, 1958). It does not reach a constant value, although it has been shown that an approximately constant rigidity can be achieved within five hours at the maturing temperature if the gel is first pre-chilled and aged at a much lower temperature (Ferry, 1948a and b). This illustrates the fact that rigidity is not simply related to the maturing temperature

and time, but also depends upon the thermal history. Pre-maturing the gel at a higher temperature than the final maturing temperature results in a higher gel strength than if the gel has been chilled directly to the maturing temperature. These observations can be explained on the basis that rapid cooling of a gelatin solution results in a less ordered arrangement of gelatin molecules because they have been 'frozen' in the configuration which existed in the solution state. This leads to only limited development of network junctions and is called a 'fine' gel network. In contrast, slow cooling leads to the formation of a 'coarse' network in which more highly organised links have had a chance to form (Stainsby, 1977b).

For a given concentration, the rigidity of a gelatin gel decreases with increasing maturing temperature. An approximately linear relationship between temperature and G/c^2 (where G is the rigidity modulus and c is the concentration) was found for low molecular weight gelatins over the range 0–30°, but the relationship has not proved to be universal for all gelatins (Ferry, 1948b). Different types of gelatin show varying dependences of rigidity upon temperature. Moreover, for gelatins of similar type (i.e. similar raw material and processing) low Bloom strength gelatins exhibit greater sensitivity to temperature.

EFFECT OF GELATIN CONCENTRATION

The rigidity modulus (G) of a gelatin gel is a function of its concentration (c) (Leich, 1904; Sheppard and Sweet, 1921; Poole, 1925; Ferry, 1948b; Ferry and Eldridge, 1949) and, in general, G is approximately proportional to the square of the concentration. Not surprisingly (in view of the differing contribution to the gel network expected for each of the different molecular species present to varying extents in commercial gelatins) deviations from the square law have been found, particularly for very dilute gels (less than 2%) (Ferry and Eldridge, 1949; Saunders and Ward, 1954), for very concentrated gels (20–30%) (Cumper and Alexander, 1952), and for highly degraded gelatins (Sheppard and Sweet, 1921). The deviation can mean that the exponent is greater or less than 2, and it has been concluded that a general relationship is unlikely to apply to all gelatins (Ward and Saunders, 1958). An average value of 1.7 has been found most useful for calculating Bloom gel strength from gel strengths determined at concentrations differing from the standard 6.67%, for

'commercial gelatins' containing moisture and ash (Kramer and Rosenthal, 1965).

EFFECT OF PH

The extent to which the strength of a gelatin gel is affected by pH varies with the type of gelatin (e.g. acid- or alkali-processed) and also with the gelation conditions. Early work on an alkali-processed gelatin at 10% concentration, following a low-temperature maturing period, indicated that rigidity was independent of pH over the range 4.4–9.0 (Gerngross, 1926). When the concentration was reduced to 1.5%, the pH range for constant rigidity was reduced to 4.4–6.7. Later work on an acid-extracted limed gelatin at a concentration of 2.7% and a constant ionic strength of 0.15, using rather weak gels obtained by maturing at 25°, showed a greater dependence upon pH (Cumper and Alexander, 1952). Over a similar pH range, an increase in rigidity was observed as the pH increased to 9, at which point the gel strength was maximal. A more marked dependence of rigidity on pH was, however, detected below about pH 4 and above pH 10. Other studies have confirmed this pattern (Steigmann, 1957; Konno and Kaneko, 1969).

Acid-processed gelatins show a more pronounced reduction in rigidity below pH 4.5 than do limed gelatins. This is a reflection of the greater degree of hydration of the gelatin molecules at pH values well away from the isoelectric point.

EFFECT OF BLENDING

Because of the relationship between G and c^2, the rigidity of a mixture of several gelatins can be calculated from the equation

$$\sqrt{G_{blend}} = a_1 \sqrt{G_1} + a_2 \sqrt{G_2} + a_3 \sqrt{G_3} + \ldots$$

where a_1 is the fraction of gelatin of rigidity G_1 in the blend, and so on.

This general relationship is useful for blending gelatins of similar types which are not widely different in gel strength, and where the exponent is fairly close to 2. However, synergistic increases in gel strength can be achieved by blending together acid- and lime-processed gelatins, when the pH of the system is such that the gelatins are oppositely charged. This will normally be the case in the region pH 5.0–6.5. This synergism has been demonstrated for 'hard capsule grade' acid ossein and limed ossein gelatins which were blended together in various proportions, the rigidities then being measured over the concentration range 5–50% w/v (Robinson et al., 1975a). Maxima in the rigidity–concentration plots occurred when the blend contained about 40–50% of limed gelatin. For the 50% w/v gels the increase in rigidity modulus was fifteenfold. In contrast, at low concentrations (3.5% or less) a decrease in gel strength occurred due to coacervate formation.

Effect of Additives

The effect of added glycerol on gelatin rigidity has been quite widely studied (Sheppard and Sweet, 1921; Hatschek, 1932; Hirai and Kishimoto, 1953; Mindru and Ceacareanu, 1966; Nixon et al., 1966; Carless and Nixon, 1970) because of the importance of the gelatin–glycerol system in the manufacture of soft capsules and suppositories. Addition of glycerol significantly increases gelatin gel rigidity: for gels containing 4–15% gelatin and up to 40% w/w of glycerol a general relationship for rigidity modulus has been derived (Nixon et al., 1966):

$$G = a + bZ^2 + (c + dZ)c$$

where Z is % gelatin concentration, c is % glycerol concentration, and a, b, c, and d are constants whose values depend upon the grade of gelatin. Other polyhydric alcohols such as sorbitol, and sugars (Sheppard and Sweet, 1921; Hatschek, 1932), such as sucrose (Sheppard and Sweet, 1921; Jones, 1977) and maltodextrins (Jones, 1977), can increase gel strength. However, at high additive levels and high total solids the rigidity can start to fall again. Also, with maltodextrins of increasing molecular weight or polyethylene glycols of increasing degrees of polymerisation, the 'critical concentration' of the additive decreases with increasing molecular weight (Holmes et al., 1985).

Ethanol produces an increase in rigidity, provided that the concentration is low enough to avoid precipitation of the gelatin from solution (Sheppard and Sweet, 1921). Formaldehyde cross-linking also increases the rigidity (Hatschek, 1932).

Reduction in rigidity can be effected by the addition of electrolytes. The addition of sodium chloride at a concentration of up to 17.5% in a dilute gel produced a decrease in rigidity which was linear with the square root of the ionic strength (I) and the following equation was obeyed (Cumper and Alexander, 1952)

$$G = G_0(1 - 0.77I^{\frac{1}{2}})$$

where G_0 is the rigidity of the gel without additives.

Compounds which destroy hydrogen bonds, such as urea, phenol, ammonium nitrate, lithium bromide, and potassium isothiocyanate at high concentration, can completely suppress gelation (Zubov et al., 1954; Watase and Arakawa, 1969).

Viscosity

Viscosity of Dilute Solutions

The relationship between viscosity and molecular weight in dilute solutions has been studied by various workers (Pouradier and Venet, 1950, 1952; Gouinlock et al., 1955; Veis and Cohen, 1957; Courts and Stainsby, 1958; Veis et al., 1960; Stainsby et al., 1969); corrections for the mutual interactions of the gelatin molecules and the contribution to the viscosity by the solvent are usually made by extrapolating viscosities, measured at a series of concentrations, to zero concentration.

If η is the viscosity of the solvent, and η_c that of the solution at a concentration c, the intrinsic viscosity is defined as

$$[\eta] = \lim_{c \to 0} (\eta/\eta_c - 1)/c$$

The Staudinger equation

$$[\eta] = KM^a$$

is generally applicable to polymer solutions, M being the average molecular weight, and K and a being constants dependent on the gelatin and the solvent.

The values of K and a vary for different gelatins, even of similar types, although constant values have been used satisfactorily to represent the behaviour of a gelatin and fractions obtained from it by coacervation or progressive thermal hydrolysis (Pouradier and Venet, 1950).

The intrinsic viscosity is affected by pH, particularly at low ionic strength. It exhibits a minimum at the iso-ionic point and maxima at approximately pH 3 and pH 10.5 (Stainsby, 1952). These effects can be accounted for by the uncoiling of the gelatin molecules due to the repulsion of ionised groups as the net charge on the molecules changes. These ionic repulsions are reduced by electrolytes, the reduction in viscosity at extremes of pH reflecting the presence of counter-ions resulting from the use of acid or alkali to adjust the pH.

Viscosity of Concentrated Solutions

Commercially, gelatin viscosities are routinely measured at 6.67% w/w at 60° using either an Ostwald or a pipette viscometer. For the gelatin used in hard capsule manufacture, measurements are frequently also made at 12.5% w/w. A relationship between viscosities at these two concentrations has been established (Stainsby, 1958, 1977a).

Over a wider range of concentration, i.e. 2–60%, a slight S-shaped deviation from the linear relationship between viscosity and concentration

$$\log \eta = kc$$

has been observed in the temperature range 50–90° (Finch and Jobling, 1977). Over the restricted concentration range of 10–50% the logarithmic relationship is quite adequate (Cumper and Alexander, 1952). Above the setting point, viscosity decreases exponentially with increasing temperature (Croome, 1953b; Finch and Jobling, 1977).

The effect of pH in concentrated solutions is similar to that for dilute solutions, with the viscosity being lowest at the iso-ionic point and highest at pH 3 and 10.5 approximately (Sheppard and Houck, 1930). However, as the gelatin concentration increases, the effect of pH becomes less significant, particularly in acid solutions (Stainsby, 1977a). This is due to the inevitable increase in ionic strength with increasing gelatin concentration, due to the presence of the counter-ions associated with the gelatin.

For any fixed gelatin concentration in the approximate range 6.67–50% and any fixed temperature in the range 50–90°, the viscosity of a blend of several gelatins can be calculated from the relationship

$$\log \eta_{blend} = a_1 \log \eta_1 + a_2 \log \eta_2 + \ldots$$

where a_1 is the weight fraction of gelatin in the blend of viscosity η_1 when tested at the same fixed concentration and temperature.

This relationship does not apply to blends of acid and limed gelatins, since synergistic increases in viscosity, analogous to the gel strength increases referred to earlier, may occur. Blends of hard capsule grade, limed ossein and acid pigskin gelatins in varying proportions exhibit marked viscosity increases. Acid ossein gelatin produces less marked synergistic viscosity increases with limed ossein gelatin (although in all cases the viscosity is higher than the calculated value) and the viscosity–blend curve is much smoother than the corresponding curve for limed ossein/acid pigskin blends. Acid ossein gelatin also produces a smooth curve for blending with either pigskin gelatin alone

or limed ossein/acid pigskin mixtures. At temperatures above the setting point, but below about 43° (depending upon gelatin concentration and viscosity), the viscosity can increase with time and become non-Newtonian in character. This is due to the association of the gelatin molecules to form aggregates.

It has also been shown that, for a 50:50 blend of hard capsule grade acid ossein gelatin and limed ossein gelatin in 30% aqueous solution at 35°, the rate of development of increased viscosity is very much greater than for either of the component gelatins alone (Robinson et al., 1975a).

Degradation of Gelatin

Gelatin in solution is susceptible to thermal or enzymatic hydrolysis, leading to a reduction in average molecular weight and a change in many of the useful properties.

The extent of thermal hydrolysis is a function of temperature, time, and pH, and is minimal at near-neutral pH (Ames, 1947). Gel strength (Ames, 1947; Croome, 1953a; Courts, 1954; Kramer and Rosenthal, 1965), viscosity, and chain average molecular weight (Courts, 1954) have each been used to monitor hydrolysis; acid-processed gelatins are more resistant to acid and more susceptible to alkaline hydrolysis than lime-processed gelatins (Ames, 1947). This difference is more obvious in the effects on gel strength than on viscosity. Studies of the terminal amino residues created during hydrolysis show that the pH dependence of peptide bond scission varies for different N-linked amino acid residues (Courts, 1954). Peptide links involving the amino groups of serine and threonine are particularly susceptible to both acid and alkaline hydrolysis, whereas those involving glutamic acid peptides are very stable. Aspartic acid peptides are particularly susceptible to acid hydrolysis.

Thermal degradation of high grade gelatin results in a more rapid reduction of viscosity than of Bloom gel strength, particularly in acid (Ames, 1947). A general formula for calculating the loss in Bloom strength on exposing gelatin solutions to various pH values in the range 3–9 and temperatures up to 100° has been reported for acid pigskin (Tiemstra, 1968), but it is not directly applicable to limed gelatins on acid hydrolysis.

One practical implication of the susceptibility of gelatin to thermal degradation is that gelatin solutions cannot be autoclaved as a means of sterilisation without suffering deterioration in physical properties. Dissolution temperatures of 55–70° can safely be used for gelatins having pH values in the normal 'commercial range' of 5.0–6.5, and solutions can be maintained at 45–60° for several hours without significant change in physical characteristics, provided that the pH is maintained in this range.

At temperatures of about 40°, the rate of thermal hydrolysis is negligible, but the rate of bacterial or enzymatic degradation increases whenever contamination by viable bacteria or enzymes exists. Gelatin in solution has a random configuration; consequently gelatin peptide segments can conform to the configurations of the active centres of enzymes with the result that gelatin is susceptible to a range of proteolytic enzymes. Gelatin hydrolysis using papain, pepsin, chymotrypsin, trypsin, and commercial bacterial enzymes has been studied (Courts, 1955; Jacobson, 1976).

It is usual for specifications for hard capsule gelatins to include a test for 'degradation rate', since the stability of solution viscosity at 45–60° over a number of hours is an important characteristic. This is commonly, but arbitrarily, carried out by measuring the percentage drop in viscosity of a 12.5% w/w solution at 60° over 17 hours. Under these conditions, a viscosity drop or more than 20% suggests bacterial or extracellular enzymatic action. It is possible to distinguish between the action of enzymes and bacteria by measuring viscosity degradation rates at 40° in the absence and presence of preservatives. The initial rate of thermal hydrolysis is greater for higher viscosity gelatins.

Setting Point and Setting Time of Gelatin Gels

The gelation temperature, or more particularly the time for the onset of gelation, is of practical importance in many applications, not least in hard capsule manufacture. Despite its practical interest, there is no universally accepted or adopted procedure for measuring setting time, as there is for viscosity and gel strength. Various methods have been described (Janus et al., 1965; Marrs and Wood, 1972; British Standard 757: 1975; Coopes, 1975; Wainewright, 1977; Itoh, 1985) which basically attempt to determine either the point at which the viscosity of the solution becomes very high, or the development of a particular degree of rigidity after the setting point has been passed. Procedures range from simple techniques, such as that of British Standard 757, which involves stirring a 10% gelatin solution with a thermometer,

whilst it is being cooled from 45° to 20°, and noting the point at which the solution no longer drips from the end of the thermometer when removed, to rather more sophisticated techniques such as that described by Marrs and Wood (1972). In this method, drops of carbon tetrachloride are released into a vertical column of gelatin solution, at a constant drop rate, and are used to detect the setting point as the system is cooled from 40° ± 0.1° to 23° ± 0.002°. The viscosity increases rapidly near the point of gelation, when the drops become almost stationary in the solution. This method has been used to show that setting time is related to the content of gelatin molecules with a very high molecular weight, i.e. greater than 500 000 (Bartley and Marrs, 1974). Similar conclusions followed from setting-rate studies using an oscillating hollow cup viscometer (Bohonek et al., 1976). It was also observed that ossein gelatins (whether limed or acid-processed) gelled more rapidly than skin gelatins (whether acid pigskin or limed) even though they had comparable contents of very high molecular weight components (Bartley and Marrs, 1974).

Although there is no published work on the relationship between setting-rate characteristics and capsule manufacture, one method which would appear to be useful for studies of hard capsule gelatins is that described by Janus et al. (1965), because it enables short gelation times of concentrated gelatin solutions to be measured. Uniform drops of gelatin solution are placed at short intervals on the polished surface of a level, hollow bar through which water at controlled temperature is circulated. Gelation time is determined by rotating the bar through 90° and observing the position of the drop which just fails to run. The bar is enclosed in a high humidity environment to prevent skin formation but no doubt the equipment could be adapted to lower fixed humidities comparable with those existing in hard capsule manufacture. Janus used this method to establish that a linear relationship exists between the logarithm of setting rate at 20° and the logarithm of gelatin concentration, up to 10% concentration. Setting rate is affected by pH; minima in the pH–setting time curves have been reported at pH 4.5–5.5 for lime-processed gelatins, and at pH 6 for acid-processed gelatins (Hopp, 1964). Similar results have been reported in a separate study but minima were also found at about pH 9 for both acid pigskin and limed hide gelatin (Marrs and Wood, 1972). Below about pH 4.5 and above about pH 9.5, the setting time increased rapidly. Itoh (1985) found a sharp minimum setting time at the iso-ionic point for limed gelatin, but a broader minimum in the region of the iso-ionic point for acid pigskin gelatin. Extremes of pH resulted in marked increases in setting time, as found by other workers.

Neutral salts such as sodium chloride and potassium chloride have only a minor effect on setting rate. In the pH range 4.5–10.8 there is a slight reduction, and outside this range a slight increase, in setting rate (Marrs and Wood, 1972).

Increasing the gel strength of the gelatin reduces setting time for both acid and limed gelatins (Itoh, 1985).

Melting Point of Gelatin Gels

The ability of gelatin gels to melt at body temperature has obvious significance for hard and soft capsules. The actual melting point depends on many factors, including concentration, molecular weight, pH, thermal history, and additives. As a gelatin gel is warmed, the rigidity decreases and then disappears relatively rapidly, but the melting point and setting point do not coincide, even when the heating and cooling rates are very slow. Indeed, holding gels at temperatures near the melting point can result in higher melting temperatures than for comparable gels heated at a constant rate (Stainsby, 1977b). For example, the melting point of a 6% gel formed at 0° rose from 31.5° to 34.5° during one day's storage at 25°. This demonstrates that the gel network is continually being reorganised to give linkages of greater thermal stability.

Increasing the gelatin concentration in the range 1–5% increases the melting point for gelatin gels matured at 0°, but for high-grade gelatins the increase is quite small once the concentration exceeds 5%. In earlier published work on fractionated gelatins of relatively low weight average molecular weights (in the range 33 000–72 100), a linear relationship was reported between the logarithm of the concentration and the reciprocal of the melting point for 2–6% gels chilled at 0°. Samples gelled at 15° had higher melting points but displayed a reduced dependence upon concentration. These gelatins also gave a linear plot of the logarithm of weight average molecular weight against the reciprocal of the melting point. Subsequent work on higher molecular weight gelatin fractions confirmed that melting point increased with molecular weight, but the relationship varied from one gelatin to another.

The effect of pH on melting point has been found to be markedly dependent upon both the gel concentration and the maturing temperature. For deionised gelatin gels of 1–5% concentration, chilled at 0° for 20 hours, the melting point was insignificantly affected by pH in the range 2–12, when compared with the effect of concentration changes (Bello et al., 1962). This was true for acid pigskin, limed ossein, and limed calfskin gelatins. A higher maturing temperature of 25°, however, gave a maximum melting point at pH 5 for limed gelatin (Kraemer and Fanselow, 1925; Pleass, 1930). At concentrations below 1%, a marked dependence upon pH was observed, which could be removed by the addition of enough sodium chloride to make the solution 0.15M (Bello et al., 1962). The acid pigskin gelatin, for example, failed to gel at 0.7% concentration over the pH range 6.0–11.0, whilst producing gels with melting points of approximately 15° at a pH of 2, 5, or 12. However, on allowing the solutions to age at 0° gels formed at all pH values and effectively became independent of pH.

Added electrolytes at high concentrations may either increase or decrease melting point: the effect of a variety of sodium salts has been examined (Bello et al., 1956). For example, 1.0 M sodium chloride depresses the melting point, whereas 1.0 M sodium sulphate raises it.

Although the general term melting point has not been precisely defined for gelatin, it will be apparent that this property, in common with setting point, is influenced by the test procedure and no universally adopted method exists. However, BS 757 describes a simple procedure which is capable of giving results to within 0.25°. In practice, it is often of more interest to know the melting point of gelatin films in water or aqueous solution, and in this situation the so-called melting point is the temperature of dissolution of the gel in water. A useful method has been described (Tabor, 1968) in which the melting point is determined by observing the temperature at which the swollen gelatin film ruptures under the weight of a standard stainless steel ball; this method has been used to study the effect of cross-linking agents.

Protective Colloid and Emulsifying Properties

The concept of 'gold number' was introduced by Zsigmondy (1901) as an arbitrary unit of measurement for the minimum amount of a protective substance required to prevent a gold sol being flocculated by sodium chloride solution. Of a number of naturally occurring macromolecular materials investigated, gelatin was found to have the lowest gold number, and its protective colloidal action was apparent irrespective of the charge on the gelatin molecule. However, when the gelatin concentration was below a critical level it actually sensitised the sols to flocculation so that they were flocculated by lower concentrations of electrolytes than in the absence of gelatin.

Gelatin is an excellent stabiliser for oil-in-water emulsions or gas–liquid systems such as foams. Apart from reducing surface tension, its stabilisation properties arise from its ability to form strong films around the disperse phase. The interfacial tension between oils and gelatin is not sufficiently low for emulsions to be formed spontaneously or by simple stirring or gentle shaking, unless the liquids are very viscous. Energy must therefore be supplied to create new surface area by using a homogeniser, colloid mill, or similar equipment.

By such mechanical methods stable emulsions can be produced with low viscosity, dilute gelatin solutions. Gelatin has been used in pharmaceutical preparations to produce stable emulsions of cod-liver oil, castor oil, lemon oil, and mineral oil, and is an effective emulsion vehicle for vitamin A and its esters, besides being a protective antioxidant carrier in the dry state (U.S. Patents 2 643 209, 1953; 2 756 177, 1956; 3 529 065, 1970; Charlson and Wiechers, 1956). The stability of gelatin-containing emulsions varies with the pH of the solution, the pH of maximum stability being a function of the type of gelatin and of its isoelectric point. Acid-processed gelatin has better emulsifying properties in acid conditions, whereas lime-processed gelatin is better in alkaline conditions (Tice, 1936). Other ionic components incorporated in the emulsion must be compatible with the gelatin to avoid the possibility of coacervation by charge neutralisation.

Properties of Gelatin Films

EFFECT OF DRYING CONDITIONS
Films formed by drying gelatin from the sol state possess different physical properties from those dried at low temperatures from the gel state. X-ray diffraction studies (Bradbury and Martin, 1952) have shown that hot-dried films give only a broad, diffuse diffraction pattern typical of liquids or glassy materials, indicating a relatively simple random coil or amorphous structure. In contrast, cold-dried films give an X-ray pattern with a series

of diffracted areas and spots, indicating a high degree of ordering, with triple-helix crystallites orientated in a direction parallel to the plane of the film. It has been estimated that up to 20% of the gelatin molecules in cold-dried films are in the triple-helix crystalline form (Jolley, 1970). The degree of orientation in the plane of the films is reduced as the drying temperature approaches the gel melting point and, as might be expected, thin (approximately 16 μm dry film thickness) gelatin films which have been rapidly dried have been shown, by optical rotation measurements, to contain more randomly orientated helices than thicker films dried more slowly (Coopes, 1976a, b).

The difference in structure between hot- and cold-dried gelatin films is reflected in their mechanical properties and their solubility characteristics in cold water (Kozlov and Burdygina, 1983). Cold-dried films have a greater tensile strength than hot-dried films, when measured at relative humidities (RH) of 45–85%, and a greater elongation at break at relative humidities up to 65%. However, at relative humidities of 75% and 85% the situation is reversed and hot-dried films exhibit marked extensibility (Bradbury and Martin, 1952). Cold-dried films swell without dissolving in cold water, whereas hot-dried films can dissolve spontaneously, at least at their surface. Again this is consistent with the picture of individual molecules of amorphous gelatin being free to dissolve whilst the ordered structure of the molecules of the crystalline film prevents dissolution. The hot-dried film may not dissolve completely, particularly if it is not very thin, because as the water diffuses into the film the amorphous structure may be converted into a crystalline gel network more rapidly than it can dissolve.

PROPERTIES OF COLD-DRIED FILMS
The properties of cold-dried gelatin films are of obvious importance in the production of hard capsules. They are intimately related to moisture content, and may be affected by pH, additives, and relative humidity.

Effect of Moisture Content
Gelatin of very low (less than 5%) moisture content is too brittle for almost all practical purposes. A higher content of moisture, which acts as a plasticiser, is necessary in hard capsules to avoid problems at the trimming stage during manufacture and in subsequent handling and filling operations.

Equilibrium moisture sorption–relative humidity isotherms for gelatin have been obtained by several workers (Sheppard *et al.*, 1940; Bell *et al.*, 1973). In the earlier study, identical isotherms were reported for acid- and lime-processed gelatins below 80–90% RH. A hysteresis effect was apparent whereby the moisture content was influenced by the previous moisture history, higher moisture content being achieved on desorption than on absorption. Equilibrium moisture content decreased with increasing gel concentration in the range 2–15% and was also slightly affected by pH; at 47% RH the moisture content decreased progressively on reducing the pH below 4.9. Hydrolysis of the original gelatin, which reduced its viscosity by a factor of three, had little effect on the moisture content; neither did varying the film thickness. The results of later work, although of a similar order, are generally not in close agreement. For example, literature data for the equilibrium moisture content of gelatin at 44% RH and 25° are compared in Table 3.2.

Table 3.2. Equilibrium moisture content of gelatin film at 44% RH and 25°

| Authors | Moisture content, % | |
	Sorption	Desorption
Sheppard *et al.* (1940)	16.5	18.5
Mason and Silcox (1943)	17.8	—
Calhoun and Leister (1959)	—	11.5
Ito *et al.* (1969)	13.5	17.0
Bell *et al.* (1973)	13.4	15.0
Melia *et al.* (1981)	—	13.46 (Limed ossein gelatin 1)
	—	13.27 (Limed ossein gelatin 2)
	—	13.24 (Acid ossein gelatin)
	—	13.09 (Acid pigskin gelatin)
Eith *et al.*, (1986)	16.0 (20°)	—
Marshall and petrie (1979)	11.3 (21°)	—

If these apparent differences in equilibrium moisture content for various gelatins were real, then they would be expected to be of significance for hard capsules. The work of Melia *et al.* (1981), indicates that there are only small but, nevertheless, statistically significant differences in the equilibrium moisture contents of gelatins. Whilst uncertainty may exist over the equilibrium moisture values for gelatin, there is evidence that the rate at which gelatins dry also varies with gelatin type. It has been reported that acid pigskin gelatin dries more rapidly than lime-processed gelatins

and that this characteristic is important in avoiding brittleness in capsule gelatin (British Patent 836082, 1960). Certainly this observation is in agreement with practical experience from hard capsule manufacture, where brittle capsules are produced when the gelatin blend contains in excess of a critical percentage (normally 40–60%) of pigskin gelatin. In contrast, it is generally found that inclusion of acid ossein gelatin into the blend reduces brittleness. However, a detailed study (Melia *et al.*, 1981) of the drying rate of films cast from acid ossein, limed ossein, and pigskin gelatins, over the range 12–85% RH and 20–35°, failed to demonstrate significant differences between the gelatins. In this work, 25% gelatin solutions were cast as thin gelled films (typically 0.40 ± 0.01 mm thickness) which were then dried at a controlled relative humidity and temperature, and fixed air flow, whilst freely suspended from a microbalance to enable moisture loss to be continuously monitored. At 25° and 44% RH, the drying rate was independent of film thickness over the range 0.24–0.56 mm, indicating that, under these conditions, diffusion of moisture through the film was not a rate-determining step. It is possible that, under different conditions, intrinsic differences in drying characteristics of gelatin may be apparent; for example, where drying occurs from only one side of the film and shrinkage of the film is restricted by the 'backing' and higher air-flow rates are experienced.

The tensile strength, hardness, and Young's modulus of thin gelatin films, measured as a function of moisture content, indicate a maximum in tensile strength at a moisture content of approximately 10%, decreasing to 90% of the maximum for moisture levels between 10% and 20% (Healey *et al.*, 1974). Other workers (Kellaway *et al.*, 1978a) have compared the mechanical properties of hard capsule grade gelatin films prepared from limed ossein and acid ossein gelatins and 1:1 blends of the two. Little difference in Young's modulus was found, at low stresses, between the acid and limed gelatins, which showed a maximum at 14–16% moisture (non-equilibrium). In contrast, the blend of the two gelatin types showed an increased modulus over the moisture range 20–50%, with a maximum at 22% moisture, although at lower moisture contents the difference was no longer apparent. At higher stresses, or when the gelatin films had been allowed to attain equilibrium moisture values in the range 10–20%, the gelatin blend behaved in a more closely similar manner to the individual types, with values of Young's modulus decreasing in the order 1:1 blend, limed and acid gelatin. Below a critical equilibrium moisture content (13–16%), all three gelatin films exhibited stress relaxation at low strains, but at higher equilibrium moisture values the stress increased with time due to contraction of the film. In contrast, more rapidly dried, non-equilibrium moisture content films did not shrink. This phenomenon was presumed to be related to the orientation of crystallites in the films.

Effect of pH
The effect of pH on the mechanical properties of low moisture content films appears not to have been studied, although the rupture properties of 10% gel strips, matured and tested at 10°, have been investigated (Marrs and Wood, 1972). Acid and limed ossein gelatins behaved similarly, exhibiting essentially constant values for rupture load and extension at break, over the pH range 4–11. For limed hide gelatins, there was a minimum in the rupture load (or extensibility)—pH curve near pH 7, with maxima at around pH 5 and pH 9.5 which were very much higher than for ossein gelatins.

Effect of Additives
Tensile strength measurements on deionised gelatin films at low relative humidity suggest that deionisation increases tensile strength (Norris and McGraw, 1964). Thus one would expect additives to reduce the strength. The addition of calcium chloride to limed hide gelatin reduced the rupture load over the pH range 4–11 for 10% gels (Marrs and Wood, 1972).

The effect of the addition of dyes (erythrosine, amaranth, brilliant blue FCF, and indigo carmine) and of titanium dioxide on the mechanical properties of thin gelatin films equilibrated to 16% moisture was studied by Robinson et al. (1975b). There was little or no effect on the Young's modulus and the tensile strength, but the dyes all influenced the stress relaxation characteristics of the gelatin. In some cases a low concentration of dye (0.1% w/v) was more effective in reducing the percentage increase in stress (i.e. the degree of contraction) of the films than a higher concentration (1.0% w/v), but amaranth had the greatest effect at the 1.0% level. Similar results were found for both limed and acid ossein gelatins.

The most important additive for soft capsules is glycerol, which exhibits strong molecular interactions with gelatin. When added as a plasticiser

at low levels (i.e. up to 10% w/w on gelatin) it reduces the affinity of gelatin for moisture (Pouradier and Hodot, 1972). The amount of water sorbed by a mixture of gelatin and glycerol is less than that sorbed at the same relative humidity by the two materials separately. This effect has been attributed to the partial or total blocking of the hydrophilic groups of gelatin by glycerol molecules.

The inclusion of glycerol in hot-dried film will transform the gelatin from a comparatively brittle, stiff material to a highly extensible rubber. Measurements of tensile relaxation modulus show that devitrification occurs at about 30% w/w glycerol, while the modulus remains almost independent of glycerol content in the ranges 0–30% w/w and 60–75% w/w. At 85–95% w/w glycerol, relatively weak gels, which tear easily, are produced (Yannas, 1972).

The viscoelastic properties of thin films formed from gelatin–glycerol–water mixtures typical of those used in soft capsule manufacture have been studied. Stress relaxation measurements showed a decrease in elasticity with increasing ageing time up to 48 hours, followed by a progressive increase. These changes appeared to reflect an initial change to a more amorphous structure followed by a gradual restoration of crystallinity.

It has been reported that gelatin films should have a minimum moisture content of approximately 12% if the inclusion of glycerol (or other low molecular weight plasticiser) is to have a plasticising action as indicated by measurement of resistance to impact (Kozlov and Burdygina, 1983). However, even at lower moisture levels, glycerol appreciably reduces internal stress when subjected to isometric heating.

Effect of Exposure to High Relative Humidity
The water solubility of hard gelatin capsules and gelatin-bound or coated tablets may progressively change with time in tropical climates where conditions of high temperature and, more particularly, high relative humidity, prevail. It has also been reported that gelatin can become insoluble under comparatively mild conditions (Pankhurst, 1947; Jopling, 1956). Gelatin heated at 45° and high relative humidity for 5 days lost some of its ability to swell in water, and had an increased melting point. At relative humidities approaching 100%, hydrothermal contraction, similar to that of collagen, occurred (Pankhurst, 1947). Similar results have been reported for films conditioned at

85–95% RH at 50°. Even at 20° some reduction in water absorption was observed, but not an increase in melting point. The effect of exposing gelatin film to various relative humidities at 50° is illustrated in Table 3.3.

Table 3.3. Melting points of isoelectric gelatin films after conditioning at 50° for eight days (Jopling, 1956)

Gelatin type	% RH	Melting point*
Lime-processed ossein	25	31.5
	60	31
	85	>97
	95	86
50% Lime-processed ossein ⎫	10	33
50% Lime-processed hide ⎭	68	34.5
	85	>97
	96	86.5
Acid-processed ossein	25	31
	60	31
	85	93
	95	53.5

* 'Melting point' (more precisely the dissolution temperature) of a gelatin film determined by placing the film in a water-bath at 20°, the temperature then being raised at a rate of 1.7° per minute until the gelatin dissolved. The initial melting point of all the samples was 32°.

The change in gelatin film properties at high RH has been explained by assuming that sufficient water is absorbed by the film to enable weaker bonds involved in gelation to reform to give crystallites of greater strength and stability. That the maximum increase occurs at 85% RH rather than at 100% is due to excessive moisture absorption at the higher level which increases the separation between molecules and makes reformation of bonds more difficult. Hydrothermal contraction of gelatin film 0.6 mm in thickness, exposed to 80% RH at 21° represented as much as 2.4% of the film length (Calhoun and Leister, 1959).

Chemical Interactions in Gelatin Solutions

The gelatin molecule possesses a number of side-chain groups capable of reacting chemically with a variety of modifying reagents, producing derivatives with their own particular chemical and physical properties. However, apart from these 'true derivatives' which involve the formation of covalent bonds, gelatin is ampholytic and is capable of ionic interaction with oppositely charged molecules. In addition to these reactions of the gelatin molecule itself, chemical impurities naturally present in the gelatin may be responsible for chemical changes observed in gelatin-containing pharmaceutical systems. As an example, soft capsule walls formed from gelatin with a high iron content may become blackened in capsules containing ascorbic acid. In other cases, the mechanism for the observed chemical change may be unknown and therefore inseparable from the gelatin. Since the impurities present in a gelatin will be a function of its manufacturing process, it is always possible that certain gelatin types from particular manufacturers may exhibit their own peculiar characteristics. Some of the chemical interactions of gelatins which are of significance in pharmacy and, more particularly, to capsules, are reviewed in this section.

REACTIVITY OF THE GELATIN MOLECULE
The reactive side-chain groups of gelatin consist of amino, carboxyl, and hydroxyl groups, of which the amino groups are the most amenable to chemical modification and the hydroxyl groups least so.

The amino groups arise from lysine and hydroxylysine residues, together with the imidazolium group from histidine and the guanidinium group from arginine. There is only about one α-amino group per 25 ε-amino groups in high-grade gelatin. Reaction generally occurs only with uncharged amino groups, which means that the highly basic guanidino group is unreactive unless a very alkaline pH is employed. The imidazolium group is also less reactive than the α- and ε-amino groups and there is evidence that its bonds, once formed, are also less stable. A wide range of modifying reagents for gelatin amino groups has been investigated and reviewed (Clark and Courts, 1977) of which acid chlorides and anhydrides, epoxides, and aldehydes are typical examples. Reagents which are capable of reacting with two amino groups can cross-link the gelatin to give increased solution viscosity and increased gel melting temperature, even to a point where the gelatin eventually becomes insoluble.

Carboxyl groups outnumber amino groups (excluding the guanidino groups) by approximately 3 to 1 in limed gelatin and approximately 2 to 1 in acid-processed gelatin, but are much less reactive. Esters can be prepared, but of much more importance is the cross-linking of carboxyl groups by metal ions such as chromium, aluminium, titanium, and zirconium.

Chemical derivatives of gelatin have found very limited application in pharmaceuticals in general, and capsules in particular, not least because of problems of legislation. The reaction of dicarboxylic acid anhydrides with acid-processed pigskin gelatin has been advocated (British Patent 836 082, 1960) as a means of reducing the brittleness and viscosity degradation of the gelatin for hard capsule manufacture, but has not been used commercially. Thiolated gelatin, prepared by reaction of N-acetylhomocysteine thiolactone or S-mercaptosuccinic anhydride with the amino groups, is capable of cross-linking itself on mild oxidation, with the formation of disulphide bridges. The controlled diffusion and release of therapeutic agents using gelatins of this type has been described (Barron and Tsuk, U.S. Patent 3 329 574, 1967).

Formaldehyde has been used to cross-link gelatin for the manufacture of enteric hard and soft capsules. It has the disadvantages of a marked pH-dependence of the reaction and difficulty in controlling its rate and its extent because it continues in the dry state for a relatively long period. The reaction mechanism is believed to involve the initial formation of hydroxymethylamino groups on lysine and arginine residues, the latter being the rate determining step. The hydroxymethyl lysine eliminates water to give a cationic imine which can react with hydroxymethyl arginine to form a dimethylene ether bridge. This subsequently reorganises to form a methylene link between amino groups of the original lysine and arginine residues. 'After-hardening' in the dry state appears to be due to slow release of formaldehyde by depolymerisation of polyoxymethylene, which is present in aqueous formaldehyde solution. (Davis and Tabor, 1963; Taylor et al., 1978) Formaldehyde also reduces helix formation (Moll et al., 1976).

IONIC INTERACTIONS OF GELATIN
Coacervation
Under certain conditions a homogeneous gelatin solution can be made to separate into two distinct liquid phases, a fairly concentrated gelatin solution and a very weak one. This technique is termed coacervation, and the concentrated protein phase is referred to as the coacervate (Bungenberg de Jong, 1949). Coacervation can be produced by the addition of a salt such as sodium sulphate ('simple coacervation') (U.S. Patent 2 800 458, 1957), or, for systems containing gelatin together with a negatively charged macromolecule such as acacia in solution, by adjustment of the pH ('complex coacervation') (U.S. Patent 2 800 457, 1957). The

latter method, which has commercial importance for the manufacture of microcapsules, is dependent upon there being a net positive charge on the gelatin molecules, at the adjusted pH, which is neutralised by the negative charge on the other polymer. For this reason, acacia will form a coacervate with acid pigskin gelatin at pH 5.0 whereas a very much lower pH is required with limed gelatins. It is possible for coacervates to be formed between lime-processed and acid-processed gelatins at pH values between their respective iso-ionic points, where the gelatins are oppositely charged (U.S. Patents 3 317 434, 1967; 3 176 001, 1965). Below the gelatin isoelectric point, coacervation can occur with agar, carrageenan, pectin, alginates, and carmellose, although it is inhibited by high sugar concentrations.

Interactions with Dyes
The interaction of eight F D & C dyes with acid- and lime-processed gelatins has been examined by measuring changes in the visible spectrum. In solution, all dyes were found to interact with acid-processed gelatin, primarily by electrostatic bonding, although erythrosine (which showed the greatest interaction) also showed hydrogen bonding, hydrophobic bonding, and even some evidence of irreversible interaction (Cooper et al., 1973). Lime-processed gelatin had no effect on the dye spectra until the very acid conditions of pH 1, when the gelatin possessed a sufficiently high net positive charge. In the dry film state, interaction was examined in the visible and infra-red regions by attenuated total reflectance spectroscopy, and was apparent for all dyes and for both gelatins. Erythrosine and Wool Violet 5BN showed the greatest effects. Dyes with the greatest changes in spectral activity had the slowest release rates from gelatin films during dissolution in simulated gastric or intestinal fluid.

In a further study (Kellaway et al., 1978b), the behaviour of erythrosine with acid- and lime-processed gelatins in solution, its effect on absorbance, and the wavelength for maximum absorbance were examined. By fractionating the gelatins by gel chromatography, a linear relationship was found between gelatin molecular weight and the quantity of bound dye, although the slopes of the plots were naturally very different for acid and limed gelatins.

Lime-processed gelatin has been reported to increase the rate of fading of indigo carmine at 60°, although there could have been a contribution by inorganic impurities present in the gelatin (Khalil and El-Gamal, 1978). At a concentration of 0.02% w/w, indigo carmine, tartrazine, and amaranth reduce gel structure formation in 3% and 6% gelatin gels (Artemova and Usova, 1964). The compatibility of amaranth, sunset yellow FCF, and indigo carmine with gelatin is influenced by the sulphur dioxide content of the gelatin, which should contain less than about 60 ppm when these dyes are used (Torrado Valeiras, 1966).

Gas Generation in Gelatin Solutions

A defect which can occur in hard capsules is the appearance in the capsule walls of very fine bubbles. This problem can often be traced back to the presence of gas bubbles in the gelatin solution circulating to the 'dip tank', at the stage in production where the capsules are formed by dipping stainless steel pins into the gelatin liquor. Gas bubbles can also develop after the gelatin solution has been bubble-free for several hours on the machines. The problem has been found to be specific to particular gelatin batches but not to particular gelatin types, and is frequently aggravated by the presence of certain dyes (e.g. amaranth and erythrosine). Gas generation can be prevented by relatively large additions of sulphur dioxide (e.g. 500–1000 ppm) although unfortunately its use is largely precluded if the dye is sensitive to it, as is indigo carmine.

Various theories have been proposed to explain gas generation, including the presence of hydrogen peroxide. At one time, it was not uncommon for hard capsule manufacturers to purchase gelatins with a sulphur dioxide content of 200–1000 ppm and to oxidise the sulphur dioxide with hydrogen peroxide when sulphur dioxide-sensitive dyes were to be used. Residual hydrogen peroxide could itself give rise to oxygen bubbles in the dipping tank by decomposition. Also, for gelatins of low (less than 40 ppm) sulphur dioxide content some correlation was found between the incidence of bubbles and the presence of trace amounts of hydrogen peroxide which were capable of coexisting with sulphur dioxide in the dry gelatin.

However, the situation is complicated by the fact that gelatins differ in their ability to catalyse the decomposition of hydrogen peroxide. For example, 10 ppm of hydrogen peroxide added to one batch of gelatin produced detectable gas generation whereas 400 ppm added to another failed to produce bubbles. The practice of controlling sulphur dioxide levels with hydrogen peroxide during capsule manufacture has now diminished and hard capsule gelatins are generally required to be free from all traces of hydrogen peroxide.

Nitrate and nitrite ions present in trace amounts in the gelatin, or derived from the water supply, have been correlated with the incidence of bubbles, particularly when nitrate-reducing thermophilic organisms such as *B. stearothermophilus* or *E. coli* are present in the system. The phenomenon can be demonstrated and investigated in the laboratory in the following manner: 200 ml of a 30% solution of gelatin in sterile water, contained in a capped, conical flask, is inoculated with a suitable thermophile culture, and a sterile magnetic follower is added. The solution is incubated at the required temperature (in the range 45–55°) for 3 days. At 24-hour intervals the flask is stirred, enabling any gas which has been generated and has supersaturated the solution to be released in the form of very fine bubbles.

Using this technique, it has been shown that, for certain gelatins, gas generation is paralleled by a net loss of nitrate plus nitrite from the system, whilst the nitrite level may increase initially and then fall. The gas generated by one particular thermophilic organism has been isolated and identified as being a mixture of carbon dioxide and nitrogen, indicating that nitrate reduction provides the energy for oxidation of the carbon source to carbon dioxide.

The action of sulphur dioxide in suppressing gas generation is not bacteriostatic since there is still a net loss of nitrate plus nitrite from the system although, in this case, the nitrite level does not rise. Nitrate reduction is accompanied by a fall in the sulphur dioxide concentration, and bubbles can occur when the level has fallen sufficiently (e.g. to 60 ppm sulphur dioxide on a dry gelatin basis) provided there is still some residual nitrate or nitrite.

In practice the extent of gas generation is influenced by the strain and activity of the particular thermophilic organism, the pH and temperature of the solution, and the level of other nutrients essential for the thermophile's activity. Consequently the presence of nitrate- and nitrite-reducing organisms in gelatin solutions does not always mean that bubbles will occur. Nor is the presence of nitrate or nitrite essential for bubbles to occur with certain organisms. It is possible for the addition of a second organism to alter the nitrate reduction pattern of a first so that the nitrite formed is not further reduced to nitrogen gas. Thus it appears possible for two gelatins which, individually, do not 'bubble', to be capable of generating gas when blended together.

Although there are no publications on this bubble mechanism for gelatin solutions, a similar phenomenon has been reported in the sugar industry (Caruthers *et al.*, private communication). In this case, the problem was not one of gas generation but the disappearance of sulphur dioxide, which had been added to prevent browning reactions, from the sugar solution by reaction with nitrite formed from nitrate by *B. stearothermophilus*. It was shown that gaseous nitrogen and carbon dioxide were metabolic end-products of nitrate reduction and, depending upon the culture, 40–80% of the gas was nitrogen. Not all of the nitrate and nitrite reduced could be accounted for as nitrogen gas, and part was found to have been converted into bacterial protein, ammonia formation being negligible. Gaseous nitrogen was shown to arise from nitrate reduction by at least two strains of *B. stearothermophilus*, the first reducing nitrate to nitrite and the second reducing nitrite to nitrogen.

Tests and Specifications for Gelatin

Standard methods for sampling and testing gelatins for chemical and physical properties are given in British Standard 757: 1975, and methods for the microbiological testing of gelatin appear in British Standard 5349: 1976–1977. Pharmacopoeias differ in their requirements for gelatin; Table 3.4 summarises the *Eur. P.* and *U.S.P.* standards.

In practice, pharmacopoeial specifications generally represent the minimal requirements; capsule manufacturers' specifications are more detailed and stringent, and may include performance tests designed to assess gelatins under conditions which more closely approximate manufacturing conditions. Thus soft capsule gelatins may be evaluated for clarity as concentrated solutions in glycerol/water, and hard capsule gelatins may be tested for viscosity at 30% concentration at 50°. Stringent microbiological standards frequently relate to the requirements of the final customer for the capsules.

Because physical properties, such as Bloom strength and viscosity, vary with the moisture content of the dry gelatin, it is common practice to correct these values to a standard moisture level of 11.5%. For hard capsules a correction of ± 5 g

Bloom or ± 0.5 mPa s viscosity (at 12.5% concentration and 60°) for each 1.0% moisture difference from 11.5% is taken as the 'rule of thumb'.

Table 3.4. Pharmacopoeial standards for gelatin

Test	Eur. P. (2nd Edn)	U.S.P. XXI
Clarity, colour (in solution)	—[a]	only slightly opalescent
Odour (2.5% solution)	—	not disagreeable
Moisture, % max.	15.0	—
pH (1% solution)	3.8–7.6	—
Gel strength, g	150–250[b]	—
Ash, % max.	3.0[c]	2.0
Sulphur dioxide, ppm max.	200	40[d]
Heavy metals, ppm max.	50	50
Arsenic, ppm max.	1.0	0.8
Hydrogen peroxide, ppm max.	100	—
Microbiological standards		
Total count, orgs per g, max.	—[e]	1000
E. coli	—[e]	absent in 10 g
Salmonellae	—[e]	absent in 10 g

[a] Comparison with specified reference solutions
[b] Gelatin intended for the preparation of pessaries, suppositories, and zinc gelatin
[c] Sulphated ash
[d] Maximum 1500 ppm permitted for capsules
[e] Limits may be specified by national authorities

Table 3.5. Typical specification for hard capsule gelatins

	Limed ossein	Acid ossein	Acid pigskin
B. S. Bloom,* g	230–255	240–265	250–275
AOAC Bloom,* g	235–260	245–270	260–285
Viscosity, 6.67%, 60°, mPa s	4.3–4.7	3.3–3.7	4.3–4.7
Viscosity, 12.5%, 60°, mPs s	18.5–20.5	12.5–14.5	18.5–20.5
% Viscosity drop max. (18 hours at 60°)	20	20	20
Moisture, % max.	13.0	13.0	13.0
Ash, % max.	1.0	1.0	1.0
pH, 1% solution	5.2–6.0	5.2–6.0	5.2–6.0
Iso-ionic point, pH	4.7–5.3	6.0–8.0	7.0–.9.0
Particle size			
% Passing 4 U.S. mesh	100	100	100
% Passing 40 U.S. mesh, max.	2	2	2
Sulphur dioxide, ppm max.	40	40	40
Heavy metals, ppm max.	50	50	50
Arsenic, ppm max.	0.8	0.8	0.8
Hydrogen peroxide	Absent	Absent	Absent
Nitrate, ppm max.	300	300	300
Nitrite, ppm max.	30	30	30
Microbiological standards			
Total count, orgs per g, max.	500	500	500
Salmonellae in 10 g	Absent	Absent	Absent
Coliforms in 0.1 g	Absent	Absent	Absent
E. coli in 10 g	Absent	Absent	Absent
Bactericides and bacteriostats	Absent	Absent	Absent

* Corrected to 11.5% moisture

Typical specifications for gelatins used for the manufacture of hard and soft capsules respectively are given in Tables 3.5 and 3.6.

Table 3.6. Typical specification for soft capsule gelatins

	Limed ossein	Acid ossein
B.S. Bloom, g	150–175	175–195
Viscosity, 6.67%, 60°, mPa s	3.6–4.0	2.7–3.2
Moisture, % max.	13.0	13.0
Ash, % max.	2.0	1.0
pH	5.0–6.0	5.0–6.0
Iso-ionic point, pH	4.7–5.3	6.0–8.0
Clarity (45% solution in 30% glycerol)	Clear, no precipitate	Clear, no precipitate
Particle size		
% Passing 10 U.S. mesh	100	100
% Passing 60 U.S. mesh, max.	5	5
Sulphur dioxide, ppm max.	60	60
Hydrogen peroxide, ppm max.	60	60
Iron, ppm max.	30	30
Heavy metals, ppm max.	50	50
Arsenic, ppm max.	0.8	0.8
Microbiological standards		
Total count, orgs per g, max.	1000	1000
Salmonellae in 10 g	Absent	Absent
Coliforms in 0.1 g	Absent	Absent
E. coli in 10 g	Absent	Absent

References

Ames, W. M., *J. Soc. chem. Ind., Lond.*, 1947, 66, 279–284.

Artemova, V. M. and Usova, E. M., *Izvestiya Vysshikh uchebnÿkh zavedenii, Pishchevaya Tekhnol.*, 1964(2), 46–48 *per Chem. Abstr.*, 1966, 64, 2659F.

AOAC, *Official Methods of Analysis*, 14th Edn, S. Williams (Ed.), Arlington, Virgina, Association of Official Analytical Chemists, 1984, p. 429.

Bartley, J. P. and Marrs, W. M., Leatherhead Food R. A., *Technical Circular No. 582*, 1974.

Bell, J. H. *et al.*, *J. Pharm. Pharmac.*, 1973, 25, Suppl., 96P–103P.

Bello, J. *et al.*, *J. phys. Chem., Ithaca*, 1956, 60, 1299–1306.

Bello, J. *et al.*, *Biochim. Biophys. Acta*, 1962, 57, 214–221.

Boedtker, H. and Doty, P., *J. phys. Chem., Ithaca*, 1954, 58, 968–983.

Bohonek, J., *Colloid Polym. Sci.*, 1974, 252, 333–334, 417–418.

Bohonek, J. *et al.*, in *Photographic Gelatin II*, Proceedings of the Royal Photographic Society Symposium, Cambridge, 1974, R. J. Cox (Ed.), London, Academic Press, 1976, pp. 37–55.

Borchard, W. *et al.*, in *Photographic Gelatin II*, Proceedings of the Royal Photographic Society Symposium, Cambridge 1974, R. J. Cox (Ed.), London, Academic Press, 1976, pp. 57–71.

Bradbury, E. and Martin, C., *Proc. R. Soc.*, 1952, A214, 183–192.

Bungenberg de Jong, H. G., in *Colloid Science*, Vol. 2, H. R. Kruyt (Ed.), New York, Elsevier, 1949.

Calhoun, J. M. and Leister, D. A., *Photogr. Sci. Engng*, 1959, 3, 8–17.

Carless, J. E. and Nixon, J. R., *J. Soc. cosmet. Chem.*, 1970, 21, 427–440.

Caruthers, A. *et al.*, British Sugar Corporation Ltd, Nottingham, private communication.

Charlson, A. H. and Wiechers, S. G., *Fd Mf.*, 1956, 516.

Clark, R. C. and Courts, A., in *The Science and Technology of Gelatin*, A. G. Ward and A. Courts (Ed.), London, Academic Press, 1977, pp. 209–247.

Cooper, J. W. *et al.*, *J. pharm. Sci.*, 1973, 62, 1156–1164.

Coopes, I. H., *J. Polym. Sci.*, 1975, 49, 97.

Coopes, I. H., *J. Polym. Sci., Polym. Symp.*, 1976a, 55, 127–138.

Coopes, I. H., in *Photographic Gelatin II*, Proceedings of the Royal Photographic Society Symposium, Cambridge, 1974, R. J. Cox (Ed.), London, Academic Press, 1976b, 121–129.

Courts, A., *Biochem. J.*, 1954, 58, 74–79.

Courts, A., *Biochem. J.*, 1955, 59, 382–386.

Courts, A., *Biochem. J.*, 1959, 73, 596–600.

Courts, A. and Stainsby, G., in *Recent Advances in Gelatin and Glue Research*, G. Stainsby (Ed.), London, Pergamon Press, 1958, pp. 100–105.

Croome, R. J., *J. appl. Chem., Lond.*, 1953a, 3, 280–286.

Croome, R. J., *J. appl. Chem., Lond.*, 1953b, 3, 330–334.

Cumper, C. W. N. and Alexander, A. E., *Aust. J. scient. Res.*, 1952, A5, 153–159.

Davis, P. and Tabor, B. E., *J. Polym. Sci.*, 1963, Part A 1, 799–815.

Eith, L. *et al.*, *The Injection Moulded Capsule*, Pharmaceutical Technology Conference, Harrogate, 1986.

Eldridge, J. E. and Ferry, J. D., *J. phys. Chem., Ithaca*, 1954, 58, 992–996.

Engel, J., *Arch. Biochem.*, 1962, 97, 150–158.

Ferry, J. D., Protein Gels, in *Advances in Protein Chemistry*, Vol. IV, M. L. Anson and J. T. Edsall (Ed.), New York, Academic Press, 1948a, pp. 20–23.

Ferry, J. D., *J. Am. chem. Soc.*, 1948b, 70, 2244–2249.

Ferry, J. D. and Eldridge, J. E., *J. phys. Colloid Chem.*, 1949, 53, 184–196.

Finch, C. A. and Jobling, A., in *The Science and Technology of Gelatin*, A. G. Ward and A. Courts (Ed.), London, Academic Press, 1977, pp. 263–271.

Flory, P. J. and Weaver, E. S., *J. Am. chem. Soc.*, 1960, 82, 4518–4525.

French, M. J. *et al.*, *Biochim. Biophys. Acta*, 1971, 251, 320–330.

Gerngross, O., *Kolloidzeitschrift*, 1926, 40, 279–286.

Gerngross, O. *et al.*, *Kolloidzeitschrift*, 1932, 60, 276–288.

Gouinlock, E. V. *et al.*, *J. Polym. Sci.*, 1955, 16, 383–395.

Gross, S. and Rose, P. I., in *Photographic Gelatin II*, Proceedings of the Royal Photographic Society Symposium, Cambridge 1974, R. J. Cox (Ed.), London, Academic Press, 1976, pp. 73–100.

Hatschek, E., *J. phys. Chem., Ithaca*, 1932, 36, 2994–3009.

Healey, J. N. C. *et al.*, *J. Pharm. Pharmac.*, 1974, 26, Suppl., 41P–46P.

Heathcock, J. F. and Jewell, G. G., Leatherhead Food R.A., *Research Report No. 213*, 1975, and *No. 239*, 1976.

Hirai, N. and Kishimoto, S., *J. chem. Soc. Japan*, Pure Chemistry Section, 1953, 74, 347–349.

Holmes, A. W. *et al.*, *Gums and Stabilisers for the Food Industry—3*, Proceedings of the Third International Conference, Wrexham 1985, London, Elsevier Applied Science Publishers, 1986, p. 249.

Hopp, V., *Leder*, 1964, *15*, 59–63.

Ito, K. *et al.*, *Chem. pharm. Bull.*, *Tokyo*, 1969, *17*, 1134–1137.

Itoh, N., in *Photographic Gelatin*, Proceedings of the Fourth IAG Conference, Fribourg 1983, H. Amman-Brass and J. Pouradier (Ed.), 1985, pp. 136–144.

Jacobson, R. E., in *Photographic Gelatin II*, Proceedings of the Royal Photographic Society Symposium, Cambridge 1974, R. J. Cox (Ed.), London, Academic Press, 1976, pp. 233–251.

Janus, J. W. *et al.*, *Kolloidzeitschrift*, 1965, *205*, 134–139.

Johnson, P. and Metcalfe, J. C., *Eur. Polym. J.*, 1967, *3*, 423–447.

Jolley, J. E., *Photogr. Sci. Engng*, 1970, *14*, 169–177.

Jones, N. R., in *The Science and Technology of Gelatin*, A. G. Ward and A. Courts (Ed.), London, Academic Press, 1977, pp. 365–394.

Jopling, D. W., *J. appl. Chem. Lond.*, 1956, *6*, 79–84.

Katz, J. R., *Recueil des travaux chimiques des Pays-Bas et de la Belgique*, 1932, *51*, 835–841.

Kellaway, I. W. *et al.*, *Can. J. pharm. Sci.*, 1978a, *13*, 83–86.

Kellaway, I. W. *et al.*, *Can. J. pharm. Sci.*, 1978b, *13*, 87–90.

Kenchington, A. W. and Ward, A. G., *Biochem. J.*, 1954, *58*, 202–207.

Khalil, S. A. H. and El-Gamal, S. S., *Mfg Chem.*, 1978, *49*(5), 52, 56 and 59.

Konno, A. and Kaneko, M., *Reports on Progress of Polymer Physics in Japan*, 1969, *12*, 65–66.

Kozlov, P. V. and Burdygina, G. I., *Polymer*, 1983, *24*, 651–666.

Kraemer, E. O. and Fanselow, J. R., *J. phys. Chem.*, *Ithaca*, 1925, *29*, 1169–1177.

Kramer, F. and Rosenthal, H., *Food Technol.*, *Champaign*, 1965, *19*, No. 9, 1417–1420.

Leich, A., *Annalen der Physik*, 1904, *14*(4), 139.

Li-juan, C. in *Photographic Gelatin*, Proceedings of the Fourth IAG Conference, Fribourg 1983, H. Amman-Brass and J. Pouradier (Ed.), 1985, pp. 136–144.

Marrs, W. M. and Wood, P. D., in *Photographic Gelatin*, Proceedings of the Royal Photographic Society Symposium, Cambridge 1970, R. J. Cox (Ed.), London, Academic Press, 1972, pp. 63–80.

Marshall, A. S. and Petrie, S. E. B., at the Royal Photographic Society Symposium on Photographic Gelatin, Oxford, 1979.

Mason, C. M. and Silcox, H. E., *Ind. Engng Chem. ind. Edn*, 1943, *35*, 726–729.

Maxey, C. R. and Palmer, M. R., in *Photographic Gelatin II*, Proceedings of the Royal Photographic Society Symposium, Cambridge 1974, R. J. Cox (Ed.), London, Academic Press, 1976, pp. 27–36.

Melia, C. D. *et al.*, 1981, unpublished work.

Mindru, I. and Ceacareanu, D., *An. Univ. Bucuresti, Ser. Stiint. Natur.*, 1966, *15*(1), 25–31.

Moll, F. *et al.*, in *Photographic Gelatin II*, Proceedings of the Royal Photographic Society Symposium, Cambridge 1974, R. J. Cox (Ed.), London, Academic Press, 1976, pp. 197–213.

Moritani, M. *et al.*, *Polym. J.*, *Tokyo*, 1971, *2*, 74.

Nixon, J. R. *et al.*, *J. Pharm. Pharmac.*, 1966, *18*, 283–288.

Norris, T. O. and McGraw, J., *J. appl. Polym. Sci.*, 1964, *8*, 2139–2145.

Pankhurst, K., *Nature*, 1947, *159*, 538.

Pines, E. and Prins, W., *Macromolecules*, 1973, *6*, 888.

Pleass, W. B., *Proc. R. Soc.*, 1930, A*126*, 406–426.

Poole, H. J., *Trans. Faraday Soc.*, 1925, *21*, 114–137.

Pouradier, J. and Hodot, A. M., *Photographic Gelatin*, Proceedings of the Royal Photographic Society Symposium, Cambridge 1970, R. J. Cox (Ed.), London, Academic Press, 1972, pp. 91–95.

Pouradier, J. and Venet, A. M., *J. Chim. phys.*, 1950, *47*, 11–20, 391–398.

Pouradier, J. and Venet, A. M., *J. Chim. phys.*, 1952, *49*, 85–92, 239–244.

Pouradier, J. *et al.*, *27th Congr. Internat. de Chimie. Ind. Bruxelles*, 1954, *3*, 769–771.

Richardson, E. G., *Trans. Faraday Soc.*, 1933, *29*, 494–502.

Robinson, J. A. J. *et al.*, *J. Pharm. Pharmac.*, 1975a, *27*, 818–824.

Robinson, J. A. J. *et al.*, *J. Pharm. Pharmac.*, 1975b, *27*, Suppl., 77P.

Saunders, P. R. and Ward, A. G., in *Proceedings of the 2nd International Congress on Rheology*, London, Butterworth, 1954, pp. 284–290.

Saunders, P. R. and Ward, A. G., in *Recent Advances in Gelatin and Glue Research*, G. Stainsby (Ed.), London, Pergamon Press, 1958, pp. 197–203.

Sheppard, S. E. and Houck, R. C., *J. phys. Chem.*, *Ithaca*, 1930, *34*, 273–298.

Sheppard, S. E. and Sweet, S. S., *J. Am. chem. Soc.*, 1921, *43*, 539–547.

Sheppard, S. E. *et al.*, *J. phys. Chem.*, *Ithaca*, 1940, *44*, 185–207.

Smith, C. R., *J. Am. chem. Soc.*, 1919, *41*, 135–150.

Stainsby, G., *Nature*, 1952, *169*, 662–663.

Stainsby, G., *Gelatine and Glue Research Association Research Report C17*, 1958.

Stainsby, G., in *The Science and Technology of Gelatin*, A. G. Ward and A. Courts (Ed.), London, Academic Press, 1977a, pp. 109–136.

Stainsby, G., in *The Science and Technology of Gelatin*, A. G. Ward and A. Courts (Ed.), London, Academic Press, 1977b, pp. 179–207.

Stainsby, G. *et al.*, in *Food Science and Technology*, Vol. 1, J. M. Leitch (Ed.), New York, Gordon and Breach, 1969.

Steigmann, A., *Science et industries photographiques*, 1957, *28*, 353–359.

Tabor, B. E., *J. appl. Polym. Sci.*, 1968, *12*, 1967–1979.

Taylor, S. K. *et al.*, *Photogr. Sci. Engng*, 1978, *22*, 134–138.

Tice, L. F., *Drug Cosmet. Ind.*, 1936, *38*, 635–636.

Tiemstra, P. J., *Food Technol.*, *Champaign*, 1968, *22*, 1151–1153.

Titova, E. F. *et al.*, *Micro Symposium, Prague*, 1973.

Toda, Y., at The Royal Photographic Society Symposium on Photographic Gelatin, Oxford, 1985.

Torrado Valeiras, J. J., *An. R. Acad. Farm. Madr.*, 1966, *32*, 353–359.

Veis, A., *The Macromolecular Chemistry of Gelatin*, London, Academic Press, 1964, Chapter 5.

Veis, A. and Cohen, J., *J. Polym. Sci.*, 1957, *26*, 113–116.

Veis, A. *et al.*, *J. Am. Leath. Chem. Ass.*, 1960, *55*, 548–563.

von Hippel, P. H. and Harrington, W. F., *Biochim. Biophys. Acta*, 1959, *36*, 427–447.

von Hippel, P. H. and Harrington, W. F., *Brookhaven Symp. Biol.*, 1960, No. *13*, 213–231.

Wainewright, F. W., in *The Science and Technology of Gelatin*,

A. G. Ward and A. Courts (Ed.), London, Academic Press 1977, pp. 507–534.

Ward, A. G. and Saunders, P. R., in *Rheology, Theory and Applications*, Vol. 2, F. R. Eirich (Ed.), London, Academic Press, 1958, p. 342.

Watase, M. and Arakawa, K., *Nippon Kagaku Zasshi*, 1969, 90(7), 658–663.

Yannas, I. V., *J. Macromol. Sci., Rev. Macromol. Chem.*, 1972, 7(1), 49–104b.

Zsigmondy, R., *Zeitschrift für analytische Chemie*, 1901, *40*, 697–719.

Zubov, P. I. *et al.*, *Kolloid. Zh.*, 1954, *16*, 109–114.

Chapter 4

Gelatin Additives, Substitutes, and Extenders

B. E. Jones

In addition to gelatin, capsule shells contain small quantities of additives which either enable the capsule to be formed more easily or improve its performance in use. The materials which are used can be put into six main categories: colouring agents, plasticisers, process and performance aids, preservatives, gelatin substitutes and extenders, and gelatin coatings.

COLOURING AGENTS

The chief reasons for colouring pharmaceutical products are the aesthetic effect, ease of identification, and the psychological effect on patients. Colouring agents may also be used for their light-screening properties to protect photolabile substances.

Aesthetic Effects
Products must have a constant standard appearance in order to be acceptable. The addition of a colouring agent effectively masks variations in the colour of the contents, and raises the confidence of the user in its quality and stability.

Identification
Coloration is the simplest and best method for quick identification of a product. It cannot be relied upon absolutely, but it does have practical advantages over methods such as embossing or printing. Colour provides a key to safety for the geriatric patient on a multiple drug regimen.

Psychological Effect on the Patient
The psychological effect of colour on the users of medicines has been recognised since the earliest times. The Egyptians used to colour their draughts (Cooper, 1956) and it is also well known that certain colours elicit specific associated effects in many people (Swartz and Cooper, 1962). This is especially true of flavours (Peacock, 1949), those most commonly used being green for peppermint and red for strawberry. However, the effect of

colour of medicines on the patient has not really been successfully evaluated. Peacock (1949) described the coloured placebo effect which is particularly relevant for the psychiatrist treating a hypochondriac patient. Madsen (1957) undertook a series of clinical trials with medicines in a variety of coloured solutions in order to test their patient acceptability. Schapira et al. (1970) studied the effect of the colour of oxazepam tablets given to patients suffering from anxiety states. They used three colours, red, yellow, and green, and found that anxiety states responded best to green whereas depressive symptoms responded best to yellow.

The specific effect of the colour of the capsule on patients has been studied by a group of Italian research workers. In their first study, which was on the effects of placebo treatments, they included capsule colour amongst their factors (Cattaneo et al., 1970). They used blue and orange capsules and found an influence of colour which appeared to be sex-related. In their second trial, which was on the hypnotic effect of heptabarbitone, again they used orange and blue capsules (Lucchelli et al., 1978), and concluded that blue capsules were better than orange for treating insomnia but that orange was a better colour for evaluating a sedative agent against a placebo.

The colour of a capsule can also influence the patient's perception of what a product will do for him. Buckalew and Coffield (1982) used a panel of students to ascertain the perceived characteristics of capsule colour and size, and their relationship to tablets. Their results indicated that certain colours were associated with the treatment of certain conditions, and that capsules were seen to be more potent than tablets.

Light Protection
The colour of the capsule governs both the amount and the wavelength of the light passing through

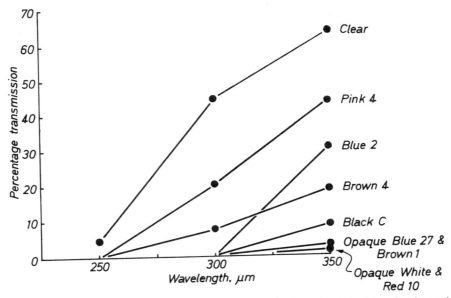

Fig. 4.1. Percentage transmission of ultraviolet light of different wavelengths through gelatin strips of various colours.

the gelatin film. The stability of photolabile substances can be improved by using capsules of an appropriate colour. Most photochemical breakdown occurs at specific wavelengths and it is possible to produce a capsule colour with the maximum screening power for the particular substance. The transmission of ultraviolet light through a series of coloured gelatin film strips (Fig. 4.1) has been measured (Hine and Robson). This shows that opaque colours generally transmit less ultraviolet light. Similar tests have been made using capsules filled with the photolabile compound menadione (Prista *et al.*, 1970).

Nomenclature for Colouring Agents

The colouring agents used in commerce usually have trivial names and there are often several synonyms for each substance. The complex chemical nature of the molecules and the fact that many of the dyes are not pure compounds militates against the use of the chemical name. To overcome this problem, several numbering systems have been introduced to assign a recognition code to each dye. The most universal system is the Colour Index Number (CI No.) which is published jointly by the Society of Dyers and Colorists and the American Association of Textile Chemists and Colorists. In this system, all food, pharmaceutical, and other dyes are grouped into chemical classes and then assigned a number on the basis of complexity and points of substitution.

Other systems include the Schultz numbers, which are similar to the Colour Index, the European Economic Community (EEC) numbers, and the American Food and Drug Administration (FDA) class. There are certain disadvantages with the latter two systems. Both set out to give recognition only to those colouring agents permitted for use. The EEC system simply assigns a number to each dye. The FDA system divides food and pharmaceutical colorants into a variety of classes depending on the uses for which they have been approved. F D & C dyes can be used in foods, drugs, and cosmetics, D & C dyes are for drugs and cosmetics only, and Ext. D & C dyes are for drugs and cosmetics used externally. However, these titles may no longer correspond to permitted uses. Table 4.1 lists colouring agents that have been reported for the coloration of capsules.

Types of Colouring Agent

The Food and Agriculture Organization of the United Nations and the World Health Organization (FAO/WHO, 1966) have classified food colours into a series of chemical groups: anthraquinone, azo (mono- and bis-), carotenoid, flavone, indigoid, inorganic, nitro, quinophthalone, triphenylmethane, and xanthene.

The colorants mainly used for colouring capsules are synthetic water-soluble dyes (azo, indigoid, quinophthalone, triphenylmethane, and xanthene), pigments (especially the opacifying

Table 4.1. Colouring agents that have been used for the coloration of capsules

CI No.	FDA Class	EEC No.	Common name	Other names
14720	—	E 122	Azorubine	Carmoisine, Food Red 3
15985	F D & C Yellow No. 6	E 110	Sunset Yellow FCF	Gelborange S, Food Yellow 3, Orange Yellow S
16035	F D & C Red No. 40	E 129	Allura Red AC	Food Red 17
16185	—	E 123	Amaranth	Acid Red 27, Bordeaux S, Food Red 9, Naphtol Rot S
16255	—	E 124	Ponceau 4R	Cochineal Red A, Food Red 7, New Coccine
18050	Ext. D & C Red No. 11	E 128	Red 2G	Acid Red 1, Azogeranine, Food Red 10, Geranine 2G, Lissamine Red 6B
19140	F D & C Yellow No. 5	E 102	Tartrazine	Food Yellow 4, Tartrazol Yellow
28440	—	E 151	Brilliant Black PN	Black PN, Food Black 1
40850	—	E 161(g)	Canthaxanthin	Food Orange 8
42051	—	E 131	Patent Blue V	Food Blue 5, Patent Blue 5
42053	F D & C Green No. 3	—	Fast Green FCF	Food Green 3
42090	F D & C Blue No. 1	E 133	Brilliant Blue FCF	Acid Blue 9, Blue EGS, Food Blue 2, Patent Blue AC
44090	—	E 142	Green S	Acid Brilliant Green BS, Acid Green S, Food Green 4, Lissamine Green, Wool Green B
45430	F D & C Red No. 3	E 127	Erythrosine	Food Red 14
47005	D & C Yellow No. 10	E 104	Quinoline Yellow	Acid Yellow 3, Canary Yellow, Food Yellow 13
73015	F D & C Blue No. 2	E 132	Indigotine	Food Blue 1, Indigo Carmine
75300	—	E 100	Curcumin	Diferoylmethane, Turmeric Yellow
77266	—	E 153	Vegetable Carbon	Carbo Medicinalis, Carbon Black, Channel Black
77491	—	E 172	Iron oxides and hydroxides	Pigment Red 101 & 102
77492	—	E 172	Iron oxides and hydroxides	Pigment Yellow 42 & 43
77499	—	E 172	Iron oxides and hydroxides	Pigment Black 11
77891	—	E 171	Titanium Dioxide	Pigment White 6

agent titanium dioxide), and certain dyes of natural origin (carotenoids and flavones).

Synthetic Dyes

The synthetic dyes are used primarily in their water-soluble forms, that is as their sodium, calcium, potassium, or ammonium salts. Sometimes they are used in the form of lakes which are produced by precipitating the water-soluble forms on to an alumina or titanium dioxide base. They are drawn from several chemical classes, the principal one being the azo group which until recently accounted for the majority of food and pharmaceutical dyes used.

Azo Dyes

These are characterised by having an azo linkage, i.e. a nitrogen-to-nitrogen double bond, —N≡N—. Chemically, their molecules contain benzene and naphthalene rings joined by the azo linkage, and containing sulphonic acid groups. There are many members which are chemical isomers of others in the same class. They are further subdivided into the monoazo and the bisazo groups, having one or two azo linkages in their molecules, respectively. Dyes in this group are the monoazo dyes Amaranth (CI No. 16185), Sunset Yellow FCF (CI No. 15985), and Tartrazine (CI No. 19140), and the bisazo dye Brilliant Black PN (CI No. 28440).

Indigoid Dyes

This group of dyes is based on indigo, which has two isatin molecules joined by a double bond. Most members of the group are produced synthetically, but indigo itself occurs in nature. Pharmaceutically, the most commonly used dye in this class is Indigo Carmine (CI No. 73015).

Quinophthalone Dyes

These dyes are based on the naphthalenequinone structure. Quinoline Yellow (CI No. 47005) is the member of this group used pharmaceutically.

Triphenylmethane Dyes

The members of this group are based on a central triphenylmethane structure, and are substituted amine derivatives, with or without sulphonic acid groups. They can be either cationic, as is Methyl Violet, a hydrochloride derivative, or anionic, like Brilliant Blue FCF, which is the disodium salt of the sulphonic acid. The dyes in this class which are used pharmaceutically are Brilliant Blue FCF (CI No. 42090), Green S (CI No. 44090), and Patent Blue V (CI No. 42051).

Xanthene Dyes

The members of this group are based chemically on the xanthene nucleus. Most of the pharmaceutical members are derived from fluorescein, being either brominated or iodinated derivatives, e.g. eosin, which is tetrabromofluorescein, and erythrosine which is tetraiodofluorescein. Several members of this class are used topically, but only Erythrosine (CI No. 45430) is used orally.

PIGMENTS

Carbon

Several forms of carbon pigment are available, produced by the incineration of animal or vegetable matter or by the controlled combustion of oil or natural gas. The most commonly used form is Vegetable Carbon (CI No. 77266).

Oxides of Iron

Iron oxide can be obtained in colours ranging from black to yellow through brown and red, the difference being due to the state of oxidation. The three oxides most commonly used pharmaceutically are Black Iron Oxide $[FeO.Fe_2O_3:Fe(OH)_2.Fe_2O_3]$ (CI No. 77499), Red Iron Oxide $[Fe_2O_3]$ (CI No. 77491), and Yellow Iron Oxide $[FeO(OH).nH_2O]$ (CI No. 77492).

Titanium Dioxide

This pigment (CI No. 77891) has been used extensively as an opacifying agent in the manufacture of capsules.

NATURAL COLOURING AGENTS

The use of naturally occurring colouring agents in capsule manufacture is restricted because many of them are light-sensitive and some are unstable in the presence of gelatin. Two types of natural dye have been successfully used to colour capsules. One is curcumin, which is an oleo-resin obtained from turmeric, the powdered rhizome of *Curcuma longa* L. The other is the carotenoids, which are widely distributed in nature, both in the plant and animal kingdoms, e.g. in carrots, tomatoes, and lobsters. Those used for foods and pharmaceuticals are β-carotene, β-apo-8′-carotenal, and canthaxanthin.

Standards for Colouring Agents

The colorants which are used in pharmaceuticals have to comply with such standards for purity as are required to protect the consumer and to enable the substance to be clearly defined by regulatory authorities. In most countries, the colorants used in capsules are those permitted for use in foods. Usually they are mixtures, and the specifications include limits on the quantities of substances, other than the main component(s), which are allowed to be present. Some substances, such as simple organic salts, may be present but are not deleterious from the functional or safety standpoint, whereas others, such as non-sulphonated amines, which may be present in the initial raw materials, must be eliminated as far as is possible.

The FAO/WHO Joint Expert Committee on Food Additives have issued specifications (Food and Nutrition Paper 31/1, 1984) which include the following tests.

Assay. This defines the total amount of colouring matter which may be present. It is usually determined by titration with titanous chloride, although in certain cases other methods, such as spectrophotometry, are used.

Loss on Drying. This limits the amount of water present.

Chlorides and Sulphates. These are calculated as sodium salts and are determined by standard analytical techniques. They are present due to their use in the 'salting-out' of the colorant at the end of the manufacturing process. The limit for them is usually combined with that for loss on drying and the total varies, according to the substance, from 15 to 30%.

Water-insoluble Matter. This indicates the quantity of extraneous materials, e.g. filter aids, which can be present and is normally not more than 2%.

Ether-extractable Matter. This indicates the quantity of organic impurities, e.g. non-sulphonated amines, which may be present and is normally not more than 0.2%.

Arsenic and Heavy Metals. These are subject to the usual type of limit tests for pharmaceutical products and are expressed in mg/kg.

Subsidiary Colouring Matters. Isomers and other related compounds are present in the raw materials, or are produced during the chemical synthesis. Those which are coloured are termed 'subsidiary colouring matters' and the limits vary from 1 to 10% depending on the colorant being examined.

Organic Compounds other than Colouring Matters. These are isomers or other related compounds which are not coloured. Limits may be given for individual specified impurities or for a combination of several impurities, and vary from 0.01 to 5% depending on the nature of the impurity and the colorant being examined.

Identification of Colouring Agents

The positive chemical identification of dyes is often difficult because of their lack of absolute chemical purity, but it can be done by comparative techniques such as chromatography or spectrophotometry. To identify the colorants which have been used to colour capsules, the first step is to extract them, free of other interfering substances. Two methods are available, the choice being dependent on the quantity of colorant in the product (Jones, 1973).

For capsules with a high level of colorant, take an empty capsule, or part of one, as required, and place in a 10-ml beaker. Add 2 ml ethanol:water (3:1) and allow to stand in the dark for 30 minutes. Decant off the supernatant liquid, and evaporate it to dryness in a stream of cool air. Redissolve in the minimum quantity of distilled water. If the capsule remains coloured after the extraction, pigments are present.

For capsules with a low level of colorant, take a sample of empty capsules as required and place in a 20-ml beaker. Add 10 ml of distilled water and warm on a water-bath at 60° until all the capsules have dissolved. Pour the solution through a set of ethylaminoethylcellulose papers (Whatman AE81) held in a mini-Buchner funnel. Wash the papers with two 10-ml quantities of boiling distilled water.

CHROMATOGRAPHY

The simplest and quickest method to identify the extracted dye is by thin-layer chromatography. Chromatographic plates coated with cellulose such as Cellulose MN 300, are the most suitable. The following solutions are applied to the plate: (a) a solution of the capsule extract, (b) a reference solution containing the dye(s) thought to be present, and (c) a combined spot of the solution of capsule extract and the reference dye(s) solution to make allowance for any co-extracted material. The chromatogram should be run in two solvent systems which are chosen to give, if possible, different R_f values for the dyes under consideration. A satisfactory pair is 2% trisodium citrate in 5% ammonia solution, and a mixture of isopropyl alcohol:strong ammonia solution (4:1). This system will distinguish between all the commonly used capsule colorants, except for the triphenylmethane dyes which have very similar R_f values and tend to produce long streaky spots on the chromatogram. To distinguish between these, a plate coated with an ion-exchange cellulose such as diethylaminoethylcellulose (Cellulose MN 300 DEAE) (Turner and Jones, 1971) can be used. This is then run in the ammoniacal sodium citrate solvent and will give a significant differentiation between the dyes (Table 4.2).

Table 4.2. hR_x (Relative R_f) values of four blue triphenylmethane dyes

Dye	Colour Index No.	hR_x
Blue VRS	42045	70
Brilliant Blue FCF	42090	45
Fast Green FCF	42053	30
Green S	44090	40
Patent Blue V	42051	100*

* Absolute R_f = 90

Legislation for Colouring Agents

The colorants which can be used to colour pharmaceutical products are governed in nearly all countries by legislation which has been drawn up on the basis of toxicity. However, the list of permitted colorants varies from country to country, and is usually subject to a regular review system. The ten most acceptable colorants worldwide are listed in Table 4.3.

Table 4.3. The ten most acceptable colorants from a survey of legislation in 101 countries (Elanco, 1986).

Dye	CI No.	Colour	No. of countries accepting
Titanium Dioxide	77891	white	101
Erythrosine	45430	red	99
Indigo Carmine	73015	blue	99
Red Iron Oxide	77491	red	95
Sunset Yellow FCF	15985	orange	93
Tartrazine*	19140	yellow	92
Yellow Iron Oxide	77492	yellow	92
Black Iron Oxide	77499	black	91
Ponceau 4R	16255	red	87
Canthaxanthin	40850	orange	84

* Many countries require a label declaration, and may exclude it from certain categories of medicines or do not accept it in new product applications.

PLASTICISERS

The difference between hard and soft gelatin capsules is that soft capsules contain appreciable quantities of a plasticiser. In fact, hard capsules have been defined as having less than 5% by weight of plasticiser present and soft capsules significantly more than this (U.S. Patent 2 491 475, 1949). The function of the plasticiser in the capsule wall is to reduce the rigidity of the gelatin and make it pliable. For soft gelatin capsules this is particularly important because the film after filling must take up the form of the mould.

A large variety of chemical materials have been suggested for this application. However, glycerol, which was the first true plasticiser used in capsule manufacture (Taetz, French Patent 106 325, 1875) is still the one most used today. The other materials which have been used are some of the polyhydric alcohols, natural gums, and sugars. Their exact function in the gelatin film does not appear to have been elucidated. Several of them are used in other applications as humectants and it is possible that they function by binding water molecules within the gelatin structure, thereby reducing rigidity.

Some materials which have been used as plasticisers in soft gelatin capsule manufacture are glycerol, sorbitol, propylene glycol, sucrose, and acacia. The proportion of plasticiser needed varies depending on the type of soft gelatin capsule being made, but is usually in the region of 20–40% by weight. Certain other materials have been claimed to enhance the effect of the main plasticiser when added in concentrations of 2–6%. These include glycine, mannitol, acetamide, formamide, and lactamide.

PROCESS AND PERFORMANCE AIDS

Hard and soft gelatin capsules are prepared from coloured gelatin solutions, with or without preservatives and plasticisers. To this mix, small quantities of other substances can be added to aid in the manufacturing process (process aids), or to aid in the subsequent performance of the capsule (performance aids). Process aids are of two types: surfactants, which enable the gelatin solution to take up the shape of the moulds better, and substances which enable the capsules to be further processed, e.g. a silicone fluid which allows formaldehyde treatment to produce an enteric product more readily. Performance aids are materials to improve the patient acceptability of the product, such as flavouring agents.

Capsules are often filled with materials such as antibiotics which have an objectionable smell and taste. Capsules containing these medicaments can be made more attractive to the patient by flavour masking. Soft gelatin capsules have been produced with walls containing either flavouring agents such as vanillin, or volatile oils such as peppermint and menthol. Similar gelatin capsules have been produced, not by adding the materials to the gelatin during the manufacturing process, but by adding them to the capsule surfaces after filling.

Sodium lauryl sulphate is a surfactant used in the production of hard gelatin capsules. Its use is specifically mentioned in the U.S.P. which allows a suitable concentration to be present. It is added to the gelatin solution during the preparation stage. The stainless steel mould pins are lubricated prior to dipping into the gelatin solution and, because of this, sodium lauryl sulphate in solution is added to reduce the surface tension of the mix and cause the mould pins to wet more uniformly. An indication of a lack of sodium lauryl sulphate is the appearance of thin areas on the capsule walls where the mould pins have not been sufficiently wetted.

Silicone fluids have been patented for use in soft gelatin capsule manufacture (R. P. Scherer, British Patent 1 252 200, 1971). The addition of a silicone fluid such as dimethylpolysiloxane (dimethicone) improves the mechanical strength, resistance to moisture, and resistance to enzymes. A typical capsule mix might contain (parts by weight) glycerol 22, water 34, dimethicone '1000' 10, and gelatin 34.

If enteric capsules are produced by treatment with formaldehyde, the disintegration time continues to increase on storage. It is claimed that silicones block functional groups within the gelatin molecule so that the formaldehyde can react only with a limited number, and so prevent further reaction on storage.

PRESERVATIVES

Gelatin is a good medium for bacterial and fungal growth, especially if sufficient moisture is available. During the capsule-manufacturing process the gelatin is in solution, and is kept warm to prevent gelling, which gives almost ideal conditions for bacterial growth. The gelatin is not initially sterile, but does have as low a bacterial count as is practicable to attain. Bacterial growth can alter the viscosity of the gelatin as well as contaminating it.

Following a code of good manufacturing practice will help to minimise contamination. During the capsule-manufacturing process, the gelatin solution should be heated to a temperature at which bacterial growth will decline significantly; by maintaining it at this temperature, circulating it constantly, and ensuring that no local cool spots exist, bacterial growth will be suppressed. If the bacterial level can be held down, through to the finished capsules, the normal moisture levels of both hard and soft capsules will be sufficiently low to prevent the growth of any organisms during storage.

However, the simplest way to control the microbiological content of capsules is to use a preservative, which is usually added during the processing of the gelatin solution. A few are bactericidal; the majority are bacteriostatic in action. The substances which can be used are limited by two considerations. Firstly, pharmaceutical legislation may restrict the substances which can be added. Secondly, the preservative may affect the capsule. For example, betanaphthol was at one time permitted but it caused the capsules to turn brown on storage.

Sulphur dioxide is the preservative which has been most widely used. It was first mentioned in French Patent 15 212, 1843. It is widely permitted for use in foodstuffs and pharmaceuticals, and in capsule manufacturing it is usually added in the form of a solution of sodium sulphite or sodium metabisulphite. The quantity used is such that the concentration in the final capsule is less than 1000 ppm, calculated as SO_2. It is volatile and is lost during the manufacturing process. It has one major drawback in that, even at low concentrations, it affects many of the commonly used colorants. As little as 60 ppm will cause colour loss with Amaranth, Sunset Yellow FCF and Indigo Carmine. Sulphur dioxide is a reducing agent, but its bleaching action is not simple. It is thought that it reacts with azo dyes by adding 1:4 across the azo-linkage, in the presence of gelatin, to produce a colourless molecule (Wyatt, 1966).

Several esters of p-hydroxybenzoic acid have been used as preservatives. They are considered to be bacteriostatic rather than bactericidal in action, and are employed in concentrations up to 0.2% w/w in the finished capsule. Each ester is effective against a different spectrum of organisms, and as a result they are usually used in combination. The most commonly used combination is methyl hydroxybenzoate (methylparaben) with propyl hydroxybenzoate (propylparaben), in a 4:1 methyl to propyl ratio.

A number of organic acids, such as benzoic, propionic, and sorbic, and their sodium salts, have been used in capsule manufacture, chiefly for their activity against moulds and yeasts, which particularly affect soft gelatin capsules. The compounds have general bacteriostatic properties, and are used at concentrations up to 1% w/w. Their activity is influenced by pH, their optimum effect being obtained at pH 4.5–5.5.

STERILISING AGENTS

It can be useful to sterilise capsules at the end of the manufacturing process, and this can be done by treatment with ethylene oxide, which is widely used to sterilise medical equipment, particularly dressings and thermolabile materials. It is used in combination with inert gases because it forms an explosive mixture with air. The most frequently employed mixtures are 10% ethylene oxide and 90% of halogenated hydrocarbons. The sterilising efficiency depends upon the exposure conditions, namely time, temperature, relative humidity, and concentration. For the treatment of capsules, only normal ambient conditions can be used, otherwise the gelatin will be affected. As a result, only count reduction can be brought about, not a complete sterilisation. The process can be applied to hard gelatin capsules after their final packaging when the appropriate dose is injected into the container, which is then sealed. The dose is such that the residual levels are less than 40 ppm in the capsules (Gold Sheet 1978). Ethylene oxide breaks down to produce ethylene glycol and ethylene chlorhydrin, and even stricter limits are placed on the residual quantities of these compounds, namely 5 ppm and 3 ppm respectively.

Like ethylene oxide treatment, γ-irradiation is widely used to sterilise surgical dressings and delicate equipment. It has been suggested for the sterilisation of capsules, but unfortunately radiation changes both the colour and the performance of capsules. The sterilising dose of γ-radiation is 3 megarads, and at this level treated capsules change colour (Robson and Allan, 1972). The gelatin itself changes from a pale translucent yellow-brown to a darker brown, almost as if charred, and several of the more commonly used dyes fade during the treatment. At exposures of 10 megarads, the disintegration times of hard gelatin capsules do not increase (Hüttenrauch, 1971) but those of soft ones do. The plasticiser content of soft gelatin capsules probably makes them more susceptible to radiation damage.

GELATIN SUBSTITUTES

The initial reason for looking for gelatin substitutes was to find ways of overcoming Mothes's original patent. In the nineteenth century, capsules were made from a variety of materials such as decoctions of starch, gluten, animal membranes, and vegetable gelatin prepared from carragheen moss. However, the only material with the correct properties was gelatin. More recently, other compounds have been tried, but only one, methylcellulose, has reached large-scale capsule manufacture, the remainder being confined to the patent literature.

The properties which are required of a gelatin substitute are, firstly, that it must be a good film former. For two-piece capsules, a film only 0.1 mm thick must be tough and flexible. For one-piece capsules, it must produce a film, when suitably plasticised, which is both pliable and easy to seal. Secondly, it must rapidly dissolve in biological fluids at 37° and, thirdly, it must exhibit a 'gelation' stage so that a capsule film can be cast or dipped, and so that existing capsule manufacturing machinery can be used. Most of the patents have this objective in mind although there have been suggestions for a radical change of method such as extrusion. Gelling must be brought about either by a temperature change or by the removal of sufficient solvent to cause a significant increase in concentration.

The cellulose ethers are the replacement materials most commonly mentioned in the literature. They can be used on standard capsule-making machines, but the process needs to be modified because of their temperature-related properties. The viscosity of the solution, when heated from room temperature, first decreases to a minimum value then increases rapidly to a gel point, which is only a few degrees above the point of minimum viscosity. This means that instead of dipping cold moulds into hot solutions as in the processing of gelatin, hot moulds are dipped into cold solutions of cellulose derivatives.

In 1950, H. W. Murphy of Eli Lilly & Co. obtained an American patent for methylcellulose capsules and the process of manufacture (U.S. Patent 2 526 683). Two-piece capsules made to this patent were produced in both the U.S.A. and the U.K. in the early 1950s. Standard hard gelatin capsule manufacturing machines were used. The patent covered all cellulose ethers and in particular methylcellulose. The grade of material used was 7–15 mPa s as determined on a 2% aqueous solution at 20°. For manufacture, a 15–20% solution was prepared by soaking the material in water at 5° for 12–24 hours. On the manufacturing machine it was heated to 18°. The gel point of this solution was 65°, and capsule pin-moulds heated substantially above this temperature were dipped into it, and then passed through the standard drying kilns. The pins cooled during this part of the cycle, contracting away from the films and allowing them to be stripped easily. The moisture content of the finished capsules was 2.5%.

A plasticiser at 5% concentration was used, the choice of which influenced not only the strength of the capsule but other properties as well. To reduce moisture uptake, mannitol, monoacetin, or triethyl phosphate were preferred, whilst for greater solubility, sucrose and sorbitol were the best choice. Disintegration could be improved by the inclusion of a small quantity of electrolyte. The capsules were claimed not to be affected by either high humidity or bacteria. They were used in significant numbers, and both the British and Italian pharmacopoeias allowed the use of capsules made from such materials. Unfortunately, in use, there was poor in vivo disintegration, so much so that capsules sometimes passed through the body unaffected. When this became known their manufacture was discontinued.

Since that time a series of patents have been granted for the production of other modified celluloses with better in vivo performance. The Dow Chemical Co. have been particularly active in this field. In 1957 they obtained a patent for thermoplastic compositions of water-soluble cellulose ethers, intended to overcome the problems caused by the limited solubilities of such compounds and their high intrinsic viscosities at low temperature (U.S. Patent 2 810 659). Mixtures such as methylcellulose or hydroxypropylcellulose with ethylene glycol as a plasticiser and triethyl citrate as a modifier, when heated to 140°, form a thermoplastic material which can be vacuum-drawn into strips and used in the rotary die process for capsule manufacture.

Improved celluloses became available during the 1960s, and in 1969, Dow were granted a patent for the preparation of medicinal capsule shells from hydroxyalkyl-alkylcellulose ethers (British Patent 1 144 225). Standard capsule equipment could be used, the capsule film being formed by draining and evaporation of a volatile solvent. Low-viscosity materials were used such as hypromellose (4–10 mPa s grade). A 15–25% solution was prepared in a mixture of 15–40% water and a C_1–C_3 alcohol, with the addition of 5–10% of a plasticiser such as glycerol or propylene glycol. A proportion of ethylcellulose could be added to delay disintegration if required.

There were obviously problems with capsule formation due to the slow speed of evaporation, and in a further patent in 1973 Dow reverted to the use of thermal gelation (British Patent 1 310 697). To obviate the problems caused by dipping a large mass of hot moulds into the preparative solution, a system of induction heating of the mould surfaces was proposed. The moulds were dipped into a solution at about 10° below its gel point, removed, and allowed to drain. The mould pins had a conductive outer surface which was induction heated to make the film gel in about 20 seconds, when the capsules were dried and stripped in the normal way.

Another solution to the problem was proposed in 1974 (U.S. Patent 3 842 242). The mould pins were pre-heated by dipping the pin bars into dipping pans which contained a fluidised bed of PTFE granules heated to 200°; 15 seconds immersion raised their temperature by 40 degrees.

In 1977, Dow obtained a patent for the use of hydroxyalkylstarch for the manufacture of capsules (U.S. Patent 4 026 986). A 20–45% solution of hydroxypropylstarch (grade 2–15 mPa s) was held at 63.5°. The moulds were dipped and slowly withdrawn to form the capsule. These hydroxyalkylstarches are compatible with other film-forming materials, and also with the standard plasticisers, and are stable at the higher temperatures that are needed to process them.

Several polymers have been patented for use in the preparation of capsules which, because of their stability at higher temperatures than can be withstood by natural materials, can be used to prepare capsules by standard plastics-manufacturing methods.

In 1970 Tanabe Seiyaku Co. Ltd obtained a patent (Japanese Patent 70 01 277) for the manufacture of soft capsules made of polyvinyl alcohol, the alcohol having a saponification value between 75 and 100%. Capsules were made using a standard seamless soft gelatin capsule machine, from a 30% aqueous solution, prepared at 90°. They were extruded at 70°, the fill being at 30°, into a bath of liquid paraffin at 0°, this low temperature

being necessary to cause gelation. The capsules were allowed to mature overnight in a liquid paraffin bath at 5°, washed in chloroethane and air-dried at 10°.

A French company, Centre de Recherches Marcel Midy, obtained patents in 1971 to prepare capsules by plastics-manufacturing techniques from a mixture of polymers, at least one of which dissolves, disintegrates, or becomes porous in contact with biological fluids (French Patent 2 073 288; British Patent 1 252 333). Polymers that have this property include copolymers of vinylpyrrolidone/vinyl acetate, polyacrylic acid, copolymers of polymethacrylates, polyoxyethylenes of molecular weights between 6×10^5 and 4×10^6, hydroxypropylcellulose and polyvinyl alcohol esters. The formulation included plasticisers as required, and the capsules were formed by injection moulding, thermoforming, or powder-deposition on a mandrel followed by fusion. The choice of method depended upon the nature of the plastic used; for example, copolymers of vinylpyrrolidone/vinyl acetate and hydroxypropylcellulose can be injection moulded, methacrylates can be extruded, and polyoxyethylenes can be thermoformed.

In 1972 Röhm GmbH were granted a patent for a soluble pharmaceutical capsule formed by polymerising vinylic monomers (Belgian Patent 785 702). The capsules produced by this method are soluble only within specific pH ranges, so that by adjusting their composition, the speed and *in vivo* location of disintegration can be controlled. An aqueous dispersion of the material was used on standard capsule-manufacturing equipment, and the polymer was made by reacting a vinylic monomer having a carboxyl group and a mono- or dialkylaminoalkyl ester group.

Another German company, Hoechst AG, applied for a patent in 1975 for the use of a modified polyvinyl alcohol (BRD Patent Application, offenlegungsschriften, 2 363 853). The material was a partially saponified graft copolymer of vinyl acetate on polyoxyethylene. It required no additional plasticiser, being self-plasticised by the polyoxyethylene. Capsules can be prepared from it either by standard dipping methods or standard plastics methods such as injection moulding or foil preparation. The material is stable at high temperatures. For making two-piece capsules, a 50% aqueous solution, dipping at 80° and drying at 100°, was recommended.

All the patents for capsules produced from synthetic polymers claim that such capsules have improved stability, being less susceptible to bacterial growth and moisture. However, the criteria on which the choice of a material to make capsules is based are the solubility in biological fluids and the oral toxicity. This latter factor is currently the most important, because gelatin has a universal acceptability and so also must any other material that is to replace it. The cost of performing the required toxicity tests is so high that the search is limited to materials that are already available. Despite the numerous patents, there have been no products successfully marketed in synthetic polymer capsules, as yet.

GELATIN EXTENDERS

These are cheap and readily available materials which can be used to reduce the quantity of gelatin needed per capsule, and to enable cheaper gelatin, with poorer physical properties, to be used.

One natural material which is now comparatively abundant is starch, and the National Starch and Chemical Corporation has obtained a patent for the use of modified starches in the production of capsules (U.S. Patent 3 758 323, 1973). The suggested material is a product of waxy maize (corn) starch, and is a dextrin which is modified either by thermal or chemical treatment, using succinic anhydride in the latter case. A weak gelatin solution is prepared, then a paste, made by heating the dextrin to 85°, is added to produce a melt from which capsules can be produced in the normal way. Another modified starch product for this purpose is hydroxyalkylstarch, patented by the Dow Chemical Co. in 1977 (U.S. Patent 4 026 986). This is both a gelatin replacement and an extender.

PROTECTIVE COATINGS

Capsules may be coated to improve the stability of the product, particularly its moisture resistance, and, for soft gelatin capsules, to prevent sticking and to prevent attack by the contents. Coatings can also modify the solution rate of the capsules, and enable enteric capsules to be produced.

Capsules contain appreciable quantities of moisture. The quantity can vary, particularly if the capsules are subject to adverse conditions. Soft gelatin capsules contain plasticisers in their shells, and when stored at high temperatures may stick together. The soft gelatin capsule is frequently used to contain liquid preparations and it is important that there is no reaction between the contents and the shell. Several types of protective coating have been patented to overcome these problems.

The American Cyanamid Co. in 1955 patented a coating consisting of a mixture of a protective resin and formaldehyde solution (U.S. Patent 2 727 833). The latter acts as a hardener and is applied for just long enough to produce case-hardening of the capsule. At the same time, the capsules are washed with the hardener solution and a resin, such as sumatra benzoin, shellac, or silicone, is applied to give a tack-free surface.

The prevention of sticking of soft capsules is also linked to heat resistance. A. Nattermann & Cie, GmbH, have patented a coating consisting of a mixture of an anionic copolymer and a plasticiser (French Patent 1 559 913, 1969). They suggested the use of a mixed copolymer of methacrylic acid and methyl methacrylate, plasticised with a mixture of dibutyl phthalate and castor oil. This is dissolved in a volatile solvent such as isopropyl alcohol or methanol and then applied in a conventional tablet-coating pan.

Soft gelatin capsules are frequently used for rectal or vaginal application and Ciba S.A. have obtained a patent for a coating which renders the capsule both tack-free and easier to use (French Patent 1 462 506, 1966). When the coating comes into contact with water it forms a gel which makes the surface slippery and the capsule easier to insert. The coating materials used include methylcellulose, magnesium aluminium silicate, vegetable gums, and polyacrylic acids (Carbopols). They are applied two or more at a time in an organic solvent, e.g. methanol/methylene chloride mixture, in a conventional tablet-coating pan.

Such coatings on the surface of hard gelatin capsules do not improve their mechanical strength. A Japanese company, Sumitomo, has a patent for coating hard gelatin capsules with materials to bring about strength improvement (Japanese Patent 68 24 048, 1968). They used a mixture of a water-soluble adhesive, such as acacia, tragacanth, or polyvinylpyrrolidone, with a carrier such as sodium chloride or sucrose. The capsules were treated with the dry mixture by tumbling, and then separated. They were next tumbled with the carrier slightly moistened, separated, and then dried. This coating is of doubtful efficacy.

A problem can occur when soft gelatin capsules packed in blister or strip packs are subjected to tropical conditions. This softens them, and they tend to burst when pushed through the foil on removal from the pack. Ciba-Geigy A.G. have patented a means of overcoming this by applying a coating to the surface of the capsule to increase the strength (British Patent 1 324 242, 1973). The coating consists chiefly of hypromellose plus a glycol such as propylene glycol and shellac or ethylcellulose. The coating is applied to the capsules as an organic solution in either a conventional coating pan or a fluidised-bed spray coater.

A method for protecting the wall of a soft gelatin capsule from its contents has been patented by the American Cyanamid Co. (U.S. Patent 2 770 571, 1956). The protective coating consists of a resin of β-pinene, formed by heating the monomer at a relatively low temperature in an aliphatic solvent with a catalyst. The resultant resin is dissolved in chloroform and applied to the gelatin film before the capsules are formed and filled.

ENTERIC CAPSULES

An enteric coating is one that resists the action of the gastric juices but dissolves under the less acid conditions in the duodenum and intestines (Schroeter, 1965). There are several reasons for using such coatings: drugs may be unstable at the pH of gastric juice, or may irritate the gastric mucosa; they may interfere with gastric metabolism, or the site of their absorption or action may be in the duodenum or intestines. Enteric capsules have been known since the end of the nineteenth century but their development has not been as prominent as that of enteric-coated tablets, largely due to the difficulties of rendering the capsule completely resistant to gastric juice. Early attempts to make enteric capsules have been described in Chapter 1.

Gelatin capsules can be made acid-resistant by treating them with an aqueous solution of formaldehyde. This causes cross-linkages to form which reduce the solubility of the gelatin. Between 100 and 350 mg/m² of formaldehyde is applied to the capsules during a set time period. After the treatment the capsules are washed with an organic solvent and dried. For this process to be used the capsules must initially be sealed, and a disadvantage of the method is that, on storage, the cross-linking reaction can continue and excessive hardening can occur. Furthermore, safety questions have been raised about the presence of trace amounts of formaldehyde in foods and pharmaceuticals.

Alternatively, the capsules can be coated with a solution of cellacephate, which was developed by Eastman Kodak in 1940 (Malm *et al.*, 1951). The first patents for the preparation of an enteric hard capsule using cellacephate were obtained by H. Bogin of Parke, Davis & Co. (U.S. Patent 2 491 475, 1949; U.S. Patent 2 575 789, 1951). His composition consisted of a mixture of gelatin and the alkali metal salt of a partial ester of a polycarboxylic acid and a suitable cellulose ether. A solution was prepared, e.g. by dissolving cellacephate in sodium carbonate solution of a strength which was just sufficient to dissolve the cellacephate; this solution was then mixed with a gelatin solution. Capsules were made from this mixture in the standard manner.

Such solutions behave differently from normal in that they do not set rapidly. To speed up the setting, cool air (below 25°) is blown across the moulds immediately after dipping. The Eastman Kodak Company in 1955 (U.S. Patent 2 718 667) prepared capsules solely from an alkali metal salt of cellacephate. Rapid gelling could be brought about by coating the moulds from a cool solution (27°) and then quickly dipping them into water at 45°.

Unfortunately, cellacephate/gelatin mixtures produce capsules which are unstable on storage because of slight decomposition of the cellacephate, which liberates acetic acid, and they become less soluble in the intestines. They are also very brittle, because of stresses in the wall caused by incompatibility between the polymers and a yield as low as 63% of acceptable capsules can occur. Thus either an alternative material, more stable and more compatible with gelatin, must be found, or else the polymers and gelatin must be kept apart by producing a two-layered capsule.

Further derivatives of cellulose with enteric properties have in fact been developed. Parke, Davis & Co. in 1974 took out a patent (U.S. Patent 3 826 666) for the preparation of enteric capsules from a mixture of gelatin and the alkali metal salt of hypromellose phthalate. The capsules were formed on the standard hard gelatin capsule machine using the same method of low temperature dipping, followed by cold air blowing, as for cellacephate/gelatin capsules, but the yield of good capsules by this process was 80–90%.

Soft single-piece capsules have been prepared by mixing both cellacephate and hypromellose phthalate with gelatin and adding casein and latex to improve the film strength. Four separate solutions are prepared which, except for the latex, contain ammonia. They are mixed to produce a liquid suitable for making soft gelatin capsules by the rotary die process.

Enteric polymers not based on cellulose are also available. Tanabe Seiyaku obtained a patent in 1973 (Japanese Patent 73 10 522) for capsules prepared from a mixture of gelatin and acrylic copolymers. In order to achieve aqueous solubility they reacted an alkali metal salt of a copolymer of methacrylic acid with alkyl methacrylate to give a methacrylate/methacrylic acid copolymer, which was plasticised with a polyhydric alcohol such as glycerol, sorbitol, polyethylene glycols or propylene glycol. This solution was mixed with gelatin solution. If less than 15% of the copolymer was used, a gastrosoluble capsule was produced; if over 30% was used, an enteric capsule was produced. Both hard two-piece and soft single-piece capsules could be produced from this mixture using the standard machines and methods.

Lilly Industries Ltd. obtained a patent in 1976 (British Patent 1 455 884) for a two-layer enteric capsule, designed to separate the gelatin from the enteric polymers. This was achieved by forming a gelatin capsule thinner than normal and then dipping the mould for a second time into a solution of the enteric polymer and an organic solvent. The resulting capsule had the same dimensions as a standard capsule. This operation could be carried out on a standard hard gelatin capsule machine which had been fitted with an additional dipping section. All of the standard pharmaceutical enteric polymers could be applied in this way.

Capsules can be coated by any of the classical pharmaceutical methods (Jones, 1970), though the method of choice is the fluidised-bed air-suspension technique. Methods using tablet-coating pans do not work very satisfactorily with capsules because their low bulk density and awkward shape means that they do not roll well in the pan and so the coating is uneven. The air-suspension technique allows coating material to be readily applied by spray over all the surface of the capsules. The polymers which can be applied in this way are the standard film coats, cellacephate, polyvinyl acetate phthalate, methacrylic acid polymers, and hypromellose phthalate. They are applied to the capsules from solution in volatile organic solvents. Plasticisers are included in the formulations in order to improve the mechanical strength and flexibility of the coat, and to decrease the transmission of water vapour through it. The most commonly used plasticisers are diethyl phthalate, dibutyl phthalate, propylene glycol, and triacetin.

The problems in applying coatings to the surface of capsules are capsule separation, and appearance. In all the coating systems, the capsules are subjected to vigorous movement and can come apart unless self-locking. One of the important features of a gelatin capsule is its high gloss finish. Anything deposited on its surface will detract from its appearance unless it is applied carefully, and even the best enteric capsules have a somewhat matt appearance.

References

Buckalew, L. W. and Coffield, K. E., *J. clin. Psychopharmac.*, 1982, *2*, 245–248.

Cattaneo, A. D. *et al.*, *Eur. J. clin. Pharmac.*, 1970, *3*, 43–45.

Cooper, J., *J. Am. pharm. Ass.*, *pract. Pharm. Edn*, 1956, *17*, 640–643.

Eighth Report of FAO/WHO Joint Expert Committee on Food Additives, *FAO Nutrition Meetings Report Series No. 38*, 1965; *Tech. Rep. Ser. Wld Hlth Org. No. 309*, 1965 and *FAO Nutrition Meetings Report Series No. 38B*, 1966; WHO/Food Add./66.25.

FAO/WHO Joint Expert Committee on Food Additives, Specifications for Identity and Purity of Food Colours, *FAO Food and Nutrition Paper No. 31/1*, 1984.

Gold Sheet, 1978, *12*, No. 7.

Hine, W. H. and Robson, A. R., personal communication.

Hüttenrauch, R., *Pharmazie*, 1971, *26*, 506–507.

Jones, B. E., *Mfg Chem.*, 1970, *41*(5), 53–54 and 57.

Jones, B. E., M. Pharm. Thesis, University of Wales, 1973.

Lucchelli, P. E. *et al.*, *Eur. J. clin. Pharmac.*, 1978, *13*, 153–155.

Madsen, E., *Dansk Tidsskrift for Farmaci*, 1957, *31*, 29–51.

Malm, C. J. *et al.*, *J. Am. pharm. Ass.*, *scient. Edn*, 1951, *40*, 520–525.

Peacock, W. H., *The Application Properties of Certified 'Coal Tar' Colorants*, Calco Technical Bulletin, No. 715, New Jersey, U.S.A., 1949.

Prista, L. N. *et al.*, *Anais Fac. Farm. Porto*, 1970, *30*, 35–46.

Robson, C. and Allan, G. A., personal communication, 1972.

Schapira, K. *et al.*, *Br. med. J.*, 1970, *2*, 446–449.

Schroeter, L. C., in *Remington's Pharmaceutical Sciences*, 13th Edn, E. W. Martin *et al.*, (Ed.), Easton, Pennsylvania, Mack Publishing Co., 1965, p. 601.

Swartz, C. J. and Cooper, J., *J. pharm. Sci.*, 1962, *51*, 89–99.

Turner, T. D. and Jones, B. E., *J. Pharm. Pharmac.*, 1971, *23*, 806–807.

Wyatt, M. A., personal communication, 1966.

Chapter 5

Capsule Standards

B. E. Jones

The standards which are applied to capsules can be divided into two categories. Pharmacopoeial standards control the quality of capsules in relation to their medicinal use, i.e. to ensure that they contain the correct drug in the correct dosage, and that it is available for absorption. Industrial standards control the quality of the capsule shell and its contents to ensure the efficiency of the manufacturing process and to produce a product which is acceptable to the consumer.

PHARMACOPOEIAL STANDARDS

The official tests are designed to ensure that capsule products comply with a minimum acceptable standard. They fall into seven groups: raw materials, content of active ingredient, uniformity of weight, disintegration of oral capsules, disintegration of enteric capsules, disintegration of rectal and vaginal capsules, and dissolution. Not all pharmacopoeias have a full set of tests, but most of them include disintegration and uniformity of weight. Standards in national pharmacopoeias vary but they are becoming more uniform, particularly because of the adoption of the *Eur. P.* by most European countries.

Raw Materials

Pharmacopoeial monographs give only brief details, if any at all, of the substances from which capsules can be made. They make the implicit assumption that all the materials shall be of pharmacopoeial quality. Apart from gelatin, materials which may be used include colouring agents, plasticisers, preservatives, and surfactants. Colouring agents and other additives are considered in Chapter 4.

Content of Active Ingredient

It is a pharmacopoeial requirement that the content of active ingredient in each dose shall be stated on the product label. The limits for content

are usually expressed in the form (for example) '90% to 110% of the prescribed or stated amount'.

Uniformity of Weight

The test for uniformity of weight is the simplest indicator of the content of active ingredient, assuming that the contents of the capsule are homogeneous. The specified weight limits, within which the capsule contents must fall, are symmetrically placed about the mean weight of the test sample in all pharmacopoeias. Details of the test in a number of pharmacopoeias are given in Table 5.1. The *Eur. P.* applies a 'double limit' test. For capsules containing less than 300 mg, not more than 2 out of a sample of 20 may be outside ±10% of the mean weight, and all must be within ±20%. For capsules with a greater weight, the *Eur. P.* specifies a stricter set of limits. In this case, not more than 2 out of a sample of 20 may be outside ±7.5%, and all must be within ±15%.

A simple test in which the decision is taken on a single sample of specified size is usually prescribed. However, the *Jpn P.* (1981) has a sequential test which is applied to soft capsules. An initial sample of 20 capsules is weighed; if they fail the test, a further sample of 40 is weighed and the results of both tests are pooled to reach a final decision. The aim is not to reduce sampling but to make allowance for the greater difficulty of handling soft capsules. The contents of a hard capsule can be tipped out, but the liquid or semi-liquid contents of a soft capsule usually have to be washed out with a suitable solvent. When removing the solvent by evaporation, it is necessary to take particularly care to avoid the loss or gain of moisture.

Capsules that are not intended to be taken orally may have different limits. An example is Sodium Cromoglycate Insufflation (*B.P.*) which contains a powder for inhalation. The quantity of powder is lower than for a normal capsule and there are technical difficulties in filling such a small dose,

Table 5.1. Test for uniformity of weight of capsule contents

Pharmacopoeia	Sample size	Fill weight mg	Inner limit %	Proportion allowed to deviate from inner limit	Outer limit %
Cz. P.	10	<200			±15
		200 to 500			±12
		500 to 1000			±10
		>1000			±8
Eur. P.[a]	20	<300	±10	2/20	±20
		≥300	±7.5	2/20	±15
E. Ger. P.	10	<50	±15	1/10	±30
		50 to 150	±10	1/10	±20
		150 to 300	±7.5	1/10	±15
		>300	±5	1/10	±10
Ind. P.	20	<300	±10	2/20	±20
		≥300	±7.5	2/20	±15
Int. P.	20		±10	2/20	±20
Jpn P.	20[b]	—			±10
	20		±10	2/20	±25
	20[c]	—	±10	2/20	±25
	60		±10	6/60	±25
Jug. P.	20		±10	2/20	±15
Pol. P.	10[d]	<150	±10	1/10	±20
		150 to 300	±7.5		±15
		>300	±5		±10
Roum. P.			*hard soft*		
	30	<200	±10 ±7.5	3/30	
	30	210 to 500	±7.5 ±6.0	3/30	
	30	510 to 1000	±6.0 ±5.0	3/30	
	30	>1000	±4.0 ±3.0	3/30	
Rus. P.	—[e]	<100			±10
		>100			±5

[a] The countries that have adopted the standards of the *Eur. P.* include Austria, Belgium, Britain, Denmark, Eire, Finland, France, Germany (West), Greece, Iceland, Italy, Luxembourg, Netherlands, Norway, Spain, Sweden, Switzerland.
[b] Hard capsules. If the first sample fails, take a further sample of 20
[c] Soft capsules. If the first sample fails, take a further sample of 60
[d] If sample fails on a sample of 10, the test is repeated on a sample of 20
[e] No sample size specified

so that a greater tolerance in weight variation is allowed. The *B.P.* also has separate limits for rectal and vaginal capsules, in each case adopting the limits applied to moulded suppositories and pessaries.

Uniformity of Dosage Units

Most pharmacopoeias prescribe separate tests for uniformity of content and uniformity of weight. However, the *U.S.P.* XXI has introduced a new type of test, the 'Uniformity of Dosage Units', which combines the two tests. It is applied to hard and soft gelatin capsules.

The weight variation test may be used on liquid-filled soft gelatin capsules, or on products which contain 50 mg or more of a single active ingredient comprising 50% or more by weight of the dosage-form unit. The test is carried out by weighing 10 intact capsules individually, emptying out the contents, and reweighing the empty shells. In the case of soft capsules, it is permitted to wash them with a suitable solvent. The amount of drug per capsule is then calculated from the net content weight, using the result of the monograph assay, and assuming that the active ingredient was homogeneously distributed in the contents.

The content uniformity test can be used for all capsule products. A sample of 10 capsules is taken, and each one is assayed individually as directed in the monograph, modifying the procedure if the amount of active ingredient per individual dose is too small for the assay method.

The test criterion for capsules is that, in no less than 9 of the 10 units, the amount of active ingredient determined by the weight variation test or the content uniformity test, lies within the range

85 to 115% of the label claim, no unit is outside the range 75 to 125%, and the relative standard deviation of the results is less than or equal to 6.0%. If this criterion is not met, and 2 or 3 capsules are outside the 85 to 115% range but inside the 75 to 125% range, or if the relative standard deviation is more than 6%, then an additional 20 capsules may be tested. Of the total 30 capsules, not more than 3 may be outside the 85 to 115% range, none must be outside the 75 to 125% range, and the relative standard deviation of the 30 units must not exceed 7.8%.

Disintegration Test for Oral Capsules

The purpose of the disintegration test is to give an indication of the time taken for the gelatin shell to release its contents into the stomach. The conditions used in the test attempt to simulate *in vivo* conditions.

EMPTY CAPSULES

The disintegration test usually refers to filled capsules but some pharmacopoeias also include a test for empty shells. These tests are simple solubility tests (Table 5.2). In the *Jpn P.*, the test is also used as a purity check, specifying that the solution must be odourless, and neutral or slightly acid.

Table 5.2. Disintegration test for empty capsules.

Pharma-copoeia	Sample size	Volume of test fluid* ml	Temperature °C	Time limit min
Hung. P.	—	—	36 to 40	10
Jpn P.	5 × 1	50	35 to 39	10
Roum. P.	0.5 g	—	37	15

* All tests specify water except for *Roum. P.* which specifies an acid pepsin solution

FILLED CAPSULES

Most pharmacopoeias attempt to simulate movement within the stomach by the use of an oscillating tube apparatus which consists of a vertically-mounted tube made of glass or Perspex, with a wire mesh base. The capsule is placed in the tube which is then raised and lowered in the test solution at a frequency of approximately 30 strokes per minute through a specified distance. The volume of the test solution is not always stated. The *Eur. P.* requires a depth of solution such that

the wire mesh is at least 25 mm below the surface of the liquid at its highest point, and 25 mm above the bottom of the container at its lowest point.

In this apparatus, those parts of the capsules which have been shed are separated from those which have not disintegrated and, theoretically, it should be possible to define an exact end-point. In practice, however, this is by no means easy. When capsules disintegrate, they split and allow the contents to escape, leaving empty capsule shells. The shell pieces may then agglomerate to form a large mass of gelatin which will take longer to dissolve because of its thickness. This situation is recognised by pharmacopoeias so that in the *Eur. P.*, for instance, the end-point is given as 'no residue remains on the screen or, if a residue remains, it consists of fragments of shell or is a soft mass with no palpable core'. The *Eur. P.* specifies a modification to this test when it is used for soft capsules. A disk, made of transparent plastic, is placed in the disintegration tube on top of the capsule. The disk may be omitted if the capsule contains a liquid which could attack it. The use of the disk is also allowed for hard capsules if they would float on the surface of the liquid.

The test in *U.S.P.* XXI applies only to hard capsules. The apparatus is modified by the addition of a 10-mesh wire cloth to the top of each tube with the object of preventing the capsules from floating on the surface of the test medium.

The usual test medium is water. However, gelatin is also soluble in acidic solutions because it hydrolyses, and the *Eur. P.* allows 0.1M hydrochloric acid to be used in certain justified and authorised cases. The *Jpn P.* uses an acid solution for all capsules. The time allowed for disintegration varies but is usually in the range 15 to 30 minutes, and the same limit is usually applied to both hard and soft capsules. The *U.S.P.* XXI specifies an individual time limit for each product. Details of the tests in various pharmacopoeias are given in Table 5.3.

However, the rate-controlling step in capsule disintegration is the formulation of the fill rather than the gelatin shell itself (Jones, 1972). The limit, therefore, is a measure of how fast the contents are released from the shell. The different limits are set because of the variable degree of agitation used in the tests and according to whether the end-point is defined as the start or the completion of disintegration. *In vivo* testing has shown that properly formulated capsule products will release their contents within 2.5 to 8

Table 5.3. Disintegration tests for filled capsules using the oscillating tube with mesh (1), or an Erlenmeyer flask with swirling (2).

Pharma-copoeia	Sample size	Method	Temperature °C	Test solution	End-point	Time limit to end-point min
Cz. P.	6 × 1	1	37 to 40	Water or acid pepsin or alkaline pancreatin	Disintegrate or dissolve	15
Eur. P.	6 × 1	1	36 to 38	Water[a]	No residue on mesh	30
E. Ger. P.	1	2	36 to 38	Acid pepsin	Start to release contents	10
Ind. P.	5	1	35 to 39	Water	No residue on mesh	15 (hard) 30 (soft)
Int. P.	5	1	35 to 39	Water	No residue on mesh	15
Jpn P.	6 × 1	1	35 to 39	Acidic sodium chloride	No residue on mesh	20[b]
Jug. P.	6 × 1	1	35 to 39	Water or acid pepsin	Release of contents	15[b]
Pol. P	5	1	35 to 39	Acid pepsin	Disintegrate or dissolve	15
Rus. P.	3 × 1	2	35 to 39	Water	Release of contents	15
U.S.P.	6 × 1[c]	1	35 to 39	Water	Disintegrate apart from shell fragments	—[d]

[a] 0.1M hydrochloric acid may be used in justified and authorised cases
[b] Allows a retest on a further sample of 6 if one fails the test. In the second sample all must pass
[c] Hard capsules
[d] Time limit specified in the individual monographs. Allows a retest on a further sample of 12 if one or two fail the test. Not less than 16 of the 18 must pass

minutes after ingestion (Eckert, 1967; Eckert *et al.*, 1969, 1971; Hunter *et al.*, 1980).

ENTERIC CAPSULES

Many pharmacopoeias include tests for enteric capsules, even though there are few products available and those are restricted to a few countries.

The official tests attempt to mimic the *in vivo* passage of the capsule through the stomach before it disintegrates in the duodenum. The capsules are first subjected to a solution which represents the conditions in the stomach, where they must not disintegrate in the time specified. They are then transferred to a solution representing the conditions in the duodenum, in which they must disintegrate and release their contents within the stated period. The *Eur. P.* specifies 0.1M hydrochloric acid for the first solution, and a pH 6.8 phosphate buffer for the second.

The transit time through the stomach can vary considerably, and depends on a number of physiological factors. The *Eur. P.* requires enteric capsules to be resistant to the first solution for 2 hours, but they must disintegrate in the second solution within 1 hour.

Disintegration Test for Non-oral Capsules

Capsules which are for rectal or vaginal administration may also have to comply with a disintegration test. The *Eur. P.* applies the test which is routinely used for suppositories and pessaries.

This consists of two perforated metal disks 30 mm apart which are held in a glass or plastic cylinder. The capsule to be tested is placed in this device which in turn is placed in a vessel containing at least 4 litres of water at 36–37°. The water is agitated with a slow stirrer. The device is inverted, without being removed from the water, every 10 minutes. Disintegration is said to be complete when the gelatin shell ruptures, allowing the release of the contents. The same limit of 30 minutes is applied to both rectal and vaginal capsules.

Dissolution Tests for Capsules

The dissolution test measures the rate at which a drug is released into solution from a dosage form and is used as an indication of the bioavailability of the product. Further information on the theoretical basis for dissolution testing is given in Chapter 13.

The apparatus used for dissolution testing varies in design, but is usually based on a rotating wire mesh basket immersed in a glass vessel containing a specified dissolution medium. The capsule is placed in the basket which is then rotated for a specified time. The *U.S.P.* XXI includes a second type of apparatus in which the liquid is agitated by a flat-bladed stirrer; the type of apparatus to be used is specified in the individual monographs.

In the *B.P.* (1980) test, a sample of the dissolution medium is withdrawn at the end of the specified time and assayed for drug content. The amount of drug released from the capsule must not be less than a specified proportion of the total. The *U.S.P.* XXI test is similar except that it is sequential, in three stages. Testing is continued through each stage unless the product conforms at a previous one.

CONTROLLED-RELEASE PRODUCTS

Products are available which release their active ingredients at a steady rate over a period of time. The *Eur. P* has a category of capsule called 'modified-release'. These are defined as hard or soft capsules in which the contents, or the shell, or both, contain added substances or are otherwise designed to modify the rate or the place at which the medicaments are released. The *U.S.P.* XXI has a similar category. For example, there are two types of phenytoin sodium capsules, referred to as 'prompt' and 'extended'. The products are differentiated by a dissolution test. 'Prompt' capsules must have released 85% of their active ingredient within 30 minutes, whereas 'extended' capsules must not have released more than 40% at 30 minutes, and must still be releasing drug at 60 and 120 minutes.

Miscellaneous Pharmacopoeial Requirements

Most pharmacopoeias include other statements in the monographs which refer to matters such as formulation of the contents, labelling of products, stability, storage conditions, and packaging.

Materials that are to be filled into capsules must conform to certain general criteria. In particular, additives should be innocuous, and should not reduce the stability of the active ingredient or interact with the capsule shell.

Pharmacopoeias do not give any indication of the physical dimensions of capsules. Hard gelatin capsules are made in a range of internationally recognised sizes which were evolved so many years ago that the rationale behind them has been lost in history.

Nearly all pharmacopoeias include statements on the storage of filled capsules. Many give a general instruction, such as that in the *Eur. P.* which states that capsules should be stored in well-closed containers at a temperature not exceeding 30°.

The *U.S.P.* XXI gives the storage requirements for empty hard gelatin capsules. They should be stored in tight containers until they are filled, and should be protected from potential sources of microbiological contamination.

INDUSTRIAL STANDARDS

Industrial standards are intended for, and are agreed between, the capsule producers and users. Usually, they do not have official legal status, but they are taken as standards on which to base good manufacturing practice.

The American Federal Standard for Capsules (for Medicinal Purposes) (Fed. Std No. 285A) is frequently used as the basis for industrial quality control. This gives the requirements for American governmental users such as the armed forces, and it applies to filled capsules. However, since the defects may arise from the empty shells, the standards are applied in the industry to the quality control of empty capsules. Because defects may arise in the filling process, there needs to be a lower level of defects in empty shells if the standard is to be achieved on filled capsules.

The Federal Standard includes references to pharmacopoeial standards but extends their scope to many other aspects of physical testing, packaging etc.

In the application of in-process quality control, standard statistical sampling and inspection methods are used. In Britain these are set out in Defence Guide DG-7-A (Sampling Inspection) and Defence Specification DEF-131-A and, in the U.S.A., in the Military Standard MIL-STD-105.

Standards for Empty Hard Capsules

DIMENSIONS

Hard gelatin capsules are made in standard sizes, although capsules made by various manufacturers are not necessarily identical in shape and size. However, they are sufficiently standard to fit all filling machines. The basic dimensions of hard capsules from three manufacturers are given in Tables 11.1, 11.2, 11.3 (Chapter 11). The lengths of the cap and the body are related to one another because when the capsule is correctly closed after filling, the cap length is exactly half of the total length (the closed joined length). The unclosed joined length is the length of the empty capsule as it leaves the manufacturer. It is important because, if the capsule is too long, it will fall apart and, if it is too short, it will fail to separate on the filling machine. This latter defect is particularly important in the case of self-locking capsules.

The diameters of the cap and the body are not constant along their lengths. Capsules are made on moulds which are tapered and as a result they are slightly conical. The diameters are important in two places. The body diameter at the open end influences how the capsule halves fit together, particularly when they are being rejoined on the capsule filling machine. The cap diameter at the end of the body, when the capsules are closed to the correct closed joined length, influences how the capsule halves stay together after closure.

SOLUBILITY

Pharmacopoeial solubility tests are usually performed on filled capsules. The results are dependent upon both the nature of the capsule wall and the formulation of the contents. Industrial tests are particularly concerned with the solubility of the capsule wall.

The American Federal Standard requires capsules to remain undissolved after immersion in water at 25° for 15 minutes, but to 'completely fall apart, dissolve, or disintegrate' after immersion in 0.5% w/w hydrochloric acid at 36°–38° for 15 minutes.

MOISTURE CONTENT AND BRITTLENESS

The moisture content of the capsule shell must be such as to prevent brittleness. It is normally 13.0 to 16.0%, determined by drying at 105°. The brittleness can be checked by applying pressure at the centre of the capsule against a smooth hard surface; the capsule must not shatter.

ODOUR

The capsule shells should not develop any foreign odour. This is usually determined by checking a sample after storage in a sealed bottle for 24 hours at 30 to 40°.

DEFECTS IN THE CAPSULE SHELL

Empty capsules can suffer from a number of defects which may be produced during manufacture. These defects are classified in three ways according to type and relative importance.

Critical defects are those which would interfere with the filling process. This category includes capsules which are too short or too long, squashed capsules, and capsules with holes, cracks, and flat areas.

Major defects are those which would cause a problem in use and reduce the effectiveness of the filled capsule. These include separated capsules, double caps, thin walls, and splits.

Minor defects are those which do not affect the performance of the capsule as a dosage form but which spoil the appearance of the product. These are surface blemishes such as pits, specks, bubbles, or other marks.

The three categories listed above are sometimes referred to as Major A, Major B, and Minor defects, respectively, although these titles are more properly applied to similar faults in filled capsules as listed in the American Federal Standard (see below).

Printing Defects. The print may be missing or totally illegible or, alternatively, it may be badly printed although still legible.

Each manufacturer supplies specifications for limits on all these defects.

Standards for Filled Hard Capsules

The American Fed. Std No. 285A lists capsule defects in three categories.[1]

Major A Defects
  Capsule not type-specified (i.e., hard shell).
  *Capsule not free of cracks, breaks, pinholes, or splits where leakage of contents may occur.
  Capsules not uniform in appearance.
  Base and/or cap of capsule not as specified.
  Capsule not uniform in colour(s).
  *Capsule empty.
  *Capsule not free of embedded surface spots and contamination.
  Capsule fill not free from foreign matter.[2]

Major B Defects[3]
  *Capsule does not maintain tight closure or seal in the immediate container, or during normal handling, or dispensing.
  *Immediate container not free from extraneous matter.
  *Capsule not intact (i.e., cap separated from body).
  *Capsule not free of foreign odour, other than characteristic odour
  *Immediate container not internally or externally clean.
  *Void space of immediate container not filled, when required.
  *Immediate container not free of excess ingredient (capsule contents).

Minor Defects
  Capsule not free of pits or dents.
  Capsule not free of thin areas.
  Capsule not free of specks, spots, or blemishes.
  *Capsule not free of cap and/or body cutting into one another.
  Capsule not smooth.
  *Capsule not free of adhering surface spots.

[1] Inspection is not restricted to classified possible defects listed above.
[2] For opaque capsules use a sample size of 20 capsules to examine contents. No capsule shall show evidence of foreign matter.
[3] Capsules obtained from the bottles used for examination of Major B defects may be used for examination of Major

A and Minor defects annotated '*'. Thus, no additional capsules need be selected.
*Applies to examination of capsules in filled, final (immediate) containers.

The acceptable quality limit (% defective) for Major A and Major B defects is 1.0% in each case, and for Minor defects is 2.5%.

References

American Federal Standard No. 285A, Capsules (for Medicinal Purposes), Washington DC 20407, General Services Administration, 1976.
Eckert, T., *Arzneimittel-Forsch.*, 1967, *17*, 645–646.
Eckert, T. *et al.*, *Arzneimittel-Forsch.*, 1969, *19*, 821–825.
Eckert, T. *et al.*, *Arzneimittel-Forsch.*, 1971, *21*, 1403–1406.
Hunter, E. *et al.*, *Int. J. Pharmaceut.*, 1980, *4*, 175-183.
Jones, B. E., *Acta pharm. suec.*, 1972, *9*, 261–263.

Chapter 6

The Manufacture of Hard Gelatin Capsules

B. E. Jones

The process for the manufacture of hard gelatin capsules has remained essentially the same as that proposed by Lehuby in his original patent in 1846, but it has been refined and automated by successive generations of pharmacists and engineers. Like many other European inventions, it was first exploited and developed in the United States of America and was then later reintroduced into Europe. The industry at present is, for historical reasons, dominated by American-based companies, the two largest being Eli Lilly & Co. of Indianapolis, and Parke, Davis & Co. of Detroit. Both of these have manufacturing plants in many other countries as well. Other American companies are active in the field, such as R. P. Scherer who now produce hard capsules as well as soft capsules, and Smith, Kline & French Laboratories, who manufacture for their own needs. Capsules are also being made in other countries including China, India, Indonesia, Jordan, Yugoslavia, Singapore, South Korea, and Taiwan. In some of these places the conventional modern machinery is used, but in others, capsules are made on a cottage industry basis using wooden hand-held moulds as described by Lehuby.

THE MANUFACTURING PROCESS

The working of a modern high-speed capsule-manufacturing machine and the necessary subsequent operations can be summarised as follows. A gelatin solution is prepared, containing the gelatin itself together with colorants and various process additives. The capsules are made by dipping, and are then dried. The dried capsules are removed from the moulds, and the caps and bodies are assembled. The assembled capsules are sorted, printed, and packaged (Hostetler and Bellard, 1976; Jones, 1982; Martyn, 1974; Norris, 1959 and 1961).

The Gelatin Solution

The materials used in the preparation of hard gelatin capsules are the gelatin itself, colorants, which may be natural or synthetic water-soluble dyes or pigments, preservatives, and surfactants. The gelatins used have been described in Chapter 3. The manufacturer purchases these against a strict specification, but it is common practice to draw material from several suppliers and blend different lots together to give the optimum combination.

A stock solution of gelatin is first prepared by dissolving the gelatin in hot (60–70°) demineralised water in stainless steel tanks (Fig. 6.1). Some manufacturers use gelatin which has been presoaked in cold water (Norris, 1961). A concentrated solution is prepared, containing from 30 to 40% w/w of gelatin. This solution is very viscous and contains bubbles of entrapped air which can be removed by applying a vacuum to the vessel in which the solution is prepared. The batch size of the mix is governed by the rate of use. Gelatin in hot solution hydrolyses, and its Bloom strength and viscosity gradually decrease. Thus the manufacturer must balance economy in work against this decline in physical properties. In practice, comparatively small batches are prepared.

When the gelatin solution has matured, aliquots are withdrawn from the manufacturing vessel and are prepared for the requirements of each individual machine. Firstly the colorants are added. These are in the form of solutions of dyes or suspensions of pigments. At the same time, other materials, such as preservatives, may be incorporated into the mix, e.g. sulphur dioxide can be added in the form of a solution of either sodium metabisulphite or sulphite. The viscosity is then adjusted, because the thickness of the capsule shell is governed by the viscosity of the initial gelatin solution. The viscosity can be measured directly

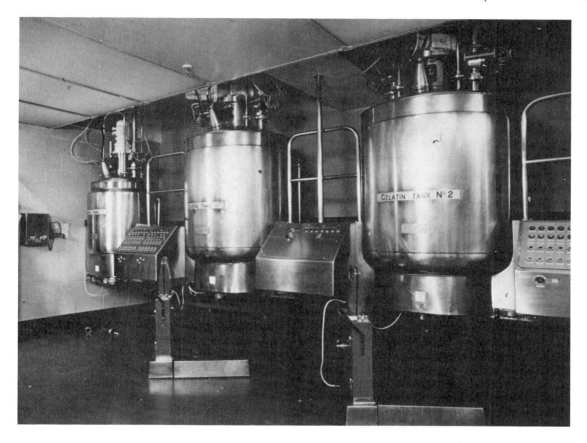

Fig. 6.1. Gelatin solution stock tanks

by a standard glass U-tube or electromechanical rotational viscometer, or inferentially by measuring the density of the solution with a Baumé hydrometer (Norris, 1961).

Solutions of more than one viscosity are supplied to each machine, the initial solution having a higher viscosity than subsequent deliveries. The reason for this is that the first solution is at the correct viscosity to make the required thickness of capsule. The temperature of the solution at dipping is from 45–55° and as a result a significant amount of water is continually being lost by evaporation. This is replaced by preparing the second and subsequent gelatin solutions for the machines at a lower viscosity.

Capsule Formation

The moulds on which capsules are formed are called pins, and groups of these are set in line on metal bars; the whole assembly is called a pin

bar. Hubel made his original moulds from iron, which resulted in capsules which became discoloured on storage. To prevent this, other metals were used, initially phosphor bronze and then stainless steel, which is the material of choice today. The moulds for both cap and body have the same general form, the body being the longer of the two. Their form is such that the capsule shell consists of two parts which are slightly but regularly tapered towards their closed ends, and the diameters are so arranged that the inner diameter of the cap near its closed end is slightly less than the outer diameter of the body at its open end (Eli Lilly & Co., British Patent 1 040 859, 1966; Parke, Davis & Co., British Patent 1 108 629, 1968). The taper, which is of the order of 0.1 to 0.3 mm/cm of length, is to ensure that the capsule parts can be removed from the mould pins after forming and drying. If the sides were parallel, a vacuum would be created which could

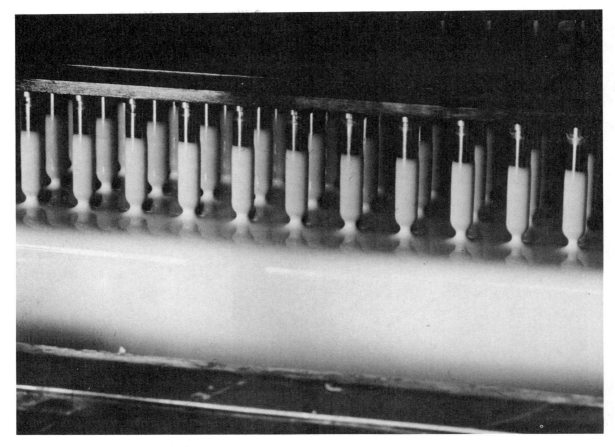

Fig. 6.2. Capsule formation: the dipping process.

cause a collapse of the capsule wall when removal was attempted.

The gelatin solution is placed in the machine in a jacketed, stirred container which is called a 'dip pan' or 'dip pot', and its level is kept constant by a reserve of fresh hot gelatin solution which is held in a jacketed container and is fed into the main container through a valve controlled by a level-sensing device. The dip pan jacket is provided with heating controls so that the temperature of the gelatin solution can be accurately maintained. The dipping section of the machine is shown in Fig. 6.2.

The pin bars are gently lowered into the gelatin solution, then slowly withdrawn. Gelatin is picked up on the mould pins, the quantity being governed by the viscosity of the solution. The viscosity also governs the way in which the gelatin solution runs down and off the mould pins. Immediately after withdrawal there is, on the tops of the pins, an accumulation of gelatin formed as the pin leaves the surface of the solution. To spread the gelatin evenly over the surface of the mould pins, the pin bars are rotated about a horizontal axis as they are transferred from the lower level to the higher level of the machine. As they rise, they pass through a stream of cool air, which helps to set the gelatin solution and fix the film on the mould. When the pin bars reach the upper level of the machine there is no further movement in the gelatin film.

Drying

The pin bars are then passed through a series of drying kilns. In these, large volumes of controlled humidity air are blown directly over the pins to dry the film. The air is heated to a few degrees

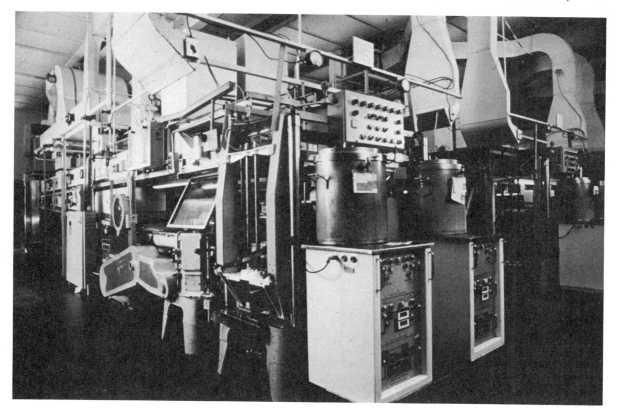

Fig. 6.3. A capsule-manufacturing machine.

above ambient (22–28°). Higher temperatures cannot be employed because the moulds have to return to the correct operating temperature for redipping, otherwise the viscosity control would be upset. At the rear of the machine the pin bars are again transferred back to the lower level of the machine and return to the front end through further drying kilns. The drying conditions are adjusted so that the drying rate is low to begin with, slowly reaches a maximum at the rear of the machine, and then slows down again as it approaches the front. Excessive drying rates will cause splits to occur in the gelatin films. When the capsule parts emerge from the last kiln they contain approximately 15–18% w/w of water. This is higher than that required in the finished capsule (13–16%), but it must be high at this stage, otherwise problems arise in removing the cast films from the moulds. A balance has to be struck between drying the film until it is strong enough to handle, and overdrying with consequent brittleness. An overall view of the machine is given in Fig. 6.3.

Capsule Removal and Assembly

The gelatin films formed on the pin moulds are longer than required for the finished capsule. This is because the lower edges of the films are 'feathery', and of variable thickness, so that they need to be trimmed to a good clean edge at the length required. Fig. 6.4 are views of the trimming section. The capsule shells are removed from the pins by sets of metal jaws, which are placed around each pin on a bar. The jaws are closed and pulled back along the pin and, in the process, transfer the shell into a metal holder or collet. The holder is rotated against a sharpened and hardened knife which is adjusted to cut the capsule part to the specified length. The trimmings are removed by suction and usually recycled, gelatin being an expensive material. The capsule parts are then transferred to a central joining block where the two halves are fitted together. The completed capsules are carried by means of a revolving belt into a receiver.

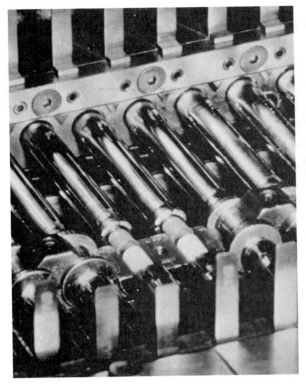 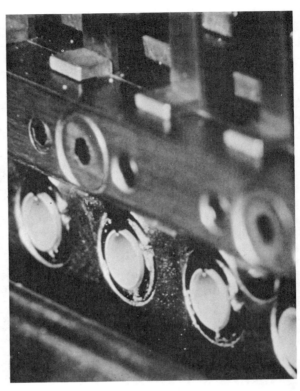

Fig. 6.4. The trimming section of a capsule-manufacturing machine. The left-hand picture gives an overall view and shows the capsule parts being joined after having been trimmed by the triangular blades between the spindles. The right-hand picture shows a capsule cap/body being trimmed.

The pin bars are passed through another section where they are cleaned with felt pads held in metal holders. At the same time a small quantity of lubricant is applied to them. The lubricant or release aid, colloquially referred to as a grease, is necessary to enable the gelatin film to be stripped from the pins. The function of this lubricant is firstly to prevent the gelatin film from adhering too strongly to the mould, and secondly to enable the gelatin film to slide easily over the surface of the metal mould. The materials used are a specific formulation of mixtures of pharmaceutical grade materials, each particular to the individual capsule manufacturer. The pin bars are then assembled in groups of five and are ready to enter into the cycle once more.

During the machine cycle the operator takes samples of capsules and checks the lengths of the cap and body, the thickness of the capsule wall, and the end wall or dome of the capsule. The thickness of the wall is usually expressed as an average or 'double wall thickness' and is measured by flat-tening the capsule between the anvils of a measuring gauge. The information obtained from the sample is used to make adjustments to the machine which can be either manual on the basis of an operator decision, or can be controlled by a computer (Martyn, 1974).

The principal manufacturer of soft gelatin capsules, R. P. Scherer, has patented the idea of applying the principle of soft gelatin capsule manufacture, filling and forming on the same machine, to the hard gelatin capsule (British Patent 1 054 977, 1967). The same basic moulds are used but instead of the cap and body moulds being mounted on separate bars, they are mounted on opposite sides of the same bar. The pin bar is first dipped to form the cap and then inverted and dipped again on the other side to form the body. The capsule shells are dried and stripped from the moulds in the conventional manner, except that the body of the capsule is passed under a filling head before it is joined up with its cap. The patent describes this machine as being in five modules, each of which can be detached for ease of maintenance or size change, and the capsule-filling portion could be omitted if not required.

The formation of the gelatin film on the surface of the mould is governed by the viscosity of the gelatin solution into which it is dipped and the intrinsic gelation time of the gelatin used. Höfliger, who also devised the well-known range of capsule-filling machines, has patented the idea of improving the formation of this film by utilising an electric current to cause electrophoretic movement of the gelatin (Senator and Höfliger, French Patent 2 302 723, 1979). Conventional stainless steel mould pins are used, and they are dipped into gelatin solutions in the standard manner. An electrical charge is applied to the system which, it is claimed, causes a positive movement of gelatin towards the mould pins with a resultant more uniform film. This improves both the physical strength of the capsules and the gelatin utilisation efficiency because it reduces variations in shell weight.

Capsule Sorting

Capsules must satisfy dimensional requirements as well as being fault-free. There are several basic dimensions of a hard gelatin capsule; these are illustrated in Chapter 11, where typical values from the three major manufacturers are given.

The lengths of the cap and the body can be measured on standard gauges. They are related to one another, in that when the capsule is closed to the correct length after filling (the closed joined length) the cap length is exactly half of the total length. The body length is chosen so that when the capsule is closed it extends into the cap as far as the base of the dome of the cap. The unclosed joined length is the length of the empty capsule as it leaves the manufacturers. It is important because, if it varies outside the allowable limits, the capsules will fall apart if they are too long, and will fail to separate on the filling machine if too short. This latter fault is particularly serious with self-locking capsules.

Capsules are made on moulds which are tapered and as a result are slightly bell-shaped. The diameters are important in two places: the body diameter at the open end because this influences how the capsule halves fit together, particularly when they are being rejoined on the capsule-filling machine, and the cap diameter at the closed end, which influences how the capsule halves stay together after closing.

The hard gelatin capsule is manufactured to tight engineering tolerances despite the fact that it is made out of natural material by a dipping process. The nature of the method causes a small percentage of defective capsules to be produced. Immediately after manufacture the empty capsules are sorted visually or by electronic equipment.

Empty capsules are placed in a hopper and are fed by means of a vibrating plate or moving band past inspectors. Their job is to remove defective capsules from the bulk. The faults which they look for are defects caused either by poor initial formation of the capsule film, such as thin areas or bubbles, or those produced as the capsules pass through the automatic section of the machine, such as poorly cut edges, splits, or holes caused by the stripper jaws. Further information on defects is given in Chapter 5.

Eli Lilly & Co. patented a system which uses an optical electronically controlled device to inspect and sort capsules. In this machine the capsules are conveyed on a chain with buckets from a hopper to a revolving disc. This orientates the capsules and spins them at high speed (10 000 rpm) in a beam of light. Defects in the capsule surface will deflect the beam; this deflection is detected by sensors which activate a rejection mechanism to remove the faulty capsules.

Capsule Printing

Hard gelatin capsules are usually printed with a variety of information such as the product name, the approved chemical name, product strength, or the company name and logo or symbol. This allows rapid identification of the contents of the capsule, which is particularly important in cases of poisoning, and it helps to promote the identity of the manufacturer. The process which is used most often is an 'offset' method using an edible pharmaceutical grade ink on an automatic machine. It is normally carried out by the manufacturer of the empty shells, although a few companies do print capsules after they have been filled.

PRINTING MACHINES

Printing machines all have the same basic parts that are essential for an 'offset' process, and differ from each other only in the way in which the capsules are handled. The legend to be printed is engraved on a highly polished metal cylinder, which is made either of stainless steel or of a softer metal such as brass which has been chromium-plated. This is called the 'rotogravure cylinder' and it revolves in a reservoir of printing ink. The ink fills the engraving and as the cylinder revolves it comes into contact with the sharp edge of a metal strip called the 'doctor blade' which removes the ink from its surface, leaving only that which fills the engraving. The ink is transferred to a rubber offset roll geared to and in contact with the roto-gravure cylinder. The capsules pass under this rub-ber roll and the image is then transferred to them. On some machines another rubber roller is used at this position, 'the pressure roll', to ensure that the capsules press against the offset roll.

There are only a few specialist manufacturers of such machines, and between them they provide models ranging in capacity from 20 000 to one mil-lion capsules per hour.

R. W. Hartnett Company produce a small-out-put machine, the Delta, in which the capsules are carried in buckets from the hopper to the printing head. This machine can be used to print legends on both sides of the capsule simultaneously. There is a 'B' series of machines with capacities up to one million per hour, on which the capsules are carried from the hopper to the printing roll in a multiple-slotted track in 16 rows.

Markem Machines Ltd produce two types of machine. The smaller and older versions use a metal disc with a slotted circumference to carry the capsules past the printing head. The larger and newer machines use a revolving cylinder with slots cut in it which are filled by centrifugal force, ena-bling higher outputs, up to 150 000 capsules per hour, to be achieved. This latter machine can also print around the capsule by using a soft rubber offset roll.

Another feature common to most machines is that the capsules are not rectified before they are printed. This means that the printing occurs ran-domly on the cap and body and also that it can run in either direction along the capsule. Thus it is not possible to print specific information solely on either the caps or the bodies. Some machines have been adapted to rectify the capsules prior to printing, but this considerably reduces their out-put. Printing a message on one half only can be achieved by using a two-coloured capsule, and choosing the colour of ink so that it exactly matches one half of the capsule; although it will still be present on both halves it will only be appar-ent on one.

PRINTING INKS

The inks which are used all have the same basic formulation, which is an insoluble colorant to-gether with a film-forming polymer dispersed in a volatile solvent system. The ingredients must be of oral pharmaceutical grade and comply with the legislation in force in the country in which the cap-sule products are used.

Two basic types of colorants are used: pigments and lake dyes. The pigments are insoluble sub-stances, most of which occur naturally. The most commonly used ones are carbon, iron oxides (red, yellow, and black), and titanium dioxide.

Lakes are dyes which have been adsorbed on a substrate of alumina or titanium dioxide. They are made from the same dyes used to colour cap-sules.

The quantity of colorant used is in the range 20–40% w/v of the ink. Using the available color-ants a large range of colours of ink could be pro-duced, but in practice this is not done, and the most common inks are the basic colours black, blue, grey, red, and white. The reason for this is that the ink is being applied to the coloured surface of a capsule, and the printing characters are very small, so that fine distinctions of colour are rather wasted.

Film formers are an important constituent of the ink, the most widely used being shellac. Other substances, such as modified celluloses, have been used, but shellac has the advantage that it is universally acceptable in medicines. It is a resinous substance produced by a scale insect, *Laccifer lacca* Kerr (Coccidae), which exudes the material onto branches of the trees on which it lives. It is collected manually, sorted, and purified before use. It is readily soluble in organic solvents, and in concentrations of 30–40% w/v gives a solution of high viscosity capable of suspending the large quantities of colorants used. When the solvents evaporate it is deposited as a tough shiny film which adheres to the gelatin surface. One draw-back in the use of shellac is that it is poorly soluble in water, which makes it difficult to clean equip-ment after use. However, one ink manufacturer, Colorcon, has patented a process for chemical modification of the shellac to make it water-misc-ible, thus considerably reducing the handling problems of the capsule printer (Piotrowski, U.S. Patent 3 694 237, 1972).

Various substances are added to the ink to improve its performance on the printing machines. These may be either surfactants or suspending agents. Surfactants improve the spreading charac-teristics of the ink by lowering its surface tension. They ensure good pick-up of the ink by the engrav-ing on the rotogravure roll, and improve its transfer to the rubber offset roll and thence to the capsule surface. Those used have included dimeth-icone and lecithin. Suspending agents improve the stability of ink on storage and ensure that the sus-pension maintains its homogeneity on the printing machines. Modified celluloses, such as hypromel-lose, have been used for this purpose.

Solvents are chosen according to their volatility as this is the most critical parameter in the perfor-mance of an ink. It must dry as soon as possible after it is transferred onto the capsules, because they come into contact with each other almost immediately when ejected from the machine. The ink, however, must not dry too fast, otherwise it adheres to the rotogravure cylinder and the rubber offset roll, and fails to be transferred to the cap-sule. The solvents are mainly mixtures of lower alcohols and are blended to give the correct evaporation rate for each particular application.

The printing ink on the machine is contained in an open reservoir in which the rotogravure cylinder rotates and there is a significant loss of solvent which needs to be replaced. An excessive loss of solvent causes the ink viscosity to increase, which worsens the ink pick-up by the engravings. This problem can be overcome by shrouding the reservoir and by providing a continuous solvent drip-feed to make good the loss. Other solvents can be added to the reservoir to modify the solvent evaporation rate and correct any printing faults which may occur.

If the ink is drying too slowly, ink transfer will occur from one capsule to another as they leave the machine. Increasing the proportion of isopro-pyl alcohol will correct this. If the ink is drying too fast, there will be poor ink transfer to the cap-sules, and addition of butan-2-ol or 2-ethoxyetha-nol is needed. If there is poor ink pick-up by the engraving, it can be overcome by the addition of ethanol to the reservoir.

DESIGN OF CAPSULE PRINT
Most typical printing involves a two-part inscrip-tion, one part on each half, laid along the long axis of the capsule. This is called axial printing. Alternatively, the inscription can be orientated perpendicularly to the long axis of the capsule. This is called radial printing. In practice, axial printing is most commonly used. The available

printing surface is limited by the curvature of the capsule, and also because the capsules are not usually orientated prior to printing. This latter fact means that the area is reduced, particularly for axial printing, because the cap/body junction of the empty capsule is not central and may be pos-itioned either way as it passes under the transfer roll. The inscription must be applied so that it does not cross the junction. The dimensions of the areas which can be used are given in Table 6.1.

Table 6.1. Dimensions, in mm, for the available printing area of capsules

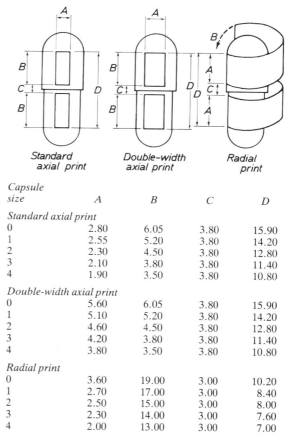

| Standard axial print | Double-width axial print | Radial print |

Capsule size	A	B	C	D
Standard axial print				
0	2.80	6.05	3.80	15.90
1	2.55	5.20	3.80	14.20
2	2.30	4.50	3.80	12.80
3	2.10	3.80	3.80	11.40
4	1.90	3.50	3.80	10.80
Double-width axial print				
0	5.60	6.05	3.80	15.90
1	5.10	5.20	3.80	14.20
2	4.60	4.50	3.80	12.80
3	4.20	3.80	3.80	11.40
4	3.80	3.50	3.80	10.80
Radial print				
0	3.60	19.00	3.00	10.20
1	2.70	17.00	3.00	8.40
2	2.50	15.00	3.00	8.00
3	2.30	14.00	3.00	7.60
4	2.00	13.00	3.00	7.00

In standard axial printing, an arcuate surface subtending an angle of 42° at the axis of the capsule is all that can be used. Elanco have devised a method of increasing this angle to 84°, which represents the maximum area of the capsule sur-face that the eye can see at one glance. In radial printing, a much larger area, subtending an angle of 360°, can be printed but can only be read by turning the capsule round.

The most important criterion in designing the print on a capsule is legibility. The engraving must be made so that it makes the best use of the available capsule surface and assists problem-free running on the printing machines. To illustrate the points which are taken into account, consider the printing of the word 'tetracycline' axially on a capsule. There are four possible arrangements, see Fig. 6.5 (Jones, 1974). The first example shows

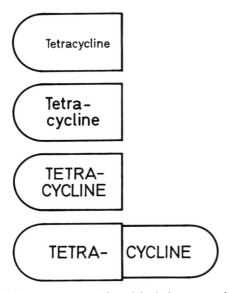

Fig. 6.5. Four arrangements for axial printing on capsules

the word in upper- and lower-case letters so that it completely fills the maximum length available on each half of the capsule. This fails to use the height of the printing area effectively. The shorter the legend the better the appearance, so that long words such as tetracycline are better hyphenated and reproduced on two lines using large print. The second and third examples illustrate this point. In the second example, upper- and lower-case letters are used and in the third example, capital letters only, which even more fully occupies the maximum printable area. If the word is suitable for division into two, one half can be printed on each half of the capsule, using the largest possible print size. This is shown in the fourth example.

It is necessary for the engraving to deposit discrete quantities of ink onto the capsule for maximum density. Two types of engraving are used

on the rotogravure cylinder. For fine lines, such as in the first example, an 'open etch' engraving is used. For thicker lines, such as in the fourth example, a screened engraving is used. This picks up less ink and as a result reduces the possibilities of ink smudging. Adequate spacing between letters is also important to reduce smudging, particularly in the case of adjacent vertical lines such as between the 'I' and 'N' in the fourth example, and where small spaces are surrounded by ink, as in the letter 'R'.

Packing and Storage

Capsules which have passed through sorting, printing, and quality control, are packaged for transport. Traditionally, they were packed into polythene-lined fibre drums which had metal or plastic lids. Because of developments in packing materials and in the design of handling systems, and also because of the economics of freight, the drum has been replaced in many cases by the cardboard box. This has the advantage that it can be stored flat when empty, thereby occupying much less storage space than drums. The capsules are placed in a liner inside the box. The liner may be a heat-sealed paper sack with Saran lining or a polythene bag, which would be quite adequate in temperate climates where proper warehouse facilities were available. However, heat-sealed aluminium foil sacks are required in severe climatic conditions.

Capsules can be stored in the unopened packs, as supplied by the manufacturers, for long periods without any undue deleterious effects, provided a few simple rules are observed. The storage areas preferably should have a temperature between 10 and 30° and a relative humidity less than 70%. If this is maintained, the only causes of capsule damage are sudden heat changes which result in localised moisture transfer effects within the container. For example, if the warehouse has windows, the sun could fall on only part of a carton and cause a high local temperature, or the container could be placed close to a heating source such as a radiator. These conditions will produce clumping of capsules inside an unopened carton due to moisture being concentrated at the spot where the highest temperature is reached.

Quality Control

During all stages of the manufacturing operation the requirements of good manufacturing practice are observed, and many quality control operations are carried out. An outline of the tests carried out in a typical manufacturing operation is given below. Further information on quality control is given in Chapter 5.

RAW MATERIALS

The gelatin is assayed for physical properties: Bloom strength, viscosity and viscosity loss; chemical properties associated with purity; limits for heavy metals, arsenic, and ash; and microbiological properties such as the total count of organisms present and the absence of coliform and pathogenic organisms.

The colorants are assayed for chemical properties: purity and limits for heavy metals and arsenic; and colour properties: dye content, subsidiary dye content and colour value.

The process aids are assayed for chemical purity, and the water for chemical and microbiological purity.

MACHINE OUTPUT

The output is continuously monitored for dimensional correctness. The colour of the capsule produced is checked visually against a standard and, if necessary, adjustments are made to the gelatin solution on the machine by adding dye solution. The capsules are monitored by thin-layer chromatography to ensure that the correct colorants are present.

SORTING FOR DEFECTS

After the capsules have been inspected, they are sampled by quality control inspectors and the results compared with an inspection plan. Capsules which fail to meet this plan can either be re-sorted or rejected depending on the type or frequency of faults found.

PRINTING INSPECTION

After the capsules have been printed they are sampled by quality inspectors. The samples are inspected for quality of print. As with capsule faults, the capsule manufacturers, in consultation with the users, have agreed upon quality levels for the nature and frequency of defective printing. The results of the examination are compared with the inspection plan. Capsules which fail this can either be re-sorted or rejected. It is difficult to remove capsules with printing faults by sorting as the faults are not easy to see.

FINAL INSPECTION

When the capsules have been placed in the final container, a further sample is taken for comparison with the inspection plan for dimensions, physical defects, and colour. Capsules can be rejected even at this late stage in the process. During the whole of the manufacturing process, capsules are being continuously monitored for microbiological quality and are only despatched if this is satisfactory.

PROPERTIES OF HARD GELATIN CAPSULES

Moisture Content

The capsule when supplied to the user should have a moisture content in the range 13–16% w/w. This moisture content can differ depending upon the atmospheric conditions to which the capsules have been exposed. Empty capsules should be supplied in moisture-proof containers and it is only when the seals of these are broken that unwanted changes in moisture content occur. The way in which water is held in the gelatin wall and the quantity which may be transferred has been the subject of study.

There is a pronounced hysteresis in the sorption–desorption isotherms for water in gelatin, which is particularly pronounced at the desorption stage (Strickland and Moss, 1962). To measure the lag time of water vapour diffusion through the capsule wall, an apparatus was devised in which sealed capsules were suspended on quartz springs in a controlled atmosphere. There was a four-hour lag time before water vapour penetrated through to the contents, which were a hygroscopic powder.

The moisture transfer between the capsule shell and its contents has been studied by examining the behaviour of several insoluble macromolecular substances, such as starch and microcrystalline cellulose, filled into capsules (Ito *et al.*, 1969). Sorption–desorption isotherms were obtained both for these materials and for empty capsules, and the final equilibrium moisture contents of the components of the filled capsules could be calculated from these values.

From this work it would appear that, to prevent moisture from passing either to or from the capsule shell or contents on storage, each component should be used at its equilibrium moisture content for the storage conditions. This has been found to be valid for most substances and, in particular, it is true for the preparation of a stable formulation for a capsule of cephalexin (Bond *et al.*, 1970). However, anomalous behaviour has also been reported (Bell *et al.*, 1973) in a study of capsules of sodium cromoglycate. When filled capsules were recycled through hygrostats at varying humidities they did not return to the initial equilibrium moisture contents. The sodium cromoglycate in the capsules was acting as a moisture sink and was continuously withdrawing water from the capsule shell.

The water present in the gelatin film is chemically bound to varying extents. Under normal ambient conditions, capsules cannot be dried to less than 4% w/w of water. This residual water is strongly bound to the gelatin molecule and if it is removed down to a level of 0.3% w/w, the gelatin will not reconstitute to the same physico-chemical state (Yannas and Tobolsky, 1967). Above 4% w/w the water molecules are less strongly bound and can easily be added to or removed.

The moisture content of the capsule wall strongly affects its physical properties, the optimum being in the 13–16% w/w range. When it falls below 10%, the capsules become brittle and will easily fracture on handling; when it rises above 18% the capsules soften and distort. The change in moisture content of the capsule is reflected by changes in its physical dimensions. There is a change of approximately 0.5% in dimensions for each 1% change in moisture content over the range 13–16% w/w (Cole, 1972).

The heat absorption, tensile strength, and moisture content of capsules exposed to different humidities have been measured simultaneously by using a specially adapted balance and thermistors (List and Schenk, 1974 and 1975). The results were affected by the type of gelatin, the overall composition, and even the colorants.

The equilibrium moisture content (EMC) of hard gelatin capsules has been determined by several groups of workers. Fig. 6.6 shows some of the results obtained. The specific equilibrium values will vary depending upon the different types of gelatin and colorants used.

The graph indicates the best conditions under which to handle capsules and from which to deduce the behaviour, particularly the stability, of a filled capsule. A capsule will have its optimum performance on high-speed filling machines if it is handled in an atmosphere with a relative humidity between 30 and 50%. If the conditions are outside this range the capsules will be adversely

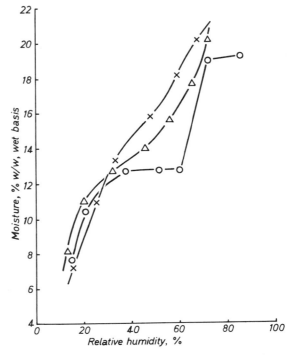

Fig. 6.6. The equilibrium moisture content of hard gelatin capsules as a function of humidity (× Bond *et al.*, 1970; △ Bell *et al.*, 1973; ○ Gore and Ashwin, 1967).

affected, but provided only the minimum number are exposed for fairly short times no practical difficulties will ensue, because the lag time to reach the EMC is several hours. Bond *et al.* (1970) used the EMC values of hard gelatin capsules and of the cephalexin which they were filling to predict both the best starting moisture contents for these raw materials and the probable stability of the finished product.

Solubility

Gelatin is readily soluble in biological fluids at body temperature, but if the temperature falls much below 37°, the rate of solution declines. Thus the temperature of solution only becomes significant for *in vitro* testing. The change in the rate of solution in the range 35° to 39° has been found to be about 30% (Jones and Cole, 1971). The solubility pattern of gelatin can be utilised to distinguish hard capsules made from cellulose polymers which are soluble in cold water.

Gas Permeability

The filled hard gelatin capsule is not gas-tight unless it has been banded, and gases can readily reach the contents by passage through the space between the cap and body in the region of overlap. They can also diffuse through the capsule wall, but the quantity of gas travelling by this route will only present a problem if the contents are very susceptible to oxidation. It is not difficult to measure the rates of diffusion of both oxygen and carbon dioxide into the contents of filled capsules (Czetsch-Lindenwald, 1967). The capsules are filled with materials which readily absorb the relevant gas, e.g. the catalyst bithional sulphoxide for oxygen, or calcium oxide for carbon dioxide. To determine the quantity of gas which passes through the wall relative to that passing through the gap between the cap and the body, normal filled capsules can be compared to separate filled capsule bodies the open ends of which are sealed. The rate of uptake will be dependent upon the concentration of gas external to the capsule. Hence, to relate the measurements to pharmaceutical practice, capsules in closed containers should also be examined, e.g. standard glass bottles with a metal screw cap. Some typical results are shown in Figs 6.7 and 6.8

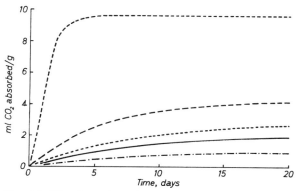

Fig. 6.8. The absorption of carbon dioxide from a normal atmosphere into capsules containing calcium oxide (lower four curves). The uppermost curve is the absorption of open capsules from an atmosphere of pure carbon dioxide.

– – – – – – – –   open capsules
· · · · · · · · · ·   closed capsules
——————   capsule bodies, sealed
– · – · – · – ·   capsules in stoppered bottles

as through the walls. Packing in a sealed container significantly reduces the problem. If the contents are still susceptible to oxygen or carbon dioxide under these conditions they must be protected by formulation procedures, such as suspending them in an oily medium.

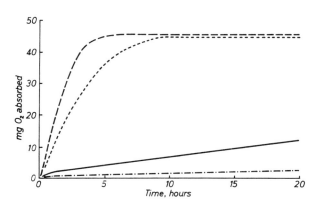

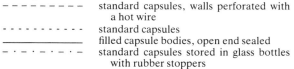

Fig. 6.7. The absorption of oxygen from a normal atmosphere into capsules containing bithional sulphoxide.

– – – – – – – –   standard capsules, walls perforated with a hot wire
· · · · · · · · · ·   standard capsules
——————   filled capsule bodies, open end sealed
– · – · – · – ·   standard capsules stored in glass bottles with rubber stoppers

The results also demonstrate that approximately three times as much passes through the overlap

References

Bell, J. H. *et al.*, *J. Pharm. Pharmac.*, 1973, *25*, Suppl., 96P–103P.
Bond, C. M. *et al.*, *Pharm. J.*, 1970, *205*, 210–214.
Cole, W. V. J., personal communication, 1972.
Czetsch-Lindenwald, H. v., *Pharm. Ind., Berl.*, 1967, *29*, 145–149.
Gore, D. N. and Ashwin, J., *J. mond. Pharm.*, 1967, *4*, 365–375.
Hostetler, V. and Bellard, J. Q., in *The Theory and Practice of Industrial Pharmacy*, 2nd Edn, L. Lachman, H. A. Lieberman, and J. L. Kanig (Ed.), Philadelphia, Lea & Febiger, 1976, pp. 389–404.
Ito, K. *et al.*, *Chem. pharm. Bull., Tokyo*, 1969, *17*, 1134–1137.
Jones, B. E., *Annls méd. Nancy*, 1974, *13*, 191–200.
Jones, B. E., *Chem. Engr, Lond.*, 1982, No. 380, 174–177.
Jones, B. E. and Cole, W. V. J., *J. Pharm. Pharmac.*, 1971, *23*, 438–443.
List, P. H. and Schenk, G. D., *Archiv der Pharmazie*, 1974, *307*, 719–726.
List, P. H. and Schenk, G. D., *Pharm. Ind., Berl.*, 1975, *37*, 91–96.
Martyn, G. W., *Drug Dev. Comm.*, 1974–75, *1*, 39–49.
Norris, W. G., *Mfg Chem.*, 1959, *30*, 233–236.
Norris, W. G., *Mfg Chem.*, 1961, *32*, 249–252 and 258.
Strickland, W. A. and Moss, M., *J. pharm. Sci.*, 1962, *51*, 1002–1005.
Yannas, I. V. and Tobolsky, A. V., *Nature*, 1967, *215*, 509–510.

Chapter 7

Powder Characteristics for Capsule Filling

G. C. Cole

It is an intrinsic property of any powdered solid that it will resist differential movement between its particles when it is subjected to external stresses. This is important in such practical contexts as flow from hoppers, relative motion in mixers, packing operations, powder drying, and consolidation processes to produce granules or compacts. The magnitude of the inherent resistance is influenced by many factors including:

(a) the surface properties of the material, particularly the effective force of attraction between particles as modified by any absorbed layers, especially moisture;
(b) the particle size distribution, the particulate shape and geometry, and the overall packing characteristics;
(c) any induced electrostatic charges.

Ideally, the powders used for capsule filling should have good flow properties, they should produce even packing density i.e. the particles of each component should have densities as close as possible to avoid segregation, and the powders should not be cohesive, although some filling machines require a certain degree of cohesiveness.

The initial object is to produce a free-flowing homogeneous powder with some cohesive properties, self-contradictory though this may sound. The powder technology problems involved in the formulation of powders for high-speed filling do not appear to have been studied. Such studies as have been made refer only to specific machines, drugs, and compounds.

A mathematical model (Reier *et al.*, 1968) was successfully developed to correlate the machine speed, capsule size, and powder properties such as particle size distribution, specific volume and flowability, with the fill-weight variation. The specific volume was obtained by placing approximately 50 ml of powder into a tared 100-ml graduated cylinder which was then tapped 15 times and the volume read off. The flowability was

obtained by allowing powder to flow through a glass funnel, using a mechanical feeder, onto a calibrated flat surface where it formed a cone. When the apex of the cone reached the funnel orifice, the powder flow was stopped and the diameter of the base of the cone determined. The area of the base was measured, rather than the angle of repose itself. This model is useful in its ability to provide information on probable fill-weight variation from simple evaluations of small samples of the formulation to be encapsulated.

POWDER FLOW

Angle of Repose

A widely used and simple method of assessing flow behaviour has been the determination of the angle of repose, γ. Experimental techniques for this measurement are based on the premise that there is a maximum possible angle between the free standing surface of a powder and the horizontal plane.

This angle is related to the coefficient of internal friction, μ_i:

$$\mu_i = \tan \gamma = \frac{2h}{D}$$

where h is the slant height of a cone of diameter D.

The angle is rarely less than 25°, and angles up to 40° indicate a reasonable flow potential; when the angle is above 50°, the powder will be induced to flow only with difficulty.

Experimental methods of determining γ may be divided into two groups, static and dynamic.

STATIC METHODS
The Fixed Funnel and Free Standing Cone. In this method (Fig. 7.1a), the powder cone is built up by lowering the horizontal plate away from the end of a funnel containing the powder. Alternatively the plate and funnel can be initially set apart

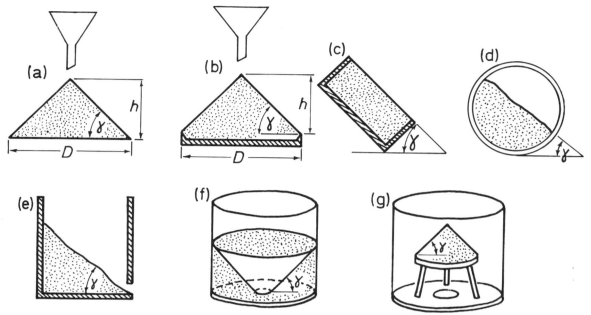

Fig. 7.1 Methods of measuring the angle of repose. (a), fixed funnel and free standing cone; (b), fixed bed cone; (c), tilting box; (d), rotating cylinder; (e), (f), and (g), apparatus to measure the drained angle of repose (ledge, crater, and circular heap, respectively).

at some suitable distance and powder added through the funnel to produce the heap. The latter technique is more prone to cause collapse of the cone of powder.

The Fixed Bed Cone. This method (Fig. 7.1b) is similar to the previous method except that the diameter of the base of the cone is fixed because the heap is poured onto a shallow cylindrical dish that has a sharp vertical rim.

DYNAMIC METHODS

It has been suggested that techniques involving measurements made under dynamic conditions are more realistic.

The Tilting Box. A rectangular box lined with sandpaper (Fig. 7.1c) is carefully filled with powder and tipped until the contents begin to slide. The geometry of the box may affect the values obtained.

The Rotating Cylinder. A hollow cylinder (Fig. 7.1d), with one end sealed by a transparent plate, is half-filled with the powder and rotated about its horizontal axis. The curved wall is covered with sandpaper to prevent preferential slip at this surface. Three values of γ can be distinguished, depending on the drum speed: 'static γ', when the drum is tilted until the powder just slips, as in the tilting box; 'surface kinetic γ', when the drum is slowly rotated with powder just continuously slipping; 'internal kinetic γ', which is the angle between the horizontal and the dividing plane between those particles which are slipping and those which are rotating when the drum is turning more rapidly.

Drained Angles of Repose. The heap is prepared by allowing the material to drain from the central or side hole of a large cylindrical container (Figs 7.1e, f). An additional value of γ can be obtained by immersing a stand fitted with a horizontal plate in the bed before draining off the material (Fig. 7.1g).

The various methods for this measurement have been critically assessed by several workers (Train, 1958; Brown, 1961; Brown and Richards, 1970) and it emerges that the value found for the angle of repose is dependent on the method of measurement: the angle decreases as the size of the bed and the particle size of the material increase. Static methods tend to give lower values than dynamic methods, although this may be due to some degree of heap collapse. Moisture plays a major role and can markedly affect the angle obtained. Thus, when quoting results, precise experimental conditions must be stated.

The Flowometer

Gold *et al.* (1966a and b) demonstrated that the angle of repose is an unreliable indicator of flow properties, and suggested the use of a flowometer that consisted of a hopper from which powder flowed on to a pan supported by a strain-gauged arm. The weight of powder could be measured so rapidly that fluctuations in the flow rate could be followed, as well as the flow rate itself. Different hoppers were available, and could be fitted with vibrators. The flowometer was used to show the effect of some glidants such as fumed silicon dioxide, corn starch, and magnesium stearate.

A recording flowometer using an electrobalance to replace the strain gauges of the original design has been applied to pharmaceutical processing (Jordan and Rhodes, 1979).

Flow from Hoppers

The flow of material from a hopper is usually accompanied by a complex pattern of movement towards the aperture as depicted in the vertical section of a cylindrical hopper shown in Figure 7.2. In the surface region, A, particles roll rapidly over region B which itself is sliding over the stationary region E. Groups of particles are fed from the above layers into region C where they move rapidly downwards and inwards to be assimilated by region D from which they rapidly discharge. This emergent stream is noticeably narrower than the aperture, due to the empty annulus, and is sinusoidal in form, suggesting that particles are fed into the aperture successively from different regions of D. This is known as 'core flow'.

The important practical implications of this are that replenishing partly emptied hoppers may result in long residence times (region E) for particular fractions of the material. The possibility of demixing in the hopper may also be increased by discharge patterns of this general form. Such flow is also subject to the stoppages known as 'bridging' and 'rat-holing'.

Alternatively, and preferably, a hopper can be designed so that 'mass flow' takes place, in which every particle is in motion and no dead spaces occur. No arches can form over the hopper outlet and the undesirable effects of segregation are minimised. Design of such hoppers can be made from a study of the failure properties, and usually depend upon making the outlet large enough and the walls, leading to it, steep enough (Williams and Birks, 1967; Jenike, 1961, 1964). In those few

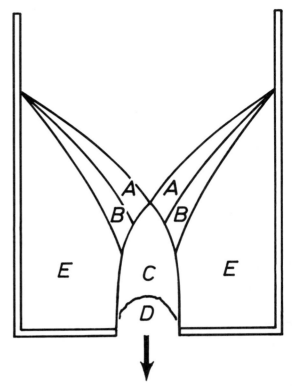

Fig. 7.2 Pattern of flow from a flat-bottomed cylindrical hopper.

cases where uniform flow is still not achieved the techniques of introducing small quantities of air into the lower hopper wall and/or the addition of glidants may have to be used. Increasing the particle size, say by granulation, will also be helpful in these circumstances.

Flow Through Apertures

For materials with low cohesion, direct measurement of the rate of flow through an aperture is possible. In practice, this is frequently carried out in systems of simple geometry, one of the most widely reported (Brown and Richards, 1959, 1960) being discharge from a cylindrical vessel through a circular aperture in its flat horizontal base, as shown in Fig. 7.3. There is an empty annulus of width $B/2$ around the aperture through which no material will pass. It is independent of the size and shape of the aperture. Twice the width of the empty annulus is the blocking aperture, B, which is the limiting size of the aperture through which material will pass. It is invariably greater than the mean particle size but dependent on it. Experiments of this type have shown that fine particles

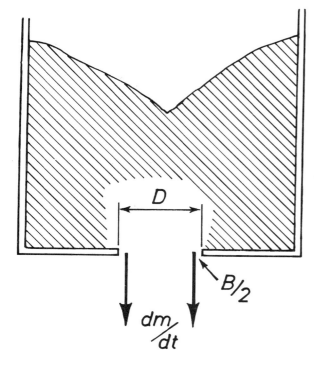

Fig. 7.3 Apparatus for the direct measurement of the rate of flow through a circular aperture.

usually discharge more more rapidly than larger ones, but the proportion of fine particles is critical. Spherical particles discharge more rapidly than irregularly shaped particles.

Moisture content is an important variable but flow rates appear to be independent of the porosity in the range 35–55% and virtually independent of the span of the cohesive arch, L, (providing $L > 3D$). Slit-like and elliptical apertures of the same cross-sectional area cause particles to discharge at about the same rate, but both give a lower rate than a circular aperture of equal cross-sectional area.

BULK DENSITY

It is necessary at an early stage in the development of a dry-filled capsule formulation to determine the density of the mixture of powders and the individual components which make up the formulation. This test should be designed with some relationship to the type of machine to be used to fill the capsules. The majority of high-speed machines rely on an even density of powder in the dosing hopper. Some machines use a mixture

of vibratory and mixing devices prior to filling and some use an initial tapping stage to ensure a consistent filling. It is therefore important that the volume the powder occupies is determined by a method which provides data that relate to the filling method.

A method using γ-ray attenuation was developed by Woodhead et al. (1979) to establish the influence of powder bed porosity variations on the capsule fill-weight. Using a rig built by Woodhead (1980) they later concluded that the degree of powder bed porosity did not appear to be reflected in the reproducibility of the capsule fill-weights.

Höfliger and Karg offer an instrument (Fig. 7.4) for determining the volume occupied by a formulation under a known pressure and relating the data to a required capsule size. A small jig, similar to a compression station, is used to determine the plug size for filling on a compression filler.

Most small hand-fillers use some vibratory action to increase the speed of filling and give an even density of powder in each capsule, though care must be used to ensure no separation of the components takes place. For such hand-machines a tapped density measurement using the same experimental procedure will ensure consistent results.

Measurement using a graduated cylinder and tapping it three times provides consistent results, although the final density is not reached until the cylinder has been tapped 500 times. The Radon unit shown in Fig. 7.5 is ideal for this measurement as it can be set automatically and it has a consistent tapping action.

COHESION

Various methods of measuring cohesion and other parameters such as shear strength and tensile strength are available. In all cases, care in preparing the samples and a knowledge of the history of the powder is important. Measurements made on the powder may not always be consistent or reliable though they may be a useful guide. Ultimately, it must be proved that the properties of the powder are such that it can be filled on the particular filling machine which is to be used.

One method, illustrated in Figure 7.6, which has been devised to measure cohesion specifically for capsule filling, uses a propeller stirrer as a modified viscometer. Cohesion is recorded as resistance to rotation of the stirrer, using a digital voltmeter.

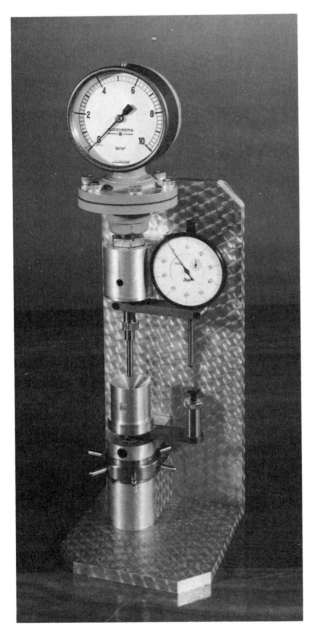

Fig. 7.4 The Höfliger and Karg powder-plug estimator.

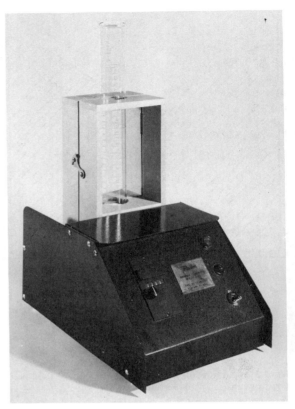

Fig. 7.5 The Radon unit for measuring bulk density.

The procedure is as follows:

A sample of powder is poured into a plastic bag and shaken vigorously for 10 seconds to remove the effects of any compaction which may have occurred on storage. The powder is poured from the bag through a funnel into a tared beaker (both funnel and beaker are kept specifically for these experiments). A fixed weight between 60 and 90 g of sample is used and, as the test is comparative, the same quantity must be used for each test. The filled beaker is then transferred, without disturbing the powder bed, to an adjustable platform, fitted with a plastic ring to locate the beaker. The viscometer is switched on and allowed to settle to a steady reading, which will usually be in the range 3.8 to 5.0 volts. The platform is raised until it is aligned with a graduation on the stand supporting the viscometer. This height is the same for each test. The powder is now stirred and readings of powder cohesion, expressed as resistance, can be made after a fixed time interval. This interval is different for each product but is normally between one and three minutes. The temperature and relative humidity must be recorded during each test.

For a more fundamental derivation of cohesion, reference may be made to the methods of measuring tensile strength using the inclined split-plate state of consolidation, which in turn is governed by the stresses acting on the powder. The development of this concept requires the use of the Jenike shear cell (Jenike, 1961, 1964), or the use of an annular shear cell (Kocova and Pilpel, 1972). The annular cell is claimed to be more convenient and rapid in use, particularly where only small quantities of powder are available. From the data derived from the shear cell experiments, the yield locus of the material can be plotted and, by extrapolation, the cohesion obtained from the intercept on the y axis.

This work has been extended to derive the flow factor of the powder by drawing a Mohr circle diagram (Gray, 1968). The smaller the value of the flow factor, the more cohesive the powder. Details of the more complex treatments of powder technology can be found in Roscoe *et al.* (1958), Williams and Birks (1965), Brown and Richards (1970), and York (1980). Cohesion has been measured as a function of the angle of internal friction, which represents the friction between individual particles (Jenike, 1961, 1964; Williams and Birks, 1967). A method for measuring the friction between the particles of the powder and the walls of the container has been devised (Pilpel, 1965), and this was defined as the angle of friction. Jenike (1961) used the general equation for the analysis of soils to characterise flow at the walls of the hopper.

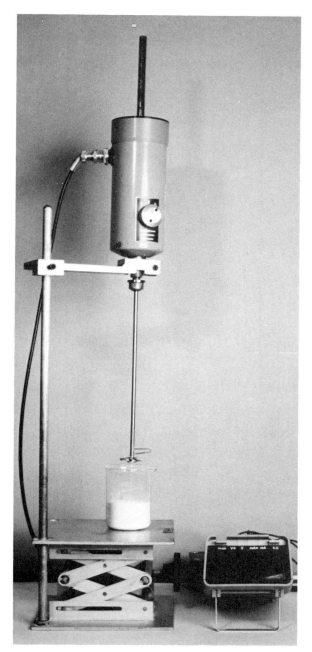

Fig. 7.6 The cohesion viscometer. The power drawn by the stirrer motor gives an indication of the cohesiveness of the powder in the beaker.

(Thouzeau and Taylor, 1961), and the horizontal split-plate (Ashton *et al.*, 1964).

For the most difficult cases where powders are not free-flowing, the flowability depends on the

References

Ashton, M. D. *et al.*, *J. scient. Instrum.*, 1964, *41*, 763–765.
Brown, R. L., Flow Properties, in *Powders in Industry, S.C.I. Monograph No. 14*, London, Society of Chemical Industry, 1961, pp. 150–166.
Brown, R. L. and Richards, J. C., *Trans. Instn chem. Engrs*, 1959, *37*, 108–119.
Brown, R. L. and Richards, J. C., *Trans. Instn chem. Engrs*, 1960, *38*, 243–256.
Brown, R. L. and Richards, J. C., *Principles of Powder Mechanics*, London, Pergamon Press, 1970.
Gold, G. *et al.*, *J. pharm. Sci.*, 1966a, *55*, 1133–1136.
Gold, G. *et al.*, *J. pharm. Sci.*, 1966b, *55*, 1291–1295.
Gray, W. A., *The Packing of Solid Particles*, London, Chapman and Hall, 1968.
Jenike, A. W., *Bull. 108*, Utah Engng Exp. Stn, 1961.
Jenike, A. W., *Bull. 123*, Utah Engng Exp. Stn, 1964.
Jordan, R. P. and Rhodes, C. T., *Drug Dev. ind. Pharm.*, 1979, *5*, 151–167.
Kocova, S. and Pilpel, N., *Powder Technol.*, 1972, *5*, 329–343.
Pilpel, N., *Chem. Process Engng*, 1965, *46*, 167–171, 179.
Reier, G. *et al.*, *J. pharm. Sci.*, 1968, *57*, 660–666.
Roscoe, K. H. *et al.*, *Géotechnique*, 1958, *8*, 22–53.
Thouzeau, G. and Taylor, T. W., *Safety in Mines Research Establishment Research Report No. 197*, February, 1961.

Train, D., *J. Pharm. Pharmac.*, 1958, *10*, *Suppl.*, 127T–135T, 143T–144T.

Williams, J. C. and Birks, A. H., *Rheol. Acta*, 1965, *4*, 170–180.

Williams, J. C. and Birks, A. H., *Powder Technol.*, 1967, *1*, 199–206.

Woodhead, P. J., Ph.D. Thesis, University of Nottingham, 1980.

Woodhead, P. J. *et al.*, *J. Pharm. Pharmac.*, 1979, *31*, *Suppl.*, 72P.

York, P., *Int. J. Pharmaceut.*, 1980, *6*, 89–117.

Chapter 8

The History of Capsule-filling Machinery

G. C. Cole

The early development of the hard gelatin capsule has been surveyed in Chapter 1. The development of the methods of filling powders into such capsules took place mainly in the U.S.A., where some 80 patents were granted between 1850 and 1900. In contrast, in Britain, only 15 patents were taken out in the same period, and only one dealt with the actual filling of capsules.

The stimulus in the U.S.A. originated from H. Planten & Son, of New York, who commenced operations in 1836 (Planten, 1914). Planten introduced the European process, and manufactured both the original Mothes capsules, and two-piece capsules filled with powder. When powder-filled capsules originated is not clear (Alpers, 1896), although Hubel (U.S. Patent 187 279, 1877) was active in their development; his entire output of hard shell capsules was sold by Parke, Davis of Detroit. Small hand-fillers for hard capsules became quite common. Some of the most widely used machines were manufactured by Whitfield (U.S. Patent 210 589, 1878), Davenport (U.S. Patent 221 534, 1879), Reymond (U.S. Patent 244 308, 1881), Schmidt (U.S. Patent 255 680, 1882), and Ihrig (U.S. Patent 596 813, 1898). Alpers (1896) improved and redesigned the Davenport and Reymond fillers. The machine invented by Walsh in 1886 was subsequently marketed by Parke, Davis.

HAND-OPERATED CAPSULE-FILLING MACHINERY

The development of hand-operated capsule-filling equipment at the end of the nineteenth and beginning of the twentieth centuries can be illustrated by comparing the Davenport, Reymond, Walsh, and Ihrig machines.

Davenport Capsule Filler

The Davenport apparatus filled only one capsule at a time, and consisted of a funnel fitted with an interchangeable tube and plunger. The funnel was flattened at one side to assist in loading the material. The tube, joined to the funnel, was fitted with a plunger and a rubber collar, and corresponded to the size of capsule to be filled. The end of this tube was cut at an angle to aid in fitting the capsule. The tube enabled powder to be pushed out of the funnel by the plunger into the capsule and compressed as necessary. In practice, a capsule body was fitted on the tube, the funnel was laid on its flat side, and a weighed amount of powder sufficient for one dose was transferred on to the flat section. The funnel was raised into a vertical position, causing the powder to fall into the tube. The plunger was used to push all of this powder into the capsule body which was then removed and capped.

Reymond Capsule Filler

The Reymond filler (Fig. 8.1) consisted of two blocks of hard wood. The lower block contained 12 sockets which were deep enough to accommodate the capsules to half their lengths. The bottom of each socket was shaped to correspond to the closed end of the capsule and had a small hole bored through the block. The upper block had 12 funnel-shaped receptacles which were large enough to hold all the powder needed to fill the capsules. The holes at the bottom of these receptacles were slightly larger than the corresponding holes in the lower block so that the protruding capsules slipped into them as the upper block was lowered. The blocks were aligned correctly and held together by means of pegs. The powder was tamped into each capsule with a plunger.

Walsh Capsule Filler

The Walsh capsule filler (Fig. 8.2) was designed to fill twelve capsules consecutively as a batch, using the Davenport operating principle. It had a metal frame and base plate. A block of wood, drilled to take the size of capsule required, could be inserted in the frame so that the capsules could

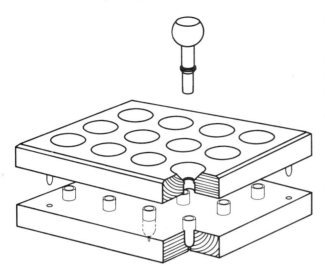

Fig. 8.1. The Reymond capsule filler.

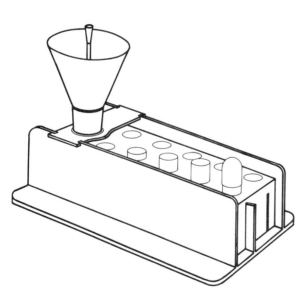

Fig. 8.2. The Walsh capsule filler.

be filled from a hopper supported overhead. The hopper was moved from one side to the other by removing and reversing the cross-member supporting it as consecutive capsules were filled. The wooden block was pushed through the apparatus and powder forced out of the hopper by the plunger when the hopper was vertically above each

capsule. The block slid along two triangular metal strips fastened to the base plate. These strips enabled the block to pass smoothly under the hopper and they forced the filled body of the capsule out of the block. When the block had completely entered the apparatus the bodies of the first two capsules filled had been forced two-thirds of the way out of their holes. At this point the caps were placed in position and the filled capsules removed. A second block, filled with empty capsule bodies, was then fed into the apparatus, gradually forcing the first block out and ejecting more filled capsules. The base section of the hopper was interchangeable to accommodate the size of the capsule to be filled. It was also possible to compress the powder by using the plunger fitted to the hopper.

Ihrig Capsule Filler

The Ihrig filler (Fig. 8.3) consisted of a stationary

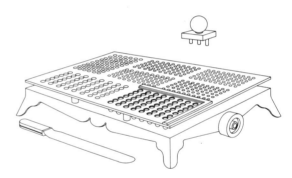

Fig. 8.3. The Ihrig capsule filler.

base with a square polished table containing holes for holding either 48 or 56 capsules, depending on their size. The table could be raised and lowered by means of a thumbscrew. The capsules were separated into their component parts, and the bodies placed in the table holes. The table was raised by means of the thumbscrew so that the tops of the capsule bodies were just below its surface. A small metal plate was supplied which was placed over any of the holes not in use. Powder was then distributed over the table and pressed down into the capsules using a metallic punch. The table was then lowered, which caused the bodies to be partially ejected so that the caps could be fitted and the assembled capsules removed and polished.

AUTOMATED CAPSULE-FILLING MACHINERY

It is probable that most pharmacists in those early days constructed their own hand-fillers for medicines dispensed extemporaneously. Further development appears to have been slow until the early twentieth century, when a few automatic machines appeared.

Colton Automatic Capsule Filler

The first and most significant automated machine was that designed and patented by Arthur Colton (U.S. Patent 1077392, 1913), which is shown in Fig. 8.4.

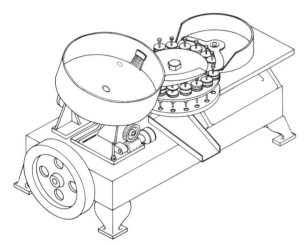

Fig. 8.4. The Colton automatic rotary capsule filler.

This machine was far in advance of anything made earlier. It consisted of a long table which carried the main drive shaft. Above this table was positioned the empty-capsule hopper, the bulk powder hopper, and the rotary filling head. The head had twenty spindles which picked up the empty capsule bodies and ejected them when full of powder. Below these rotating spindles was a circular plate which supported and retained the capsule cap.

A number of ideas were incorporated in this machine which demonstrated Colton's inventiveness. Compressed air and vacuum were used to transport empty capsules from one section to another, and a wheel was designed to allow the body of the capsule to pass but not the cap, thus ensuring correct orientation of the capsule before separation and filling.

The correctly orientated capsules, having left the empty-capsule hopper, were transferred body uppermost by means of an applied vacuum through a tube to a holding plate, situated below the rotating filling head. This vacuum was applied through the capsule holding plate from a small box situated on top of the plate. The body of the capsule protruded above this plate and a small door in the side of the box allowed the capsule to pass outside when the plate rotated. The spindles mounted on the filling head were raised and lowered by a shaped cam on the top of the head. After the capsule left the vacuum box, a spindle descended and the body of the capsule was pushed into an opening in the base of the spindle. This was then raised by a cam, and the body was separated from the cap. The cap was retained in the plate due to its larger diameter and the design of the hole in the plate. The spindle containing the body rotated around the head approximately ninety degrees before it was lowered into a shallow part of the hopper containing the powder. The level of the powder in this section of the hopper was adjusted by cross pieces which removed excess powder. It was also compressed by means of a tamping bar to ensure even filling.

Further action of the cam raised the spindle and body from the powder hopper and reunited the body with its cap. A piston activated by a small spring inside the spindle pushed the body into the cap and ejected the filled capsule down a chute. This machine was claimed to have an output of 20000 capsules per day (Cook and LaWall, 1926).

The Development of Automated Machinery

Colton was the first to produce an automatic feed and separating mechanism for hard shell capsules based on the difference in diameter of the cap and the body. Small hand machines, such as that manufactured by Winchester (British Patent 22522, 1906) would separate 40 capsules into bodies and caps, but these had to be fed and orientated correctly into the top plate by hand.

Many of the machines would handle capsules after they had been separated. One of these, designed by Mahler and Fischer (British Patent 17773, 1908), resembled a cachet-filling machine, although it was described as a capsule-closing machine. An automatic machine, operated by turning a handle manually, was developed by Genat (British Patent 205064, 1924). It required separated caps and bodies to be fed to it, and the filling speed depended on the operator. Powder was compressed before being pushed into the capsule body. A similar machine was produced in Nurnburg (Schmidt, British Patent 266 323, 1928) but, although a mechanical drive was used to rotate the various parts, the caps and bodies still had to be separated before they were fed to the apparatus. Compressed air was used to retain the caps and bodies in the cavities on the machine. Later, modifications to this machine were made by Schmidt to improve the closing of the capsules (British Patents 274 414, 296 046, 1928). It would appear from these later modifications that the capsules would be more accurately described as cachets.

By this time Colton had also developed a semi-automatic capsule filler which was the forerunner of the Colton 8 machine; this is still very widely used. This had a claimed output of between 70 000 and 90 000 capsules per day (Cook and LaWall, 1926).

There appears to be little on record regarding the development of machines in England and Europe prior to 1940. Following the Second World War the most significant machines have come from Höfliger and Karg in Germany, Pedini, Zanasi and mG2 in Italy, and a number of smaller manufacturers such as Wierzbinski in France, Leidsche Apparatenfabriek N.V. (LAF) in The Netherlands, and Bonapace/Zuma in Italy.

The first capsule-filling machine to be manufactured by Zanasi was the LZ-55 (Fig. 8.5). It was used with separate caps and bodies, which were readily available in the Italian market during this period, and an output of 3600 capsules per hour was claimed. It was quickly superseded by the LZ-57 (Fig. 8.6) which used complete capsules, separating each one for the filling operation. Both these machines operated with intermittent motion and both used a compression method for dosing the powder.

Empty capsules were placed in a bulk hopper and were then rectified, opened, filled, closed, and ejected. The machine chamfered the lip of the body to make fitting of the cap easier. Faulty capsules were rejected without stopping the machine. All sizes of capsules could be filled providing that suitable change parts were fitted. The output was 3600 capsules per hour.

Since 1970 a number of other companies, such as Macofar and Farmatic in Italy and Osaka in Japan, have entered the market with machines capable of filling at speeds up to 160 000 capsules per hour. Descriptions of some of these machines

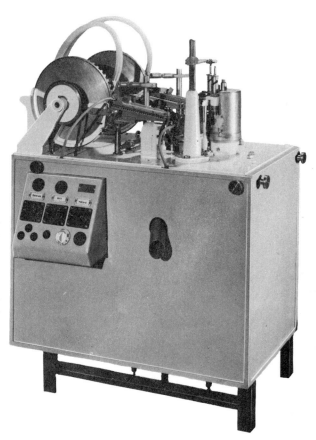

Fig. 8.5. The Zanasi LZ-55 capsule filler.

appear in Chapter 10. It was in this period that different techniques in filling capsules were developed for large-scale automatic machines.

The general principles of filling a small number of capsules, either singly or on a small hand machine, have not altered, though the level of sophistication of the operation has improved. For instance, the Davenport filler, 1879, filled single capsules, and a plunger was provided for compressing the powder into the body of the capsule as necessary. The capsules also had to be separated into cap and body by hand. Nowadays the same idea is used on the Tevopharm machine, but the capsules are separated and reunited automatically, and a plate with a number of plungers is provided, though the powder still has to be weighed and divided equally into the number of capsules. Col-

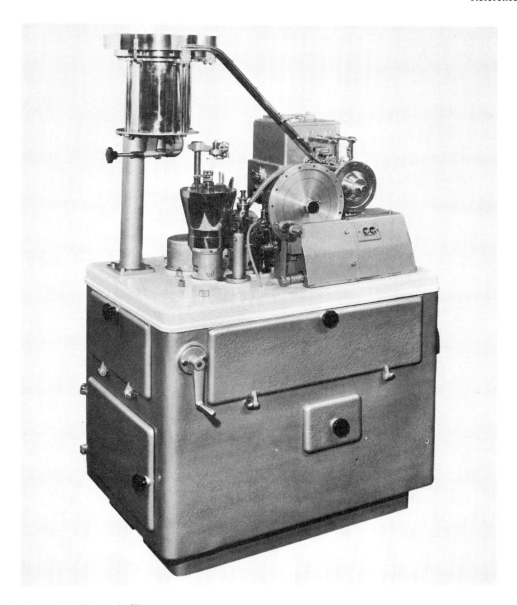

Fig. 8.6. The Zanasi LZ-57 capsule filler.

ton developed this method to its limits in the design of the Colton 8 machine described in Chapter 10. The limitations of this machine have only become apparent in recent years with the need for closer weight tolerances, high outputs, labour economy, and a dust-free finished product.

References

Alpers, W. C., *Am. J. Pharm.*, 1896, *68*, 481–494.

Cook, E. F. and LaWall, C. H., *Remington's Practice of Pharmacy,* 7th Edn, Philadelphia, J. B. Lippincott Co., 1926, pp. 1679–81.

Planten, H. R., *The Art of Capsulating,* New York, H. Planten & Son, 1914.

Chapter 9

The Mechanical Operations of Filling Hard Capsules

G. C. Cole

Hard capsules are normally filled with a powder containing the active ingredient(s). However, other preparations or combinations of preparations may also be filled into capsules, using special dosing devices. Various possibilities are illustrated in Fig. 9.1. The range can be extended by changing the form of enclosed tablets which may be enteric-coated, sugar-coated, or compression-coated. Sustained-release enteric-coated pellets may also be filled.

The filling machine must carry out four operations. It must rectify the capsules, separate the body from the cap, fill the body, and replace the cap. Rectification means that all the capsules are positioned cap uppermost in the machine ready for separation. Fig. 9.2 illustrates the filling process.

The following problems may arise during the basic process. Firstly, a damaged capsule may block the feed system. Rectification may not take place, again resulting in a blocked feed system. Separation may not occur, so that the powder or other dosage form is available but cannot be put into the capsule body. Transfer or selection of the dosage form may fail to take place. The powder may be wrongly delivered, or the alternative dosage form may be damaged during its entry into the capsule body. The cap or the body, or both, may be damaged when reunited. The body may be damaged on ejection from the machine. Finally, empty capsules may be ejected from the machine along with the filled ones. All fully automatic equipment is fitted with devices that will eliminate some or all of these problems as the capsules pass through the machine. If new equipment is being evaluated, an examination of the

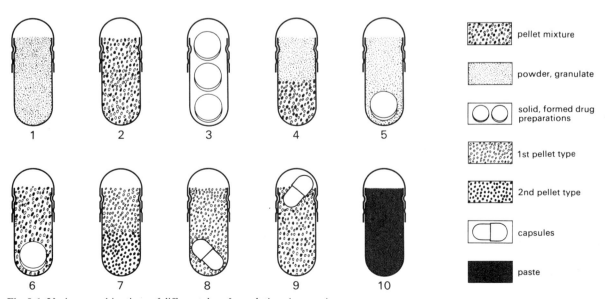

	pellet mixture
	powder, granulate
	solid, formed drug preparations
	1st pellet type
	2nd pellet type
	capsules
	paste

Fig. 9.1. Various combinations of different drug formulations in capsules.

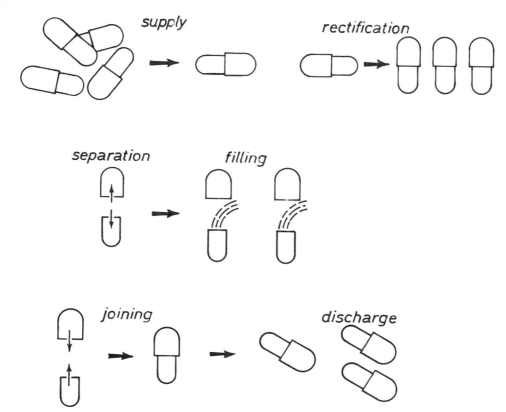

Fig. 9.2. The capsule filling process.

above problems must be included in the test programme.

Filling Hard Capsules with Powders

Capsule filling suffers from the disadvantage, compared with tablet making, that the method of putting powder into the capsule varies greatly from one manufacturer of filling equipment to another.

THE PLATE METHOD

The plate or single capsule method is the traditional method used for filling hard shell capsules. It developed from the hand filling of single capsules in the middle of the 19th century to its present form and it is still widely used in pharmacies and development laboratories.

Figure 9.3 illustrates a block containing three capsule bodies, a quantity of material filling them, and an excess covering the top of the block. If all the material is to be filled into the bodies then the tamping device (shown above the block) will have to be used. According to the density of the powder several tamping actions may be required. The powder will have been pre-weighed to give a required weight of fill and spread evenly over the block. However, when the powder has been formulated for a certain size of capsule and is of reasonably uniform density, it is possible to use the plate method without pre-weighing. In this case, excess material is spread over the capsule bodies until they are full and the excess removed before replacing the caps. Some form of vibration on the block is useful, despite the possibility of inducing segregation. Good formulation will minimise this. Various machines have been developed that use this principle, such as the Tevopharm and the Bonapace.

A development of the plate method is the use of a hopper fitted with an agitator and an auger. An example is shown in Fig. 9.4. The agitator is used to feed material into the auger which in turn feeds it into the capsule body.

Höfliger and Karg produced a machine using this type of feed system which filled at the rate

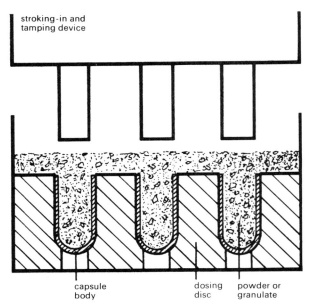

Fig. 9.3. Filling capsules by the plate or single capsule method.

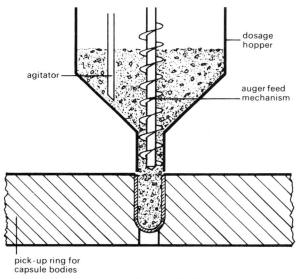

Fig. 9.4. Filling capsules by the auger feed system.

of 3000 capsules per hour. It operated only while the hopper was positioned above the capsule body, and the timing control on the auger drive regulated the fill-weight. The hopper was fixed and the capsule bodies were moved by the plate. In the Colton 8 machine, a similar hopper was moved over a rotating ring containing the capsule bodies, which enabled a skilled operator to fill up to 20 000 capsules per hour.

Höfliger and Karg have also developed a method, illustrated in Fig. 9.5, based on the use of free flow of material into the body, combined with a tamping punch. Powder initially flows into the holes in a dosage disk, which is machined to thickness to provide a certain fill-weight in the capsule. A tamping punch compresses the powder against the base plate and then rises. Filling and retamping takes place in five successive stages. After the fifth stage the dosage hole moves off the base plate and the plug of powder is ejected into the capsule body. Difficulties can occur when using this method of filling if the batch-to-batch variation in density of the powder is very wide. The dose is controlled primarily by the thickness of the transfer disk, the adjustment of the tamping punches, and the depth of powder in the dosage hopper.

INTERMITTENT COMPRESSION FILLING
The compression method shown in Fig. 9.6 is used by Zanasi and latterly has been introduced by mG2; the illustration is the dosator of a Zanasi LZ-64 intermittent machine. Powder is fed into the dosage hopper and its level adjusted to about twice the depth of the compressed plug. The dosage tube enters the powder bed and the powder inside it is pressed by the dosage punch just sufficiently to form a coherent plug that can be lifted by the dosator, carried to the capsule body, and ejected into it by the piston. If the powder has been correctly formulated the use of the compression head is not necessary. The compression force used should be just sufficient to allow clean transfer to the capsule body and to ensure that the plug does not break up on ejection from the dosage tube. The plug should also fit into the capsule body without protruding too far above the top.

Jolliffe (1980) established that for differing particle sizes of lactose there was an optimum compression setting for a particular particle size. His concept of optimum compression settings was verified using a capsule simulator and substantiated in a production machine when cohesive powders did not respond to a compressive force.

The dosator assembly is shown in more detail in Fig. 9.7. The calibration scale is used to set up each dosator assembly to an identical point at the commencement of a filling operation. On larger

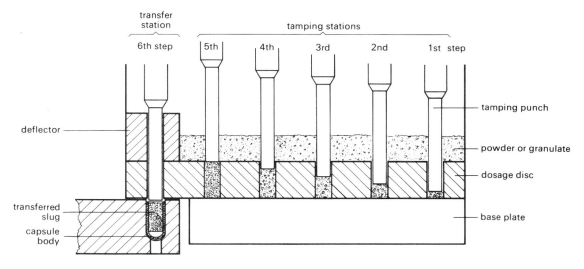

Fig. 9.5. Filling capsules by the tamping method.

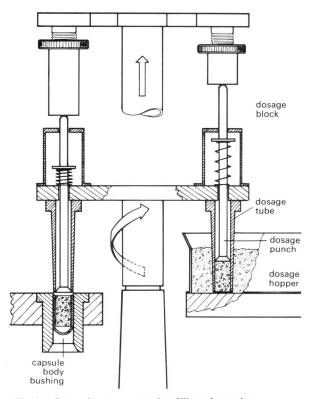

Fig. 9.6. Intermittent compression filling of capsules.

machines there are multiple dosators: on the AZ-60, for instance, there are 24. The fill-weight is adjusted by regulating the height of the dosing piston inside the dosing tube. The depth of powder in the dosage hopper will also affect the fill-weight. Extra compression may be achieved by using the compression head, which is adjusted to come into contact with the top of the piston when the dosator assembly is at the bottom of its stroke and forming the plug.

To minimise fill-weight variation a lubricant such as magnesium stearate and a flow aid such as Aerosil are usually used, to ensure that the plug does not bind on ejection from the dosing tube or stick to the end of the piston. A uniform density is necessary in the dosage hopper and a flow aid helps in this respect. Lubricants are often hydrophobic, which is a reason for using minimal compression. The harder the compact, the more difficult it is to wet, and the more likely that the bioavailability of the product will be reduced.

CONTINUOUS COMPRESSION FILLING

The use of compression filling on a continuous machine was first developed by the mG2 Company. Essentially there is little difference between the application of the principle on a continuous machine and on an intermittent machine. The method is illustrated in Fig. 9.8. The dosage trough here is annular, rotates, and is fed from a bulk hopper. The dosators dip into it whilst it is in motion.

It is possible to obtain much higher filling speeds using a much simpler mechanical design, providing

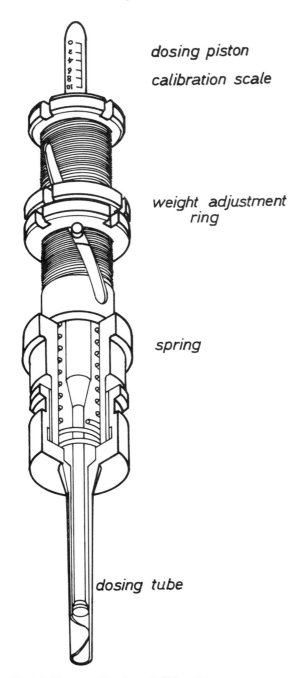

dosing piston

calibration scale

weight adjustment ring

spring

dosing tube

Fig. 9.7. The assembly of a typical Zanasi dosator.

that the turret carrying the dosators can be arranged so that there is no relative movement between it and the powder during the short time that the dosator is being dipped. For example the

Zanasi BZ-150 (claimed output 150 000 capsules per hour) has only one weight control and one pressure control, whereas the AZ-60 (claimed output 60 000 capsules per hour) has 24 dosators which all need individual adjustment. A comparison of the mechanical drive of the two machines shows similar advantages for the continuous-motion machine.

As the speed of filling increases, the dwell time (i.e. the time taken for the dosage tube to dip into the powder and compress the plug of material) becomes shorter. This means that the powder must be of uniform density, easily compressible, and not too elastic. The formulation must be free-flowing, but yet possess some cohesiveness.

It can be seen that the speed of the machine, the level of fill, and the density of the substance to be filled all have an influence on the dosage accuracy. One factor which considerably affects the fill-weight variation is the behaviour of the powder left in the hopper after a plug of material has been removed. Where the powder is free-flowing and non-cohesive the cavity will collapse, and a simple stirring device will produce a homogeneous mixture before the next plug is removed. When the material is very cohesive the powder must be thoroughly mixed before the next entry of the dosator.

VACUUM FILLING
Perry Industries Inc. developed a method based on their own idea of using vacuum to dose vials with volumetric quantities of powders. The machine is continuous in operation and similar in action to the mG2 models. The principle, illustrated in Fig. 9.9, is to draw the powder into the dosator by suction, applied through a filter pad. Some compression takes place but not as much as in the Zanasi piston dosator. The material is held in place by the vacuum until the dosage tube is in position over the capsule body, when the powder is ejected by releasing the vacuum and applying positive pressure. This method has interesting possibilities because it does not rely on the movement of mechanical parts during the filling operation. Lubricants are not needed in the formulation. It is also possible to fill single substances, especially where the drug has a high dose level, although it is claimed that doses as low as 10 mg can be dispensed. This machine incorporates a 'no capsule, no dose' feature. This is activated when capsules have not been separated or when an empty-capsule feed tube becomes

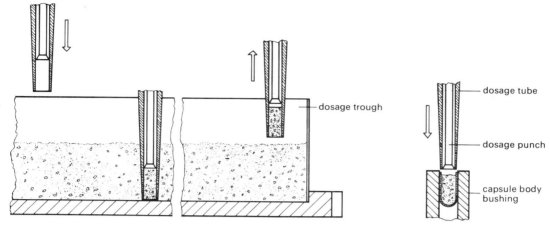

Fig. 9.8. Continuous compression filling of capsules.

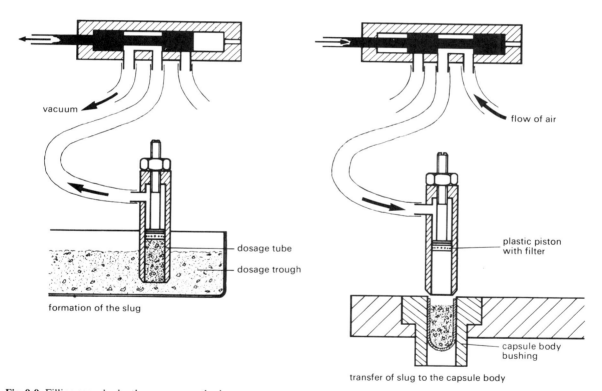

Fig. 9.9. Filling capsules by the vacuum method.

blocked and prevents a capsule entering the holding bush. The powder which has been taken into the dosage tube is blown out, by a blast of compressed air, activated by an electronic sensor and relay, back into the dosage trough, preventing loss of material and ensuring a clean machine.

The dosage tubes consist of two parts, a cylinder and an adjustable piston, made of polyethylene fitted with a nylon filter. Adjusting the piston alters the volume of powder that is picked up. The assembly is connected to the vacuum and air pressure system by a snap-closure connector. Each of the individual dosage tubes has to be independently calibrated as central adjustment is not possible. The instrumentation allows a sample to be taken from any individual dosage tube without stopping the machine.

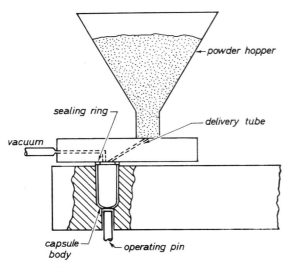

Fig. 9.10. Filling capsules by the Drugpack system.

The Zanasi, mG2, and Perry machines all depend on presenting a powder with a uniform density to the dosator. All three use an annular trough which is fed from a larger hopper, so it is important to know what the behaviour of the powder will be under the conditions that exist in these three machines.

An alternative method of filling capsules is illustrated in Fig. 9.10. A vacuum is used to remove air from the capsule body through an exhaust passage. This causes powder to flow from the hopper down an inclined delivery tube into the capsule. The flow of material ceases following restoration of normal atmospheric pressure. The vacuum system is adjusted to cause a predetermined quantity of material to be dispensed into the capsule.

The points at which the vacuum and powder delivery passages open on the underside of the top plate are sufficiently close together to come within the mouth of capsules larger than size 5. The sealing ring ensures that no leakage occurs during the filling process. The operating pin raises the capsule body from the carrier against this sealing ring and activates the filling. A machine has been built using this principle with an output of up to 20 000 capsules per hour. There are a number

of advantages of this method. It is possible to fill single substances, which reduces the amount of formulation work required, and it eliminates the need for powder lubricants.

Filling Hard Capsules with Pellets

Certain products are designed to provide prolonged therapeutic action. They are variously described as 'prolonged action', 'sustained release', or 'controlled release'. One way of producing this type of product is to make coated pellets (time pills or time beads).

Figure 9.11 shows a simple means of filling pellets into capsules, either directly or by using a hopper. All the hand-operated machines may be converted to fill pellets using one of these methods, but difficulties may be experienced in obtaining dose uniformity due to the variations in the size of the pellets and the volume of the capsule body. If a mixture of pellets is used, for example neutral pellets together with those coated so as to have different release characteristics, the difficulty of maintaining homogeneity is increased. Damage to the pellet coating may also occur, especially with the hopper method, which will alter the drug-release characteristics of the pellets. In an attempt to prevent this, several indirect methods of feeding have been developed; they are illustrated in Figs 9.12 to 9.15. There are problems associated with each of these methods. Separation of individual pellets may occur due to differences in size, shape, or susceptibility to electrostatic attraction. Separation can also be due to poor hopper design, resulting in so-called rat-holing, core flow, or bridging. The pellets may agglomerate in the storage hopper, and damage to the pellets may be exacerbated by the multiplicity of slides, resulting in variations in the drug-release characteristics.

The piston method (Fig. 9.12) and the double slide method (Fig. 9.13) give good results for weight variation and dosage accuracy, although they have now largely been replaced by the piston and slide method (Fig. 9.14) which gives better mechanical reliability.

The continuous method illustrated in Fig. 9.15 shows two different types of pellet being filled on the same machine. The danger with this type of equipment is that it relies on a very accurate measurement of dose at the first station, otherwise an overfill or underfill occurs at the second station. Apart from this, cross-contamination of the two types of pellet can occur at the dividing wall, and when refilling the storage hopper. Damage to the

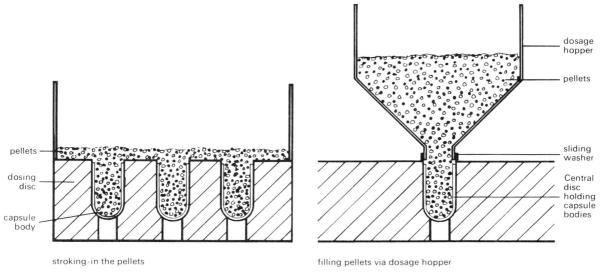

Fig. 9.11. Methods for filling capsules with pellets, either directly or using a hopper.

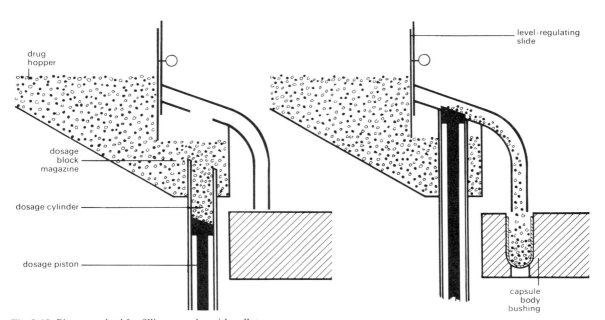

Fig. 9.12. Piston method for filling capsules with pellets.

pellet coat may also occur at this dividing wall because the pellets roll and wear in contact with it.

In general, when evaluating a pellet-filling device the most important points to consider are the dosage accuracy (Marquardt and Clement, 1970), the extent to which pellets are damaged at various filling rates, the degree of segregation if a mixture is used, the effect of batch variations in pellets on attainable filling speeds, the type of flow from the storage hopper which ideally should be mass flow, the effect of ambient conditions on the filling characteristics, and the filling speeds at which partial fills start to occur.

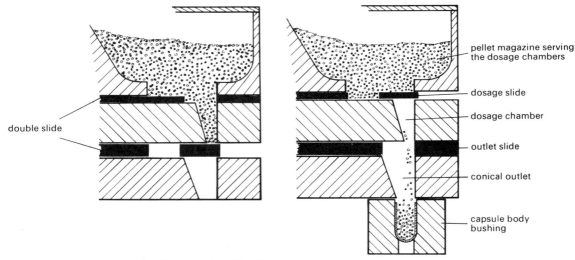

Fig. 9.13. Double slide method for filling capsules with pellets.

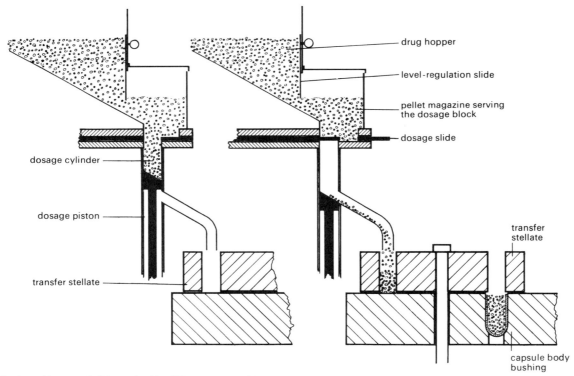

Fig. 9.14. Piston and slide method for filling capsules with pellets.

Filling Hard Capsules with Tablets

The reasons for the use of pellets also apply to the use of tablets. Ordinary compressed tablets, sugar-coated tablets, compressed rods, enteric-coated tablets, small capsules, and soft gelatin capsules can all be filled into capsules, although there

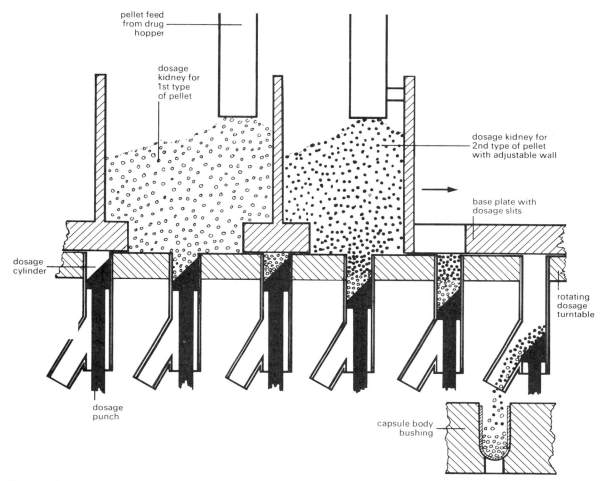

Fig. 9.15. Continuous method for filling capsules with pellets.

is a limit on the size of the inserted tablet relative to the diameter of the capsule into which it is to be put. The tolerances allowable for various types of tablet, when using Zanasi equipment, are as follows:

spherical shape minimum diameter of 3 mm;
dragée minimum diameter 4.5 mm and minimum height 2.5 mm (minimum ratio 1.8);
core minimum diameter 4 mm with minimum height of 2.5 mm (maximum difference 1.5 mm), or minimum diameter of 3 mm and minimum height 3 mm (ratio 1).

In all cases, the tolerance on these measurements is ±0.1 mm. For the spherical shape or the dragée, the diameter must be 0.4 to 0.5 mm less than the internal diameter of the capsule to be filled. In the case of the core, the same limit applies across the maximum dimension.

This method of presentation eliminates the problem of incompatibility of drugs since one of the drugs can be tabletted and the other can be a powder or a pellet. However, the problem of filling this combination on a machine at high rates may well outweigh the advantages of extra stability (Heufel, 1978). Some examples of filling tablets into capsules are shown in Figs 9.16, 9.17, and 9.18. One distinct advantage of this idea is in the preparation of materials for clinical trials, since small tablets may be concealed inside capsules and products may be compared for therapeutic response without the knowledge of the patient.

The Zanasi LZ-64 is capable of filling tablets into capsules. The RM-63, RV-59R, AZ-25/R,

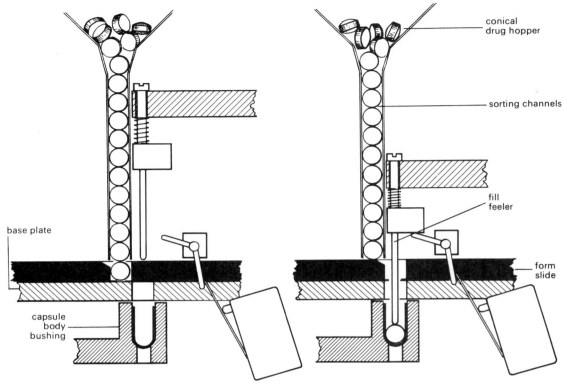

Fig. 9.16. Slide dosage, method 1, for filling tablets into capsules.

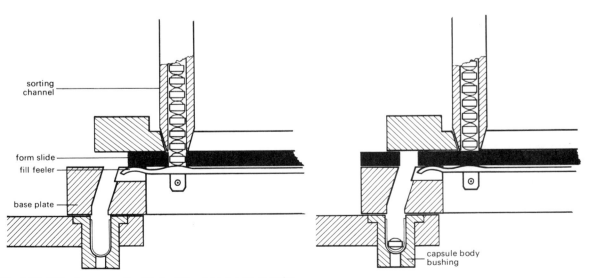

Fig. 9.17. Slide dosage, method 2, for filling tablets into capsules.

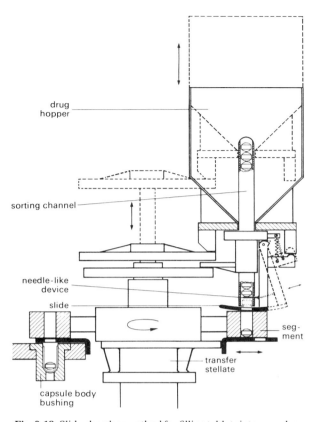

Fig. 9.18. Slide chamber method for filling tablets into capsules.

AZ-20, AZ-30, and AZ-60 can fill both tablets and capsules into capsules.

Hard shell capsules, size 3, may be filled into a size 000 hard shell capsule. A size 4 capsule may be put into sizes 00 and 000, and a size 5 capsule into sizes 0, 00, and 000.

References

Heufel, *Elanco Capsules Technology Symposium*, 1978.
Jolliffe, I. G., Ph.D. Thesis, University of Nottingham, 1980.
Marquardt, H. G. and Clement, H., *Drugs Germ., 1970, 13,* 21-33.

Chapter 10

Capsule-filling Machinery

G. C. Cole

The machinery described in this chapter has been divided into three types: hand-operated equipment, semi-automatic machinery, and fully automatic units.

HAND-OPERATED EQUIPMENT

The machines described in this section are those made by Feton Chemical and Pharmaceutical Industry (ChemiPharm), Tevopharm-Schiedam, and Bonapace/Zuma. A model similar to the Feton is supplied by Davcaps.

THE FETON MACHINE

This machine (Fig. 10.1) is made to accept capsule sizes from 000 to 4, holding 30, 60, or 100 of each, though the rectifier will only accept sizes 2 to 3 in numbers of either 60 or 100. A special unit is required for Coni-Snap or Posilok capsules and is only available for sizes 0 to 3. No claim is made by the makers that the equipment can be used to fill pellets or tablets into the capsules, but to do so presents little difficulty. The dosing accuracy claimed for this filler is ±2.5%. For each size of capsule to be handled, a separate unit is needed.

CHEMIPHARM CAPSULE FILLERS

ChemiPharm make several capsule fillers; the Universal Model is shown in Fig. 10.2. It has a filling plate with four parallel rows of 24 holes, each row being machined for a different capsule size. A daily output of 2000 capsules is claimed.

The larger Model 300, shown in Fig. 10.3, can take 144 capsules in sizes from 1 to 5, although it can handle sizes 0 and 00 at a reduced plate capacity of 100 capsules. The machine is built for one size of capsule only, and is capable of an output of 2000 capsules per hour.

Two other models exist, the 200 and the 200A. These can both accept 96 capsules up to size 1, and for 0 and 00 have a reduced capacity of 57. The Model 200 is built for one side of capsule only,

but the Model 200A, with the necessary change parts, can be used for three sizes. Both these models have an output of 1000 capsules per hour.

THE TEVOPHARM MACHINE

This machine is a more sophisticated hand-operated filler than either the Feton or the Chemi-Pharm models. It has extra features which enable the operator to achieve a more even density of fill by vibrating and tamping the powder in the capsule.

A general view is shown in Fig. 10.4. The CAP III model holds 60 capsules in its plate, whilst the CAP IV holds 90, so that their respective outputs, for capsule sizes over the whole range from 000 to 5, are 2000 and 3000 capsules per hour.

The Tevopharm filling machine is designed for the small-scale filling of hard shell capsules, and is simple enough for even inexperienced personnel to use. The capsules are simply poured in bulk on to a filling plate. A special 'nesting' mechanism positions each capsule in the filler plate holes. The capsules are then opened, filled, tamped, closed, and ejected by manipulating two hand-levers and a foot-pedal. The tamping device is to ensure that each capsule is filled uniformly. There are no high-frequency vibrators to cause separation of the ingredients. Interchangeable filler plates adapt the machine for handling any size of capsule. All parts which come into contact with the product are made of chrome-plated brass, plastic, and other corrosion-resistant materials.

Figure 10.5 shows the essential parts of the Tevopharm filler. To fill capsules using this machine the following detailed procedure should be followed. Lift the lid (C) to a vertical position by releasing the locking bar (D) and pressing backwards. Mount the required size of plate (J) on the two supports (A), on top of the machine, taking care that the plate is pressed as far back as possible. Turn the handle (E) carefully clockwise in order to ensure that the pins (B) slide freely into the corresponding holes. Place an excess of capsules into the capsule loader. Shake slightly until all the holes are filled and return the surplus capsules to the bulk container.

Place the sorting device on top of the filling plate, and press its upper half forward. The capsules will now drop down into the corresponding holes of the filling plate. When loading the empty capsules into the plate, the capsule body locking knob (F) must be loosened in order to permit the capsules to drop into the bottom plate. They are then pressed down lightly with the plastic plate. Now tighten the knob (F) and take off the top plate (J). The tops of the bodies are now level with the surface of the plate, so that powder can be spread over it and will fall into the bodies. After the powder has been filled into the capsule bodies, replace the top plate holding the capsule caps.

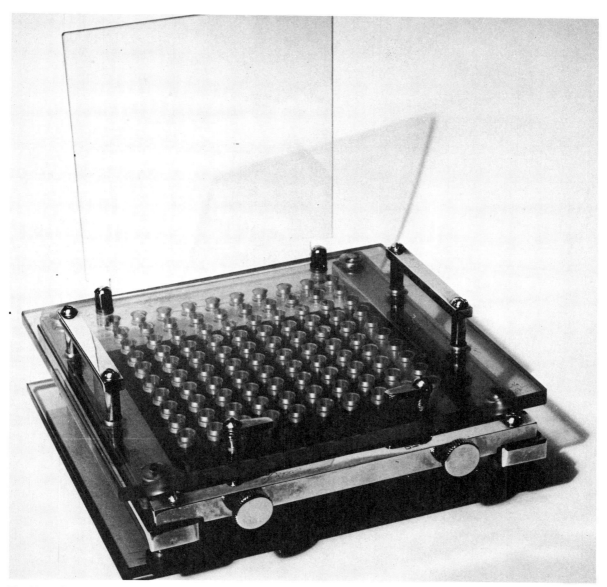

Fig. 10.1. The Feton hand-operated capsule filler.

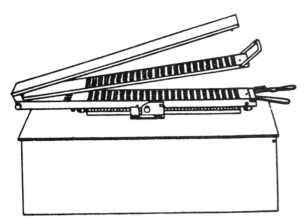

Fig. 10.2. The ChemiPharm Universal Model hand-operated capsule filler.

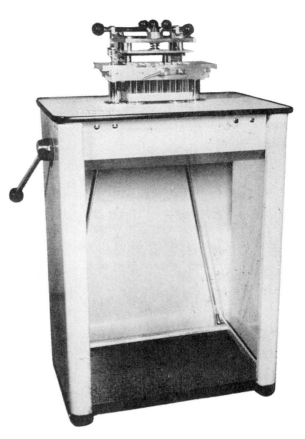

Fig. 10.4. The Tevopharm hand-operated capsule filler.

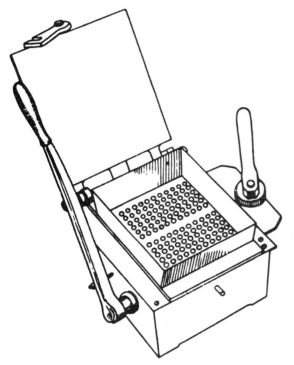

Fig. 10.3. The ChemiPharm Model 300 hand-operated capsule filler.

Cover the top plate with the plastic plate to prevent the capsule caps being blown out by the trapped air.

Turn the lid (C) down to its horizontal position. This lid is constructed with a separate plate (H),

which can be adjusted using knob (I). The adjustment does not need to be very accurate. Springs between plates (C) and (H) then ensure that when the capsule bodies are pressed into the caps, the same pressure is applied to all the capsules. When the handle (E) is turned clockwise the pins (B), are lifted and press the bodies into the caps. The bodies are lifted further than is necessary to close the capsules, so that the bodies press the caps upwards against the tension of the springs and thus ensure a firm closure.

By moving handle (E) further the pins will return to their original position. Lid (C) is now lifted into the vertical position, the top plate (J) taken off the machine, and the closed capsules removed from it. The plates must be cleaned from time to time to ensure smooth operation. By removing knob (F) and the screws on the front side, the plates which hold the capsule bodies can be taken apart.

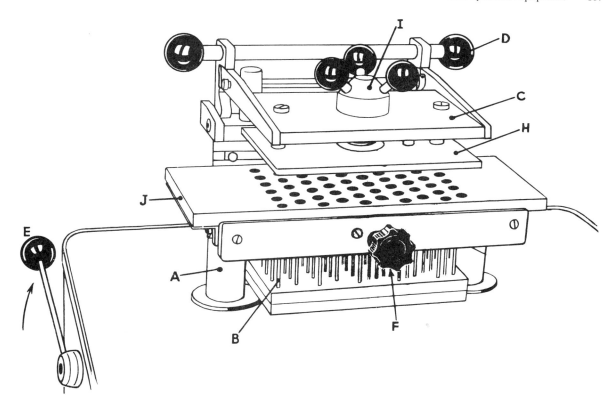

Fig. 10.5. The filling head of the Tevopharm capsule filler. A, supports; B, pins; C, lid; D, locking bar; E, handle; F, capsule body locking knob; H, fixed top plate; I, top plate adjustment; J, removable top plate.

Some powder may remain on the surface of the plate even though all the bodies are apparently filled, but on depressing a foot-pedal, the bodies can be lowered and it may be seen that not all of them are equally filled. In some the powder will sink much lower than in others, but by brushing in further powder, the difference can be reduced. The more the powder is tamped into the capsule bodies, the smaller the weight difference will usually be and normally it will be well within the accepted limits.

For powders which are very cohesive and of low bulk density, a pressing apparatus with 60 pins corresponding to the holes in the plates is available and should be used. With this additional device the power is easily pressed into the capsules to produce an even fill.

THE BONAPACE/ZUMA MACHINES
These range from a simple type, rather like the Feton, to a fully-automatic machine capable of filling 20 000 capsules per hour. It is possible to

increase the output of the smaller capacity equipment by using semi-automatic separation of the empty capsules. Some examples are shown in Table 10.1.

Table 10.1. Bonapace/Zuma machines

Bonapace model	Zuma model	Output (max.) capsules/ hour
	150 B/3	1500
B/B-3		3000
B/B-6		4000
	150 B/3 + multiform A/4	5000
B/B-3 + sorter A/B-4		6000
	300 B6 + multiform A/7	8000
B/B-6 + sorter A/B-7		8000
	300 B6 + Zumatic A/1	12 000
B/B-6 + sorter A/B-1		14 000
	Mex B/7 + Zumatic A/1	20 000

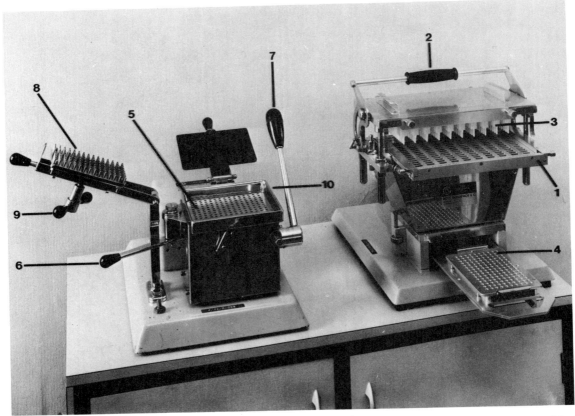

Fig. 10.6. The Bonapace capsule filler B/B-6/S and capsule sorter A/B-4/S. 1, orientation tray; 2, orientation tray positioning handle; 3, direction prongs; 4, receiver plate; 5, filling plate; 6, locking handle; 7, closure and ejection handle; 8, closing prongs; 9, pressure closing handle; 10, surround.

Some of these fillers should be classified as semi-automatic, but for simplicity it is better to consider all the Bonapace machines together.

The Bonapace capsule filler B/B-6 and capsule sorter A/B-4 are shown in Fig. 10.6. The tray (1) is filled with empty shells by dipping it into the bulk supply and rejecting the excess. The tray is located in the top of the sorter and by activating the handle (2), the tray is positioned under the prongs (3) and the capsules pushed vertically downwards, correctly orientated, into the receiver plate (4). This is then removed and transferred to the filler and located on the filling plate (5). Moving the handle (6) locks the bodies of the capsules and enables the caps to be removed in the plate (4). The handle (6) is now released and the top of the body falls below the surface of the plate (5); the surround (10) is placed on this plate to prevent material being lost. The powder, which has previously been weighed out and is sufficient for 150 capsules, is placed on top of the plate (5) and evenly distributed into the bodies. The surround is then removed and the plate (4) replaced over the bodies in plate (5). The closing prongs (8) are then located over plates (4) and (5). The handle (7) is activated, forcing the bodies into the caps. Extra pressure may be applied by screw (9) to ensure a firm closure. The filled capsules are then ejected from the machine by removing the closing prongs (8) and activating handle (7).

The Zuma—Mex B/7 and Zumatic A/1 combination is a later development of this type of operation. Here 300 capsules are filled in one cycle. The A/1 is used to orientate the capsules and the B/7 to fill them. The capsules are opened automatically and then filled by sliding the hopper over the plate containing the bodies. The powder is fed out of this hopper by three augers and the required dosage is obtained by varying the speed of these augers. The capsules are closed and ejected from the machine automatically.

SEMI-AUTOMATIC MACHINES

The machines described in this section are listed in Table 10.2.

THE PEDINI MODEL 21B

This machine is now obsolete and the company do not now manufacture capsule-filling equipment. About 40–60 capsules could be filled in one operation, depending on the size. The output claimed for a number 2 size capsule was 2000 capsules per hour. Change parts were available for all sizes. The empty capsules were loaded by hand, and the powder was filled into a hopper which was vibrated by a motor. The same motor also served to move the hopper over the empty capsule bodies, the powder flowing into the bodies by both gravity and vibration. A filled weight variation of ± 1–3% was claimed for this machine, but the powder had to be free-flowing and homogeneous, particularly with regard to density, to ensure consistent results. The filled capsules had to be polished after ejection from this machine.

LAF MULTIFILL MACHINE

This multi-purpose machine (Fig. 10.7) was manufactured by Leidsche Apparatenfabriek N.V., but no capsule-filling machines are now made by them. It has the advantage that four different operations can be achieved with virtually the same unit: powder or liquid can be filled into either vials or hard capsules. It has a claimed output of up to 5000 capsules per hour depending on the size of the capsules and the physical characteristics of the powder.

The capsules are filled with powder by means of an auger, and while this method is suitable for free-flowing powders, difficulties arise when the powder is cohesive. Capsules from size 000 to size 4 may be filled, depending on the parts fitted, and changing to another size is simple.

THE COLTON MACHINE

The Colton 8 machine, and the Parke, Davis and Lilly versions of it, are probably the most widely used semi-automatic capsule fillers in the world. These machines have been extensively sold or rented, and their introduction into industry was

Table 10.2. Some semi-automatic filling machines

Model	Capsule sizes filled	Output (max.) capsules/hour	Method of filling
Pedini 21B	000–5	2000	direct
LAF Multifill	000–4	5000	auger
Colton 8*	000–5	20 000	auger

* Also known as the Lilly or Parke, Davis capsule-filling machine. Outputs of 250 000 capsules per day have been claimed.

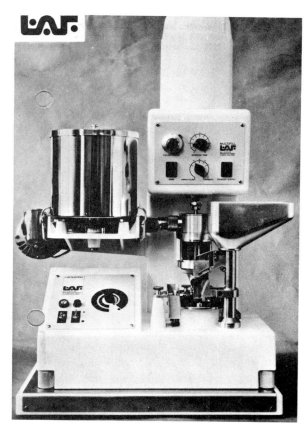

Fig. 10.7. The LAF Multifill capsule filler.

a major step forward in capsule-filling technology. There are, however, serious limitations. The speed and success depend upon the skill of the operator; the capsules produced are very dusty, so that a separate cleaning and polishing operation is required; difficulties in meeting the weight variation limits demanded by the *U.S.P.* and *B.P.* make its operation uneconomic for certain products, and pellets are easily damaged during the filling cycle.

The Lilly version of the Colton 8 machine is shown in Fig. 10.8. To fill capsules on this

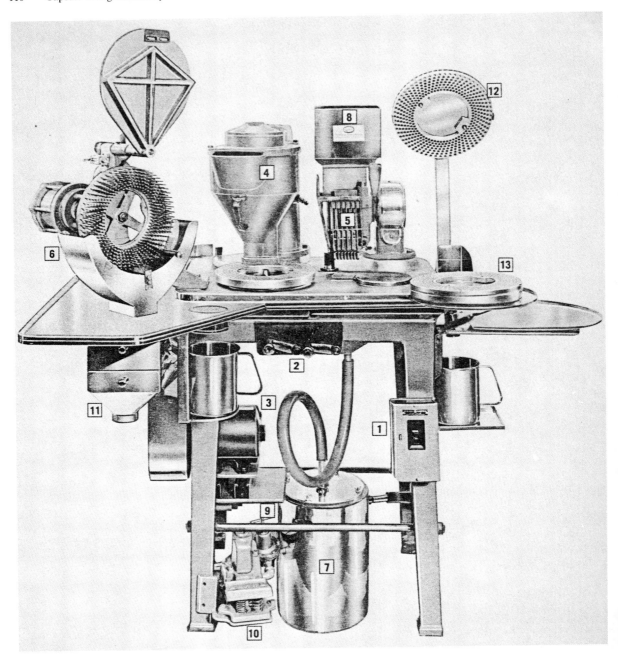

Fig. 10.8. The Lilly version of the Colton 8 semi-automatic capsule-filling machine. 1, motor switch; 2, weight control levers; 3, drive motor; 4, powder hopper; 5, rectifier head; 6, capsule-closing assembly; 7, filter can; 8, empty-capsule hopper; 9, air line regulator and pressure gauge; 10, foot-control valve for closing; 11, receptacle box; 12, filling ring (cap section); 13, filling ring (cap and body section).

machine, the filling ring (13), which consists of a cap and body section, is placed under the rectifier head assembly (5). The filling ring is designed so that the caps cannot pass into the body section when vacuum is applied. The ring positions the capsules, one row at a time, under the rectifier head (5) and over a slot in a leather gasket through which vacuum is applied. As the holes pass over the slot, capsules are dropped from the rectifier head and are drawn into the holes in the ring.

The rectifier head assembly (5) consists of several parts. At the top is the empty-capsule hopper (8), and immediately beneath it is the magazine through which the capsules are fed from the hopper and down tubes. The diameter of these tubes is approximately the same as that of the capsule bodies and the number of tubes is the same as the number of holes in the ring.

At the front of the magazine there is attached a spring gate, and beneath this is the raceway, which is a block into which are cut grooves, each the width of a capsule. The raceway is pronged at the end facing the front of the machine. Attached to the guide block, which lies directly under the raceway and coming up over it, is the gate lifter, a thin bar of metal which operates the spring gate on the magazine. When the magazine is lowered to the raceway, the gate lifter parts the spring gate enough to allow one capsule to be released from each tube of the magazine. The capsules fall into the grooves in the raceway and are pushed forward to its open end by a pusher blade, a thin casting that passes forward and backward over the top of the raceway. Under the raceway is the guide block, designed to feed the capsules into the filling ring.

The rectifier block comes down over the pronged end of the raceway and pushes the capsules down through the openings in the guide block into the holes in the capsule ring. Since the raceway openings are wider at the top than at the bottom, the rectifier block forces the capsules through to the capsule ring with the body of the capsule down. The rectifier head assembly should operate at 82 strokes per minute for proper production. If the pulleys on either the motor or machine are changed in order to increase the speed at which the head operates, it will be found that capsules fly off the end of the raceway, as the pusher blade will not merely push the capsule, but will strike it so hard that it will travel too far.

When the capsule is in the filling ring the vacuum separates the body from the cap, and when all the holes in the filling ring are full of capsules, the filling operation may be commenced. The capsule ring is taken from the turntable and placed on the round tray at the right front of the machine.

The top and bottom rings are separated by lifting the cap ring and placing it in the easel to the right and above the machine, the body ring being left in the tray. All capsule bodies which have remained in their caps should be pulled out of the cap ring (12) and placed in the body ring, and the operator should make sure that every hole has a capsule body in it. The body ring is then placed on the left turntable, and the powder hopper (4) is pulled over it for one revolution of the ring. The speed of the turntable will determine the amount of material pressed into each capsule. The cap ring is then placed on the body ring, and the capsules are ready for joining.

At the left side of the machine is the closing assembly (6), at the bottom of which is a semicircular structure, the ring support, which holds the capsule ring in position. Above this is a ring with pegs on it called the peg ring, the pegs being arranged to register with the holes of the capsule ring. It is attached to a shaft which has a flat steel washer on the end, and the action of the air air cylinder piston shaft against this washer drives the pegs into the capsule ring. A circular plate, which is counterbalanced at the back and locks at a neutral position above the ring support, is pulled down during the closing process and is used as a closing plate to brace the capsule ring against the peg ring.

The filled capsule is then taken from the filling table, placed on the ring support and the capsules closed, either by hand or automatically.

If the capsules are to be closed by hand, the operator pulls the closing plate down, aligns the pegs in the peg ring with the holes in the capsule ring, and slams the peg ring against the capsule ring. This will have to be done several times with great pressure to ensure the closing of the capsules.

If the machine has an automatic closing device, the operator closes the capsules by bracing the capsule ring against the closing plate, aligning the pegs in the peg ring with the holes in the capsule ring, and tripping the foot-pedal two or three times. More than three times should never be necessary.

The capsule ring is then pushed against the peg ring to eject the capsules, which fall down the chute under the joining mechanism into a container.

The speed of the left-hand turntable, the power-filling table, and the level of powder in the hopper, control the weight of powder filled into each capsule. There are eight speeds for the turntable, selection being made using two levers on the front of the machine. The left-hand lever has two positions, A and B, A being the fastest speed. With each setting of this lever is combined a setting of the right-hand lever, which is numbered 1 to 4, 1 being the fastest and 4 the slowest speed. Generally, the slower the rotational speed the heavier the fill-weight. It is possible to rotate a ring twice under the powder-filling hopper to increase the fill-weight but this is not recommended practice as it reduces output and can cause mechanical problems. When changing the size of capsule to be filled, it is usually necessary to change the magazine, raceway, push blade, rectifier block, guide block, capsule ring, and peg ring, although some of these items span two or three capsule sizes.

AUTOMATIC MACHINES

Automatic machines can be classified according to whether the movement of the capsules is intermittent or continuous. In the former case, capsules are moved by carrier mechanisms which move rapidly, usually by rotation about an axis, and then stop whilst a separation or filling operation occurs at a fixed station. In the latter, the capsules are transported by some form of flexible conveyor and the separation and filling operations are carried out whilst they are moving.

Intermittent Motion Machines

THE ZANASI LZ-64

This machine has an output in the range of 3600–4200 capsules per hour. It is an ideal pilot-plant machine for small batches of material and can be used to test formulations before scaling up to the larger production size machines. The main features are shown in Fig. 10.9.

Empty hard gelatin capsules are placed in the hopper (1). The action of the feed tube (2) inside the hopper ensures that capsules flow down the tube into the alignment block, and the capsule stop can be used to shut off the flow when necessary. Because the cap and body of the capsule have different diameters, the capsules become orientated so that they always arrive cap uppermost in the upper bush. The machine then indexes rapidly round to the opening station, where the cap and body are separated. At this point the upper bush is aligned with the lower bush, which is held in the turntable (5). The upper bush is moved out of its holder by a push-rod, and the body of the capsule is drawn into the lower bush by an applied vacuum. On indexing round to the next station, the upper bush, which has returned to its holder,

and the lower bush, separate to allow the powder to be filled into the capsule body. A microswitch is fitted between these two last-mentioned stations to stop the machine if a damaged capsule is present.

Powder is supplied from a hopper (3) which is divided into three segments, the powder being taken from the segment closest to the turntable by the dosator filling heads in the form of small plugs or pellets, which are ejected by the pistons of the dosators into the capsule bodies. If a capsule has failed to separate into body and cap the plug passes straight through the lower bush hole into a receptacle located underneath the turntable. The unopened capsule, which will have been retained in the upper bush is then ejected by means of a rod into a container. The length of the rod is such that when it enters an upper bush containing only a cap it will reach inside but not dislodge it, so that it is not ejected. The next step is to reunite the cap with the filled body and to eject the filled capsule down the chute (6).

The weight of fill can be adjusted by means of the two compression piston-height rings which are screwed on the outside of the compression piston holders in the upper part of the dosator filling head. By raising or lowering the piston the dose is either increased or decreased. A small scale is provided which enables each filling head to be set to approximately the same level. To obtain a compacted pellet it is necessary to adjust the large screw (4) immediately above the filling head. In operation, it is advisable to start with this screw set at zero compression i.e. 000 on the scale, particularly when using a new material. The level of the powder in the powder hopper can affect the physical characteristics of the pellet. The level on the dosator filling side should be adjusted to its maximum at the beginning of a run, which should be twice the depth of the dosage volume in the dosator.

The change parts which are required in order to handle different capsule sizes are: upper and lower bushes, dosator heads and pistons, empty-capsule feed tube, ejection bush, alignment block, reject capsule bush, and various push and ejection rods.

There are four other Zanasi machines that operate on the same principle, with outputs (capsules per hour) as follows: RM-63, 8000–12 000; AZ-20, 10 000–20 000; AZ-25R, 25 000–35 000; AZ-60, 30 000–60 000.

An improved version of the LZ-64 machine is

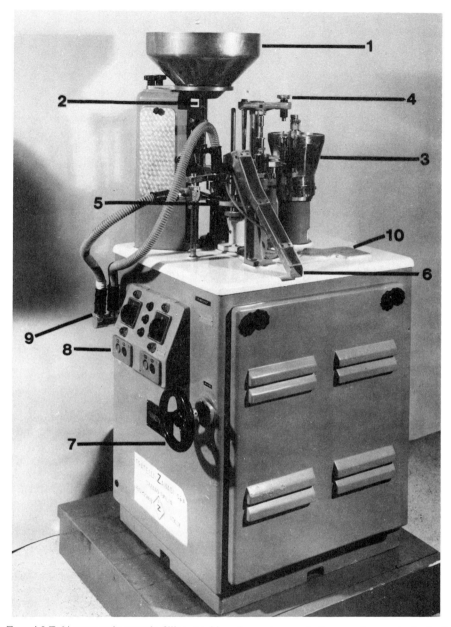

Fig. 10.9. The Zanasi LZ-64 automatic capsule-filling machine. 1, empty-capsule hopper; 2, capsule feed tube located inside the hopper; 3, powder feed hopper; 4, pressure adjustment; 5, turntable holding eight bushes; 6, ejection chute; 7, hand-wheel; 8, control panel; 9, cleaning system; 10, pellet or tablet dosing unit site.

manufactured by Macofar s.a.s. The model MT-13/1 with an output of 5000 capsules per hour is shown in Fig. 10.10. The procedure for capsule filling is essentially the same as for the LZ-64, but with the following important differences:

1. Only one dosator is used.
2. The dosator is situated above the powder hopper and does not rotate.
3. The plug is formed in the dosator and is raised above the turntable in a vertical movement.

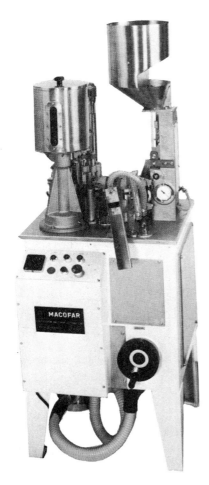

Fig. 10.10. The Macofar Model MT-13/1 automatic capsule-filling machine.

4. The empty capsule body is moved below the dosator for filling.

5. The amount of residual powder required is reduced from approximately 300 g to 150 g.

6. The machine is simpler than the LZ-64 to operate.

7. To double the output a second dosator can be fitted.

THE ZANASI AZ-60

This is the largest of the range of machines with intermittent operation manufactured by Nuova Zanasi s.p.A. There are two intermediate machines, the AZ-20 and the AZ-25, which have outputs of between 10 000 and 35 000 capsules per hour, respectively.

Fig. 10.11. The Zanasi AZ-60 automatic capsule-filling machine. 1, empty-capsule reservoir; 2, empty-capsule feed hopper; 3, alignment and capsule guide channels; 4, turntable; 5, powder hopper; 6, powder feed tubes; 7, dosator hopper; 8, dosator filling heads; 9, weight control; 10, pressure control; 11, ejection point and chute; 12, control console; 13, isolating key.

The AZ-60, illustrated in Figs 10.11 and 10.12, has a maximum output of 60 000 capsules per hour.

Capsules are fed into the larger of the two hoppers (1). Powder is placed inside the powder hopper (5), from where it flows into the three dosator hoppers (7); the machine is operated for about five minutes to allow it to fill up and for the conditions to become steady. Powder flow is assisted by a stirrer inside the powder hopper (5) and mixing vanes inside each of the dosator hoppers. Each of the 24 dosator filling heads (8) will initially require adjusting to obtain the correct dosage. When this has been achieved, eight dosators may be adjusted from a single control.

Empty capsules leave the capsule reservoir (1) and fall into the empty-capsule feed hopper (2) and then into the alignment and capsule guide channels (3). This ensures the correct alignment of the capsules. Between this position and the first of the dosating points the capsule is separated by applying vacuum to the lower bush when it is in contact with the upper bush. After separation, the upper slide, containing the twelve upper bushes holding the caps, is withdrawn, allowing the slide in the turntable (4) containing the twelve lower bushes holding twelve bodies to be exposed. At the first dosator hopper, four of the bodies are filled: the remainder are filled at the second and third dosators. After the third dosator, a microswitch stops the machine if a capsule body or pellet is protruding above the lower bush. At this point also, capsules which have failed to separate are ejected into the appropriate receptacle, in the same way as on the LZ-64 machine. The upper and lower bushes meet again at this point and when they move to the final station the capsules are closed and immediately ejected, passing up the ejection tube and falling down the chute (11). The ejection tube (Fig. 10.13) consists of a number of components designed to ensure that the closed capsule has a uniform length. Between the ejection point and the recharging point there is a cleaning unit which removes surplus dust and powder by means of an applied suction, followed by a blast of compressed air. There is also a small brush to free tenacious particles.

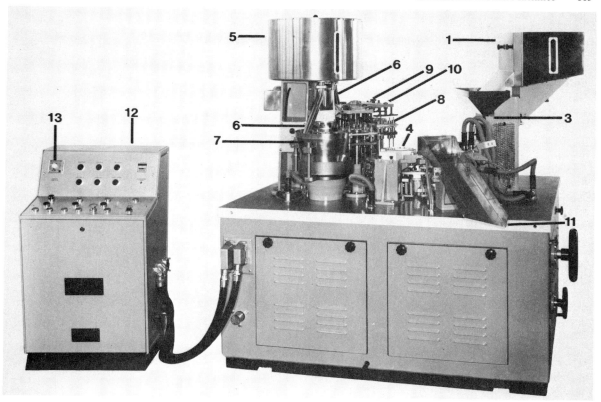

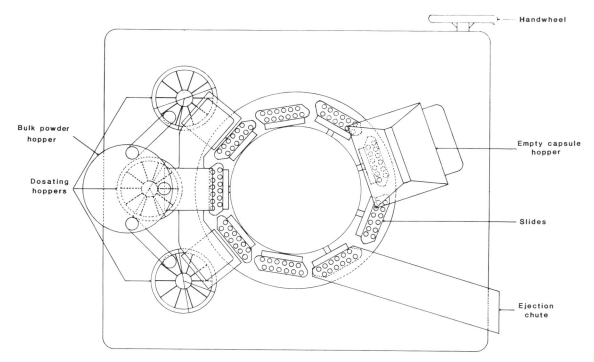

Fig. 10.12. Plan view of the Zanasi AZ-60.

The operating controls are built into a separate console (12) which also controls the lubricating system, vacuum pump, and compressor. There is an isolating key (13), similar to an ignition key, without which the controls cannot be switched on.

The lubrication system is completely automatic. A process timer in the control console governs the intervals at which lubricant is pumped around the system. It is important that the correct time interval is used otherwise surplus oil will work back along the guide channels and onto the capsules during the filling operation.

Cleaning the machine is a lengthy process and the time required to change from one size of capsule to another is between four and six hours. Cleaning involves the removal of the powder hopper, three feed tubes, three dosator hoppers and 24 dosators; there are 84 upper and lower bushes which, fortunately, can then be cleaned *in situ*. The dosator hoppers are heavy, especially when they contain powder, and need two operators to remove them. They can then be dismantled for cleaning, the top being removed from the base plate and the rotating vanes taken out. It is very important that these parts are correctly reassembled and seated in position, otherwise serious damage will occur during the operation of the machine. The drive requires a 3-phase electricity supply. It is also useful to have a means of extracting compressor and vacuum pump fumes from the working area.

The results of some weight variability tests are given in Tables 10.3 and 10.4. Table 10.3 gives the individual weight variation obtained at production rates of 35 000, 48 000, and 60 000 capsules per hour, using a placebo formulation consisting of 246 mg of lactose, 2.5 mg of magnesium stearate, and 1.5 mg of Aerosil, filled into size 3 capsules to a fill weight of 290 mg.

Table 10.4 shows the weight variations from individual dosators at an output of 60 000 capsules per hour. The variation is well within the *B.P.* limits (10% deviation with only two deviating more than 10% and none more than 20% for a sample of 20 capsules).

There are a number of problems associated with the AZ-60 machines.

1. The quantity of powder remaining unused inside each of the dosator hoppers is approximately 3 kg, so that there is a considerable wastage at the end of each batch. The desirability of mixing several such lots to produce one batch for subse-

Table 10.3. Weight variation obtained from Zanasi AZ-25 and AZ-60 machines at various output levels for a target weight of 290 mg

Model	Output capsules/ hour	Mean weight mg	Standard deviation mg	Coefficient of variation %
AZ-25	35 000	289.6	4.58	1.60
AZ-60	48 000	290.3	5.54	1.91
AZ-60	60 000	286.1	2.23	0.78

Table 10.4. Weight variation for individual dosators on the Zanasi AZ-60 machine at 60 000 capsules per hour, for a target weight of 290 mg

Dosator	Mean weight mg	Standard deviation mg	Coefficient of variation %
1	287.7	5.50	1.91
2	287.9	5.28	1.83
3	290.4	6.35	2.19
4	289.3	5.85	2.02
5	289.2	5.61	1.94
6	288.3	7.30	2.53
7	292.4	3.24	1.11
8	290.2	4.13	1.42
9	290.0	3.02	1.04
10	289.8	5.14	1.77
11	287.5	4.30	1.50
12	290.0	2.62	0.91
13	288.1	4.63	1.61
14	292.5	2.32	0.79
15	288.9	2.33	0.81
16	288.6	2.41	0.88
17	288.0	2.31	0.80
18	288.1	3.54	1.23
19	285.1	5.13	1.80
20	284.6	3.84	1.35
21	294.7	3.33	1.13
22	286.1	2.23	0.78
23	285.6	7.35	2.57
24	288.2	7.81	2.71

quent filling is debatable. Careful statistical sampling is necessary to provide the analytical test samples.

2. The size and weight of the machine have been increased so that it requires 25% more production area than the AZ-25, and the control console is a separate unit.

3. A single control is provided for altering the weight delivered by eight of the dosators, and, once the batch has been set up, this is theoretically the only control which needs to be adjusted. However, experience has shown that during the filling of a batch some individual dosators need adjustment.

4. When Snap-Fit or Lok-Cap capsules are used,

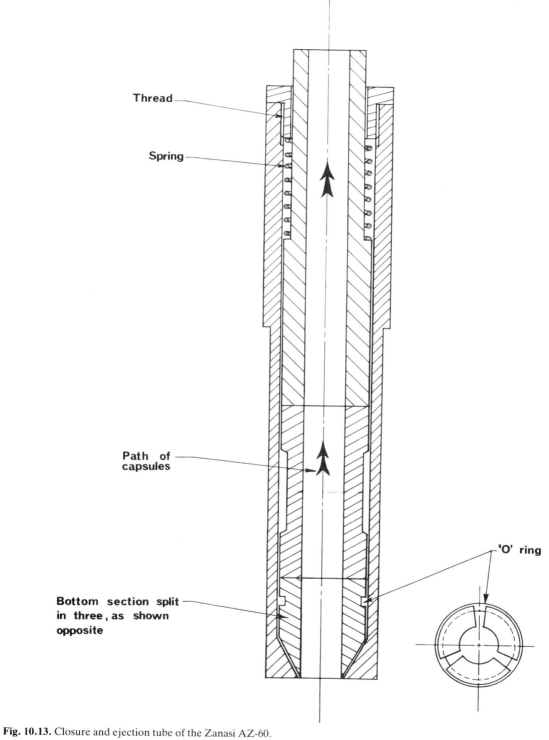

Thread

Spring

Path of capsules

Bottom section split in three, as shown opposite

'O' ring

Fig. 10.13. Closure and ejection tube of the Zanasi AZ-60.

the proportion of unopened capsules rises considerably. In one particular production run this averaged between one and two per cent, resulting in the loss of a large amount of powder.

5. The loading of the powder hopper and the capsule hopper is difficult due to their height above the machine.

6. Close supervision is required, as it is not possible to check each individual dosator weight without stopping the machine.

7. At 60 000 capsules per hour a constant rate of flow of powder must be maintained to each of the dosator hoppers. In a test programme, bridging occurred in the feed tubes, which caused excessive weight variation. This underlines the need for powder formulations to be free-flowing, and for

the feed hopper design to be improved.

The hopper has a horizontal base and vertical sides; powder flows out of three openings in the base and the stirrer maintains a level powder surface. Without the stirrer there would be virtually no flow, and even with it the flow leaves much to be desired.

8. The main powder hopper was originally provided with a flat-bladed stirrer to improve the flow properties, but this was gear-driven from the main drive shaft at a single speed. In later models an independent variable-speed motor is fitted which allows adjustments to be made for the falling level of the powder in the hopper and for the different flow characteristics of different materials.

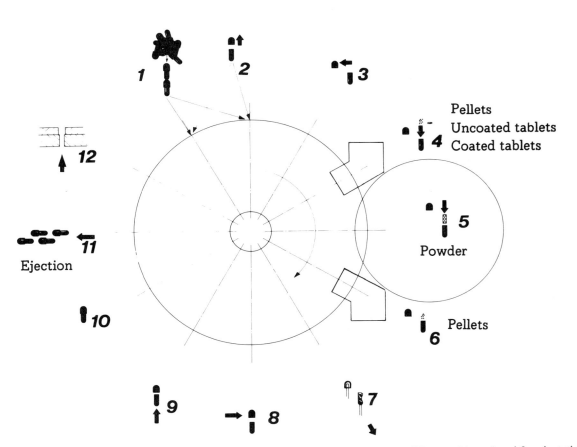

Fig. 10.14. Schematic diagram of the operation of the Höfliger and Karg GKF capsule-filling machines. 1 and 2, orientation and separation of capsules; 3, removal of capsule body; 4, metering station for insertion of pellets, coated tablets, or uncoated tablets; 5, metering station for powder; 6, metering station for pellets; 7, faulty-capsule ejection; 8, realignment of the capsule caps and bodies; 9 and 10, preliminary and final closing of the capsules; 11, ejection of the filled capsules 12, vacuum-cleaning the capsule segments.

HÖFLIGER AND KARG MACHINES

All the machines produced by this company have an intermittent action. The range available is listed in Table 10.5. Capsule sizes from 0 to 4, either regular or self-locking, can be filled on the standard machines, and sizes 00 and 5 can be filled to special order.

The GKF 2400 is a twin GKF 1200 with two filling heads. The GKF 70 is no longer available.

A schematic diagram of the general arrangement of all the machines is shown in Fig. 10.14, and the tamping method for forming the plug and filling the capsule body is shown in Fig. 10.15. The empty capsules are loaded into the storage hopper. They are mechanically orientated and then transferred to the segments on the machine by suction. They are forced slowly downwards by plungers which give a slow effective rate of insertion of the capsules into the segment, and prevent damage

Table 10.5. Höfliger and Karg machines

Model	Output capsules/minute	Number of holes per segment
GKF 70	70	1
GKF 330	330	3
GKF 602	635	6
GKF 1200	1270	12
GKF 2400	2540	2×12

to the bodies. Separation occurs in the segment at station 2. At station 3 the upper segments are lifted away and moved inward to prevent over-long capsule bodies from being damaged. The fourth station is for use with a filling unit to insert tablets, pellets, or coated tablets into the capsules.

The powder is fed from a reservoir hopper to a vertical feed-screw which transports it to the actual filling hopper (station 5). A proximity switch keeps the level in the filling hopper constant

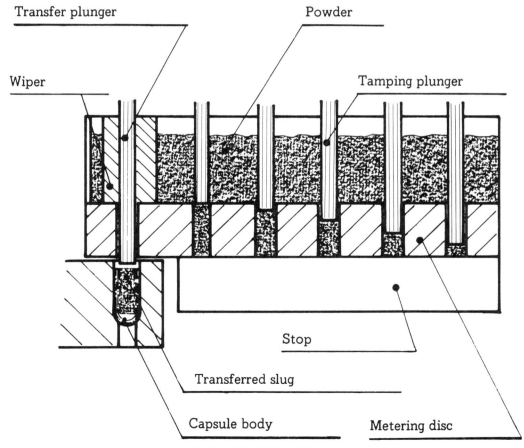

Fig. 10.15. Schematic diagram of the tamping principle of the GKF machines.

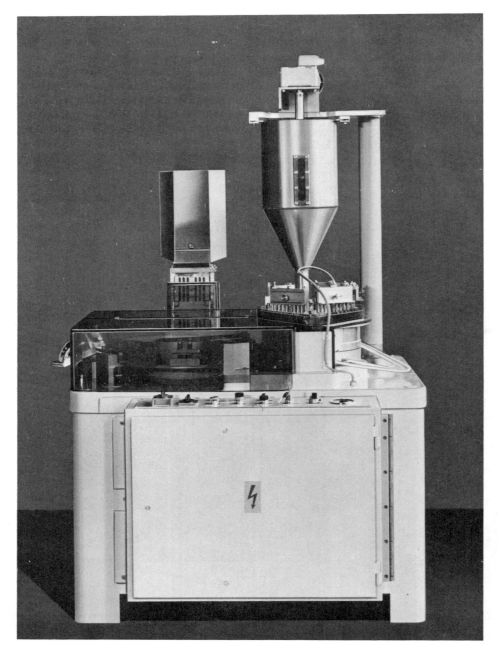

Fig. 10.16. The GKF 602 automatic capsule-filling machine.

by switching the feed-screw on and off. The filling hopper base surrounds the entire filling disk, which contains holes corresponding to the volume to be filled.

Five sets of filling plungers compact the powder slowly, using one tamp per cycle. The plunger pressure is variable, but is generally between 1 and 5 kg. The filling plunger sets can be adjusted individually by using the scales marked on the plungers. Two vertically moving columns with ball bushings support the bridge with the five sets of filling and transfer plungers, the latter being sealed inside the filling hopper by a pressure guide. The filling plungers and their guides can easily be removed for cleaning. At the fifth station of the capsule transport wheel, the filled holes in the disk pass over the capsule bodies, and the product is then transferred to the bodies by the transfer plungers. If a capsule body is missing at this point, the powder goes into a collecting container. More powder can be added, if required, at station 6. The caps, held in the segments, are inspected at station 7. If a capsule has not been opened, or was inserted incorrectly, it is automatically rejected here. At station 8 the segments holding the caps are located over the capsule bodies, and capsule closure occurs at stations 9 and 10, where

push rods raise the capsule bodies into the caps. The closed capsules are ejected at station 11, and the segments are vacuum-cleaned before receiving empty capsules at station 12 to repeat the cycle.

Figures 10.16 and 10.17 illustrate the GKF 602 and GKF 2400 capsule fillers, respectively. The methods used for inserting tablets or pellets into the bodies are shown in Figs 10.18 and 10.19, and a general view of a GKF machine equipped to fill two different types of pellet is shown in Fig. 10.20.

When tablets are to be inserted into capsules (Fig. 10.18), they leave the product hopper (1) and pass through the filling shaft for singling-out. They arrive in front of the slide (2) which pushes them over the capsule body (3), which is held in the segment (4). The tablet is detected by the pro-

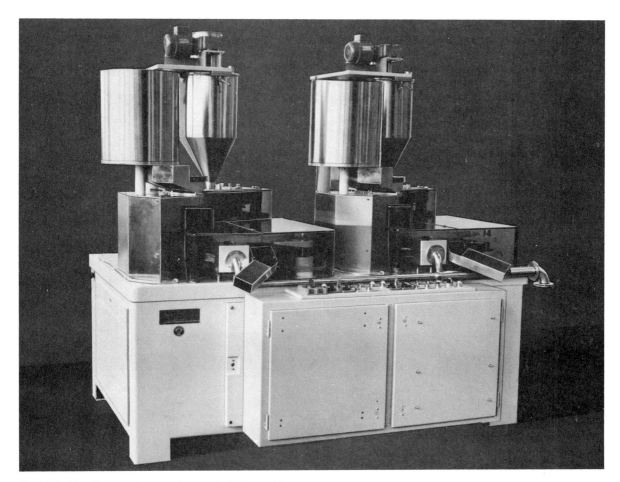

Fig. 10.17. The GKF 2400 automatic capsule-filling machine.

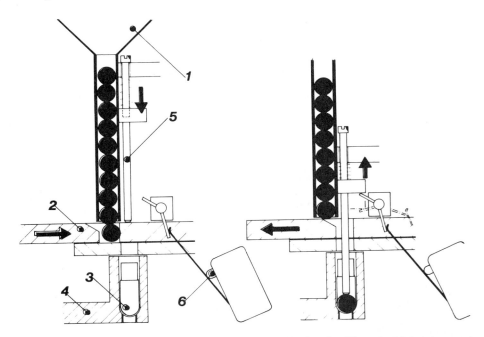

Fig. 10.18. Schematic diagram of the metering station of the GKF series for the filling of tablets into capsules. 1, product hopper; 2, slide; 3, capsule body; 4, capsule segment; 5, product sensor; 6, product-sensing microswitch.

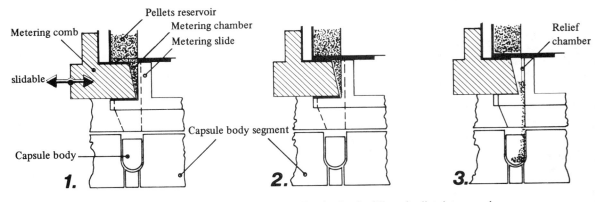

Fig. 10.19. Schematic diagram of the metering station of the GKF series for the filling of pellets into capsules.

duct sensor (5), which, in the absence of a tablet, operates the product-sensing microswitch (6). Capsules can be inserted by the same method.

The sequence for filling pellets is shown in Fig. 10.19, 1, 2, and 3. In the initial position, the storage hopper is located directly above the metering chamber, which is closed at the bottom end to prevent pellets entering the capsule or escaping before the correct dose is monitored. The meter-ing slide then closes the chamber entrance thus isolating it from the storage hopper.

In the third stage, the top of the closing chamber remains closed whilst the metering segment is moved, thus opening the outlet and permitting pellets to enter the capsule body. A small air relief chamber allows air to escape from the capsule body and permits unhindered dosing.

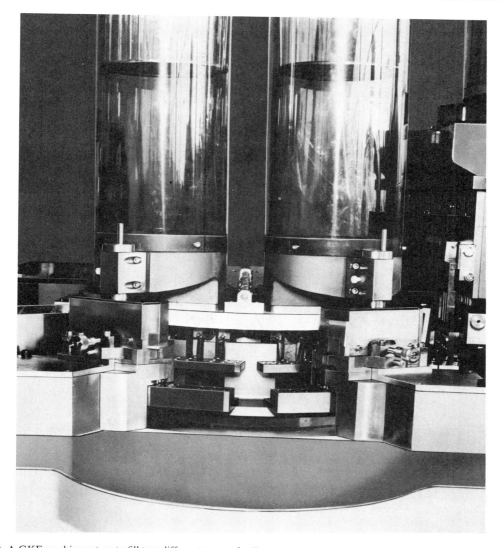

Fig. 10.20. A GKF machine set up to fill two different types of pellet.

THE HARRO HÖFLIGER MACHINE

A small machine based on the same filling principle as the GKF range is manufactured by Harro Höfliger. This machine, the KFM III, is useful for development and formulation work. It is illustrated in Fig. 10.21, and can fill powder, pellets, tablets, and liquids, or a combination of dosage forms, up to a filling speed of 50 capsules per minute.

Continuous Motion Machines

The mG2 Company is generally credited with the production of the first commercially available continuous motion capsule filler. Arthur Colton's first attempt, described in U.S. Patent 1 077 392 (1913), does not appear to have been developed, probably due to his preoccupation with the semi-automatic Colton 8 machine.

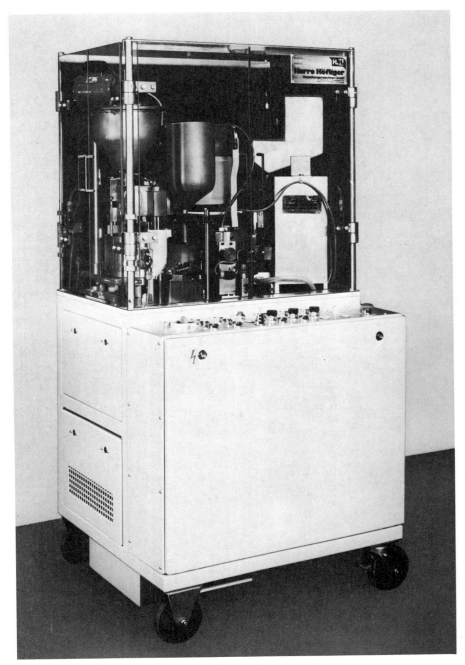

Fig. 10.21. The Harro Höfliger KFM III automatic capsule-filling machine.

The mG2 range of models is based on their highly successful G36, available in three versions designated G36/4, G36/2, and G36, with respective outputs of 9000, 18 000, and 36 000 capsules per hour. The output doubles from one model to the next, but there is the designed-in advantage that the same drive, control panel, and body can be used, and theoretically it is possible to increase

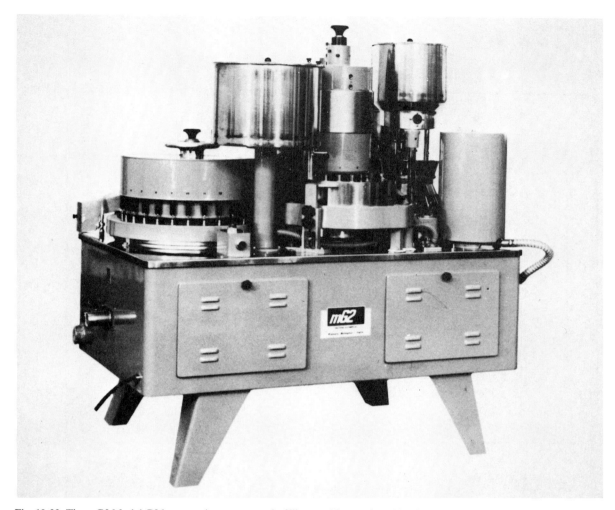

Fig. 10.22. The mG2 Model G36 automatic rotary capsule-filling machine equipped for filling granules and powder.

output simply by replacing units on the machine. Models with higher output, G37 and G38, are also made, and provide output capacities of up to 100 000 capsules per hour.

The mG2 Model G36

A general view of the G36 is shown in Fig. 10.22, and the basic layout is illustrated in Fig. 10.23. Each of the numbered units is linked by a continuous chain which supports and transports the capsule holders. Capsules are tipped into the empty-capsule feed hopper (1), which has been designed for easy cleaning and change-over. It has two parts, one fixed and one moveable, and can be adjusted in height to enable different-sized capsules to enter the feed tubes. The capsules are

orientated by using a drum of the type shown in Fig. 10.24. This uses the centrifugal force to ensure that the bodies of the capsules always enter the capsule holders first.

The drum is split into two halves, and on its underside are transfer tubes which must be lined up with the capsule holders, only one capsule being fed into the drum at a time. A lever, attached to a pillar outside the drum, can be used to stop the flow of empty capsules into the orientation drum.

The capsules are fed into the capsule holders (Fig. 10.25) which transport them to each of the functional stations in succession. Once the shell is in the holder it can be separated by vacuum into body and cap. The holder consists of two

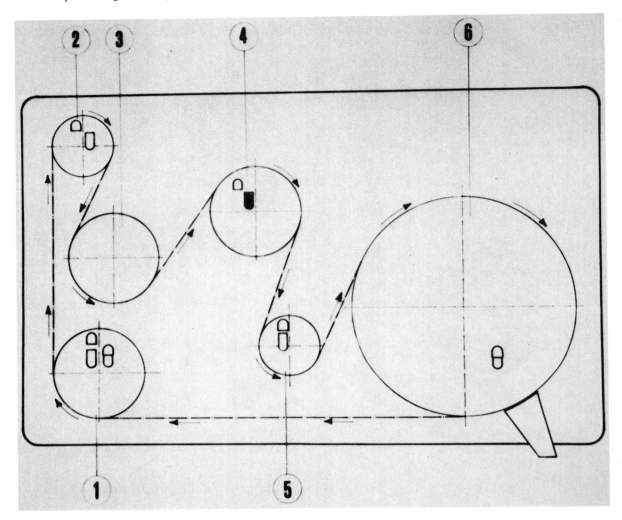

Fig. 10.23. Schematic diagram of the operation of the mG2 Model G36 machine. 1, empty-capsule feed hopper; 2, capsule separation; 3, pellet- or tablet-dosing unit; 4, powder-dosing unit; 5, reunion of capsules; 6, closing of capsules.

parts, the upper punch bush (2), which holds the cap, and the lower bush (1) which holds the body. By removing the upper bush and placing it on the opposite side of the chain, the capsule is separated into the two parts, which takes place at station (2) (Fig. 10.23). At the next station, (3), tablets or pellets are inserted into the capsule.

At station 4, powder is filled into the capsule body using the compression dosator method of filling. The rotating-ring type of powder hopper is shown in Fig. 10.26.

The hopper rotates at the same speed as the dosators, which take powder from it to fill the capsules. To maintain a constant depth, additional powder is fed from a bulk container positioned above the machine.

The adjustment of the dosage depends on two factors: firstly, the depth of powder in the filling hopper and, secondly, the setting of the piston within the dosator. The dosator setting is controlled by a single wheel, shown on top of the unit in Fig. 10.30, whilst the depth of the powder in the hopper is controlled by a levelling device similar to a weir, Fig. 10.27 (B).

The powder depth may be varied by loosening the two knobs shown in Fig. 10.27 (A) and raising or lowering the block depending on whether an increase or decrease in the weight is required. A

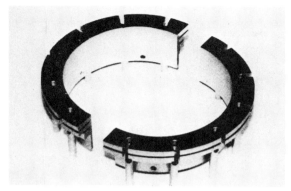

Fig. 10.24. The orientation drum of the mG2 Model G36 machine.

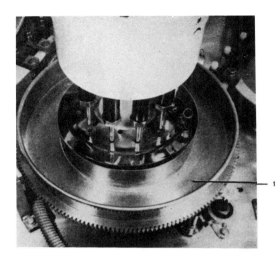

Fig. 10.26. The powder hopper of the mG2 Model G36 machine.

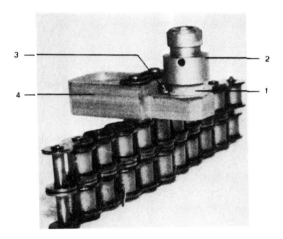

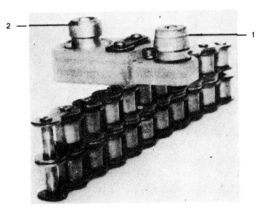

Fig. 10.25. The capsule holders of the mG2 model G36 machine. 1, lower bush; 2, upper punch bush; 3, screw; 4, block.

scale is provided, and there is another on the dosator piston control. A mixing device is provided inside the hopper which ensures a homogeneous mixture, and also that freshly added powder is mixed into that already present. Also, if the powder has poor flow properties, areas of reduced density will occur and tend to persist where the dosator has removed a plug of powder. The agitator eliminates these.

From the filling station the capsules pass to the unification station (5, Fig. 10.23) where the top bush holding the cap is placed back on the body-holding section. The body is then pushed into the cap by a rod from beneath. The height to which this rod rises may be adjusted to ensure a tightly fitted capsule of the correct overall length. The filled capsule is then ejected from the machine. Any capsule which has failed to separate initially and so has remained empty is diverted away from the main capsule receiver by an air jet and a suction device.

The capsule holder and chain now pass through a cleaning section which removes dust and capsules which have failed to be ejected from the machine. When using granules or pellets in the rotating hopper the mixing device should be removed.

If pellets are to be filled, a special unit is fitted at position (3) of Fig. 10.23, which is illustrated in Fig. 10.28, and can be used on all versions of the G36. The principle of the operation is shown in Fig. 10.29. Two chambers are provided which

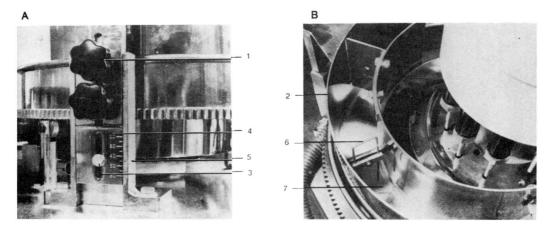

Fig. 10.27. Powder-depth control in the hopper of the mG2 Model G36 machine. A, the adjustment knobs; B, the levelling device. 1, weir-adjustment locking knob; 2, powder hopper; 3, locking nut; 4, powder-adjustment block; 5, adjustment and locking support; 6, weir mixing device; 7, base of hopper.

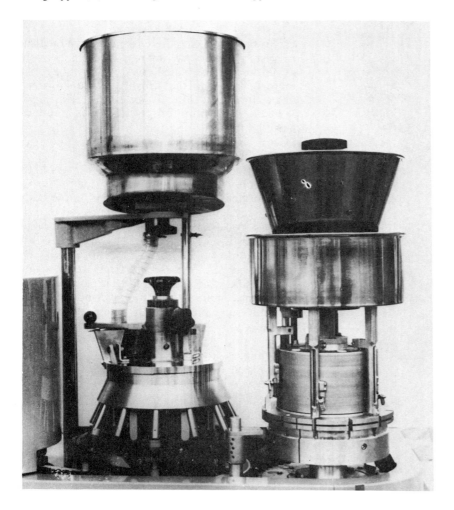

Fig. 10.28. The dosing unit for granules and pellets of the mG2 Model G36.

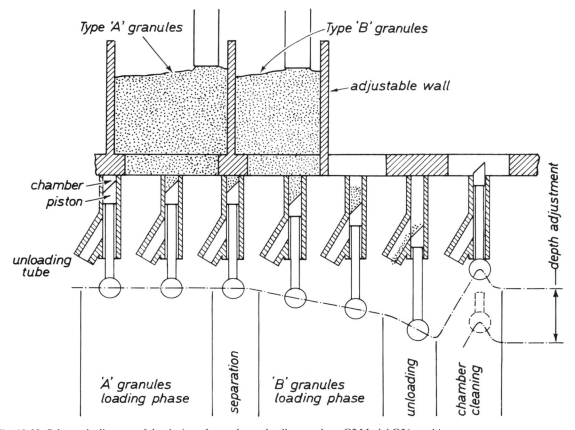

Fig. 10.29. Schematic diagram of the dosing of granules and pellets on the mG2 Model G36 machine.

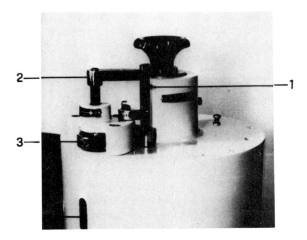

Fig. 10.30. The weight and pressure controls of the mG2 model G36 machine. 1, scale; 2, compression index; 3, adjuster.

allow two different types of pellet to be filled. Various combinations of pellets may be filled by putting mixed granules in one or both chambers. Graduated scales are provided to ensure accurate measurement of the dosage, and the unit can also be used in conjunction with a powder unit. Units are available for the following size combinations. For ready-mixed pellets: capsule size (000–00–0–1), (0–1–2–3), or (2–3–4–5).

For separated pellets: capsule size (000), (00–0), (1), (2–3), (4), or (5).

One of the main advantages of the continuous motion principle is the ease with which weight and pressure adjustments can be made. Fig. 10.30 shows the controls that are positioned at the top of the machine.

The pressure applied to the dosator piston may be regulated, using the adjuster (3), on a scale (1). The compression should never exceed 8 mm on this scale. Fine adjustments to the weight may be made using the single wheel on top and major

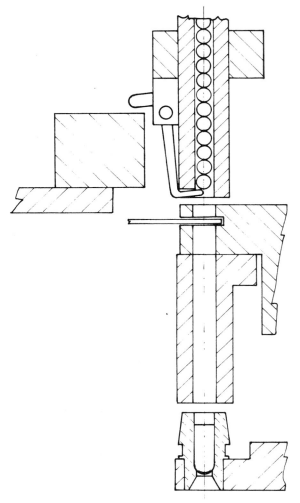

Fig. 10.31. Schematic diagram of the method of filling tablets into capsules on the mG2 Model machine.

of the upper or lower closing stations, in which case the capsule feed tubes may be at fault. The orientation plate at the bottom of the feed tube must be set so that it presses the body of the capsule approximately 1 mm from the bottom edge of the cap. Faulty opening of capsules at the capsule feed station is usually indicated by an irregular noise which is normally caused by a fragment of a capsule being stuck in the holder. The same effect is caused by the jamming of dirty capsule feed stop springs. A leaky vacuum system may be a contributory factor.

The most frequent cause of problems is the feeding of empty capsules. It may be that there has been damage to the empty shell, which is more common when the capsules have been printed. The capsule release lever may have become jammed, or there may be fragments of broken capsules in the feed tubes. Faulty separation is usually due to a blocked vacuum cleaning nozzle, the need to clean the vacuum filter, or simply that the capsules are too tight to be separated efficiently.

In the dosing system, it is quite possible that the small hole at the top of the dosator may become blocked. This is easily remedied by a blast of compressed air. The springs inside the dosator may break, or there may be damage to the tip of the dosator. This is usually caused by incorrect settings resulting in the tip touching another part of the powder hopper. One consequence of this is breakage of the plug of powder as it leaves the dosator so that the fill-weight is inaccurate.

The level of powder in the dosage hopper and uniformity of the powder density are of major importance in maintaining weight consistency. The correct positions for the level and mixing devices for each individual powder can only be found by trial.

THE mG2 MODEL G38
This machine is shown in Fig. 10.34. It has 20 dosing nozzles of the compression type, with vacuum transfer and suction opening of capsules. The machine head can be raised and lowered mechanically to make cleaning and capsule size changing easier. Adjustments to the compression and the fill-weight may be made from controls on the top of the machine. A screw feeder automatically feeds powder from a large reservoir container to the rotary hopper. Unopened capsules and empty bushes are detected and rejected automatically. The machine is totally enclosed in

changes in weight are best made by altering the depth of powder in the rotation trough.

The method used to insert tablets into capsules is shown in Fig. 10.31, and Fig. 10.32 illustrates some of the combinations that may be used. Fig. 10.33 shows a unit used to fill four tablets into a capsule.

There are a number of problems which can arise with mG2 machines. For instance, a capsule may be crushed. This may be due to the use of capsule cap holders which have too large a diameter hole, so that the body edge can meet the cap edge, and the obvious remedy is to replace the holders. Crushing may also be caused by incorrect settings

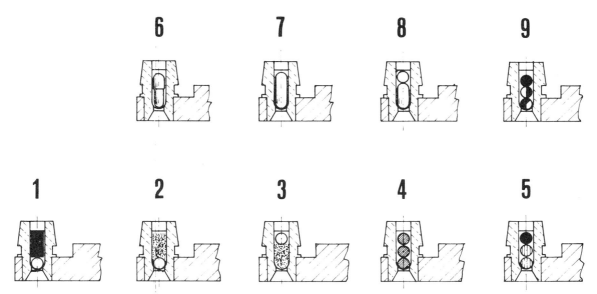

Fig. 10.32. Various combinations of products that can be filled into capsules on mG2 equipment. 1, one tablet and powder; 2, one tablet and pellets; 3, pellets and one tablet; 4, three identical tablets; 5, three tablets of which two are identical; 6, one small capsule inside larger body; 7, one capsule-shaped tablet; 8, one capsule-shaped and one round tablet; 9, three different tablets.

Fig. 10.33. An mG2 Model G36 machine equipped to fill four different tablets.

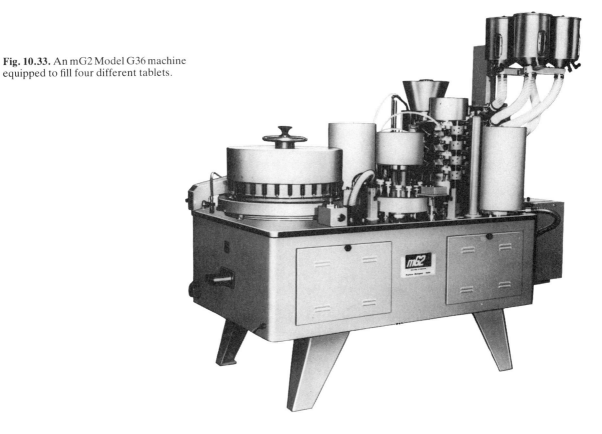

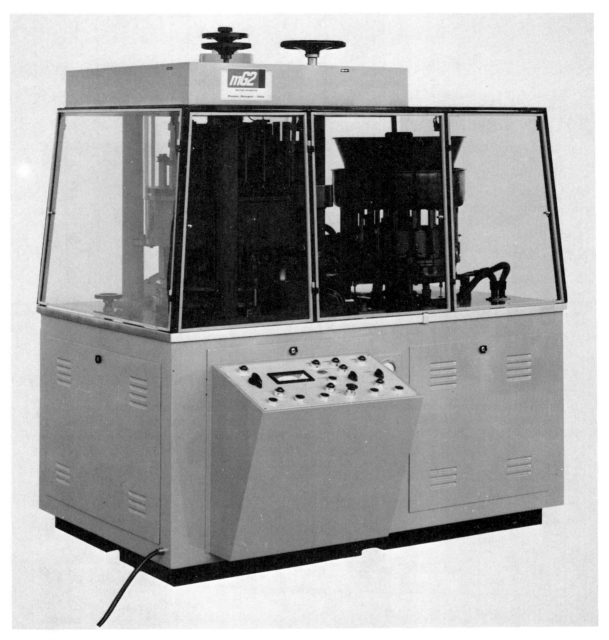

Fig. 10.34. The mG2 Model G38 automatic rotary capsule-filling machine.

a transparent plexiglass unit, and its operation will now be described.

Empty capsules are fed into the large hopper (1) shown in Fig. 10.35. They move under gravity into the tubes (2), and are orientated by two blades to the body-downwards position, and are dropped into the orientation drum (3) below, which retains each capsule in the drum by means of the vacuum applied by two suction nozzles (4). The flow of capsules can be stopped by operating the lever (5).

The drum (3) holds the empty capsules until

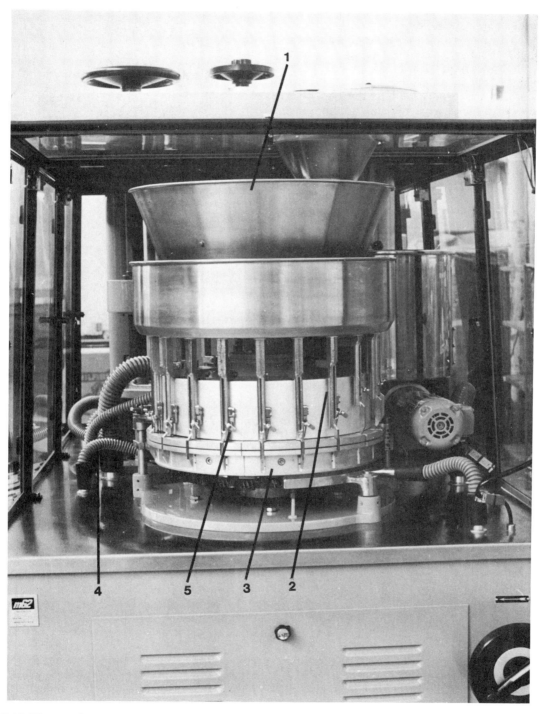

Fig. 10.35. The capsule storage and supply unit of the mG2 Model G38 machine. 1, empty-capsule hopper; 2, capsule feed tubes; 3, orientation drum; 4, suction nozzles; 5, lever.

they are required and then, by means of vacuum directed through the suction nozzles (4), feeds them into an appropriate bush.

The separation of the capsule into body and cap is brought about by vacuum. The capsule body partly falls and is partly drawn into the body-holding bush, which is supported by a transparent block, whilst the cap is held in the cap bush. Unopened capsules are ejected and their presence is indicated by a warning light on the machine control panel. Ejected faulty capsules are collected in a container, together with any that have two caps. In this last case the bottom closing pins eject the faulty capsules on their upward stroke. After separation, the transport blocks, carrying the bushes holding the capsule bodies, are aligned with a filling nozzle which takes powder from the rotary hopper and puts it into the body. After the filling operation each capsule body is reunited with its cap. An overhead stop pin holds the cap securely while the bottom closing pin pushes the body into the cap. This latter pin is adjustable so that the closed capsules are all brought to a uniform overall length. To eject the filled capsules from the machine the overhead stop is raised and the bottom closing pin allowed to continue on its up-stroke, thus lifting the capsule clear of the bush. The transport bushes are then cleaned by suction to remove any residual powder and capsule fragments before the next operating cycle commences.

There is an automatic mechanism to keep the rotary hopper full of powder. The powder is placed in the main hopper (1) (Fig. 10.36). At the bottom of this hopper there is a mixing blade which stirs the powder continuously, and it is fed to the rotary hopper using a screw feeder in a box (2) operated by a geared motor (3). Figure 10.37 shows that inside the rotary hopper there is a levelling unit (2) which provides a constant depth of powder. It is made up of a float gauge (3), connected to two magnetic sensors acting as high- and low-level probes, and operated by the vertical movement of the float. If the level of powder falls below the bottom probe the machine will stop.

The operation of changing the machine to accommodate another size of capsule is easy to perform, and involves replacing the following parts: the capsule feeding tubes, orientation drum, transfer drum, and cap and body bushes, together with the filling nozzles and their pistons and springs.

Different types of capsule, such as regular, and those with special locking and handling mecha-

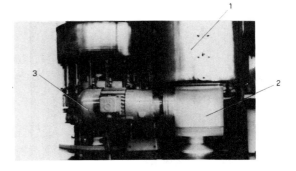

Fig. 10.36. The main powder hopper of the mG2 model G38 machine. 1, main powder hopper; 2, box containing screw feeder; 3, motor.

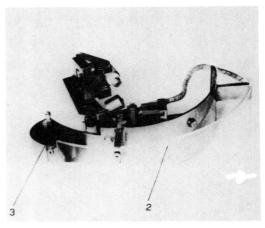

Fig. 10.37. The levelling unit inside the rotary powder hopper of the mG2 Model G38 machine. 2, levelling unit; 3, float gauge.

nisms, in their different sizes, require different degrees of vacuum to separate them into bodies and caps. The machine is supplied with a vacuum gauge, linked to the vacuum pump filter, so that the appropriate adjustments can be made. The vacuum is indicated on a dial in cm Hg (Fig. 10.38). To determine the current setting press the button (1), when the vacuum level will be registered on the dial (2).

For short or slow movements, such as might be needed during setting-up of the machine, two hand-wheels are provided (Fig. 10.39), which must only be rotated in the direction indicated. The hand-wheel (1) rotates the upper unit while the second hand-wheel on the side of the machine rotates the lower unit. If powder is present in the

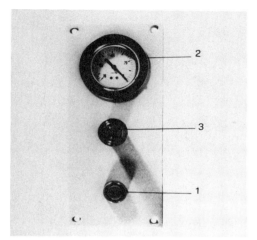

Fig. 10.38. The vacuum dial and adjustment control of the mG2 model G38 machine. 1, button; 2, dial 3, vacuum adjuster.

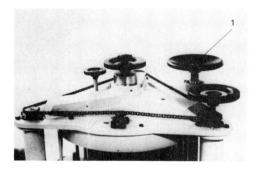

Fig. 10.39. The hand-wheels for rotating the upper and lower units of the mG2 Model G38 machine. 1, hand-wheel rotating the upper unit.

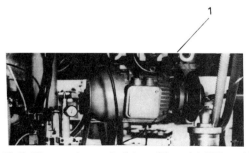

Fig. 10.40. The speed control of the mG2 model G38 machine, 1, speed adjuster.

hopper and dosators are fitted the vacuum pump should also be operated. It is important to note that if the machine is rotated in the wrong direction damage may occur to some parts.

A thyristor speed control is fitted, which permits the best operating speed to be selected for a particular product (Fig. 10.40). Sometimes a slight variation in fill-weight may result from a change in speed, and the dosators may need to be adjusted to restore the correct dosage.

The G38 may be fitted with a granule or pellet dosing unit, as illustrated in Fig. 10.41, which can

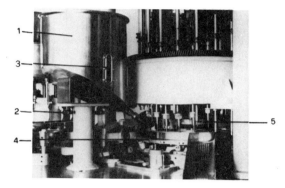

Fig. 10.41. The granule feed hopper of the mG2 model G38 machine, 1, granule feed hopper; 2, hand-knobs; 3, hopper sight glass; 4, rotary hopper; 5, dosators.

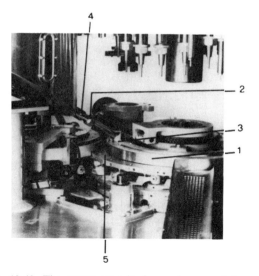

Fig. 10.42. The rotary granule dosage hopper of the mG2 Model G38 machine, 1, rotary hopper; 2, granule feed tube; 3, product exit hole; 4 winged screw; 5, turntable.

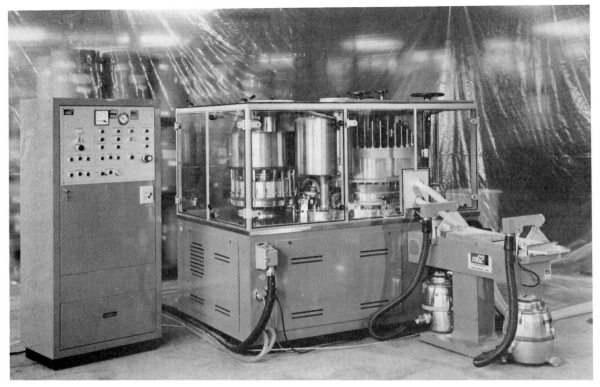

Fig. 10.43. The mG2 Model G37/N automatic rotary capsule-filling machine together with control console and filled-capsule selector.

be used in place of the powder dosing system. The granules or pellets are placed in a large hopper (1), secured by two large hand-knobs (2), to the frame of the machine. From the hopper they fall under gravity into the rotary hopper (1), Fig. 10.42.

The cylinder (3) (Fig. 10.42) through which the product leaves the rotary hopper is designed to give a measured dose. The feed into the rotary hopper may be stopped or started by using the winged screw (4). The level of granules may be checked by using the hopper sight glass (3) (Fig. 10.41). The dosing chambers are filled under gravity and closed by a set of plates.

During the capsule-filling operation, further granules are prevented from entering the dosing chamber by a scraper plate. The bottom plate on the dosing chamber is then moved and granules enter the capsule body. The filled capsule body then passes to the capsule joining and closing station. Granules which are not filled because of the absence of a body are collected by a vacuum-operated nozzle.

mG2 Model G37/N

This is a rotary continuous motion machine with an output of up to 100 000 capsules per hour. It is equipped with attachments for the automatic filling of powders, pellets, and tablets or a combination of dosage forms. The machine is suitable for use with a centralised 'in-house' vacuum and compressed air system. It is equipped with a fully interlocked hardened glass protective screen, sound-proofed to 80 dB(A).

Various views of the machine are shown in Figs 10.43–10.47. Figure 10.43 is a general view of the G37/N with control console and filled-capsule selector; Fig. 10.44 shows the panel of the control console; Fig. 10.45 shows the empty-capsule feed station; Fig. 10.46 shows the dosing station with the dosators in the raised position, and Fig. 10.47 shows some detail of filled capsules ready for ejection, and the annular powder-dosing hopper.

The numbering sequence of the mG2 machines is rather illogical, since the G37 is a larger-capacity machine than the G38. The G37 has an output of 60 000 to 100 000 capsules per hour and can

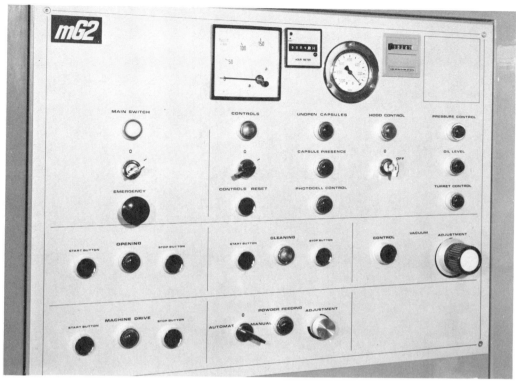

Fig. 10.44. The panel of the control console of the mG2 Model G37/N machine.

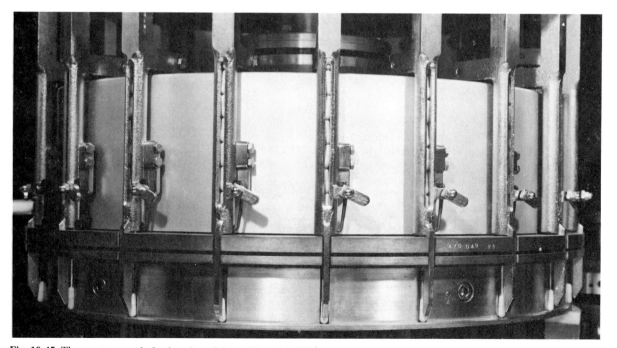

Fig. 10.45. The empty-capsule feed station of the mG2 model G37/N machine.

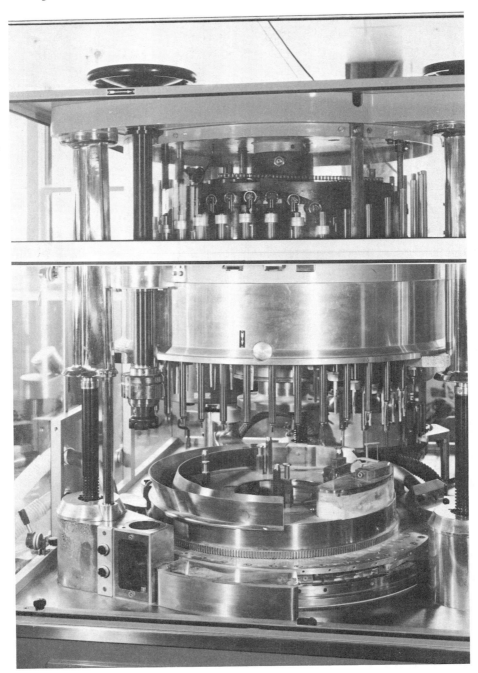

Fig. 10.46. The dosing station of the mG2 model G37/N machine. The dosators are shown in the raised position.

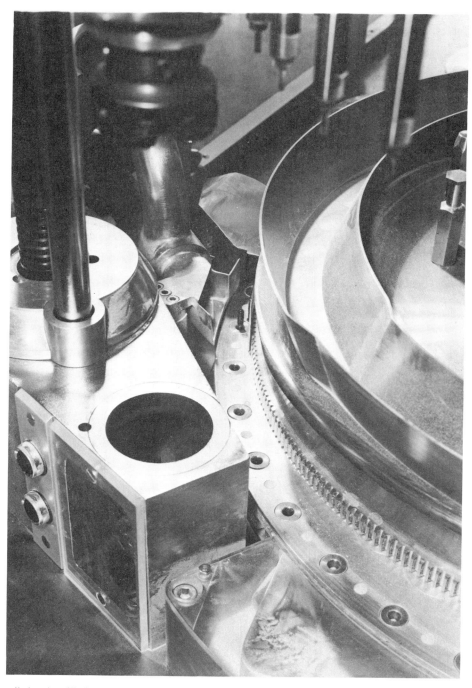

Fig. 10.47. Detail showing filled capsules ready for ejection and the annular powder-dosing hopper on the mG2 model G37/N machine.

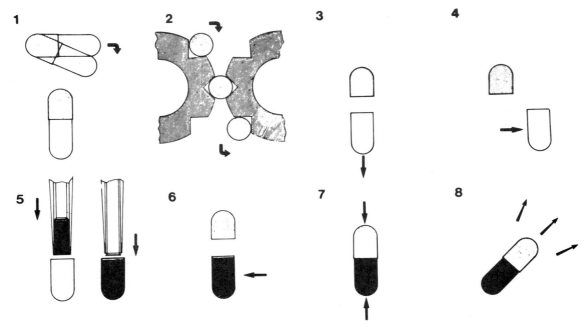

Fig. 10.48. The operating cycle of the mG2 Model G37/N machine. 1, capsule rectification; 2, transfer; 3, separation; 4, alignment for filling; 5, filling; 6, alignment for closing; 7, closing; 8, ejection.

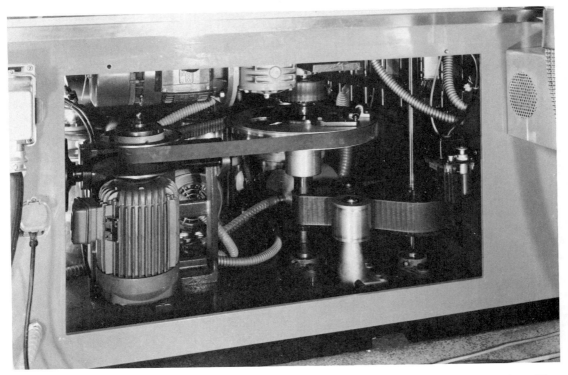

Fig. 10.49. The main drive motor, situated below the empty-capsule feed station and powder hopper, on the mG2 model G37/N machine.

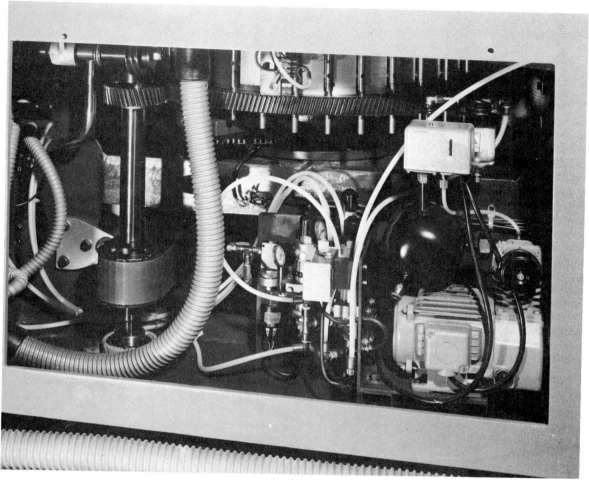

Fig. 10.50. The drive system for the annular powder-dosing hopper on the mG2 model G37/N machine.

handle capsules of sizes 00 to 5.

The operating cycle is shown in Fig. 10.48. During the capsule rectification stage, open capsules, capsules with two caps, and capsules which fail to orientate are automatically ejected without interruption of the filling cycle. Capsules are retained in a slot in the transfer disk by vacuum applied through a hole in the slot. This reduces the possibility of crushed capsules during the transfer to the filling hopper. Powder is maintained at a constant level in the central filling hopper by the high- and low-level probes fixed in the wall of the hopper. Unopened capsules are automatically rejected.

The annular powder-dosing hopper is designed

in such a way that the dosator picks up powder from a fresh position in the powder bed on each cycle. This enables the density of the powder bed to be kept uniform, which reduces the weight variation of the filled capsules. The NT/1 computer station enables samples of capsules from individual dosators to be selected and weighed. Two views of the main drive motor and drive mechanism are shown in Figs 10.49 and 10.50.

The model G37 capsule filler may be used in conjunction with several pieces of equipment which improve its overall performance, such as the empty-capsule pre-sorter, model SV/LV1 (Fig. 10.51).

This unit can be equipped with an automatic

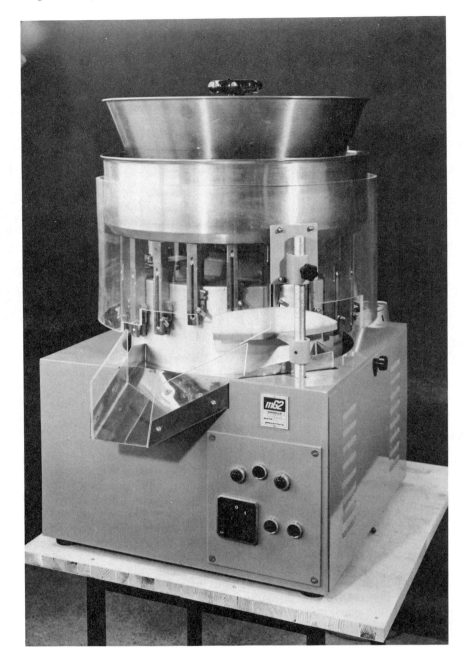

Fig. 10.51. The Model SV/LV1 empty-capsule pre-sorter which may be connected to the mG2 Model G37/N machine.

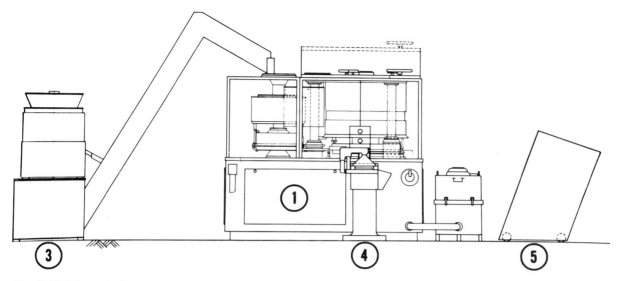

Fig. 10.52. Schematic diagram showing the attachment of ancillary equipment to the mG2 Model G37/N capsule-filling machine. 1, G37/N; 3, SV/LV1 empty-capsule pre-sorter with automatic loader to the capsule filler; 4, SC filled-capsule selector; 5, VR/1 computer which incorporates the NT/1 dosator sampling device.

loader to the capsule filler, which is not illustrated, but is schematically shown in the layout plan in Fig. 10.52.

Figure 10.53 shows the model SC filled-capsule selecting machine. This enables the filled capsules to be inspected when they are ejected from the capsule filler, so that they can be de-dusted and any empty and broken capsules can be removed.

Figure 10.54 shows a typical print-out. The VR/1 statistically controls the capsule weight during the working cycle of the capsule filler. It is programmable, and individual weights from each dosator are included in the print-out. These weights are summarised as required by the programme and the number of samples weighed can be quoted, together with the average weight, coefficient of variation, and standard deviation. Each sub-lot is recorded and the total for the day summarised. A feedback to the machine can also be provided to control the weight and the pressure exerted to form the plug during the filling cycle.

The importance of this unit lies in the print-out produced, which shows the weight of individual capsules and the mean weight of random selected samples. This print-out, and the summary of the day's production, could be used for analytical batch records. The balance used to weigh samples is a conventional analytical balance modified to provide an output to a desk-top computer.

When the system is started, the programme, supplied by the manufacturer, requires the operator to insert a series of data (date, time, batch number, theoretical weight, tolerances, etc.) used both for the processing of the gathered data and for the printing of the record document (sub-container and container records). When the operator inserts the last required datum, the system automatically commands the sequential selection and weighing of the capsules from individual dosators until the weighing cycle is completed.

The computer prints out the weight of each individual capsule and the number of the dosator from which it was filled, and indicates out-of-tolerance weights. The system processes the gathered information and compares the results with the chosen acceptance criteria.

An alarm system and automatic stopping mechanism of the capsule filler may be fitted. The system gives an alarm signal whenever a capsule is outside the tolerance limits. The capsule filler is automatically stopped when the production quality is outside the pre-set limits for weight variation. The frequency of the record print-out is variable and is decided when the system is started; the frequency will vary according to the operative conditions and the limits imposed by the control programme.

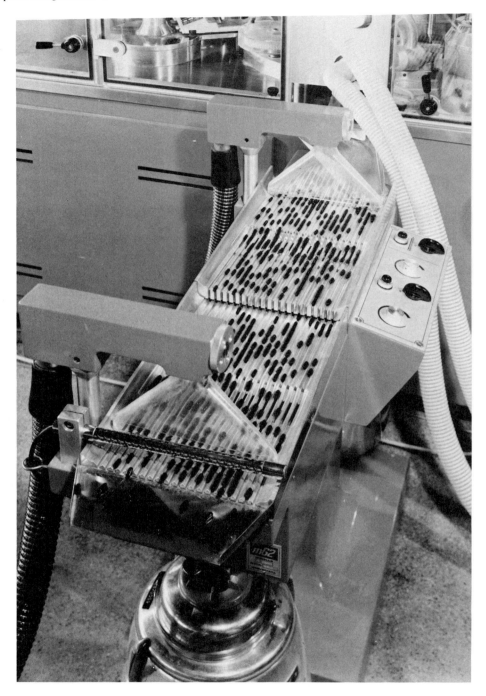

Fig. 10.53. The Model SC filled-capsule selector which may be connected to the mG2 Model G37/N machine.

```
DATE                        15
DAY/MONTH              0.433
        5.02                16
HOUR                   0.438
        9.00                17
LOT N.                 0.431
        0                   18
CODE N.                0.441
        8805                19
THEORIC WEIGHT         0.441
        0.435               20
TARE                   0.435
        0.099               21
UPPER TOLERANCE        0.434
LIMIT                       22
        0.453          0.439
LOWER TOLERANCE             23
LIMIT                  0.436
        0.417               24
UPPER SAFETY           0.441
LIMIT                       25
        0.468          0.436
LOWER SAFETY                26
LIMIT                  0.441
        0.402               27
DOSERS N.              0.443
        40                  28
SUB-LOTS/RECORD        0.441
(4 MAX.)                    29
        4              0.442
TIME UNIT                   30
        4              0.443
                 MISSING    31
YES=1                       31
NOT=0                  0.443
                            32
WEIGHT PRINTING        0.428
        1        REPORT       4
AUTOMATIC        AVERAGE  0.4367
CONTROLS         SD       0.0044
        1        CV%      0.997
                 MAX      0.446
AVERAGE CONTROL  MIN      0.426
                 RANGE    0.020
UPPER SAFETY     N            89
LIMIT (AVERAGE)
        0.438    F        0.01
LOWER SAFETY     C
LIMIT (AVERAGE)
        0.432

SAMPLING PLAN
PARAMETERS
(SUB-LOT)            * * * *
                    LOT RECORD
ALPHA%              * * * *
        5.00
P=ZERO%             TOTAL SUB-LOTS
        3.89
BETA%               DATE       5.02
        5.00        LOT N.        0
P-ONE%              CODE N.    8805
        10.00       AVERAGE   0.436
SAMPLE SIZE- N=     STD. DEV. 0.0047
        101         C. V. %   1.075
ACCEPT. CRIT. %-F=
        6.39        DEFECTIV.  0.02
***************     ACCEPT. CRIT. 8.02
UPPER AVERAGE
WARNING             WEIGHINGS   392
        0.437
LOWER AVERAGE       ================
WARNING
        0.433         ACCEPTED LOT
***************     ================
```

Fig. 10.54. A print-out from the Model VR/1 computer console.

THE PERRY ACCOFIL MODEL CF

The Perry Accofil (Perry Industries Inc.) has an output of 36 000, 48 000, or 60 000 capsules per hour according to which drive is selected from a three-pulley system. It is illustrated in Fig. 10.55.

The Accofil CF is built on a nickel-plated steel modular frame. The aluminium top plate is sheathed in a stainless steel skin, and the doors and machine side covers are stainless steel. There are no painted surfaces on the exterior of the machine, and all parts in contact with the product are made from stainless steel. The remaining parts that are exposed above the table top are made from either stainless steel, aluminium, or other materials approved by the FDA.

The machine has four rotating assemblies. These are the rectification, filling, and closing turrets, and the rotary powder hopper. The three turrets are linked together by a unique swing-like capsule-conveying system. The filling turret, closing turret, and powder pan are synchronously driven by a sprocket and timing-chain system located in the machine base. The rectifier has no moving parts but rotates because it is driven by the capsule-conveying system.

Capsules are fed into a bulk hopper mounted above the rotating rectifier turret. In the turret they meet a ring which oscillates as the whole rectifier rotates. This slight motion helps capsules to feed into 24 vertical tubes which lead them down towards the conveying chain. Around each of the vertical tubes are two large 'O' rings, which permit the timed escape of single capsules into the lower rectifying or orientation rings. At this point the capsules are not orientated: that is, either the cap or the body may be uppermost.

The lower rectifying rings have slots of such a size that only the body of the capsule can pivot through the outer part of the slot. The pivoting of the capsules is effected by the moving capsule being brought into contact with a stationary horizontal blade. As the capsules pass this blade, they pivot so that their bodies point away from the rectifier axis although they may lie either above or below the plane of the horizontal blade. When they have passed the blade they lie in an approximately horizontal position, bodies out, and they can then be gradually forced down by cams into a vertical, body-down, position.

A series of disks now move the capsules into a free position in the lower rectifying rings, where they sit on a drop plate. At this time in the cycle,

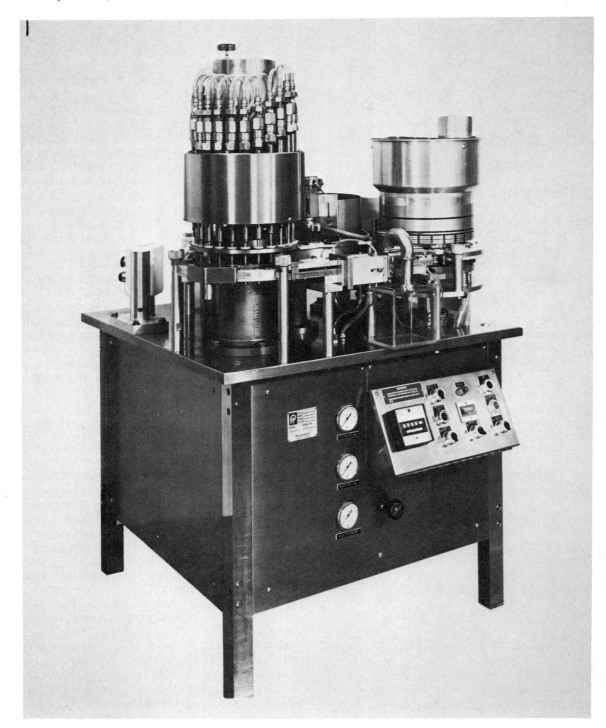

Fig. 10.55. The Perry Accofil model CF automatic rotary capsule-filling machine.

the capsules are drawn from the plate and picked up by the vacuum applied through each position in the capsule conveyor.

The conveyor is a stainless steel roller chain, which utilises the centre of the rollers as carriers for capsule-conveying bushings or pockets. Around each main bush is located a swing link, which contains another bushing and carrier pocket. The main bushing carries the capsule body, and the swing bushing, the capsule cap, the latter being automatically positioned in or of line by a guide-rail system.

The capsules can thus be separated, after which the cap bushing swings out of line for filling, then back into line for closing. This system ensures that each cap is reunited with the same body that it was with originally.

After the capsules have been transferred from the rectifier onto the conveyor and separated, they pass through the monitoring area, where a sensor checks that the capsule has been separated. This sensor is simply a spring-loaded cam which normally pushes the cap-carrying swing link to one side. Should the capsule not have been separated, the cam itself is displaced, allowing the cap bushing to approach a proximity sensor, which in turn activates a pneumatic circuit and ejects the non-separated capsule from the conveyor. Production can be maintained even though some damaged capsules may be found in the bulk supply.

A second sensor in the monitoring area tests for the presence of the capsule body. Should the capsule have been ejected due to non-separation, or should a bushing in the conveyor be empty due to a blockage in one of the rectifier tubes, this sensor will cause a signal to be relayed to the particular filling dosator which would normally have dosed powder into the empty bushing. That specific filling dose is then returned to the powder hopper before the dosator moves away from it. The machine thus has the useful property of 'no capsule, no fill'.

The powder-filling system consists of the rotary powder hopper and the filling turret. The basic machine has a bulk powder supply hopper, mounted on the left side of the machine. Its top is only 44 inches (1117.6 mm) from floor level, which means it can be replenished easily. The feed from the bulk supply to the rotary powder hopper is a fully-automatic screw type, actuated by a level-sensing paddle in the rotary hopper, which starts and stops the bulk feed supply as the need arises. This method of powder level control is as effective

with cohesive powders as it is with more free-flowing products.

The powder hopper rotates in a counter-clockwise direction, its path intersecting that of the filling head, which rotates in a clockwise direction. At the intersection point, the dosators descend into the powder hopper and pick up a predetermined amount of powder. As each dosator ascends to its exit position from the powder hopper, the excess product is cleaned from the end of the dosator and falls back into the powder hopper, eliminating waste. The dosator then moves to the dosing position. The powder hopper is designed to handle a wide range of powders of varying flow characteristics and densities. The hopper cover is stationary, which allows an inverted ramp to be positioned so as to pre-compact low-density products.

The filling turret has the 24 vertically operating, cam-controlled dosators already mentioned, rotating continuously. Vacuum and pressure are applied as required through a stationary valve plate. Beginning with an empty dosator, the cycle is as follows. (a) The dosator descends into the powder hopper, and vacuum is applied through a porous filter to pick up the powder by suction. This method is characteristic of the Accofil machine. (b) The application of vacuum is continued, to hold the dose during its ascent from the powder hopper. (c) The excess product is removed from the end of the dosator, whilst still maintaining the holding vacuum. (d) The dosator is moved until it is in position over the capsule to be filled. (e) The vacuum is cut and low-pressure air is applied to transfer the powder into the capsule. (f) High-pressure air is applied to purge the porous filter ready to begin the cycle again. The cycle is only interrupted if there is no capsule present in the conveyor, when the vacuum is cut and pressure applied between (b) and (c) which returns the dose into the powder hopper.

The dosator has three parts: outer needle, inner needle, and filter. The filter is attached to the end of the inner needle by a tongue-and-groove fitting. The inner needle screws into the outer needle and the adjustment of this thread gives the required filter depth setting. The whole assembly fits easily into a quick-release fitting secured to the needle carrier; another similar fitting allows the vacuum/pressure hose to be connected to the top of each inner needle. Removal of all 24 dosators can be effected in about four minutes. The dosator filters are pre-set to the required depth, and an adjustable gauge is provided with the machine to aid the setting up procedure.

The filters are made of a monofilament material and are comparatively free from blinding, especially since the applied purge pressure on every cycle ensures that the filter has a back-flow to keep the powder out. The filters are easily removable for cleaning at the end of a production batch, the simplest and preferred method of cleaning being the use of an ultrasonic bath.

After the capsule body has received the required dose of powder, it advances to the closing turret. During this advance, the swing link and cap bushing are gradually moved by a cam into position above the body bushing until, at the closing station, the capsule body busing and cap bushing are in vertical alignment. Cam-controlled closing pins gradually raise the body of the capsule through the lower portion of the cap bushing, until closure occurs, the upper plate of the closing turret retaining the capsule cap during this operation.

The filled, closed capsule now advances to the ejection station, where it is removed from the conveyor by means of air pressure. As it passes through the ejection tube, it is counted photo-electrically, and the total count is displayed digitally on the front control panel. Immediately following capsule ejection, the now empty swing link is moved to one side, and passes over a series of angled air jets which have a cyclonic cleaning effect on the bushings and links. After passing through the cleaning area, the conveyor bushing has completed one machine cycle.

Prior to dosator pick-up, the action of the pre-compaction ramp mounted on the powder pan cover, combined with the removal of entrapped air during the vacuum holding of powder in the dosator, stabilises the product density. This provides consistent fill-weights, after the initial pre-production calibration of each dosator by means of its screw.

There is an option available which enables capsules to be selected and automatically ejected from the machine for quality control purposes. The number of the dosator to be evaluated is push-button selected on the control panel, and a sample from it is then automatically ejected into a separate collector. Single samples from any of the 24 dosators may be taken, or 24 consecutive samples may also be taken in the same manner, all without stopping or interfering with normal production running.

In order to change from one product to another,

assuming that the same size capsule is to be used, it is necessary to remove the capsule conveyor, remove and disassemble the filling needles and filters, and remove the powder hopper and cover, the dust collector manifolds, and the bulk supply hopper. This procedure takes about 45 minutes.

All these components must be washed and dried. The guide rail system, rectifier turret, filling head wiper ring and bushings may all be cleaned in position. Replacement of the listed parts takes approximately the same amount of time as their removal.

The following parts need to be changed if the size of capsule is changed: the capsule conveyor, the rectifier turret, the dosators (although for sizes 2 and 3 capsules they are the same size), the closing pins and the wiper bushings, although these too are the same size for capsule sizes 2 and 3.

The Zanasi BZ-72

This machine will fill capsule sizes from 00 to 5, and has an output of 72 000 capsules per hour. It is small and compact for its output, designed to be readily accessible for cleaning and for the change-over of parts for different capsule sizes.

The machine as a whole, with its control console, is shown in Fig. 10.56. The principle used on this machine is a departure from the standard technique ysed by Zanasi. Its operation is very similar to the method used on the Perry Accofil machine and is shown in Fig. 10.57.

In (1), the capsule is shown on the left, having been separated into cap and body. The dosator has commenced its descent into the powder hopper. The end of the filling operation is shown in (2). The dosator has completed its downward motion and has compressed the powder between the dosator piston and the bottom of the powder hopper. In the next stage, (3), the dosator is raised out of the powder hopper, constant suction being applied inside the dosator to retain the powder during transfer to the empty capsule body. The cap is shown moving laterally to the left. Any excess powder is removed, (4), by a small scraper attached to the bush holding the capsule body. It is claimed that this ensures a dosage accuracy of within $\pm 2\%$. Suction is maintained during this transfer. When the dosator is located above the capsule body (5), the suction is removed and a very small positive pressure applied. At this point the piston has completed its downward stroke and ejected the powder into the capsule body. The positive pressure reduces the risk of losses and

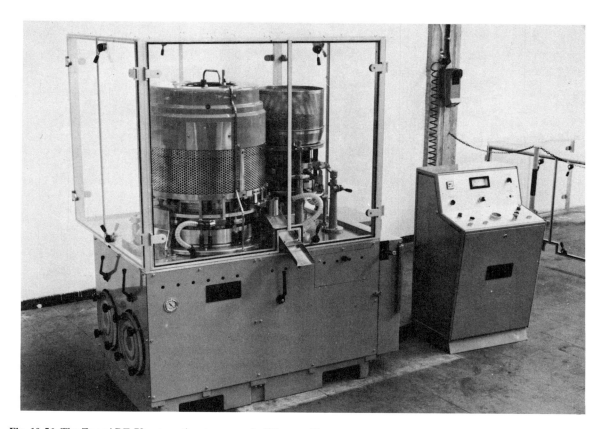

Fig. 10.56. The Zanasi BZ-72 automatic rotary capsule-filling machine.

of weight variation. The body and cap are then aligned and closed (6).

Pellets can be filled in a similar way. This vacuum-assisted method gives good weight consistency.

THE ZANASI BZ-150

This machine, illustrated in Fig. 10.58, has an output of up to 150 000 capsules per hour. It is a continuous motion machine, and is claimed to be suitable for powders, granules, and tablets.

A plan of the layout of the machine is shown in Fig. 10.59. The operating sequence is similar in some respects to the method of compressing tablets on a rotary tablet machine. The mechanisms of opening, filling, and closing the capsules are similar to those of the BZ-72. There is a central turret (1), an empty-capsule feed hopper (2), and a powder supply hopper (3), all supported on a rectangular base (4). The turret houses the annular powder trough into which powder is fed from the powder hopper, 72 bushes into which empty capsules are fed from the empty-capsule hopper, and 72 dosators to fill the capsules.

Powder flows from the powder hopper, aided by a single flat-bladed stirrer similar to that used in the AZ-60, into the central powder trough through a tube fitted with a screw feeder. The powder flow can be controlled (a) by a valve fitted in the tube, and (b) by the screw feeder being activated by high- and low-level probes fitted with a mixing device which ensures the uniformity of composition and density of the powder in the trough, despite the disturbance due to withdrawal of the powder plug. It is necessary to raise the turret to allow the trough to be emptied for cleaning, and also for fitting different bushes, pistons and dosators when a different size of capsule is to be filled.

The turret rotates at a maximum speed of 35 rpm, whilst the empty-capsule hopper rotates at 70 rpm as it has only 36 empty-capsule filling

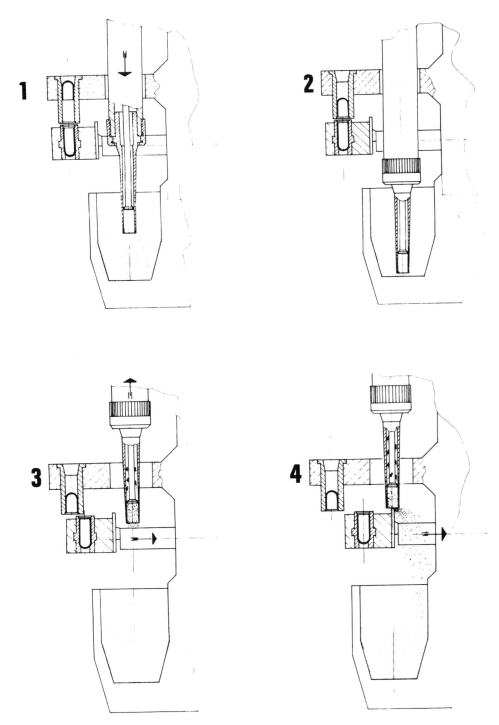

Fig. 10.57. Schematic diagram of the operation of the Zanasi BZ-72 capsule-filling machine. 1, capsule separation; 2, filling of the dosator; 3, removal of powder plug; 4, removal of excess fill; 5, ejection of powder into capsule body; 6, closing of the capsule.

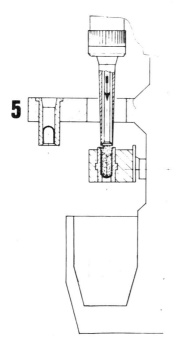

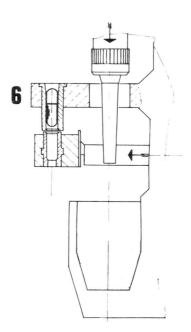

tubes. The hopper has a very low effective capacity considering its size, because the capsules tend to be thrown outwards by centrifugal force, which poses a problem of supply when the machine is running at full speed. The level of capsules in this hopper must be kept fairly low so that the operator can remove damaged capsules quickly when blockages occur in the feed tubes.

The following problems may occur in operating the machine.

1. The capacity of the empty-capsule hopper is low so that it requires replenishing too frequently.
2. The effect of damaged empty capsules is much more apparent on this machine than on, for example, the AZ-60. Since 2500 capsules are filled every minute, a defect level of only 0.04% will cause a feed tube blockage every minute.
3. The dust extraction and the number of cleaning points on the machine are not fully capable of dealing with the excess powder and the dust that are created during filling.
4. It is basically a single capsule-size machine. The estimated time for change-over to another size of capsule is of the order of one to two days. The change parts required are 72 dosators, pistons, bushes and push rods for ejecting the filled capsules, and 36 empty-capsule feed tubes.

Tables 10.6 and 10.7 show typical results obtained from filling a placebo formulation and an in-line product.

Figure 10.60 shows the layout of three BZ-150 machines at the Merck Sharp and Dohme plant at Cramlington, England.

Table 10.6. Statistical analysis of weight variation of two batches of capsules filled on the Zanasi BZ-150 encapsulation machine at 152 000 capsules per hour, taking three samples of each batch. The target weight was 300 mg.

Batch number	1	1	1	2	2	2
Mean weight (mg)	309.7	311.4	312.1	297.9	299.5	299.3
Degrees of freedom	62	57	59	58	55	55
Variance	37.64	25.82	54.65	128.21	77.47	56.51
Standard deviation (mg)	6.13	5.08	7.39	11.32	8.80	7.52
Coefficient of variation (%)	1.98	1.63	2.36	3.80	2.93	2.51

Table 10.7. Statistical analysis of one batch of capsules filled on the Zanasi BZ-150 encapsulation machine at a speed of 152 000 capsules per hour. The target weight was 290 mg.

Batch number	3	3	3
Mean weight (mg)	284.5	286.7	287.8
Degrees of freedom	60	60	60
Variance	65.91	44.65	70.45
Standard deviation (mg)	8.12	6.68	8.40
Coefficient of variation (%)	2.85	2.33	2.91

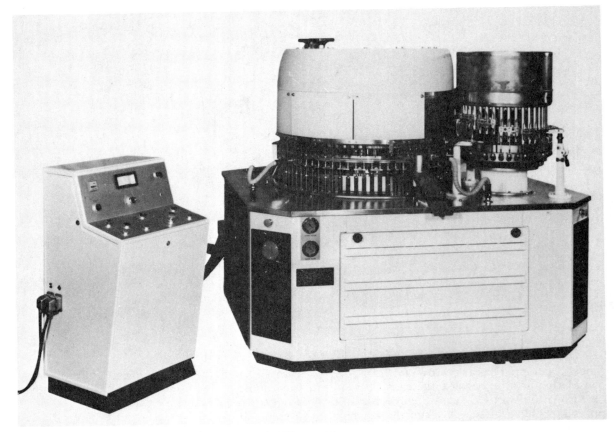

Fig. 10.58. The Zanasi BZ-150 automatic rotary capsule-filling machine.

THE ZANASI Z 5000 RANGE

The Zanasi BZ range of fillers has been replaced by the Z 5000-R series. One of these machines is illustrated in Fig. 10.61. There are three models, the Z 5000-R1, Z 5000-R2, and Z 5000-R3, with maximum outputs in capsules per hour of 70 000, 110 000, and 150 000, respectively.

The dimensions of the machines in this series have been reduced, and the control console has been attached to the main frame of the machine. A reduction in noise level to 79–85 dB(A) has been achieved. The d.c. motor of the BZ series has been replaced by an a.c. motor which requires less maintenance and is more reliable. A schematic diagram of the operation of the Z 5000 is shown in Fig. 10.62.

The control console incorporates a small built-in computer control system for a more detailed analysis of capsule weight. Any part of the machine which has a fault can be quickly identified by this system. The Siemens fan has been replaced by compressed air for the capsule transfer system, which has led to a reduction in noise level and in heat generation during capsule filling. A better guarding system is fitted, which is lighter, and which allows adjustment of weight and compression without removing the guard and stopping the machine. The two vacuum pumps have been replaced by one, with savings in noise, size, dimensions, and maintenance. Improvements have been made to the method of fitting the lower pins which assist in the opening, closing, and ejection of unseparated capsules. These pins cannot now free themselves during the operation of the machine and yet a quick change from one size to another can be accomplished without tools. A modification has also been made to the location of the upper and lower pins at the point where the cap and

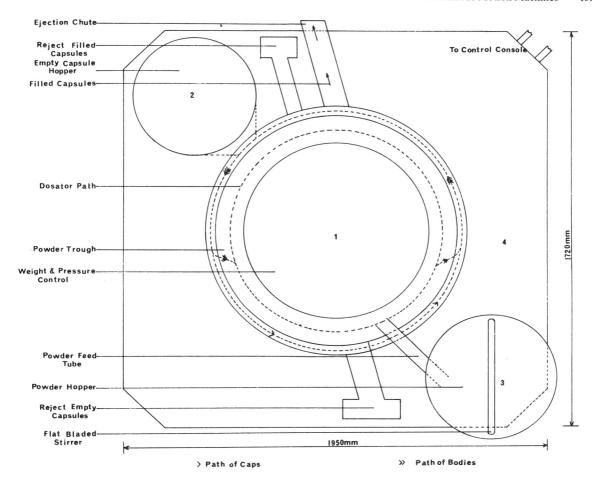

Fig. 10.59. Plan of the Zanasi BZ-150 capsule-filling machine. 1, central turret; 2, empty-capsule feed hopper; 3, powder supply hopper; 4, rectangular base.

filled body are reunited. The two bushes are now better aligned, which reduces the likelihood of splitting in the body or cap.

The annular hopper from which the dosators pick up powder has been separated from the main drive of the machine and its speed relative to the turret has been altered. This ensures that the dosator does not enter the powder at the same point on each revolution, resulting in better dosage weight uniformity.

The sequence of operations is illustrated in Fig. 10.63. Powder dosing is effected by means of a cylindrical tube in which a piston is used to regulate volume. The dosator enters the powder bed then rises holding the volume volume of powder. The capsule body is brought under the dosator

and the powder charge is ejected by means of the piston.

For the filling of pellets, the volumetric principle is again employed with the assistance of vacuum for transfer of the product. By this means, even micro-capsules containing liquid or pellets with soft coatings such as wax can be handled without damage. High-accuracy filling is achieved by means of a dosator levelling system which operates after the dosator enters the product bed. Employment of this principle, rather than gravity filling, enables pellets with poor electrostatic qualities to be handled without affecting accuracy.

An attachment which is available for the Z 5000-R1 allows feeding of a tablet into the capsule body followed by a powder dose (Fig. 10.64). Every

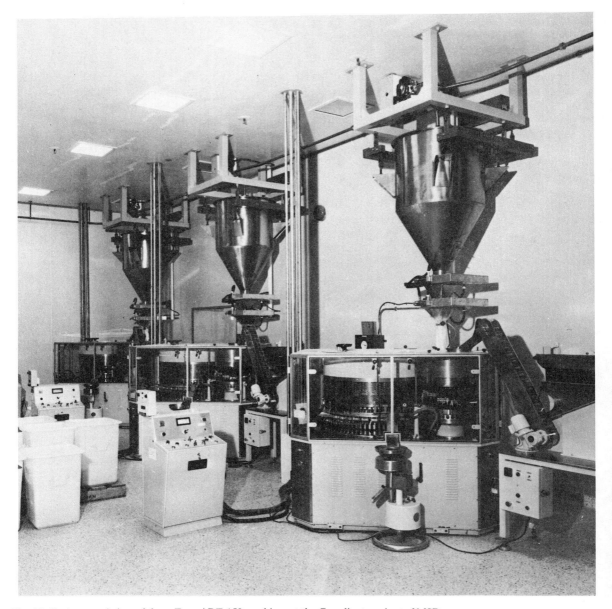

Fig. 10.60. A general view of three Zanasi BZ-150 machines at the Cramlington plant of MSD.

capsule is checked for the presence of a tablet. Capsules without tablets are automatically ejected. Regulation of the dosing volume and the compression of the plug are effected by single controls operating on all dosators simultaneously. Control can be effected while the machine is in motion without nullifying the safety interlocks. In the event of excessive compression, a safety interlock protects the working parts against mechanical damage.

The overall design of the equipment and parts is to the highest standard of good manufacturing practice, and allows simple, effective, and speedy cleaning. Most components are smooth shapes

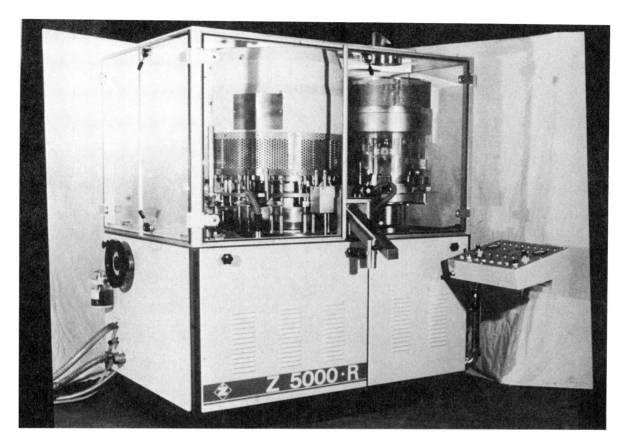

Fig. 10.61. The Zanasi Z 5000-R automatic rotary capsule-filling machine.

without corners or joins where the product might lodge. The manufacturers claim that a change in the size of capsules to be filled can be accomplished in less than one hour.

FARMATIC MACHINES
This series consists of 3 machines, the 2000/15, 2000/30, and 2000/60, with maximum outputs of 40 000, 80 000, and 160 000 capsules per hour, respectively.

These machines have a single operating tower (Fig. 10.65), with a separate turret to hold the powder. A central hopper holds the empty capsules which are fed into special scoops for intercepting and rejecting damaged and distorted capsules. In a lower part of this central turret, the capsules are rectified, separated, filled, and re-

united. If a capsule is missing from a dosing station, the powder plug is ejected from the machine. Selection of samples for check-weighing is accomplished by an electronic pneumatic device which monitors the dosator.

THE ELANCO ROTOFIL
The Elanco Rotofil (Eli Lilly & Co.), shown in Fig. 10.66, is a continuous motion pellet filler capable of a maximum rate of 60 000 capsules per hour. A weight variation of ±2% is claimed. It is essentially a volume filler, and the product has to be formulated specifically for the volume of the capsule to be filled. Capsule sizes 0 to 4 can be filled and it is claimed that the size change-over and cleaning take 2 hours. Excess pellets can be recycled to the filling hopper.

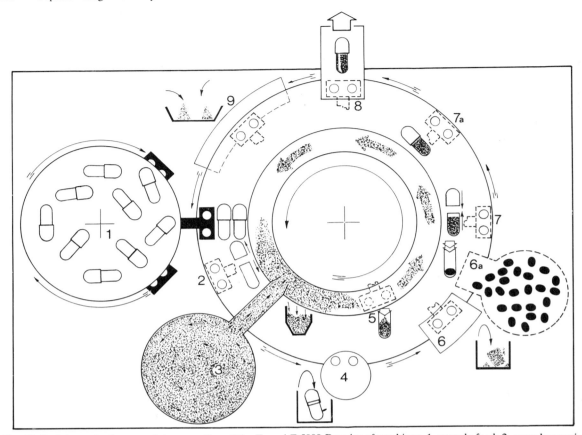

Fig. 10.62. Schematic diagram of the operation of the Zanasi Z 5000-R series of machines. 1, capsule feed; 2, capsule opening; 3, powder or pellet feeding; 4, unopened-capsule rejection; 5, dosing; 6, product ejection in case of empty bushings; 6a, tablet feeding; 7, commencement of capsule closure; 7a, end of capsule closure; 8, finished-capsule ejection; 9, cleaning of bushings.

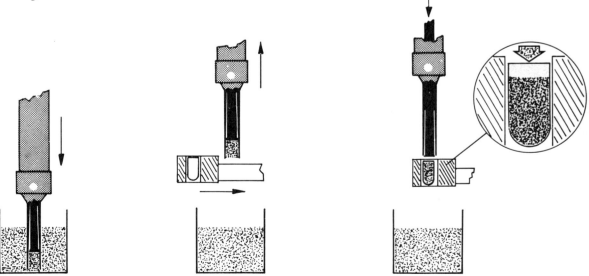

Fig. 10.63. Schematic diagram of powder dosing in the Zanasi Z5000-R series.

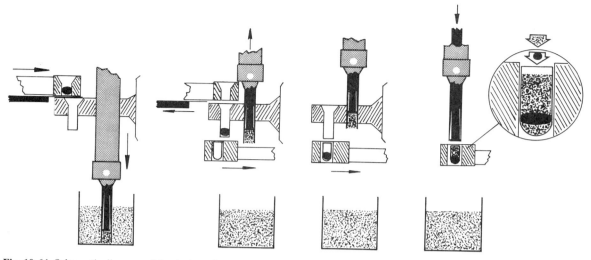

Fig. 10.64. Schematic diagram of the dosing of a tablet and powder on the Zanasi Z5000-R1.

The Filling of Liquids and Pastes into Hard Capsules

There have been a number of significant developments in the use of hard shell two-piece capsules for liquids, pastes, and thixotropic formulations. Both Nuova Zanasi, and Höfliger and Karg have produced machines based on their existing model range which are capable of this technique. Walker *et al.* (1980) and Francois and Jones (1979) describe the process and its requirements in detail. The important physical properties of the formulated mass are its viscosity, surface tension, and melting point, which govern how the product can withstand handling and storage. If the thixotropic effect is low then the problems of leakage will be greater.

A variety of medicines which are normally filled into soft gelatin capsules can now be presented in hard capsules. The limitations to this technique are the interactions of the materials with hard gelatin; materials with low moisture content, and oils, are preferable. One advantage of this process is that a simple machine can be placed at the formulator's bench and relatively small amounts of material are sufficient for filling trials. Greater accuracy can also be claimed for this method compared to normal powder filling and, since the amount of gelatin used for a hard shell capsule is less than for a soft shell one, it is cheaper as well.

Machines which are available for filling liquids into hard capsules include the Zanasi RM/L-75, Zanasi RM/P-75, a series of machines from Höfliger and Karg, and the Harro Höfliger unit.

The Zanasi RM/L-75

The basic machine, illustrated in Fig. 10.67, can carry out six sequential operations: feeding of empty capsules, and rectification; opening of capsules by vacuum; sorting and ejection of faulty capsules; filling of capsules with liquid products by means of dosing pistons and liquid-injecting needles; closing of capsules, and the ejection of filled capsules. The machine must be fitted with the size-parts relating to both the capsules and the product.

The two-piece hard shell capsules must meet the standard dimensional requirements, but can be either the standard or the self-locking type. The range of sizes that can be handled is listed below, and the contained volumes are also given here for ease of reference: size 000 (1.37 ml), size 00 (0.95 ml), size 0 (0.68 ml), size 1 (0.50 ml), size 2 (0.37 ml), size 3 (0.30 ml), size 4 (0.21 ml), and size 5 (0.13 ml).

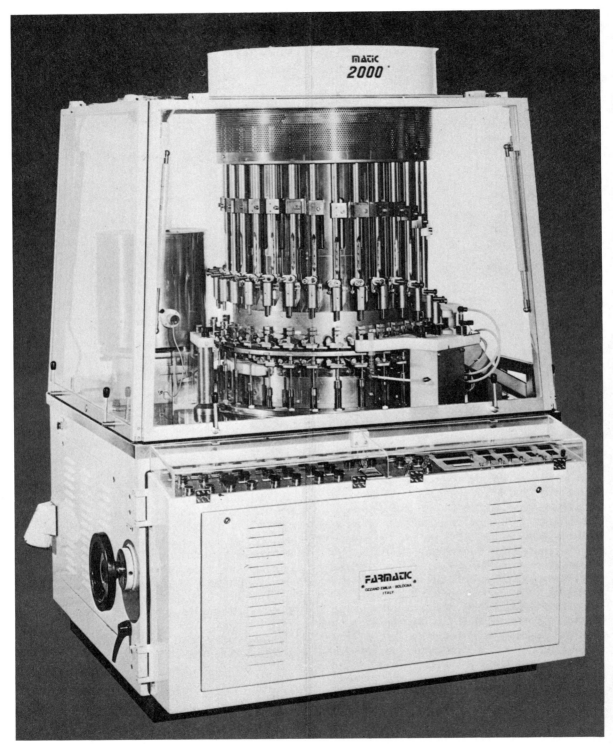

Fig. 10.65. The Farmatic model 2000 automatic rotary capsule-filling machine.

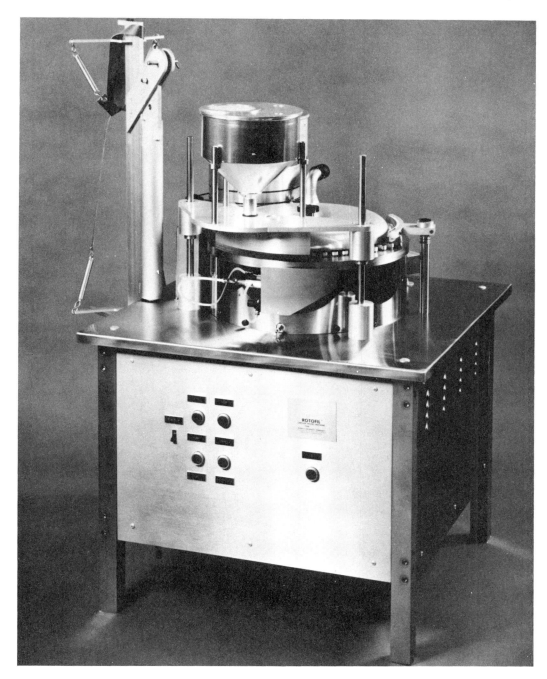

Fig. 10.66. The Elanco Rotofil automatic pellet filler.

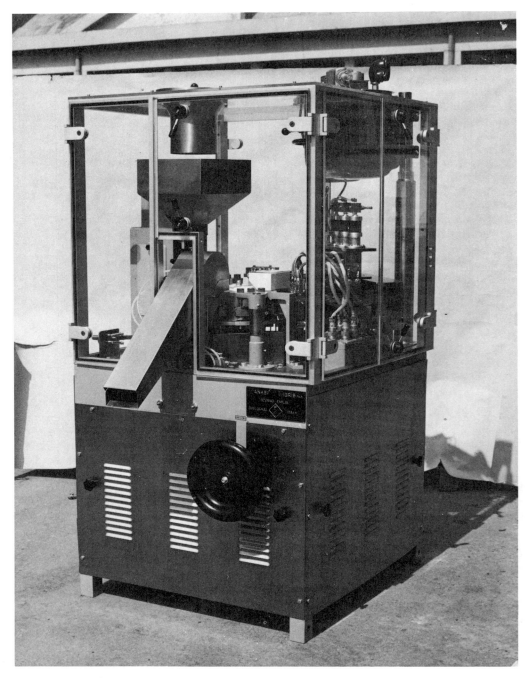

Fig. 10.67. The Zanasi RM/L-75 automatic machine for filling liquids into hard capsules.

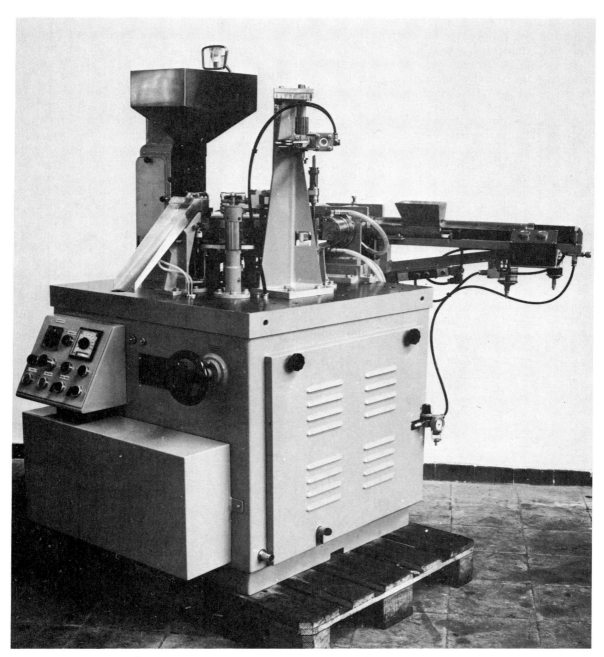

Fig. 10.68. The Zanasi RM/P-75 automatic machine for filling pastes into hard capsules.

The machine has a general rotary motion but is intermittent. Empty capsules are fed into a high-capacity container inside which is a plate, with two vertical channels each having a slightly larger diameter than the capsules. The capsules fall through these channels and are rectified, body downwards. The turntable then transfers the capsules to the opening station for the separation of the cap from the body. This operation is performed by pins and vacuum. In their passage from the opening station to the sorting station, all the bodies are positioned at the same height, and at the sorting station all those capsules which have not opened are rejected.

The bodies then move to the filling station which has a container for the liquid, two dosing pistons with micrometric adjustments, two filling needles, and two valves for suction and delivery of the product. When the bodies are under the filling station, they are checked by a 'no capsule body—no filling' device which allows the needle to be lowered only when a capsule body is present. The whole filling unit is made of stainless steel. After completion of the filling operation, the capsules are transferred to the closing station where the cap and body are reunited. The filled and closed capsules are transferred to the last station, where ejection

is brought about by two hollow pins, which push the capsules out and down a chute into a container.

The output is up to 12 000 capsules per hour.

The Zanasi RM/P-75

The Zanasi model RM/P-75, illustrated in Fig. 10.68, will fill pastes into hard shell capsules by means of special dosators fitted with a micrometric adjustment. The basic machine is the same as the RM/L-75, but the filling station consists of a hopper, paste-extruding unit, and four dosators with micrometric adjustment. When the bodies are under the filling station, they are filled by two dosators, whilst the other two dosators pick up the paste as formed by the extruder to repeat the filling cycle. The paste is extruded in the desired shape and size by a piston and screw feeder, working inside a cylinder which has a cavity and cooling-water jacket. Waste material is retained on a plate, and can be recycled. After filling, the capsules are transferred to the closing station where the cap and body are reunited.

All moving parts on both these Zanasi machines are located within a single base and are surrounded on all sides by safety guards with safety devices on the doors. The working table can be protected by means of a transparent anti-dust and anti-noise

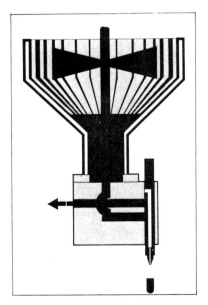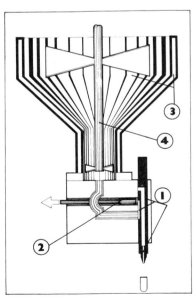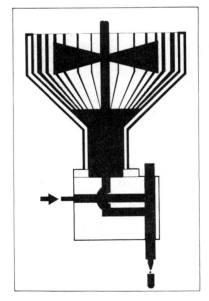

Fig. 10.69. The mechanism of filling liquids into hard capsules on the Höfliger and Karg machines. 1. control valve, outlet valve, and filling needle; 2, dosing piston; 3, jacketted product container; 4, stirrer.

protection hood, which is also fitted with safety devices on the doors.

HÖFLIGER AND KARG MACHINES

Höfliger and Karg offer three versions of their standard range of capsule fillers equipped to fill liquids into hard shell capsules. Table 10.8 shows the variations that are possible. The dosing mechanism is shown in Fig. 10.69. In the left-hand illustration, the control valve is in the upper position and product is drawn into the dosing cylinder.

The stroke of the piston is adjustable. The dosing stroke is shown in the right-hand illustration. The downward movement of the control valve causes the outlet valve to shut off the product flow. Simultaneously, the dosing piston forces the measured dose through the dosing needle into the capsule.

References

Francois, D. and Jones, B. E., *Mfg Chem.*, 1979, *50*(3), 37, 38, 41.

Walker, S. E. *et al.*, *J. Pharm. Pharmac.*, 1980, *32*, 389–393.

Table 10.8. Applications for liquid pumps on Höfliger and Karg machines

Model	No. of holes in carrier segment	Dosing possibilities (in order of sequence with the stations on the machine)	Description of liquid pump	Output (caps/min) tablets pellets powder	liquids
330L*	3	liquids only	3-Head pump with drive motor in place of powder filling station (brake-clutch combination). Dosing impulse comes from cam-operated switches. Dosing disk can be stopped manually, whilst the dosing piston continues to operate.	—	50–60
330	3	pellets-powder-pellets tablets-powder-pellets pellets-liquids-pellets tablets-liquids-pellets	As for 330L	110	50–60
603	6	liquids-powder-pellets pellets-powder-pellets tablets-powder-pellets	6-Head pump, drive synchronised with main drive shaft. Dosing disk can be manually stopped, whilst the dosing piston continues to operate.	105	70
603L*	6	liquids only	As for 603	—	70
1200L*	12	liquids only	Two 6-head pumps in place of pellet stations. Otherwise same as for 603.	—	70

* These models cannot be equipped with additional dosing systems

Chapter 11

Capsule Types, Filling Tests, and Formulation

G. C. Cole

Capsule Sizes and Types

There are eight sizes of hard gelatin capsules commercially available:

Capsule size	000	00	0	1	2	3	4	5
Volume in ml	1.37	0.95	0.68	0.50	0.37	0.30	0.21	0.13

For pharmaceutical products it is unusual to use a size larger than 0 because of the difficulty in swallowing larger sizes, whilst size 5 is rarely used due to difficulties in the automatic filling process. Other sizes are available to order but are used mainly in veterinary practice.

The main suppliers of capsules are the Elanco Qualicaps division of Eli Lilly & Co., the Capsugel Division of Parke, Davis & Co. Ltd, and R. P. Scherer Ltd. The sizes and specifications adopted by the three manufacturers are very similar, which allows any of their sizes to be used on standard automatic filling machines. Each manufacturer produces a range of standard capsules which are designed so that the body and the cap do not separate before the filling operation takes place. They each also make a range of capsules which are locked after filling to ensure that the contents do not leak during packaging and distribution. Each company uses its own brand name to market its regular and locking capsules.

SELF-LOCKING CAPSULES

The self-locking capsule was developed as an alternative to the dot-sealing or banding of capsules which was used by Parke, Davis & Co. for a number of their products and was a costly, difficult, and lengthy process. To eliminate this process, Eli Lilly produce the Lok-Cap and Posilok capsules, Parke, Davis the Snap-Fit and Coni-Snap capsules, and R. P. Scherer the Star-Lock and Lox-It capsules. These are described and illustrated below.

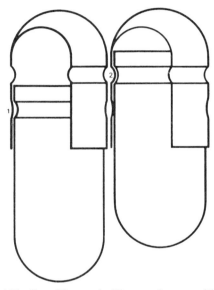

Fig. 11.1 The Snap-Fit capsule. The protuberances (1) prevent premature opening; the grooves (2) lock the two halves together once the capsule has been filled.

The Snap-Fit principle is shown in Fig. 11.1. A development of this design is the Coni-Snap (Fig. 11.2) which is claimed to reduce defects during the filling operation. In 1983, Parke, Davis introduced the Coni-Snap Supro capsule, claiming it to be virtually tamper proof. To achieve this, the dimensions of the capsule have been changed and given new designated sizes from A to E. The capacity is related to the standard Coni-Snap capsules as shown in Table 11.1(b) The cap is so designed that after filling and closing only the rounded end of the body is visible. Due to this change in dimensions, additional machine change parts are required for the filling and packaging operations. The dimensions of capsules made by Parke, Davis are given in Table 11.1(a) and (b).

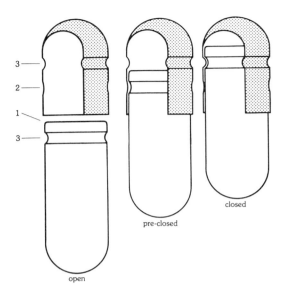

Fig. 11.2 The Coni-Snap capsule. The tapered rim (1) avoids telescoping; the protuberances (2) prevent premature opening; the grooves (3) lock the two halves together once the capsule has been filled.

Table 11.1(a). Dimensions of Coni-Snap capsules made by Parke, Davis, measured at a moisture content of 12–16%

Capsule size	Cap length mm	Body length mm	Cap diam. mm	Body diam. mm
00	11.74*	20.22*	8.53	8.18
0	10.72*	18.44*	7.64	7.33
1	9.78	16.61	6.91	6.63
2	8.94	15.27	6.35	6.07
3	8.08	13.59	5.83	5.57
4	7.21	12.19	5.32	5.05
Tolerance	*±0.51 ±0.46	*±0.51 ±0.46	—	—

Table 11.1(b). Dimensions of Coni-Snap Supro capsules compared with standard Coni-Snap capsules.
Coni-Snap Supro capsules

Size	External diam. body/cap mm	Volume ml	Standard capsule size with same volume	diameter
A	8.18/8.53	0.68	0	00
B	8.18/8.53	0.50	1	00
C	7.33/7.64	0.37	2	0
D	6.63/6.91	0.30	3	1
E	6.07/6.35	0.21	4	2

Standard and Lox-It capsules are illustrated in Fig. 11.3. R. P. Scherer also manufacture capsules with the registered name 'Star-Lock'. The dimensions of capsules made by Scherer are shown in

Table 11.2. The manufacturers recommend storage at 24°C and about 50% relative humidity.

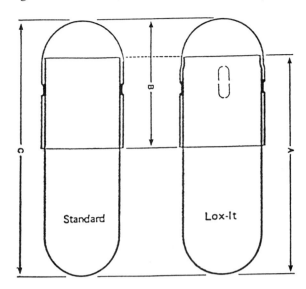

Fig. 11.3 Standard (or Star-Lock) and Lox-It capsules.

A Posilok capsule is illustrated in Fig. 11.4. The pre-lock feature is designed to prevent the cap and body from separating during transit from the manufacturer to the purchaser. Air is released through vents during closure with a resultant increase in the final holding force between the cap and the body. The dimensions of capsules made by Elanco Qualicaps are shown in Table 11.3. Target weights for empty shells are shown in Table 11.4.

Capsules can be manufactured with elongated bodies to meet specific requirements, and specifications for these capsules are supplied to individual customers. Capsule diameters are not a directly controlled parameter and various factors, e.g. moisture content, wall thickness, length, etc., can influence them.

Hard gelatin capsules with a larger volume than size 000 (1.37 ml) are available (e.g. from Kruger, Willi K. G.). In the United Kingdom they are supplied by Davcaps. The sizes range from 3.5 ml to 51.5 ml; dimensions of these capsules are shown in Fig. 11.5.

Experimental Filling Tests

The results of a number of filling trials, comparing Coni-Snap and conventional capsules, are given in Table 11.5 (Latchem, 1979; Mallory, 1980).

Table 11.2. Dimensions of capsules made by Scherer, measured at a moisture content of 12–16%

Capsule size	Body length (A) mm	Cap length (B) mm	Body diameter mm	Cap diameter mm	Filled length (C) mm	Volume of standard length ml	Volume of elongated length ml
0	18.69	11.05	7.35	7.65	22.0	0.7	0.76
1	16.55	9.82	6.65	6.90	19.6	0.5	0.54
2	15.29	9.04	6.10	6.36	18.0	0.4	0.45
3	13.66	8.12	5.60	5.85	16.2	0.3	0.34
4	12.39	7.36	5.09	5.34	14.7	0.21	0.22
Tolerance	±0.3	±0.3	±0.05	±0.05	—	—	—

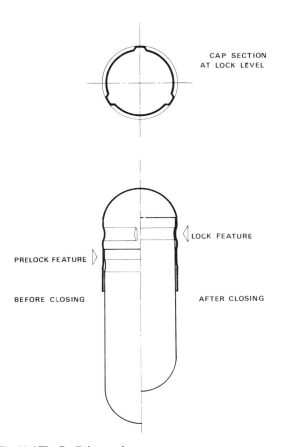

CAP SECTION
AT LOCK LEVEL

LOCK FEATURE

PRELOCK FEATURE

BEFORE CLOSING

AFTER CLOSING

Fig. 11.4 The Posilok capsule.

Table 11.3. Dimensions of capsules made by Elanco Quali-caps, measured at a moisture content of 13 to 16% w/w

Capsule size	Cap length mm	Body length mm	Cap diameter mm	Body diameter mm	Closed joined length mm
00	11.4	20.2	8.51	8.16	22.9
0	10.9	18.5	7.63	7.33	21.8
1	9.7	16.5	6.90	6.62	19.5
2	8.9	15.1	6.35	6.07	17.8
3	7.9	13.5	5.82	5.56	15.9
4	7.2	12.3	5.32	5.06	14.5
Tolerance	±0.3	±0.3	±0.05	±0.05	±0.3

Table 11.4. Average weights of 100 capsules manufactured by Elanco Qualicaps

Capsule size	Average weight mg	Limit mg
00	126	±12
0	98	±9
1	76	±7
2	63	±6
3	50	±5
4	40	±4

These results show a reduction in the number of filling defects when the Coni-Snap design is used.

The results from a series of fillings of Elanco Qualicaps capsules followed by controlled inspections are shown in Tables 11.6, 11.7, and 11.8.

An examination of the results shown in these tables will illustrate that the fault levels are reasonably constant for each machine. One reason for this may be the age of the capsule bushings. If they are very worn, the number of telescoped capsules increases, whilst if the bushings are new the tightness of fit results in more cracked ends. Generally, the level of defects in the empty capsules from all manufacturers is very low and the quality high. There can be considerable batch-to-batch variation in capsules from the same supplier, and the conditions of storage can affect the quality significantly. For instance, in a trial to examine the performance of capsules from two different suppliers, one manufacturer supplied capsules containing only 8% moisture, which were very brittle.

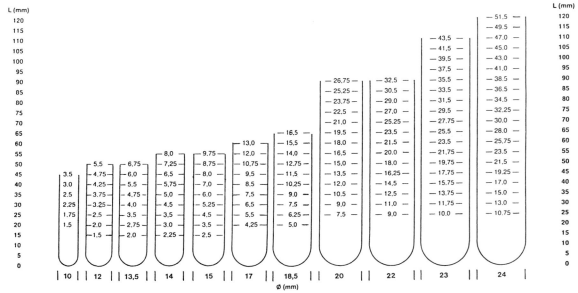

Fig. 11.5 The dimensions of capsule bodies larger than size 000, showing diameter (ø), length (L), and the volume (ml) contained at various filling levels.

Table 11.5. Summary of trials comparing filling defects between Coni-Snap and conventional capsules on different capsule-filling machines

| | Filling rate | Defects per 100 000 capsules | | | |
| | | Split capsules | | Punched ends | |
Machine	c.p.h.	Conventional	Coni-Snap	Conventional	Coni-Snap
AZ-25[a]	32 000	37	0	6	0
AZ-30[a]		167	3	49	2
AZ-30[a]	32 000	19	0	0	0
AZ-60[a]	58 000	9	0	4.5	0
AZ-60[a]	60 000	11	2	1	1
GFK-600[b]	36 000	30	5	105	55
GFK-700[b]	38 000	20	2	1	1
GFK-1000[b]		11	2	36	16
GFK-1200[b]	73 000	1	0.1	14	0.3
GFK-1200[b]	70 000 to 80 000	18	0.2	2	0
G-37[c]	70 000 to 80 000	6	0	17	0

[a]Zanasi
[b]Höfliger and Karg
[c]mG2

The type of capsule-filling machine may also have a significant effect on the level of defects. In a trial which compared Coni-Snap capsules with Posilok capsules, the former fared better when filled on a Zanasi BZ-72 machine, whereas the Posilok capsules showed a lower level of defects when filled on an mG2 G37/N machine.

When pellets are being filled into Coni-Snap capsules, material can lodge on the lip of the body and hinder closure. This is also true if the powder plugs are loosely packed. The body-edge chamfer also reduces the area of contact between the body and the cap when the capsules are empty, which causes a higher than normal level of separated

Table 11.6. Faults in a batch of filled capsules (Opaque Yellow, size 3), from three Zanasi BZ-150 fillers; sample size, 1200 capsules

	Sample 1	Sample 2	Sample 3	Total (%)
Machine No. 1				
Telescopes	9	4	8	0.58
Crush cracks	1	2	2	0.14
Other faults	2	1	3	0.17
Total	12	7	13	0.89
Machine No. 2				
Telescopes	1	4	2	0.19
Crush cracks	22	18	16	1.56
Other faults	0	2	2	0.11
Total	23	24	20	1.86
Machine No. 3				
Telescopes	2	2	12	0.44
Crush cracks	5	10	8	0.64
Other faults	5	1	1	0.19
Total	12	13	21	1.27

Table 11.7. Faults in two samples, each of 10 000 capsules (Opaque Yellow, size 3), from one Zanasi BZ-150 filler

	Sample 1	%	Sample 2	%
Telescopes	63	0.63	22	0.22
Dented	6	0.06	4	0.04
Crush cracks	16	0.16	6	0.06
Split	4	0.04	3	0.03
Holed body	1	0.01	0	0
Overclosure	0	0	0	0
Thin spot	0	0	1	0.1
Halves	12	0.12	0	0
Empty	1	0.01	0	0
Dirty	10	0.10	0	0
Total	113	1.13	36	0.36
Print defects	8	0	0	0

Table 11.8. Summary of defects found after inspections of 50 different batches of capsules from three different Zanasi BZ-150 fillers

Defect	Highest %	Lowest %	Mean %
Machine 1			
(36 inspections) Telescopes	0.70	0.09	0.25
Crush cracks	0.44	0	0.13
Others	0.21	0	0.09
Total			0.47
Machine 2			
(33 inspections) Telescopes	0.64	0	0.16
Crush cracks	0.35	0	0.10
Others	0.18	0	0.07
Total			0.33
Machine 3			
(33 inspections) Telescopes	0.70	0	0.13
Crush cracks	0.26	0	0.10
Others	0.32	0	0.11
Total			0.34

Overall mean defects from 102 inspections = 0.38%

empty capsules. However, some tests have shown a considerable reduction in the number of splits and telescoped capsules when Coni-Snap capsules have been used.

The Formulation of Capsule Products

There are a number of factors to be considered in the formulation of capsules. These include the size and colour of the shell, powder characteristics, stability, bioavailability, filling method, and packaging, storage, and marketing.

The size of the shell is governed largely by the bulk density of the contents (see Chapter 7). The colour of the shell must be different from that used for other capsules and must be acceptable in the country to be supplied (see Chapter 4). Powder characteristics (Chapter 7) are a significant factor in the filling process and it must be remembered that a formulation which is suitable for a hand-operated filling machine may need to be changed when an automatic machine using compression filling is to be used. The particle size and other formulation factors may affect bioavailability (Chapter 13).

FORMULATION FOR HIGH-SPEED FILLING

A lubricant, such as magnesium stearate, is essential for high-speed filling. One difficulty that arises is that there is no generally accepted method for quantitatively assessing lubrication capability. It has been suggested (Butcher and Jones, 1972) that particle densities, packing characteristics, tensile strength measurements, surface area measurements, and shear strength measurements may give a clearer indication of the lubrication properties of batches of magnesium stearate. Considerable batch-to-batch variation has been shown to exist, sufficient to produce large differences in compression properties (Hanssen *et al.*, 1970). Some materials, such as corn starch, that are commonly used as excipients in formulation work, possess some lubricating properties, whilst others, like lactose, do not.

The concentration of glidants is also important as quantities above 1% tend to decrease the flow rate; about 0.1% is usually adequate. Not all authors agree that glidants and lubricants are separate, different, classes of compound (King, 1970). Magnesium stearate can certainly act as both a glidant and lubricant.

Investigation of Factors Affecting Filling

In an attempt to define the formulation process more accurately, Cole and May (1975) used an instrumented Zanasi LZ-64 capsule-filling machine to investigate the filling characteristics of some commonly used excipients by measuring the forces exerted in the transfer of powder. The machine was fitted with a modified dosator assembly, shown in Fig. 11.6.

The capsule fill-weight depends on (a) the position of the dosator in the dosator nozzle (distance X in Fig. 11.6), (b) the powder depth in the dosator hopper, (c) the bulk density of the material in the dosator hopper, and (d) the filling speed of the machine.

In this machine, the tubular nozzle was dipped into a powder bed of constant depth and, during plug formation, the distance X was always less than the depth of powder in the hopper. To eject the powder plug into the capsule body, the piston was moved to the end of the dosator nozzle, pushing the plug before it, after which the spring returned it to its original position. In these studies, the axial forces exerted by the powder on the end of the dosator piston were measured during formation, carry-over, and ejection of the powder plug.

The small values of the forces made measurement difficult. On a tablet machine the punch forces during compression are typically 3×10^4 N, whereas in capsule filling the values rarely exceed 400 N, and are more typically in the range 20–30 N. To measure forces of this order with strain gauges, a large degree of amplification is necessary, with its attendant drift and signal-to-noise ratio problems.

The piston of the dosator assembly was fitted with four strain gauges, two active and two passive, the active pair being fitted on opposite sides of the stem so that only axial forces were recorded: lateral bending forces were automatically compensated and had no effect. To prevent the leads becoming twisted during operation, the dosator was driven so that it turned in the opposite direction to, and at the same angular velocity as, the rotating head on which it was carried. The system was calibrated in compression and in tension.

Experiments were made using size 00 capsules at a filling speed of 50 per minute. The materials used were microcrystalline cellulose (Avicel), a modified corn starch (Starch 1500, formerly Sta-Rx 1500), and two grades of lactose, 50T and 80 mesh. These were all used either alone or after the addition of 0.5% w/w magnesium stearate as

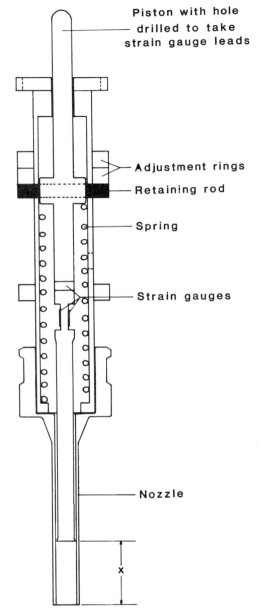

Fig. 11.6 The modified dosator assembly used on an instrumented Zanasi LZ-64 capsule-filling machine (Cole and May, 1975).

a lubricant. The machine was run for several revolutions before fitting the dosator nozzle to stabilise the powder level in the dosator hopper. When using the lubricated materials, several capsules were filled before taking recordings of pressure, but with the unlubricated materials recordings were started immediately to enable the onset of binding to be studied. A recording was made with the machine running but with the powder hopper removed, to ascertain the effects of machine movement on the oscillograph trace.

The particle sizes and bulk densities of the materials examined are shown in Tables 11.9 and 11.10, and the traces in Fig. 11.7. The first event

Table 11.9. Particle size distribution (% retained on sieves) of powders used in experimental filling tests

Sieve mesh no.	Lactose 80-mesh %	Lactose 50T %	Avicel pH 101 %	Sta-Rx 1500 %
60	0	0	0	1.2
100	3.8	18.3	1.5	6.0
150	12.6	38.0	6.5	11.7
200	14.8	20.0	12.4	14.6
350	30.3	18.5	33.4	22.6
through 350	39.3	4.2	46.2	43.6

Table 11.10. Bulk density of powders used in experimental filling tests

	Untapped g/cm³	Tapped g/cm³
Lactose 80-mesh	0.500	0.877
+0.5% magnesium stearate	0.658	0.926
Lactose 50T	0.758	0.909
+0.5% magnesium stearate	0.840	0.917
Avicel pH 101	0.309	0.455
+0.5% magnesium stearate	0.373	0.463
Sta-Rx 1500	0.625	0.840
+0.5% magnesium stearate	0.690	0.877

marker on each trace shows when the powder plug was picked up, and the second when it was ejected into the capsule.

Figure 11.7C is a typical trace, which is modified in detail by the characteristics of the material being filled. An initial compaction force was produced at *a*, as the plug was formed, and was partially retained, *b*, during carry-over of the plug to the capsule body. A second force was produced at *c*, as the powder plug was ejected into the capsule body. This second force changed considerably according to the extent of lubrication of the material.

The amount of compression which is given to the powder during plug formation is governed by the combined effects of the depth of powder in the filling hopper and the distance of the end of

the dosator piston from the end of the nozzle. These were both kept constant so that any differences in the resulting forces were attributable to the nature of the powder.

Lactose requires lubrication before tablets can be produced. That this is also true of capsule filling when using the plug method can be seen from the rapid ejection force build up in lactose 50T. Figure 11.7C is the trace taken after about 20 capsules had been filled, and Fig. 11.7D after about 50 (note the change of vertical scale). At this stage the noise from the machine was sufficient to indicate that a binding problem existed. The cause was the entrapment of small particles between the inner wall of the dosator nozzle and the flared end of the dosator push rod. Magnesium stearate, added at a concentration of 0.5%, overcame this (Fig. 11.7E).

Addition of magnesium stearate to lactose 80 mesh resulted in an increase in compaction pressure, a possible explanation for which is that the pressure increase is due to the 5.5% increase in bulk density caused by the glidant effect of the lubricant. Addition of magnesium stearate to the lactose 50T produced little change in either compaction pressure or bulk density, probably because the coarser and more evenly sized particles of this grade of lactose are more free-flowing than those of the lactose 80 mesh, and rapidly assume a maximum packing density in the dosator hopper, whether lubricated or not. Sta-Rx showed an increase in bulk density of similar magnitude to that of lactose 80 mesh after lubrication (4.4%) but did not show the same increase in compaction pressure. It is possible that the Sta-Rx particles deform more easily under compaction than the lactose particles and so absorb the energy of compaction more easily.

The effect of 0.5% magnesium stearate on the Avicel was slight. The compression force was not reduced, and the carry-over or retention force was only slightly reduced, as was the ejection force. This material would fill satisfactorily without lubrication, which supports the claim by Fox *et al.* (1963), that Avicel has some lubricant properties. The bulk density of the material did not increase appreciably after lubrication (1.73%).

Mehta and Augsburger (1981) suggested that increased levels of lubricant might be required to improve the dissolution characteristics of the capsule when an insoluble filler such as Avicel is used. This could probably be explained by the reduction in hardness of the plug more than offsetting the

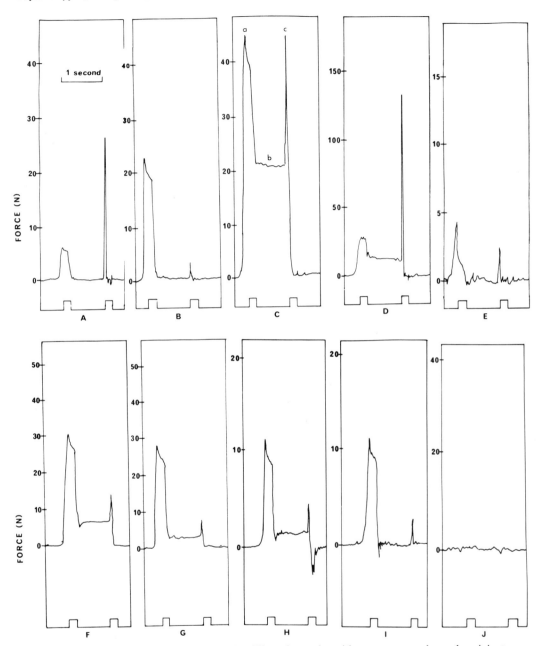

Fig. 11.7 Recorder traces of the forces operative in the filling of capsules with some commonly-used excipients, on a Zanasi LZ-64 machine. A, lactose 80-mesh; B, lactose 80-mesh with 0.5% magnesium stearate; C, lactose 50T after 20 capsules; D, lactose 50T after 50 capsules; E, lactose 50T with 0.5% magnesium stearate; F, Avicel; G, Avicel with 0.5% magnesium stearate; H, Sta-Rx 1500; I, Sta-Rx 1500 with 0.5% magnesium stearate; J, machine noise.

hydrophobic properties of the magnesium stearate. Where the filler is soluble (e.g. lactose) some increase in dissolution with increased lubrication level was shown.

The retention and ejection forces seen on the Sta-Rx trace (Fig. 11.7H) were almost eliminated after the addition of 0.5% magnesium stearate (Fig. 11.7I), as was the tensile force, which can be seen just after ejection in the trace of the un-lubricated material. This was due to tension in the dosator rod, arising from the frictional resistance to its return caused by particles of powder getting between it and the inner surface of the nozzle. This happened only with Sta-Rx.

Measurements such as these can help in the determination of minimum lubricant levels during the formulation of powders for encapsulation, and of the optimum mixing time for the powders.

Another method, using the piezo-electric princi-ple of measuring force (Money *et al.*, 1976), is shown in Fig. 11.8. The device was fitted to a

excipients and lubricants were examined: lactose, extra-fine and fine; microcrystalline and granu-lated cellulose; maize, rice, and potato starch, and sodium starch glycolate; talc; and magnesium stearate. No details were given of such parameters as particle size or surface area. The type of trace produced is shown in Fig. 11.9.

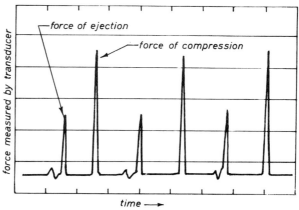

Fig. 11.9 Trace of the forces operative in the filling of capsules, measured by the piezo-electric transducer.

Further work in this field was conducted by Small and Augsburger (1977) who essentially repeated the work of Cole and May (1972, 1975) but used a slip ring between the instrumented dosator and monitoring equipment. They also used a mercury contact swivel to minimise the pos-sibility of noise in the output. Their results sup-ported the conclusions reached earlier by Cole and May.

Small and Augsburger (1978) extended their work to study in detail the behaviour of a number of lubricants commonly used for capsule formula-tions. They used an instrumented Zanasi LZ-64 capsule filler to study the behaviour of a number of fillers (compressible starch, microcrystalline cellulose, and anhydrous lactose) with several lubricants such as magnesium stearate, stearic acid, and magnesium lauryl sulphate. The results for compressible starch are shown in Fig. 11.10.

Comparative Evaluation of Capsule-filling Machines

When testing a new machine's suitability for a new product, or even for an old product that is required in greater quantity, certain basic information can be obtained by using placebo formulations. But it is not possible to estimate mechanical reliability

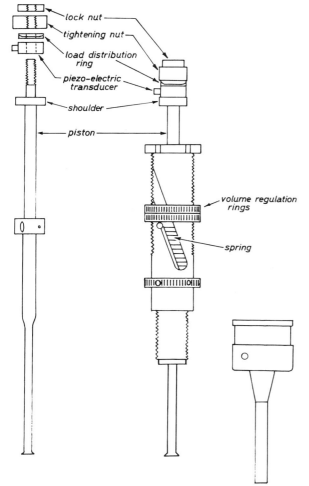

Fig. 11.8 The dosator assembly with piezo-electric transducer, used on a Zanasi RV-59 capsule-filling machine.

Zanasi RV-59 capsule filler, and the following

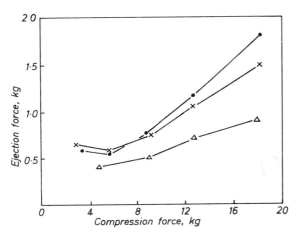

Fig. 11.10 The effect of lubricant type on the ejection force of compressible starch blends containing 0.1% of lubricant. Depth of powder bed, 50 mm, piston height, 15 mm. ● magnesium lauryl sulphate, × stearic acid, △ magnesium stearate.

using this method, because it is necessary to run it over a long period in a production area. The tests which are described here are designed for high-speed equipment capable of filling from 30 000 to 150 000 capsules per hour. For smaller output, the quantities of materials may be adjusted accordingly.

When evaluating a new machine, the following points should be considered.

1. Overall comparison of the new model with the existing machines of similar capacity.
2. The time needed to set up the machine, and the degree of technical competence required.
3. The time needed to dismantle and/or to change over from one capsule size to another.
4. Ease of maintenance, quantity of spare parts required for maintenance and for handling different capsule sizes.
5. Extent of services required.
6. Delivery and cost.

TESTING THE PERFORMANCE OF A MACHINE
At least three different powders are needed for satisfactory evaluation. Suitable mixtures are as follows.

Coarse powder (fill-weight 250.0 mg): lactose 50T, hydrous, dense, 246.0 mg + colloidal silicon dioxide, 1.5 mg + magnesium stearate, 2.5 mg.
Fine powder I (fill-weight 250.0 mg): lactose 80-mesh, 246.0 mg + colloidal silicon dioxide, 1.5 mg + magnesium stearate, 2.5 mg.

Fine powder II (fill-weight 200.0 mg): lactose 80 mesh, 160.0 mg + maize starch, 38.0 mg + magnesium stearate, 2.0 mg.

The test will require 2 000 000 Posilok capsules, 2 000 000 Coni-Snap (Star-Lock could be used as an alternative) and 200 kg of the Company's product.

To carry out the test, set up the machine with each type of powder in turn, and run under ideal conditions, applying the following criteria for the appraisal of the machine.

1. Uniformity of weight between individual capsules.
2. Uniformity of weight between groups of capsules.
3. Uniformity of closure of capsules.
4. Need for polishing capsules.
5. General appearance of capsules.
6. Proportion of rejects.
7. Time spent clearing operating faults.
8. Output of capsules.
9. In-process control of fill-weights.

The machine should then be run under non-ideal conditions.

1. Allow the powder to fall to a low level in the hopper, and check the weight variation of the filled capsules.
2. Examine the effects of changing the temperature and, if possible, the humidity.
3. Vary the speed of the machine over as wide a range as is possible.
4. Estimate the amount of dust produced, the smooth running or vibration of the machine, and examine for overheating.
5. List any modifications that are going to be needed.
6. Consider the noise level near the machine, the extent to which moving parts are protected, and how easy it is to load the machine with empty capsules and material for filling.

To compare the weight variation at various speeds of the Zanasi AZ-60 and the BZ-150, the following scheme was used by the author.

1. Run both machines at 60 000 capsules per hour, using a single batch of 700 000 capsules divided in two. After the machines have been adjusted for a specific target weight, the gross individual

weights of samples of 50 capsules taken at intervals of 25 minutes of actual encapsulation time from each machine (including an initial and final sample) are measured for statistical analysis. A timed log detailing events occurring during the run (e.g. capsule blockage, shutdowns, weight adjustments made, etc.) should be kept.

2. Compare the performance of the BZ-150 at a speed of 60 000 capsules per hour with that at a speed of 100 000 capsules per hour, using a single 700 000 capsule batch divided in two. Estimate the total process time and divide into 10 equal intervals to give the sampling times. At each sampling time withdraw 100 capsules and weigh 20 of these capsules using a suitable balance. If the data can be stored in a retrieval system then progressive analysis during the evaluation may be possible.

3. Compare the performance of the BZ-150 at filling speeds of 60 000 capsules per hour with that at a speed of 150 000 capsules per hour in a similar way to run 2.

4. Compare the performance of the BZ-150 at a speed of 100 000 capsules per hour with that at a speed of 150 000 capsules per hour in a similar way to run 2.

Determine the effect of sampling time on weight uniformity, i.e. is the weight variation occurring between samples taken at different times greater than the weight variation of samples at those times? This is a one-way ANalysis Of VAriance, and such an ANOVA table for each group of data shows whether sampling time is important. This table gives a significance value for the F-ratio which, when compared with tabulated values, shows whether the batch is homogeneous for statistical purposes.

If there is no effect of sampling time then the batch can be considered as a whole and a single parameter (variance) generated which can be examined to show the effect of machine speed, batch, type of machine, production conditions, etc. If the batch is not homogeneous (i.e. sampling time has an effect), then the direct comparison of two variables, e.g. sampling time and machine speed, is required. This is a two-way ANalysis Of VAriance and produces a two-way ANOVA table.

Determination of more elementary statistics, such as the mean weight, standard deviation, and coefficient of variation is also conducted on each sample.

References

Butcher, A. E. and Jones, T. M., *J. Pharm. Pharmac.*, 1972, *24, Suppl.*, 1P–9P.

Cole, G. C. and May, G., *J. Pharm. Pharmac.*, 1972, *24, Suppl.*, 122P–123P.

Cole, G. C. and May, G., *J. Pharm. Pharmac.*, 1975, *27*, 353–358.

Fox, C. D. *et al.*, *Drug Cosmet. Ind.*, 1963, *92*, 161–164, 258–261.

Hanssen, D. *et al.*, *Pharm. Ind., Berl.*, 1970, *32*, 97–101.

King, R. E., in *Remington's Pharmaceutical Sciences*, 14th Edn, A. Osol *et al.* (Ed.), Easton, Pennsylvania, Mack Publishing Co., 1970, p. 1652.

Latchem, P., *Capsugel Newsheet*, May, 1979.

Mallory, M., *Capsugel Newsheet*, BAS-104-UK, 1980.

Mehta, A. M. and Augsburger, L. L., *Int. J. Pharmaceut.*, 1981, *7*, 327–334.

Money, C. *et al.*, *Capsugel Newsheet*, BAS–86–UK, 1976.

Small, L. E. and Augsburger, L. L., *J. pharm. Sci.*, 1977, *66*, 504–509.

Small, L. E. and Augsburger, L. L., *Drug Dev. ind. Pharm.*, 1978, *4*, 345–372.

Chapter 12

Capsule Handling Systems

G. C. Cole

CAPSULE WEIGHING EQUIPMENT

This section contains a description of equipment used to monitor the weight of capsules after the filling process, and to sort batches that are likely to be rejected due to wider variation than is acceptable. There are a number of pieces of equipment that can sort capsules into pass and reject fractions, but generally they operate at a much lower speed than the filling equipment.

Capsule Balances for Rapid Check-weighing

THE INQUISITOR CAPSULE BALANCE
This may be used for either in-process control or in a quality control function.

The Inquisitor balance (C.I. Electronics Ltd) is shown in Fig. 12.1. This balance automatically check-weighs samples of capsules from production batches to give a print-out of any or all of the following information: the number of samples weighed, the target weight, the mean weight, the percentage drift of the mean weight from the target weight, the standard deviation, the coefficient of variation, all the individual weights in ascending order with an indication of any that are outside the set limits, and a histogram to show the weight distribution.

It consists of a weighing unit with a vibratory feeder, weighing head with opening pan, and a

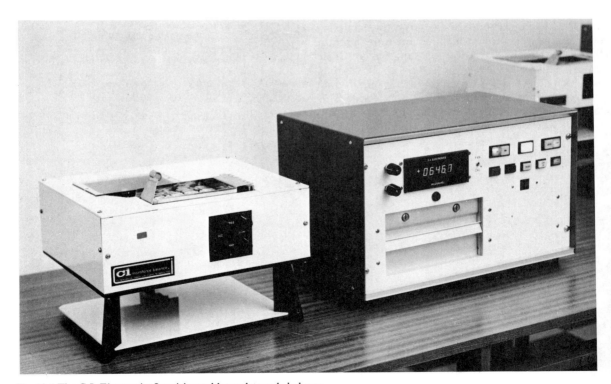

Fig. 12.1 The C.I. Electronics Inquisitor tablet and capsule balance.

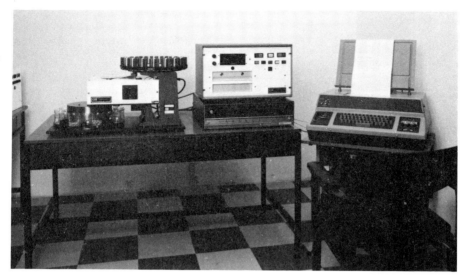

Fig. 12.2 The C.I. Electronics Carousel tablet and capsule balance.

semi-automatic calibration mechanism. The balance control unit has a digital weight display, on/off switch, zero control, calibration control, and a set/run switch. The mini-computer has a core memory of 16K. As an optional extra, a teletype to produce hard copy and eight-hole punched paper tape may be fitted.

The balance is checked, set to zero, and calibrated at the start of the day. Batch identification, product code, etc., are entered into the system on the teletype, together with the sample quantity required. The samples are placed on the vibrator and the balance started. Thereafter the operation is fully automatic. When the required number have been weighed, the surplus of capsules is flushed through the system and a print-out given of the results. The weighing rate is 20 capsules per minute with a precision of ± 1 mg, and the maximum individual capsule weight is 1.5 g.

A typical print-out shows: product name, date, number of batches, individual weights, histogram of weight distribution, target weight, mean weight, number of samples, time of sample, limits, and number outside limits.

THE CAROUSEL CAPSULE BALANCE
An alternative to the Inquisitor is the Carousel balance (C.I. Electronics Ltd) shown in Fig. 12.2 The print-out is similar to that from the Inquisitor. This balance will automatically check-weigh samples of capsules from up to 16 batches, sequentially. It has 16 acceptance and delivery units with

a vibratory feeder. It will weigh at either 12 or 20 capsules per minute from a minimum weight of 15 mg up to a maximum of 1.5 g. The delivery unit holds up to 50 capsules, the unit being programmed to weigh an exact number from each position and then reject the excess. The control unit has a digital display, the mini-computer has a 16K memory, and data transfer is to an ASR 33 teletype.

THE VIGILANTE WEIGHT CONTROL SYSTEM
The Vigilante system (C.I. Electronics Ltd) is designed for the control of a number of filling machines. It has the following features: fast initial set-up, regular or continuous weight monitoring for each production machine, immediate analysis during or at the end of each production batch, daily production records and comprehensive weight data for quality control.

The coupling of the Vigilante to weighing units and sampling stations is shown schematically in Fig. 12.3. Capsules can be taken from production machines either automatically or manually. Sampling is supervised by the system which records the time at which each sample is taken. Samples are taken from the exit chute of each capsule machine in a coded scoop which is identified with that machine by a series of coded slots on one edge. The scoop is inserted into a verification unit, shown in Fig. 12.4, near the filling machine and this unit relays, via a cable to the system control, the time and the identity of the machine from

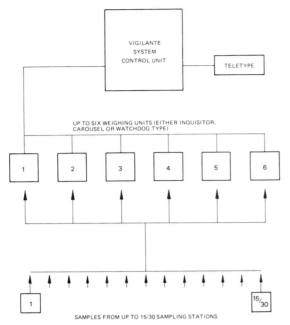

Fig. 12.3 Schematic diagram of the optimum usages of the Vigilante weight control system.

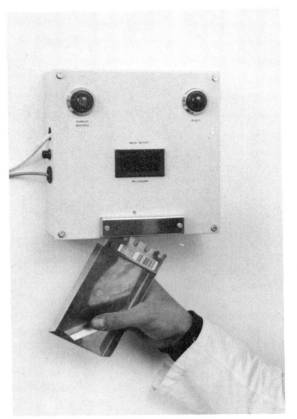

Fig. 12.4 The C.I. Electronics verification system.

which the sample has been taken. A small lamp on the control unit indicates that the scoop has been identified.

The capsules contained in the scoop are then fed, by the operator, into a weighing unit. When this has been done, the verification unit will digitally display the mean weight of the sample, and will light a red lamp if the mean weight or any individual capsule weight is outside the pre-set limits. For resampling, or for normal sampling after the next appropriate time interval, the unit lights a green lamp. There is a reset button to restore the unit to normal operation after it has given an alarm signal.

Capsule Weighing and Sorting

This section describes equipment which is designed for sorting batches of capsules, which have been rejected for excessive weight variation, into 'accept' and 'reject' batches, or for tightening up the weight control. Such units can also be used to divide capsule lots into various weight fractions.

The SADE Balance

The Sorting Automatic Device Electronic (SADE) balance (C.I. Electronics Ltd) is illustrated in Fig. 12.5. This balance will weigh and

sort capsules at the rate of 2400 per hour into 'accept' and 'reject' fractions between 0 and 2.0 g with a precision of ±1 mg. The capsules pass from the large 100-litre hopper into a rotary bowl which divides them into two streams. The capsules in each stream are then passed singly into a bucket-type pan on one of the two electronic balances that make up the unit. The digital panel meter displays the weight and, after weighing, the bucket opens and allows the capsule to fall into one of two chutes, for acceptance or rejection. The unit has an automatic self-calibrating facility which permits it to operate unattended for long periods. An audio-alarm sounds when attention is required.

The Anritsu-Zanasi Check-weigher

This check-weigher, illustrated in Fig. 12.6, can sort capsules of sizes 0–4 into three fractions according to upper and lower pre-set limits which are adjustable up to ±50 mg from a mean value. The machine has five weighing channels, each of which operates at speeds of up to 7200 capsules

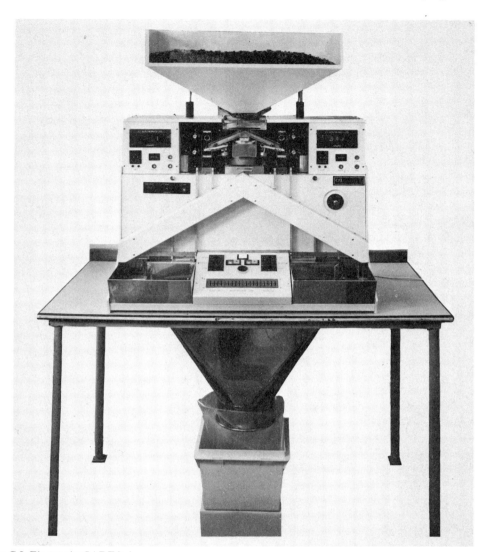

Fig. 12.5 The C.I. Electronics SADE balance.

per hour, giving a total throughput of 36 000 capsules per hour. Three counters provide read-outs of the number of capsules in each fraction.

Capsules are fed from a hopper through conventional capsule handling techniques onto the weighing head (Figs 12.7 and 12.8). This head is a linear variable differential transformer (LVDT) the output of which is proportional to the linear displacement and hence to the capsule weight. The capsule is ejected from the weighing head by the succeeding capsule, and falls down a chute, past a photoelectric counter. The counter is an electromagnetic type, and counts one digit for every ten capsules.

After passing the photoelectric counter the capsule takes one of three paths depending on its weight and the calibrated machine settings. Capsules within the set limits pass straight along the chute into a receiving container, whilst the overweight or underweight capsules fall through one of two flaps which are connected to the counting mechanism, so that separate counts are recorded for overweight, underweight, and normal capsules.

If any of the five channels become blocked by a damaged capsule, or if the hopper becomes empty, an alarm is sounded and the machine stops.

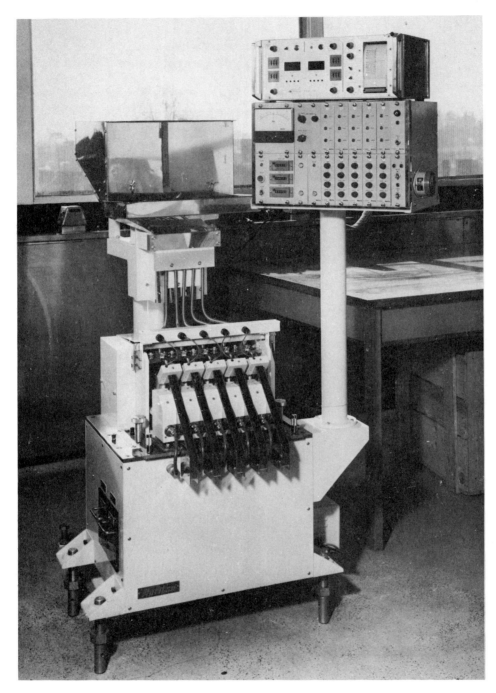

Fig. 12.6 The Anritsu-Zanasi K515B check-weigher.

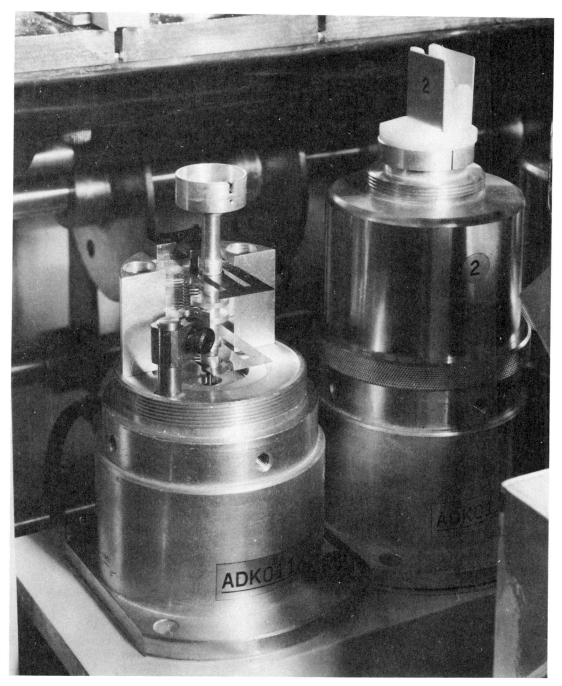

Fig. 12.7 The weighing head (with cover removed) on the Anritsu-Zanasi K515B.

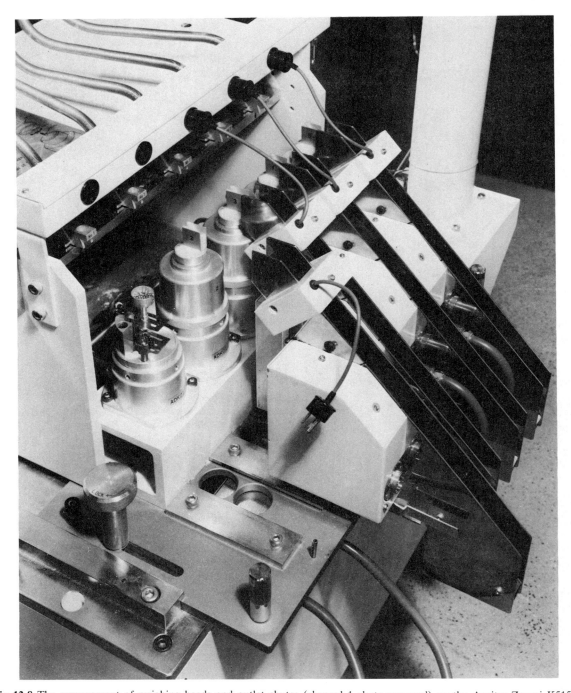

Fig. 12.8 The arrangement of weighing heads and outlet chutes (channel 1 chute removed) on the Anritsu-Zanasi K515B.

The change from one capsule size to another takes approximately 10–15 minutes and is effected by changing (a) the hopper feed mechanism, which is fixed by two hexagonal socket screws and five bayonet fasteners, where the ends of five tubes enter the transfer mechanism to the weighing heads, (b) five transfer arm pieces, each of which is fixed by one hexagonal socket screw, and (c) five weighing heads which rest on top of the LVDT mechanisms.

The performance of one of these machines is indicated in Table 12.1.

Table 12.1. The drift (mg) away from the set weight of a capsule sorting machine, measured after each 1000 capsules

| | Channel number | | | | |
	1	2	3	4	5
Initial	0	0	0	0	0
1000	+5	0	0	+1	0
2000	+6	+1	+2	+2	+1
3000	+9	+1	+2	+4	+2
4000	+10	0	+2	+3	+1
5000	+7	+1	+2	+3	+2
6000	+10	+1	+3	+5	+2
7000	+10	+2	+3	+5	+3
After cleaning	+8	0	−1	0	+1

Drift after 15 000 capsules had been sorted

Total drift	+3	+5	+6	+2	+6
Electronic drift	+2	+1	+3	+1	+2
Dust	+1	+4	+3	+1	+4

Drift after 30 000 capsules had been sorted

Total drift	+12	+5	+7	+1	+1
Electronic drift	+6	+2	+4	0	−2
Dust	+6	+3	+3	+1	+3

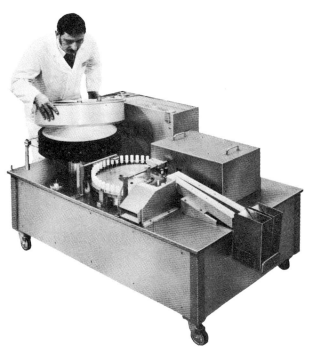

Fig. 12.9 The Elanco Rotoweigh check-weigher.

THE ELANCO ROTOWEIGH CHECK-WEIGHER

This machine is illustrated in Fig. 12.9 and is available from Manesty Machines Ltd under licence from Eli Lilly & Co. It operates by measuring the back-scattered X-ray intensity from a capsule and its contents. The claimed throughput is 73 000 capsules per hour, with an accuracy of ±3%. A schematic diagram is shown in Fig. 12.10.

Filled capsules are placed in the hopper (1). They move under gravity into the chamfered holes in plate (2) and are fed into the tubes in the rotating turret (3). The capsules drop one at a time from the tubes into sleeves (4) mounted on pins in the perimeter of an inspection wheel. The wheel carries the capsules past a low-energy X-ray beam (5). The energy back-scattered by the capsule is in direct proportion to the mass of its contents. This energy is detected by a scintillation crystal (6) which is read by a photomultiplier tube to provide a voltage in proportion to the intensity of the reflected energy.

If the mass of a capsule is lower than a pre-set standard, the voltage is processed so as to activate a valve, releasing an air jet which blows the underweight capsule into low-mass chute (7). If the mass is higher than a pre-set standard, another valve is opened which blows the capsule into the high-mass rejection chute (8). If the mass of the capsule falls within the accepted range, a third air jet blows the capsule into a hopper for packaging (9).

The inspection wheel carrying the capsules past the inspection beam rotates 26 times per minute and there are 47 inspection pins in the wheel. Thus, 1222 capsules will pass through the unit in one minute. A 48th pin (10) carries a standard mass which passes the inspection beam 26 times per minute. The purpose of this mass is to restabilise the detection system to offset any drift in sensitivity which may be caused by changes in temperature, component age, line voltage, or other factors. Some typical test results are shown in Table 12.2.

The results in Table 12.2 show that out of a total of 171 000 capsules, only 17 (0.01%) would

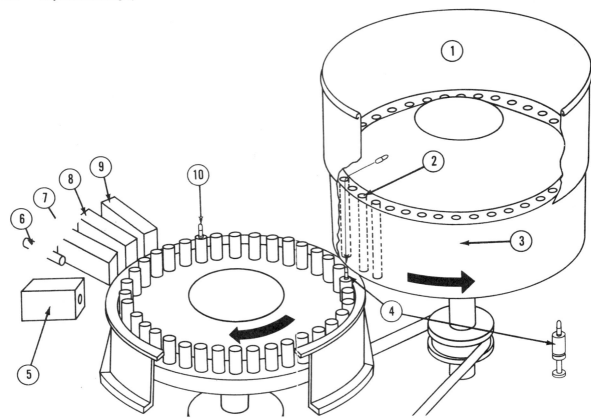

Fig. 12.10 Schematic diagram of the operation of the Elanco Rotoweigh. 1, hopper; 2, plate containing chamfered holes; 3, rotating turret; 4, capsule sleeves; 5, low-energy X-ray beam; 6, scintillation crystal; 7, low-mass rejection chute; 8, high-mass rejection chute; 9, acceptance chute to hopper; 10, 48th pin carrying a standard mass.

Table 12.2. Test results from five sub-batches, each containing 34 200 capsules, obtained from the Rotoweigh check-weigher

				Number of rejects	
Sub-batch	Weight category	Total rejects	Within set limits	Outside set limits	Outside U.S.P. XX limits
1	high	144	106	38	0
	low	22	0	22	5
2	high	64	51	13	0
	low	203	188	15	2
3	high	77	55	22	0
	low	28	14	14	4
4	high	159	131	28	0
	low	45	38	7	4
5	high	30	18	12	1
	low	37	31	6	1

fail the *U.S.P.* XX weight variation test. To determine the reliability of these results, several capsules known to be outside the pre-set limits were inserted into the batches; they were all rejected by the machine. Two of the sub-batches were passed through the machine a second time; no further rejects were recovered.

The average time for each sub-batch to pass through the Rotoweigh was 30 minutes, which is equivalent to 68 400 capsules per hour. Fine tuning of the calibration at the start of the batch reduced the number of capsules rejected without affecting those rejects which were outside the normal limits. The majority of capsules rejected were on the borderline of the pre-set limits but did not amount to more than 1% of the total.

THE VERICAP 1800 CHECK-WEIGHER

A schematic diagram of the Vericap 1800 (MOCON/Modern Controls Inc.) is shown in Fig. 12.11. The system is based on the change in capacitance which occurs when a non-conducting object, such as a capsule, is placed between two oppositely-charged plates. The average dielectric

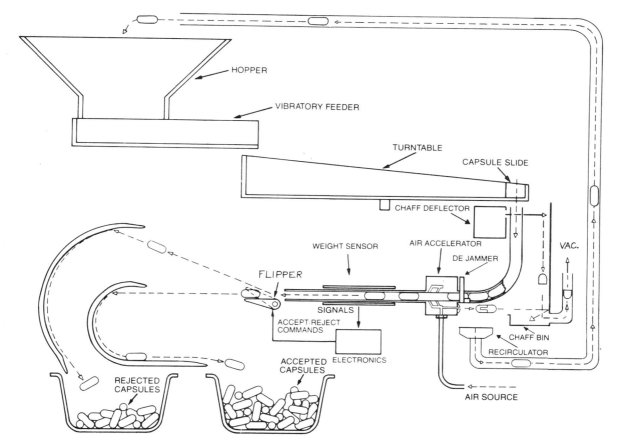

Fig. 12.11 Schematic diagram of the operation of the Vericap 1800 check-weigher.

constant between the plates when separated by air is 1, and a significant and measureable change takes place when a capsule is passed through the electric field. The system is calibrated so that the weight of the capsule can be related to the change in capacitance. A detailed description of this type of system has been given by Demorest (1980). The machine is claimed to have a throughput of 72 000 to 108 000 capsules per hour. An advantage of this system is that the air used to propel the capsules has a de-dusting effect.

CAPSULE HANDLING EQUIPMENT

THE PARKE, DAVIS CAPSULE-FINISHING SYSTEM

In this system, the constituent units clean, polish, inspect and count the capsules, and may be arranged in various combinations to suit different requirements. One arrangement is shown in Fig. 12.12.

The drum dumper is designed to handle a 24-gallon (100-litre) cylindrical drum, 655 mm long × 440 mm diameter, weighing approximately 300 kg when full. The operator loads a drum into the drum carrier and raises it to an inverted position above the capsule cleaner/polisher. When the drum reaches the upper limit of its travel, the operating motor is automatically stopped.

As part of this dumping process, after a few millimetres of upward movement, the drum contacts a spring-loaded conical cover which clamps tightly to the drum and serves as a retaining cover for it and its contents. The cone prevents the capsules from leaving the drum when the drum is inverted. When the drum has reached its final position, the operator opens a valve on the cone to release the capsules into the cleaner unit. The drum remains in its inverted position until it is empty.

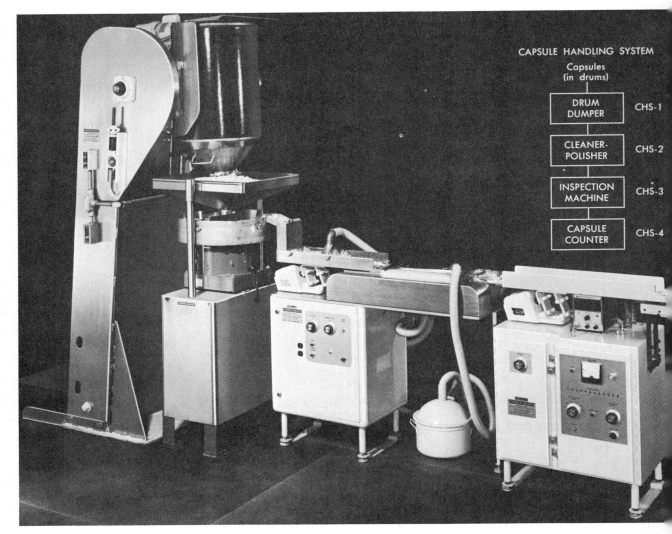

Fig. 12.12 The Parke, Davis capsule-finishing system showing, in order, the drum dumper, the cleaner-polisher, the inspection machine, and the capsule counter.

When the drum is empty, the operator presses a pushbutton to return it to floor level, the spring-loaded cone being automatically released from the drum as it descends. The cone is made of stainless steel and is easily cleaned between batches to eliminate cross-contamination of products. To save time, extra cones are available so that washing can be off-line.

The dumper is driven by an electric motor with a spring-operated mechanical brake: when power is removed, the brake locks the drum carriage, preventing further travel. Limit switches prevent inadvertent manual operation that might drive the drum carrier too far in the wrong direction, and a slip clutch prevents damage to the equipment if the drum carrier sticks at any point within its normal travel.

The cleaner/polisher is designed to clean and polish capsules by tumbling them in moisturised salt or other cleaning agent. It consists of a hopper, feeding capsules into a bowl mounted on a vibratory drive, all supported on a heavy steel base. The vibrating bowl is the heart of the cleaning system. There are several blades in the bottom of the bowl that serve to tumble and rotate the salt and capsule mixture. The capsules are cleaned by this tumbling process because the powder on the capsule exterior has a greater affinity for the damp salt than it has for the gelatin of the capsules. In addition, the capsules are polished by the vibration. Salt is separated from the capsules as they ascend a perforated metal ramp to discharge from the cleaning bowl into an empty capsule extractor and thence into a drum or an inspection machine.

The capsule feed rate is controlled by varying the distance between the bottom of the hopper and the feed chute of the bowl, though minor feed rate adjustments can be made with the vibrator potentiometer. When used in conjunction with the inspection machine, the throughput of the cleaner/polisher is held to between 40 000 and 80 000 capsules per hour by the operator's inspection rate.

The hopper is designed to hold at least 150 litres of capsules. Used with the inspection line, the drum remains inverted in the drum dumper where it is used as a supply hopper for the cleaner, with only a minimum quantity of capsules in the cleaner hopper. The salt has to be changed periodically, depending on the amount of powder on the capsules. This is accomplished by stopping the inflow of capsules to the bowl and raising a slide valve that connects the drain at the bottom of the bowl to the central vacuum system. As soon as the dirty salt has been sucked out, the valve is closed, new salt placed in the bowl, and the capsule feed restarted. This takes only 20 to 30 seconds.

If moisturised salt is used, the capsule feed must be stopped and all the capsules removed from the bowl whenever the machine stops operating for ten minutes or more. If this is not done, the damp salt will fuse to the capsules and will not be removed by further tumbling or vibrating.

The hopper and the bowl are made of stainless steel, and are removable for cleaning to prevent product cross-contamination. Such cleaning is required between different batches of the same or different products, but not between drums of the same batch. When used after filling, it is manually stopped and started by a built-in switch, but when used as part of an inspection line, a relay in the inspection machine stops and starts the cleaner at the end of a predetermined count or whenever the operator manually stops the inspection machine.

Capsules are fed into the inspection machine by a linear vibrating feeder consisting of a grooved orientating plate that feeds capsules in single file into a 12-track grille slanting across a moving conveyor belt. Since the grille guides the capsules at an angle to the conveyor belt, they rotate as they move past the operator, enabling the entire capsule to be seen. The operator sits in front of the grille to inspect the capsules, removing defective ones with a hand-held vacuum pick-up tube. The remainder are conveyed by the belt into the capsule counter. Built into the input feeder of this machine is a vacuum-operated hood that removes empty capsules and any loose dust, and the belt itself is vacuum-cleaned by a brush and vacuum connection located underneath it.

The rate at which capsules leave the capsule cleaner and discharge directly into the inspection section is set according to capsule size, capsule quality, and the operator's inspection rate. It ranges from about 40 000 capsules per hour for size 0 to 70 000 capsules per hour for size 4. There is a belt speed-control on the machine, a vibrator control, and an on/off switch. This latter is used by the operator to stop and start the cleaner/polisher, the inspection machine, and the capsule counter during operation. When the predetermined count is reached, the counter automatically stops the system.

All metal parts that come into contact with the product are made of stainless steel, anodised aluminium, or are nickel-plated. The conveyor belt is removable for washing, as is the grille. The only change parts are the two grilles, each of which accommodates three sizes of capsule.

The final unit in the inspection system is a 12-channel electronic pre-set counter. Capsules leaving the inspection machine are conveyed through the counter by a vibrating grooved pan which aligns the capsules in 12 rows and feeds them through the 12-channel electronic detector. Signals from the detector are fed through an electronic system that counts the capsules and shuts off the counter, the inspection machine, and cleaner/polisher when the pre-selected count is reached. These counts are manually selected, according to capsule size and drum capacity, by means of a rotary switch. The counter will count capsules passing the detector whether they pass one or twelve at a time. The counter has a six-digit visual display counter that indicates the actual count at all times. Its primary purpose is to enable non-standard amounts of capsules to be counted.

The counter is designed so that if a detector lamp fails, the system will stop, but the lamp can be changed and the system restarted without losing the stored count. A reset button is provided to clear and reset the counter when necessary. The operator, using a switch on the inspection machine, can stop the whole system, including the counter, without the counter losing its stored count. Mounted on the front panel are 12 small lamps. As a capsule passes a particular detector, its lamp momentarily blinks, as the capsule is sensed. These lights are useful for quickly checking the performance of the counter. Finally, a rate meter and an associated rate-alarm signal are provided. The rate per hour can be read directly from the rate meter, and the alarm circuit can be pre-set so that a piercing audio alarm will sound at a count rate slightly above the desired production rate. This prevents the counter from being flooded with capsules without the operator knowing it. Too many capsules attempting to pass the detector will 'piggyback' and cause miscounts, and the alarm is provided to alert the operator to this condition.

All parts in contact with the capsules are nickel- or chrome-plated. The counter itself is built with sophisticated but robust solid-state circuitry, providing extremely long life. Most of the critical circuitry is mounted on plug-in circuit boards, and procedures exist for rapid trouble-shooting by non-technical personnel for locating a defective board and replacing it with a new one.

The following predetermined count settings are provided for various capsule sizes: size 0, 65 000; size 1, 80 000; size 2, 100 000; size 3, 150 000; size 4, 200 000; size 5, 250 000. Other counts, such as those at the end of a run or for special lots, can be made by reading and recording numbers on the built-in visual display counter. The counter cannot run independently of the inspection machine.

The Perry CCP/2 Polisher and BFD/2 Descagger

These two machines (Perry Industries Inc.) may be used as a combination unit or independently. The polisher is a saltless cleaner, designed to ensure the maximum cleaning of two problem areas, the ends of the capsule and the ledge where the cap forms a trap with the body. The descagger removes all empty shells and broken pieces of shell before the cleaning and polishing operation. The polisher is shown in Fig. 12.13 and incorporates a two-stage process.

The first stage consists of a pre-cleaning section to remove heavy deposits or the results of a capsule opening and spilling its contents. The pre-cleaning is followed by a final buffing operation to remove any remaining dust. The system is variable in speed, with two adjustments, and is designed as a continuous-flow machine which can be operated at the outlet of a filling machine or can be fed from a belt or vibratory feed system.

The object of pre-cleaning is to reduce contamination of the buffing medium and to extend the time before changing or cleaning it is required. The pre-cleaner also enhances the cleaning of the trap areas. The pre-cleaner utilises a combination of reduced pressure (partial vacuum), air propulsion, and impact with a high-voltage screen. Each of these brings about some cleaning, and in combination they remove between 85 and 95% of the dust.

In operation, capsules are fed into an input chute and carried into an air jet which propels the capsules and dust forward through a tube. At the end of the short air path, the capsules hit a stainless steel screen at a potential of 5000 volts. The high voltage, the high-velocity air stream, and the impact, cause dust to be released. The dust-collection suction is applied behind the high-voltage screen, accelerating particles of dust through the screen and on to the dust collection system. The combination of suction and air jet create a negative pressure within the system from the input chute to the output. The pre-cleaning system is designed for easy dismantling and cleaning.

The capsules pass through the pre-cleaner and drop from a chute into a rotating tube for final cleaning and buffing. The stainless steel rotating tube is fitted with a synthetic fabric liner to clean and polish the capsules. The tube liner and the entire tube assembly is quickly and easily removed; changing a liner requires about two minutes, and they are both washable for re-use, and are long-lasting. This final buffing section has two adjustments: a dial speed control adjustment, and an angle adjustment.

The services that the system requires are, besides electricity, clean air at about 60 litres/minute at 0.2 MPa for size 0 capsules, and a negative pressure equivalent to a vacuum cleaner, approximately 1 metre water gauge, for dust collection. There must be a negative pressure at both the inlet and the outlet chutes.

Capsule-inspecting Machines from mG2

The mG2 model SC filled-capsule selecting machine (see Chapter 10, Fig. 10.53), is designed to process up to 100 000 capsules per hour at the ejection side of a capsule-filling machine, and it

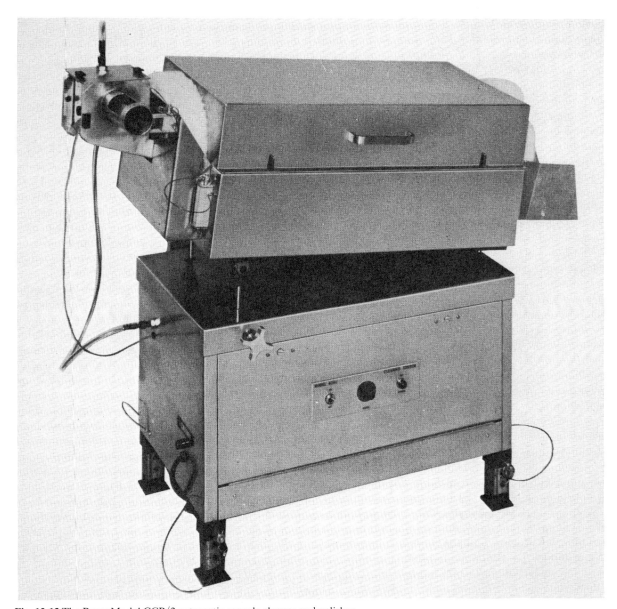

Fig. 12.13 The Perry Model CCP/2 automatic capsule cleaner and polisher.

can be used in conjunction with the cleaning and inspecting machine, also manufactured by mG2, Fig. 12.14. The selecting machine removes capsule fragments and open or empty capsules from the filled capsules. It has two independently-driven vibrating grooved plates, each controlled by its own rheostat; the capsules pass across one of them and then the other, travelling in the grooves and being propelled by the vibration. Loose powder, dust, and capsule fragments are removed by suction. If several capsule sizes are to be selected, the second vibrating plate is replaced. A static charge eliminator can be fitted for neutralising the charge on the capsules.

The mG2 cleaning and inspecting machine, model P1, is shown in Fig. 12.14 and is intended

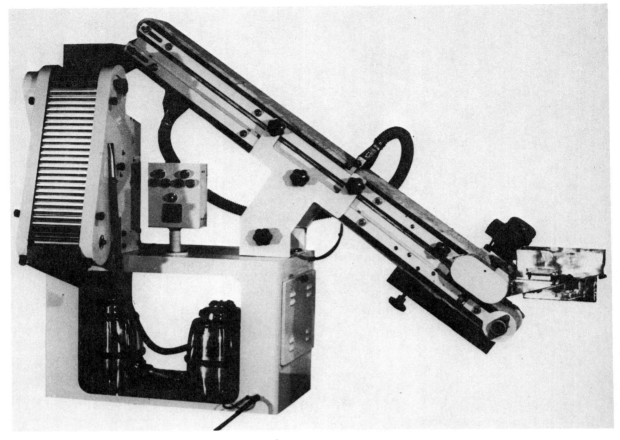

Fig. 12.14 The mG2 Model P1 capsule cleaning and inspecting machine.

for use with any capsule filling machine. Its function is to remove powder from the outside of capsules, to polish them, and to detect broken or ill-shaped capsules. The latter are manually selected for removal through a suction nozzle. The machine can handle over 100 000 capsules per hour. For a better performance, the machine can be linked to the exit of the filled-capsule selecting machine model SC.

Capsules are introduced into the hopper and are conveyed on to two lambswool belts, where powder is removed and the capsules are polished by the relative movement of the belts. Capsules are subsequently moved on to the inspection unit where they can be checked by the operator as they move downwards on rollers, passing over a luminous surface. The convenient height of the inspection unit and its oblique orientation enable the operator to check and to remove faulty capsules with the suction nozzle.

THE ELANCO ROTOSORT CAPSULE-SORTING MACHINE

This machine is available from Manesty Machines Ltd under licence from Eli Lilly & Co. It can remove the following defective items: uncapped capsule bodies containing powder, uncapped empty capsule bodies, loose capsule caps, unfilled joined capsules, and loose powder.

The gentle conveying motion is produced by a crank and rod mechanism. The crank is driven by a variable speed motor which allows the output rate to be set for optimum sorting. The capsules travel through three sections (Fig. 12.15): powder separation (A), dual-plate sorter (B), and vacuum pick-up (C).

The powder-separation screen removes and contains the loose powder from unjoined capsules and other sources. The dual-plate sorter allows the joined capsules to pass, but removes the unjoined caps and bodies. The vacuum pick-up

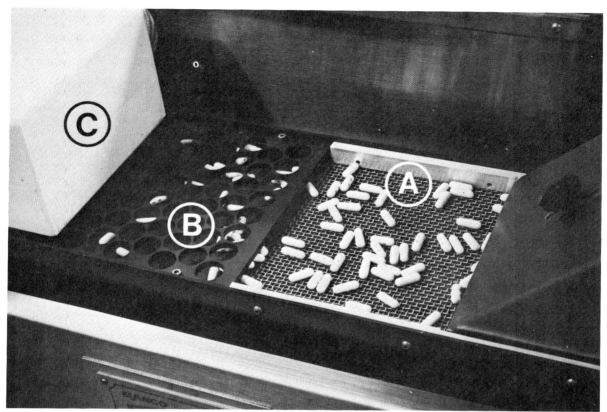

Fig. 12.15 The three sections on the Elanco Rotosort capsule-sorting machine. A, powder separation; B, dual-plate sorter; C, vacuum pick-up.

removes joined capsules which are empty or contain very little powder. A removable empty-capsule catch-basket is located in the vacuum line. All contact parts of the machine are washable and are made of aluminium alloy, stainless steel, or polyurethane. It is a compact automatic unit requiring only one operator.

ZANASI CAPSULE SORTERS

The Zanasi DS/71 capsule selection device (Fig. 12.16) removes empty capsules, partially-filled capsules, and bodies or caps from amongst the filled capsules on ejection from the filling machine. It has no moving parts. The capsules are balanced on a fluidised bed and the difference in weight between empty and filled capsules enables separation to take place. Excess dust on the capsule surface is removed. Generally the only maintenance required is the periodic cleaning of the filter.

The Zanasi empty-capsule preselector, model L/34, has been designed to prevent faulty capsules from obstructing the feed channels of any capsule filler. It is illustrated in Fig. 12.17. It does not eliminate capsules with every kind of fault, but only those whose diameter is different from the norm. The channels of the feed plate of the L/34 machine are the same as those mounted in all the capsule fillers made by Zanasi Nigris.

The empty capsules contained in the feed hopper pass into the channels of the feed plate, by the continuous vibratory motion of the hopper towards the plate. If the capsules are of the size intended for the filling machine and if their cylindrical section is not deformed, they will pass through the plate channels under gravity and will fall into the underlying collecting funnel, which will discharge them into the buckets of the conveyor.

Any fault in the cylindrical section of the

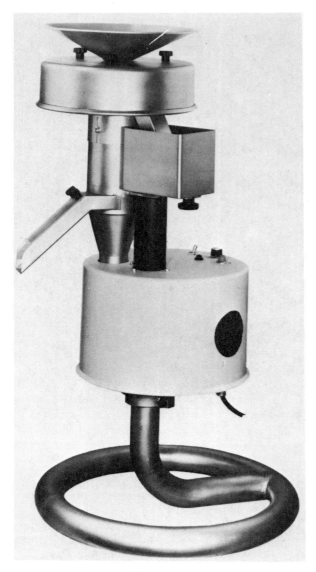

Fig. 12.16 The Zanasi DS/71 capsule selection device.

capsule, which would cause it to obstruct the feed channels of the capsule filler, will only cause the blocking of one of the plate channels of the L/34 machine, which is much easier to clear. The operator checks the plate and removes the faulty capsules, thus keeping the feed channels clear.

Banding and Sealing of Capsules

The sealing of capsules has several advantages. It can ensure that filled capsules do not open, thereby releasing powder, it can protect the contents

against the atmosphere to some degree, and can protect against substitution. The main methods of sealing capsules are banding with gelatin, sealing the overlapping section of the capsule, and spot welding the gelatin.

Until the early 1980s the increased use of self-locking capsules had largely eliminated the use of banding machines for sealing the two halves of the hard gelatin capsule. In recent years interest in banding and sealing has grown following some cases of deliberate contamination of paracetamol capsules in the U.S.A. Sealing of a self-locking capsule provides a product that is virtually tamper proof. Sealing has also become more important for use with liquid or semisolid formulations to avoid leakage and to contain substances with a strong odour.

For many years, Parke, Davis have used a band of gelatin (which may be coloured) around their capsules as an identification, under the trade-mark Kap-Seal.

Banding capsules is a time-consuming and messy operation, but it is 100% effective. Where Zanasi equipment is used, the filled capsules are transferred directly from the filler into the banding unit. Here the capsules are fed into a revolving plate and onto the banding station. The gelatin solution is contained in a heated tank underneath the plate holding the capsules. Banding wheels rotate half immersed in the gelatin solution and take up a quantity of gelatin which is deposited around the junction of the gelatin capsule. The width and thickness of the band may be adjusted. The turntable then deposits the capsule in the cradles of a drying chamber through which a current of cold air is blown. The capsules remain in the cradles long enough to ensure complete drying of the gelatin. Other polymers may be used in place of the gelatin, e.g. cellulose acetate phthalate in a suitable solvent such as methyl ethyl ketone.

More recently, the Capsugel division of Parke, Davis have introduced a sealing process under the trademark Licaps, and Elanco Qualicaps have introduced the Qualiseal process, which is effectively a refinement of the older banding process.

The Licaps process has three stages which ensure that the contact areas of the cap and body are thermally bonded by using a solution, such as water and alcohol, which lowers the melting point of gelatin. Capillary action ensures that in stage 1 the solution is uniformly distributed in the area of overlap between the cap and body. In stage 2 the excess liquid is removed by draining and air

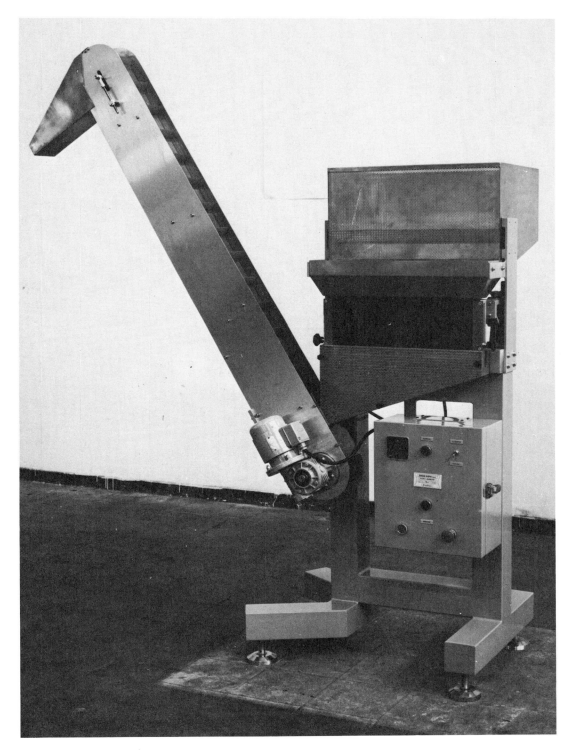

Fig. 12.17 The Zanasi Model L/34 empty-capsule preselector.

drying of the capsule. Stage 3 strengthens the bond between the cap and body by heating in a fluidised bed. A laboratory model is described by Withered (1986) for sealing 16 capsules, and this model duplicates the cycle time of the production equipment for which outputs of up to 150 000 capsules per hour are claimed.

Elanco Qualicaps have developed and improved the gelatin banding process to seal the open edge of the cap to the body of filled capsules in the Qualiseal process.

The process consists of applying two bands of gelatin onto the open edge of the cap and body sequentially. This eliminates any imperfections such as air bubbles, an uneven band, or a discontinuous band and generally ensures a stronger seal than one thick application. Capsule seals are then dried using filtered air at 25° and 50% RH. The advantage of this method is the use of an aqueous solution of gelatin, which does not introduce any new material or solvent into the process.

There are three stages to the Qualiseal process. In stage 1, the filled capsules from a storage hopper are passed through the feed roller, the rectifier roller, and the transfer roller, and fed continuously into the pockets of the conveyor belt slats. In stage 2, the capsules are positioned uniformly in the slat pockets regardless of the joined length of the capsule, and sealed once around their circumference while being rotated by the roller of the first sealing unit. The second seal is applied by the second sealing unit in a similar manner to the first. The sealing solutions are maintained under constant conditions by circulating water at a thermostatically controlled temperature through the jackets of the holding tanks. In stage 3, the sealed capsules are transferred by carriers from the conveyor belt to the drying unit, where filtered air is used to dry the gelatin seals.

Laboratory equipment is available with an output of 100 capsules per hour, and production equipment with an output of 80 000–100 000 capsules per hour.

In addition to these two methods there is a process for ultrasonic welding which uses high-frequency sound waves as an energy source to generate heat for fusing body and cap together.

References

Capsugel Newsheet, BAS-124-UK; 1984.
Demorest, R. L., *Pharm. Technol.*, 1980, *4*(12), 41–44.
Withered, D. F., *Pharm. Engng*, 1986, *6*(4), 22–23.

Chapter 13

Drug Release from Capsules

J. M. Newton

Concepts of Bioavailability

After administration of an oral preparation, the active substance is delivered to the site of pharmacological activity by a complex process which involves solution of the drug in the gastro-intestinal fluid, absorption, usually by passive diffusion across the membrane of the gastro-intestinal wall into the capillary blood supply, and distribution via the portal circulation to the systemic circulation and the site of action. The dissolution of the drug at the site of absorption is frequently, though not always, the rate-limiting factor in the distribution process. It has been established that the formulation of the dosage form and the physicochemical characteristics of the drug may have a marked influence on the dissolution process and hence on the pharmacological performance of the drug. The rate at which, and the extent to which, the active ingredient is delivered to the circulation is referred to as the bioavailability.

To evaluate the performance of a formulated product, the bioavailability can be assessed by measuring the concentration of the drug in plasma or serum over a period of time after administration. The variation in the plasma concentration with time gives an indication of the amount and rate of absorption of the drug. Increasing the rate of absorption will increase the peak concentration, and decrease the time taken to reach it, but will not change the total area under the plasma concentration-time curve (total amount absorbed). Changing the extent of the absorption will change both the peak height and the total area under the curve.

Alternatively, the rate and extent of urinary excretion of the drug or its metabolites can be measured.

Another approach, which is less time-consuming, is to use *in vitro* tests which attempt to simulate the *in vivo* performance of the dosage form.

Such tests are based on the ability of the dosage form to disintegrate in a fluid under given conditions (disintegration test), or upon the amount of drug that is released into solution in a specified fluid under given conditions (dissolution test). These tests are used in official standards for certain preparations in the *B.P.* and the *U.S.P.* Dissolution tests provide reproducible conditions for the solution process and can indicate the way in which formulation variables influence the solution rate process. However, some caution is necessary in the interpretation of *in vitro* tests in terms of *in vivo* performance as they do not always correlate.

No single test procedure has been devised which can simulate accurately what happens to a dosage form after administration, mainly because individuals vary in their responses. The apparent simplicity of capsule formulations as a blend of powders which will be readily available for dissolution promotes the belief that hard gelatin capsules are a readily bioavailable oral dosage form.

However, evidence that capsule formulations may be subject to problems of bioavailability can be obtained by comparison of the plasma concentration-time curve with that of other preparations containing the drug. These may be other commercial products, such as capsules or tablets, which have been found to be clinically acceptable. Alternatively, an intravenous injection or other type of preparation such as a solution or a suspension may be used as a reference.

Comparison with an intravenous injection will give a measure of the absolute bioavailability because it eliminates the absorptive phase. Comparison with other types of preparation only indicates the relative bioavailability of the formulation.

A solution of the drug is considered to be the most useful oral reference preparation as it eliminates the dissolution phase. Hence, comparison with a solution should indicate whether dissolution is the rate-limiting factor.

Intravenous injections and solutions may not be

feasible for insoluble drugs, yet these are the ones that are more likely to give rise to bioavailability problems. Solutions in non-aqueous polar solvents or in oils may offer an alternative as reference formulations for such drugs.

A drug which is clinically effective over a wide range of blood concentrations would provide products which may not differ significantly in bioavailability. However, if there is a narrow range between the minimum therapeutic concentration and the minimum toxic concentration, then changes in bioavailability may have serious clinical consequences. For example, phenytoin has dose-dependent elimination kinetics and a narrow therapeutic range, and even small differences in bioavailability may be hazardous. The earliest reports (Eadie et al., 1968; Martin, 1968; Rail, 1968) indicated that patients had shown the toxic effects of phenytoin overdosage when the capsule formulation of an established brand was changed. In this particular example, the difficulty was shown to be due to the substitution of lactose for calcium sulphate dihydrate as the excipient. Since then, numerous studies of this drug have shown that different formulations may not be bioequivalent. The bioavailability of phenytoin has been reviewed by Neuvonen (1979).

Consideration of published papers should provide an answer to the question as to whether hard gelatin capsules do present problems in terms of ensuring bioequivalence. Unfortunately, individual papers taken in isolation may provide conflicting evidence. For example, Tannenbaum et al. (1968) concluded that a commercial capsule formulation of triamterene and hydrochlorothiazide was less effectively absorbed than an experimentally formulated tablet. Randolph et al. (1985), however, found that a capsule formulation of the same two drugs was bioequivalent to an aqueous solution, suggesting that the capsule formulation of the earlier study was probably not optimised.

Since many published papers lack details of formulation, it is generally impossible to make an accurate assessment of which formulation factors are important. It is also important to realise that reports of capsule formulations being less bioavailable than other preparations could be due to a particular drug being poorly absorbed by the oral route for various reasons. For example, Sasahara et al. (1980) concluded that the relatively low absolute bioavailability of levodopa in capsules is probably due to first pass metabolism.

An alternative source of difference between the various preparations of the same drug is the use of non-optimum formulations in the comparison. Wagner et al. (1966) provided clear evidence that a capsule formulation of indoxole was inferior to emulsion, soft gelatin capsule and suspension formulations. Whether this was the best hard gelatin capsule formulation cannot be judged from the evidence available in the paper. Thus comparison of capsules with other formulations must be judged with caution.

Another factor to be considered in assessing the comparison of formulations is the physiology of the gastro-intestinal tract and its involvement in drug absorption. For example, Stewart and others (1979) compared an experimental capsule formulation with a solution of riboflavine as a standard. The higher urinary excretion observed after administration of capsule formulations could be associated with the rapid transit of the solution past the limited area of the intestine capable of absorbing riboflavine.

Comparison of different capsule formulations of the same drug should provide better evidence that formulation needs to be considered to ensure comparable bioavailability of capsule formulations, but even here caution must be used in interpretation of some of the papers listed in the Bibliography. In several instances conclusions are drawn from poor in vivo experimental data, e.g. Brice and Hammer (1969), where serum levels produced by commercial formulations of oxytetracycline were compared at only four time intervals, providing insufficient data for a reasonable pharmacokinetic analysis.

The evidence of the papers contained in the Bibliography, while not being unequivocal, does lead to the conclusion that it is necessary to consider formulation to ensure an adequate in vivo performance of certain drugs.

Formulation and the Release of Drugs from Capsules

Because the release of drugs from hard gelatin capsules can be influenced by the formulation, it is important to consider the ways in which maximisation and/or consistency of drug release can be achieved. For this purpose, it is necessary to understand the mechanism of absorption of the drug to be formulated, and especially to know which stage is the rate-controlling step in the process. Much time can be wasted in attempting to improve the formulation, in terms of drug release, if this is only a minor aspect of the absorption process. In the present account, it will be assumed that the drug is in the correct crystalline form; there will be no consideration of the influence of crystal structure, nor the existence of solvates or hydrates.

An important feature of formulation is to ensure that the capsule contains the correct, uniform dose of the drug. The formulation will only exist as a single-component system if the drug completely and reproducibly fills the capsule volume. Small dose levels of drug require prior blending with an inert diluent. Similarly, larger doses can be blended with a diluent if, by this addition, a greater reproducibility of bulk volume can be achieved. High-speed filling machines, which operate by pre-forming a plug of powder prior to transferring it to the capsule, often involve a degree of consolidation of the powder bed, and friction between this plug and metal makes necessary the addition of a powder/metal lubricant. Glidants may also be needed to improve powder flow and ensure reproducible bulk volume.

The work involved in studying formulation variables by *in vivo* techniques is costly and time consuming, hence many studies involving formulation factors use *in vitro* testing, particularly dissolution. This makes two important assumptions: that dissolution is the rate-controlling step in the absorption process, and that the particular *in vitro* dissolution test reflects the *in vivo* performance of the formulation.

Unfortunately, these two restrictions are only rarely assessed. Any deductions made from dissolution results should be used only as guidelines to formulation, not as absolute values.

In order to ensure adequate bioavailability when formulating hard gelatin capsules, it is necessary to consider various factors. These include the solubility, particle size, and wettability of the drug, together with the combination of possible additives, the filling process to be used, and the requirement to produce a granulation. An essential feature is to ensure that the capsule disintegrates both *in vitro* and *in vivo*. Whilst the application of the *in vitro* test may not be a conclusive indicator of a bioavailable capsule formulation, a capsule which does not disintegrate is very unlikely to be effective. These factors will now be considered.

DRUG SOLUBILITY

Unless other factors dominate, the rate-controlling step in the absorption process is the rate at which the drug is transferred from the solid state into solution. For a wide range of compounds, the intrinsic rate of dissolution is directly proportional to the solubility (Hamlin *et al.*, 1965). Hence the lower the drug solubility, the lower will be the rate of dissolution and so absorption. The combined effects of drug solubility and of additives within the capsule on the dissolution rate of a range of drugs were studied by making measurements at two levels (20 and 80%) of three diluents, and in the presence or absence of magnesium stearate and sodium lauryl sulphate (Newton and Razzo, 1977a). There was a strong indication that the rate was proportional to the logarithm of the drug solubility (Fig. 13.1). Thus one can anticipate

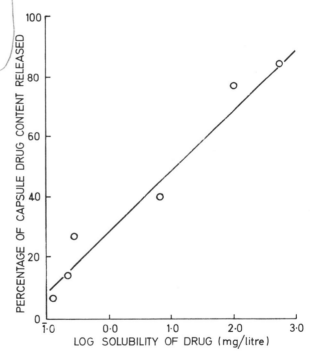

Fig. 13.1. The influence of drug solubility on the *in vitro* release of drugs from capsules.

problems when presenting drugs with low water solubility in capsules. Blending of simple additives did not overcome the formulation problems.

PARTICLE SIZE

The standard method of increasing the rate of solution of a drug is to increase the surface area in contact with the solvent by reducing the particle size. However, the effectiveness of this method will depend on the contact between liquid and solid.

When nitrofurantoin, a relatively insoluble substance, was administered to rats in a hard gelatin capsule, the proportion of the dose excreted in the urine increased as the particle size was decreased (Fig. 13.2) (Paul *et al.*, 1967). Capsules

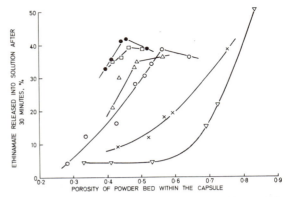

Fig. 13.3. The percentage of ethinamate released into solution after 30 minutes from capsules containing different particle size fractions packed to give different porosities.

● 251–420 μm	○ 125–152 μm
□ 177–251 μm	✕ 66–76 μm
△ 152–177 μm	▽ 8.3 μm

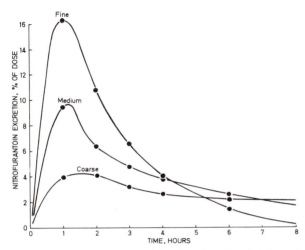

Fig. 13.2. The effect of particle size of orally-administered nitrofurantoin on urinary excretion in rats.

containing sulphafurazole of mean particle size 1.7, 39, and 95 μm were tested in dogs by Fincher *et al.*, (1965); the peak blood concentration increased with decreasing particle size.

Results such as these for relatively water-insoluble drugs make it appear that reduction of the particle size of the drug should solve the bioavailability problems of capsules. However, the opposite effect can occur. Capsules of ethinamate, a drug with a solubility of 1 in 400, were tested for dissolution *in vitro*, using various particle sizes packed to give different porosities. For equivalent packing densities as judged by porosity, a greater drug release was obtained with the largest particle size fraction (Fig. 13.3) (Newton and Rowley, 1970). This was because the powder bed with smaller particle sizes was less permeable to liquid. Similar effects were obtained with aspirin (Newton and Bader, 1980).

When four different particle size fractions of the same drug, <6, <10, <50 and <100 μm in size, were administered in capsules to dogs, there was no significant difference in absorption, but when

the powder was more closely classified to give better-defined size ranges, namely between 6 and 12 μm, and between 60 and 100 μm, higher blood concentrations resulted from the administration of the capsules containing the larger particle size fraction (Ljungberg and Otto, 1970). Ridolfo *et al.* (1979) established that for capsules containing particles of 67 μm or 640 μm mean equivalent diameter of a relatively water-insoluble drug, benoxaprofen, the capsules containing the smaller size particles dissolved more rapidly and gave a higher *in vivo* bioavailability, judged by plasma concentration/time curves and urinary excretion. The capsules, however, contained nearly twice as much starch as drug. This could ensure water penetration between the fine particles, and thus adequate contact with their larger surface area. Confirmation of this result was reported from the same laboratories (Wolen *et al.*, 1979). Again, the drug was incorporated into a large quantity of starch within the capsules.

WETTING

As discussed in the previous section, decreasing the particle size of a drug, although it increases the surface area for dissolution, does not necessarily increase the dissolution rate because there may be a reduction in the contact between the liquid and the solid. This is particularly likely if the liquid does not wet the solid. Whether a liquid will spread over the surface of a solid is determined by the relative values of the attraction of the molecules of the liquid for those of the surface, and of those of the liquid molecules for each other. If the former exceed the latter, spreading of the liquid over the solid surface will occur. The ease of wetting is best expressed by the contact angle between the edge of the liquid meniscus and the solid surface. A zero value implies ready and complete wetting`of the solid by the liquid while a value of 180° would correspond to absolute non-wetting. Water-insoluble drugs usually have a low affinity for aqueous fluids, and hence have high values of the contact angle, indicative of non-wetting (Lerk *et al.*, 1977). Similarly the addition of the hydrophobic lubricant, magnesium stearate, can also prevent wetting of powders and hence retard dissolution. Wetting, as indicated by the liquid penetration test of Studebaker and Snow (1955), and drug release as indicated by dissolution, have been shown to correlate inversely. The interesting behaviour of magnesium stearate is shown in Fig. 13.4 (Samyn and Jung, 1970).

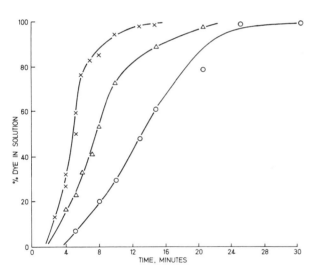

Fig. 13.4. The dissolution of dye from capsules containing lactose (×), and capsules containing lactose with 2% (△) or 5% (○) of magnesium stearate.

However, for more complex formulations, systems giving poor wetting do not necessarily give poor dissolution (Fig. 13.5) (Rowley and Newton, 1970). Sodium lauryl sulphate dissolves with swelling and it may retard penetration in the wetting test, yet aid disruption of the capsule in the dissolution test. Most surfactants produced only small increases in the dissolution rate of ethinamate in

capsule formulations (Newton, 1972). An alternative method of increasing the wettability of a capsule formulation is to incorporate a hydrophilic material such as starch or lactose. Such additives may of course act by disintegration as well as wetting, and their effectiveness is not reliably disclosed by dissolution techniques (Newton, 1972). Large proportions (up to 80%) of the diluent may be needed to be effective and do not always guarantee complete drug release, especially of highly insoluble drugs (Newton and Razzo, 1974).

The inability of physical mixing to ensure wetting and drug release was confirmed by mixing hexobarbitone with hydroxymethyl or hydroxyethyl cellulose, which failed to reduce the contact angle or increase dissolution rate (Lerk *et al.*, 1978). However, by intimate mixing of the drug with a solution of the hydrophilic material, followed by drying to give minigranules, a reduction in the contact angle and a marked improvement in dissolution were achieved. The contact angles, although reduced, remained relatively high, so that the improved dissolution should perhaps be attributed to the structure introduced by granulation. Treating griseofulvin with hydroxypropyl cellulose, by a similar process, improved the drug release, as assessed by dissolution and urinary excretion of the major metabolite (Fell *et al.*, 1978). As no measurements of contact angles were reported, it could again be the granulation as well as the wetting process which is involved in improving drug release. The same process has been shown by Lerk *et al.* (1979) to improve the rate of absorption, relative to pure drug, when phenytoin capsule formulations were administered to human volunteers. The authors were able to show that the process improved water uptake into the powder plug, employing penetration tests. *In vitro* dissolution tests were found to reflect the improved liquid penetration, irrespective of the presence of surfactant in the dissolution fluid.

GRANULATION

Granulation provides a method of assembling the individual particles in a regular manner, as opposed to the random aggregation which occurs under the influence of the natural interparticulate forces between small particles, and it is known that granulation can increase the dissolution rate of fine particles (Finholt *et al.*, 1968). The technique is applicable to capsule formulations (Newton and Rowley, 1970). In this case a solvent is the only binder, so there is no change in contact angle;

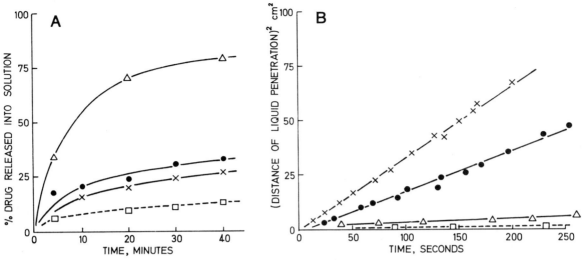

Fig. 13.5. A, the dissolution of a drug for four different capsule formulations. B, the liquid penetration test for the same formulations.

　□　drug with 0.5% magnesium stearate
　×　drug with 0.5% magnesium stearate, 1% sodium lauryl sulphate, and 5% lactose
　●　drug with 0.5% magnesium stearate, 1% sodium lauryl sulphate, and 20% lactose
　△　drug with 1% magnesium stearate, 1% sodium lauryl sulphate, and 50% lactose

only the particle arrangement is altered. The improvement in dissolution rate is related to the permeability of the structure produced (Fig. 13.6).

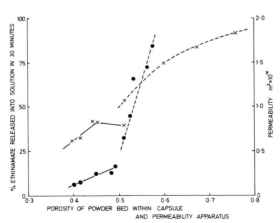

Fig. 13.6. The dissolution of drug from capsules containing crystals and granules of micronised ethinamate, packed to give different porosities, compared with the liquid permeability of beds of the same samples.

　———— crystals, 251–420 μm　×　dissolution
　-------- granules, 251–420 μm　●　liquid permeability

Granulation appears to be an extremely beneficial process in capsule formulation; it should improve flow and uniformity of bulk density in addition to assisting drug release.

DISINTEGRATION
Disintegration of the capsule into primary particles is a necessary requirement, especially for high-dose drugs.

Deaggregation performance and serum level have been shown to be related for four chloramphenicol capsule formulations (Aguiar *et al.*, 1968). Incorporation of twice the drug weight of sodium bicarbonate into tetracycline capsules ensured disruption of the capsule and improved dissolution, (Nelson, 1960) but the incorporation of an equal weight of citric acid did not affect the drug release at all (O'Reilly and Nelson, 1961). Improved drug release, as indicated by dissolution testing, was claimed to follow the incorporation of sodium starch glycolate (Primojel, a tablet disintegrant) into capsule formulations, but as no disintegration test results are reported, improved drug release may also be a function of improved wetting as well as of disintegration (Newton and Rowley, 1975). This is also true of a comparison of capsule disintegrants by dissolution testing (Ryder and Thomas, 1977). A ranking order of starch glycolate (Primojel) > Nymcel > no disintegrant was established, and the results also suggested that maize starch is not an effective disintegrant.

To assess the *in vivo* disintegration of capsules, Eckert (1967) used capsules filled with sodium bicarbonate and determined the disintegration time by the change in pH of the gastric juice, measured by a radio-endoscope.

Casey *et al.* (1976) reported the use of external scintigraphy, using a gamma camera to estimate the dispersion of a gamma-emitting isotope (^{99m}Tc) contained in capsule formulations. They found that a more rapid disintegration occurred when the capsule contents were soluble (6 minutes) than when they were insoluble (30–40 minutes). Using the same technique, Hunter *et al.* (1980) found that the condition of the subjects was important. Capsules containing resin beads labelled with ^{99m}Tc provided little dispersion when administered to fasting subjects, whereas after food the dispersion was more rapid and reflected *in vitro* disintegration times. A profile scanning technique was used by Alpsten *et al.* (1979) to compare the *in vivo* and *in vitro* disintegration of granule formulations of aspirin labelled with ^{51}Cr. Subjects were scanned with a movable detector whilst sitting in a well-defined position in an armchair within a low-activity laboratory. The disintegration times were considerably longer *in vivo* for both formulations than those obtained from *in vitro* disintegration tests.

COMBINATIONS OF ADDITIVES
The presentation of drugs in hard gelatin capsules is usually considered to be a relatively simple matter, but it is seldom possible to provide formulations which meet the needs of filling machines without resorting to a multicomponent system. The added components, however, do not always result in a simple additive effect on drug release (Newton *et al.*, 1971a and b; Newton and Razzo, 1974). The effect of changing the quantity of additives has been modelled for a single drug by fitting a second-degree equation to relate capsule composition to dissolution (Newton and Razzo, 1977b). Such a relationship is the simplest model that allows the interactions between pairs of factors to be represented. The results also include the influence of formulation combinations on the filling performance, allowing the feasibility of filling a particular combination of ingredients into the capsule to be assessed.

CAPSULE FILLING
The method by which the capsules are filled is also important. The available processes vary in complexity, and hence the resultant powder-bed structures will be very different. For fine particles, decreasing the porosity resulted in a decrease in drug release (Newton and Rowley, 1970). This effect applied equally for capsules containing a drug with 10 or 50 per cent of lactose (Newton, 1972). For more complex formulations, packing seemed to be less important than other formulation factors (Newton *et al.*, 1971b). Loose and tight filling of capsules of cephalexin did not influence serum levels (O'Callaghan *et al.*, 1971), but it has been claimed that a high salicylate plasma level was obtained when the same quantity of aspirin and dibasic calcium phosphate was packed into a smaller size shell (McGee *et al.*, 1970). It would seem, however, desirable to ensure that the ingredients are filled into a capsule in such a manner as to allow rapid deaggregation of the particles, which means that they should be filled with a minimum of compression, or incorporate a disintegrant which will ensure deaggregation.

Drug Release from Soft Gelatin Capsules

There are only a few drugs which are of the correct consistency and dose level to form the total content of the capsule. Thus the vehicle used to present the drug within the shell is important. In general, the system must have the correct rheological characteristics to be handled by the filling process, and must be compatible with the gelatin shell. Water-immiscible oils are the most important type of vehicle although water-miscible polyethylene glycols and non-ionic surfactants have also been used.

CAPSULES CONTAINING THE DRUG AS THE MAJOR COMPONENT
Drugs which are oils or which are highly soluble in oils can be readily presented as a unit dose in a soft gelatin capsule, e.g. cod liver oil, clofibrate, ethchlorvynol, and paramethadione. There appears to be little published work establishing the 'absolute bioavailability' of such drugs, and indeed the low water solubility would present difficulties for formulation of an intravenous preparation.

Taylor and Chasseaud (1977) compared the bioavailability of clofibrate in a soft capsule with that of calcium clofibrate in a hard gelatin capsule formulation; the results indicated the bioequivalence of the two formulations. In a later paper, Taylor *et al.* (1978) compared the bioavailability of a soft gelatin clofibrate capsule with that of a film-coated tablet containing calcium clofibrate and calcium carbonate (1:1 mixture), under conditions approaching steady state. The results suggested that the two formulations did not differ significantly.

Fischler *et al.* (1973) compared soft gelatin capsule formulations containing chlormethiazole base with a tablet formulation containing chlormethiazole edisylate. They established that there was a more rapid and complete absorption from the capsules than from the tablets, due to drug forms of different solubility. The addition of arachis oil to the capsule formulation was found to result in a further increase in the peak drug concentration. As the dissolution rate was not improved by the addition of arachis oil, the authors suggested that a change in the absorptive conditions of the gastro-intestinal tract might take place in the presence of the arachis oil.

Angelucci *et al.* (1976) compared the bioavailability of flufenamic acid formulated as hard or soft gelatin capsules. The soft capsule contained vegetable oil, hydrogenated vegetable oils, beeswax, and soya lecithin in addition to the drug. Results using both dogs and humans indicated that the soft gelatin formulation produced consistently higher plasma concentration-time curves.

Capsules Containing the Drug as a Minor Component

The solution of a drug in a solvent allows the use of accurate methods to sub-divide the drug into unit-dose systems. If the solubility of the drug is high and the dose relatively low, it is possible to contain the dose within the volume of a soft gelatin capsule. Alternatively, the drug, especially if low-dose, may be dispersed in a fluid to provide an emulsion or a suspension. Such a dispersion must have suitable rheological properties.

Water-immiscible oils, which are compatible with the shell, provide only limited dissolving power. There is also the question of whether the drug is absorbed with the oily vehicle, an unlikely possibility, or has to transfer to the aqueous phase before absorption can take place. Water-miscible solvents which are compatible with the shell, e.g. polyethylene glycols or non-ionic surfactants, have solvent properties for a large range of drugs.

Mallis *et al.* (1975) administered soft gelatin capsules containing 0.2 mg of digoxin dissolved in polyethylene glycol and propylene glycol and compared them with a rapidly dissolving tablet containing 0.2 mg and two commercially available tablets containing 0.25 mg, in a single- and a multiple-dose study. Serum-digoxin concentrations achieved with the capsules were similar to those obtained with both the 0.25 mg tablets, and better than those achieved with the 0.2 mg tablets. The time to achieve peak concentration was equivalent for all four preparations, but the area under the curve was significantly greater for the capsules than for the equivalent dose of a rapidly-dissolving tablet, and equivalent to that achieved with the 0.25 mg tablets. There were no significant differences between any formulations in the serum concentrations on the 2nd, 8th or 10th days, nor in the steady-state urinary excretion.

In a second study, the capsules were compared with a solution of the capsule contents and with a commercially available elixir; results indicated that the mean area under the serum concentration-time curve was greater for the capsule than for either of the two liquids. The mean time to reach peak concentration was similar for all three preparations. These results imply that presenting the drug in a capsule has a beneficial influence on bioavailability, possibly due to changes in the rate of movement within the gastro-intestinal tract.

Marcus *et al.* (1976) compared the bioavailability of a soft gelatin capsule of digoxin (in ethanol, water, propylene glycol, and polyethylene glycol 400) with an oral alcoholic solution and a standard commercial tablet, relative to an intravenous solution (0.25 mg/ml in 40% propylene glycol, 10% ethanol, 0.3% sodium phosphate, and 0.08% anhydrous citric acid). The intravenous infusion was administered over 1 hour and 3 hours. The serum concentration peaked at 5 ng/ml at the end of the 1-hour infusion, and at 3.5 ng/ml after the second hour of the 3-hour infusion. The 6-day urinary excretion after the 3-hour infusion was 21% more than for the same dose given over 1 hour. Hence, the assessment of the absolute bioavailability will be affected by the choice of infusion rate. In general, the soft gelatin capsule had the highest level of bioavailability.

Lindenbaum (1977) compared a soft gelatin capsule formulation of digoxin (in polyethylene glycol 400, ethanol, water, and propylene glycol) with an equivalent dose in 10% aqueous ethanol, and with a tablet formulation. It was established that the area under the serum concentration-time curve, and the 6-day cumulative urinary excretion, were greater after administration of the capsule than for the other two formulations.

Wagner *et al.* (1979) compared the *in vivo* bio-availability of four commercial soft capsule formulations of digoxin, but no details of formulation were given. There were no significant differences in the amount of digoxin absorbed from each formulation, as judged by urinary excretion or area under the plasma concentration-time curve. There were significant differences in the time to reach peak plasma concentration, in the *in vitro* 'burst time', and in the time required to release 50 or 85% of digoxin in a dissolution test.

The possible involvement of the shell in the absorption process can present problems if the shell characteristics change on storage. Johnson *et al.* (1977) studied freshly-prepared digoxin capsules and capsules which had been stored at 5° and 37° for 10 months. There was some evidence that storage delayed the onset of peak plasma concentrations but there was no evidence that the extent of absorption was reduced.

Further indications of the enhanced bioavailability of digoxin when presented as soft gelatin capsules come from papers reporting the administration of commercially available formulations, e.g. Binnion (1976), Longhini *et al.* (1977), O'Grady *et al.* (1978) and Alvisi *et al.* (1979). Padeletti and Brat (1978), however, compared equivalent doses of commercially available soft capsules and tablets and reported that they were bioequivalent.

The use of polyhydric alcohols with non-ionic surfactants to provide solutions or dispersions in soft gelatin capsules was proposed as a method of improving the bioavailability of water-insoluble drugs by Hom and Miskel (1970). The suggestion was based on the *in vitro* dissolution performance of soft gelatin capsules of dicoumarol, stilboestrol, digitoxin, ethinyloestradiol, hydrocortisone, phenobarbitone, phenylbutazone, propylthiouracil, and sulphadiazine. In all cases, the drug appeared in solution at least as quickly and often at a faster rate from capsules than from commercial tablets.

However, an improvement in bioavailability with this type of formulation does not always occur. Albert *et al.* (1974) found that soft capsule formulations of paracetamol and nitrofurantoin containing surfactants were only equivalent in bioavailability and not superior to commercial tablets. Gundert-Remy *et al.* (1975a) found that soft

capsule formulations of diphenhydramine hydro-chloride based on polyethylene glycol and surfactants were no more bioavailable than commercial sugar-coated tablets or hard capsule formulations. When the same drug was presented in soft capsule formulations in oil/wax surfactant mixtures, no reduction in bioavailability occurred. Similarly, oil/wax surfactant formulations of phenobarbitone were found to be bioequivalent to tablet formulations (Gundert-Remy *et al.*, 1975b). In these latter cases, the drugs were relatively water-soluble and the rate of drug release could be retarded by the presence of oil.

Further indications of the improved bioavailability of soft capsules come from the work of Fuccella *et al.* (1977) and Fuccella (1979), although no details of formulation are given. Comparison of commercial hard and soft capsules of temazepam in a single-dose study established that the soft capsule produced faster absorption, with earlier and higher peak plasma concentrations. However, there was no difference in the relative bioavailability as judged by the total area under the plasma concentration-time curve.

Liquid Filling of Hard Gelatin Capsules

Walker *et al.* (1980) have described a method whereby molten and thixotropic formulations can be filled into hard capsules on a conventional filling machine. Such a process allows all the advantages previously claimed for soft gelatin preparations such as the use of an accurate liquid feed, and the inclusion of polyethylene glycols and surfactants to improve the bioavailability of highly water-soluble drugs. Similarly, formulations containing waxes, which retard drug release, can be filled into hard capsules by this process, e.g. Francois *et al.* (1983). Thus the formulation techniques for both hard and soft capsules are now similar, and this widens the scope for controlling the release of drugs from capsule formulations and the range of dosage forms available.

References

Aguiar, A. J. *et al.*, *J. pharm. Sci.*, 1968, *57*, 1844–1850.
Albert, K. S. *et al.*, *J. clin. Pharmac.*, 1974, *14*, 264–270.
Alpsten, M. *et al.*, *J. Pharm. Pharmac.*, 1979, *31*, 480–481.
Alvisi, V. *et al.*, *Arzneimittel-Forsch.*, 1979, *29*, 1047–1050.
Angelucci, L. *et al.*, *J. pharm. Sci.*, 1976, *65*, 455–456.
Binnion, P. F., *J. clin. Pharmac.*, 1976, *16*, 461–467.
Brice, G. W. and Hammer, H. F., *J. Am. med. Ass.*, 1969, *208*, 1189–1190.
Casey, D. L. *et al.*, *J. pharm. Sci.*, 1976, *65*, 1412–1413.
Eadie, M. J. *et al.*, *Med. J. Aust.*, 1968, *2*, 515.
Eckert, T., *Arzneimittel-Forsch*, 1967, *17*, 645–646.

Fell, J. T. *et al.*, *J. Pharm. Pharmac.*, 1978, *30*, 479–482.

Fincher, J. H. *et al.*, *J. pharm. Sci.*, 1965, *54*, 704–708.

Finholt, P. *et al.*, *Meddeleser fra Norsk Farmaceutisk Selskap*, 1968, *28*, 238–252.

Fischler, M. *et al.*, *Acta pharm. suec.*, 1973, *10*, 483–492.

Francois, D., *Labo-Pharma Probl. Tech.*, 1983, *31*, 944–949.

Fuccella, L. M., *Br. J. clin. Pharmac.*, 1979, *8, Suppl.* 1, 31S–35S.

Fuccella, L. M. *et al.*, *Eur. J. clin. Pharmac.*, 1977, *12*, 383–386.

Gundert-Remy, U. *et al.*, *Drugs Germ.*, 1975a, *18*, 99–104.

Gundert-Remy, U. *et al.*, *Pharm. Ind., Berl.*, 1975b, *37*, 905–909.

Hamlin, W. E., *et al.*, *J. pharm. Sci.*, 1965, *54*, 1651–1653.

Hom, F. S. and Miskel, J. J., *J. pharm. Sci.*, 1970, *59*, 827–830.

Hunter, E. *et al.*, *Int. J. Pharmaceut.*, 1980, *4*, 175–183.

Johnson, B. F. *et al.*, *J. Pharm. Pharmac.*, 1977, *29*, 576–578.

Lerk, C. F. *et al.*, *J. pharm. Sci.*, 1977, *66*, 1480–1481.

Lerk, C. F. *et al.*, *J. pharm. Sci.*, 1978, *67*, 935–939.

Lerk, C. F. *et al.*, *J. pharm. Sci.*, 1979, *68*, 634–638.

Lindenbaum, J., *Clin. Pharmac. Ther.*, 1977, *21*, 278–282.

Ljungberg, S. and Otto, G., *Acta pharm. suec.*, 1970, *7*, 449–456.

Longhini, C. *et al.*, *Curr. ther. Res.*, 1977, *21*, 909–912.

Mallis, G. I. *et al.*, *Clin. Pharmac. Ther.*, 1975, *18*, 761–768.

Marcus, F. I. *et al.*, *Clin. Pharmac. Ther.*, 1976, *20*, 253–259.

Martin, C. M., *J. Am. med. Ass.*, 1968, *205*(9), 23–24 and 30.

McGee, B. J. *et al.*, *J. pharm. Sci.*, 1970, *59*, 1430–1433.

Nelson, E., *J. pharm. Sci.*, 1960, *49*, 54–56.

Neuvonen, P. J., *Clin. Pharmacokinet.*, 1979, *4*, 91–103.

Newton, J. M., *Pharm. Weekbl. Ned.*, 1972, *107*, 485–498.

Newton, J. M. and Bader, F., *J. Pharm. Pharmac.*, 1980, *32*, 167–171.

Newton, J. M. and Razzo, F. N., *J. Pharm. Pharmac.*, 1974, *26, Suppl.*, 30P–36P.

Newton, J. M. and Razzo, F. N., *J. Pharm. Pharmac.*, 1977a, *29*, 205–208.

Newton, J. M. and Razzo, F. N., *J. Pharm. Pharmac.*, 1977b, *29*, 294–297.

Newton, J. M. and Rowley, G., *J. Pharm. Pharmac.*, 1970, *22, Suppl.*, 163S–168S.

Newton, J. M. and Rowley, G., U.S. Patent 3 859 431, 1975.

Newton, J. M. *et al.*, *J. Pharm. Pharmac.*, 1971a, *23*, 452–453.

Newton, J. M. *et al.*, *J. Pharm. Pharmac.*, 1971b, *23, Suppl.*, 156S–160S.

O'Callaghan, C. H. *et al.*, *J. Pharm. Pharmac.*, 1971, *23*, 50–57.

O'Grady, J. *et al.*, *Eur. J. clin. Pharmac.*, 1978, *14*, 357–360.

O'Reilly, I. and Nelson, E., *J. pharm. Sci.*, 1961, *50*, 413–416.

Padeletti, L. and Brat, A., *Int. J. clin. Pharmac. Biopharm.*, 1978, *16*, 320–322.

Paul, H. E. *et al.*, *J. pharm. Sci.*, 1967, *56*, 882–885.

Rail, L., *Med. J. Aust.*, 1968, *2*, 339.

Randolph, W. C., *Curr. ther. Res.*, 1985, *38*, 990–996.

Ridolfo, A. S. *et al.*, *J. pharm. Sci.*, 1979, *68*, 850–852.

Rowley, G. and Newton, J. M., *J. Pharm. Pharmac.*, 1970, *22*, 966–967.

Ryder, J. and Thomas, A., *J. Pharm. Pharmac.*, 1977, *29, Suppl.*, 63P.

Samyn, J. C. and Jung, W. Y., *J. pharm. Sci.*, 1970, *59*, 169–175.

Sasahara, K. *et al.*, *J. pharm. Sci.*, 1980, *69*, 261–265.

Stewart, A. G. *et al.*, *J. Pharm. Pharmac.*, 1979, *31*, 1–6.

Studebaker, M. L. and Snow, C. W., *J. phys. Chem., Ithaca*, 1955, *59*, 973–976.

Tannenbaum, P. J. *et al.*, *Clin. Pharmac. Ther.*, 1968, *9*, 598–604.

Taylor, T. and Chasseaud, L. F., *J. pharm. Sci.*, 1977, *66*, 1638–1639.

Taylor, T. *et al.*, *Eur. J. clin. Pharmac.*, 1978, *13*, 49–53.

Wagner, J. G. *et al.*, *Clin. Pharmac. Ther.*, 1966, *7*, 610–619.

Wagner, J. G. *et al.*, *J. Pharmacokinet. Biopharm.*, 1979, *7*, 147–158.

Walker, S. E. *et al.*, *J. Pharm. Pharmac.*, 1980, *32*, 389–393.

Wolen, R. L. *et al.*, *Biomed. Mass Spectrom.*, 1979, *6*, 173–178.

Bibliography of Capsules

B. E. Jones and J. M. Newton

The compilation of this bibliography was started in 1968 as a means of providing a literature source similar to that provided by Evans and Train in their 'Bibliography of the tabletting of medicinal substances' (Pharmaceutical Press, 1963). The aim was to cover the literature on hard and soft capsules, because information sources were few or non-existent. Although capsules have a long history, the number of references to them from before the 1950s is very small. This bibliography contains mainly those published since 1960 (although there are some from before that date). Earlier references will be found in Chapters 1 and 8. References have been added to the bibliography up to the second half of 1986.

A decimal classification system was devised to bring together similar references and make their information more accessible. The work is divided into four main sections:

1. Historical and General
2. Gelatin
3. Capsule Practice and Manufacture
4. Drug Availability from Capsules.

The main sections are further sub-divided into 103 smaller sets of information as shown in the Classification below.

Arrangement

The references within each subsection are arranged
1. chronologically by year of appearance,
2. alphabetically by first author within each year,
3. alphabetically by title of journal within each year for the same author,
4. numerically by volume within each year, and
5. numerically by page within each volume.

The journal (or book) reference and the title of the paper are followed, in smaller print, by a simple keyword abstract which has the information arranged in the following fashion:

1. The dosage forms described, except where the items appear in a section specific to either hard or soft gelatin capsules. This is followed by a colon.
2. A series of keywords or phrases separated by semicolons and commas and arranged in the order:
   (a) the drug name,
   (b) for *in vivo* studies the sample in which drug level was measured, i.e. plasma, urine, etc.,
   (c) the remainder of the information in alphabetical order.
3. If the reference appears in more than one subsection, the number(s) of the other subsection(s) in which it is included are listed at the end. For these entries, keywords or phrases are not repeated in each entry and only appear when relevant to the subsections.

Only the major subjects included in this bibliography have been indexed. Once the user becomes familiar with the classification headings set out below it should become a simple matter to locate the relevant references.

CLASSIFICATION

1 Historical and General

1.1 Historical

1.2 Books

1.3 Miscellaneous Applications

2 Gelatin

2.1 Official Standards

2.2 Gelatin Testing

2.3 Gelatin Manufacture and Applications

2.4 Gelatin Substitutes

1 Historical and General

1.1 Historical

Alpers, W.C., *Am. J. Pharm.*, 1896, *68*, 481–94

Gelatin Capsules

capsules, hard and soft gelatin: filling, hard gelatin, powders and pill masses, manual device; manufacture, hard and soft, history

Wilkie, W., *Bull. Pharm.*, Detroit, 1913, *27*, 382–4.

The manufacture of gelatin capsules

capsules, hard and soft gelatin: manufacturing method, hard gelatin capsules

Feldhaus, F.M., *Dt. ApothZtg*, 1954, *94*, 321

On the history of medical capsules (in German)

capsules, hard and soft gelatin: review

Griffenhagen, G., *J. Am. pharm. Ass., pract. Pharm. Edn*, 1956, *17*, 810–13

Tools of the apothecary. 10. lozenges, tablets and capsules

capsules, hard gelatin, lozenges, pastilles and tablets: filling, small scale; manufacture, small scale

Stadler, L.B., *J. Am. pharm. Ass., pract. Pharm. Edn*, 1959, *20*, 723–4

The gelatin capsule

capsules, hard gelatin: manufacture, industrial scale

Jones, B.E. and Turner, T.D., *Pharm. J.*, 1974, *213*, 614–17

A century of commercial hard gelatin capsules

capsules, hard gelatin: enteric capsules; manufacture, industrial scale

Jones, B.E., *M & B pharm. Bull.*, 1980, *27*, 76–80

The hard gelatin capsule, a modern dosage form

capsules, hard gelatin: colorants; enteric capsules; filling, industrial scale, self-locking capsules; manufacture, industrial scale

1.2 Books

Lee, C.O., *The Official Preparations of Pharmacy*, 2nd Edn, St. Louis, C.V. Mosby Company, 1953, pp. 400–12

Capsules

Lyman, R.A. and Sprowls, J.B., *Textbook of Pharmaceutical Compounding and Dispensing*, 2nd Edn, Philadelphia, J.B. Lippincott Company, 1955, pp. 58–67

Capsules

Kern, W., *Hagers Handbuchen der Pharmazeutischen Praxis*, 2nd Suppl., Vol. 1, Berlin, Springer-Verlag, 1958, pp. 806–36

Capsulae gelatinosae (in German)

Münzel, K., Büchi, J. and Schultz, O.-E., *Galenisches Praktikum*, Stuttgart, Wissenschaftliche Verlagsgesellschaft mbH, 1959, pp. 501–5

Capsules (in German)

Czetsch-Lindenwald, H. and Fahrig, W., *Arzneikapseln*, Aulendorf i. Württ, Editio Cantor, 1962 (in German)

Fishburn, A.G., *An Introduction to Pharmaceutical Formulation*, London, Pergamon Press, 1965, pp. 90–3

Capsules

Jenkins, G.L., Sperandio, G.L. and Latiolais, C.J., *Clinical Pharmacy: A Text for Dispensing Pharmacy*, New York, McGraw-Hill, 1966, pp. 69–79

Capsules

Sprowls, J.B. and Beal, H.M., *American Pharmacy, an Introduction to Pharmaceutical Technics and Dosage Forms*, 6th Edn, Philadelphia, J.B. Lippincott Company, 1966, pp. 348–59

Capsules

Guichard, C., *Eléments de Technologie Pharmaceutique*, Editions Médicales Flammarion, 1967, pp. 342–51

Capsules (in French)

Prista, L., Noguiera and Alves, A. Correia, *Técnica Farmacêutica a Farmácia Galénica*, Lisbon, Fundacão Calouste Gulbenkian, 1967, pp. 950–94

Capsules (in Portugese)

Mangeot, A. and Poisson, J., *Notions de Pharmacie Galénique*, Paris, Masson et Cie, 1968, pp. 112–14

Capsules (in French)

Sandell, E., *Pharmaceutics, Galenical Pharmacy*, Stockholm, Boktrycheri AB Thule, 1968, pp. 272–9

Capsules

Parrott, E.L., *Pharmaceutical Technology, Fundamental Pharmaceutics*, Minneapolis, Burgess Publishing Company, 1970, pp. 66–9

Capsules

Geçgil, Ş. and Geçgil, T., *Galenik Farmasiye Başlangiç*, Istanbul, Yörük Matbaasi, 1972, pp. 296–300

Capsules (in Turkish)

Gstirner, F., *Einführung in die Verfahrenstechnik der Arzneiformung*, Stuttgart, Wissenschaftliche Verlagsgesellschaft mbH, 1972, pp. 177–84

Capsules (in German)

Gutcho, M., *Capsule Technology and Microencapsulation*, New Jersey, Noyes Data Corporation, 1972

Patents

Le Hir, A., *Abrégé de Pharmacie Galénique*, Paris, Masson et Cie, 1974, pp. 231–42

Capsules (in French)

Sprowl's American Pharmacy, Dittert, L.W. (Ed.), 7th Edn, Philadelphia, J.B. Lippincott Company, 1974, pp. 318–43

Capsules

Cooper and Gunn's Dispensing for Pharmaceutical Students, Carter, S.J. (Ed.), 12th Edn, London. Pitman Medical, 1975, pp. 182–6

Capsules

Dispensing of Medication, Hoover, J.E., 8th Edn, Pennsylvania, Mack Publishing Company, 1976, pp. 85–97

Capsules

Lachman, L., Lieberman, H.A. and Kanig, J.L., *Theory and Practice of Industrial Pharmacy*, 2nd Edn, Philadelphia, Lea & Febiger, 1976, pp. 398–438

Capsules

Bentley's Textbook of Pharmaceutics, Rawlins, E.A. (Ed.), 8th Edn, London, Baillière Tindall, 1977, pp. 310–14 and 339–40

Capsules

Wailes, R.A., *Ethical Tablet and Capsule Handbook*, Sydney, Australia, PVP Publications, 1980

Capsules and Tablets: colour and markings

The Capsule, Basics, Technology and Biopharmacy, a Modern Dosage Form (in German), Fahrig, W. and Hofer, U., (Eds), Stuttgart, Wissenschaftliche Verlagsgesellschaft mbH, 1983

Reports from symposium 'The capsule in the pharmacy and in industry', 27th APV annual congress, 1981, Braunschweig, FRG (in German)

Remington's Pharmaceutical Sciences, Gennaro, A.R. (Ed.), 17th Edn, Pennsylvania, Mack Printing Company, 1985, pp. 1625–31

Capsules

1.3 Miscellaneous Applications

Natale, F. and Arrivabene, G., *Scienza Aliment.*, 1967, *13*(3), 45–7

The use of gelatin capsule trimmings to augment the protein ration of livestock (in Italian)

capsules, hard gelatin: animal feedstuffs, protein source; gelatin, amino acid composition; manufacture, gelatin waste

McGeer, E.G., *Analyt. Biochem.*, 1970, *35*, 300–1

Gelatin capsules as disposable wells for $^{14}CO_2$ absorption

capsules, hard gelatin: carbon dioxide, radioactive isotope; assays, glutamic decarboxylase; assays, reproducibility; capsule, use as container

Maddox, V.H., assigned to Parke, Davis & Co., *U.S. Patent* 3 620 759, 1971

Food capsule

capsules, hard gelatin: capsule shells, perforated wall; capsule contents, soluble food extract

Borgmann, G., *French Patent* 2 155 286, 1973, through *Derwent Accession No.* 404130–B, 1972

Gelatin capsule for oral administration

capsules, hard and soft gelatin and pills: coating soluble in saliva; coating materials for flavour and taste

Controulis, J., Larsen, K.N. and Wheeler, L.M., assigned to Parke, Davis & Co., *U.S. Patent* 3 823 816, 1974

Water-soluble package

capsules, hard gelatin: capsule, perforated wall, holes sealed with readily soluble strip; capsule, as water-soluble package

Noren, O.B., Garland, C.C. and Kwarsick, E.J., assigned to Parke, Davis & Co., *U.S. Patent* 3 831 476, 1974

Capsule handling apparatus

capsules, hard gelatin: equipment, to produce capsules with holes in sides

Sandoz, S.A.R.L., *French Patent* 2 241 291, 1975, through *Derwent Accession No.* 36356W/22, 1973

Flavouring (non) pharmaceutical shapes by impregnation

cachets and capsules, hard and soft gelatin: capsule shell composition, gelatin, natural or synthetic polymers; coating composition, flavouring/sweetening agent; coating method, by dipping

Padfield, J.M., Moss, S.H., Norton, D.A. and Gill, M.S., *Pharm. J.*, 1976, *216*, 212–15

An interactive drug information system

capsule, hard gelatin: imipramine hydrochloride; computer information retrieval system

Rock, G.A., Decary, F. and Cole, R.S., *Lancet*, 1981, *1*, 1419–20

Orange plasma from tanning capsules

capsules, hard gelatin: oral tanning, cosmetic use

2 Gelatin

2.1 Official Standards

Argentina: Farmacopea Nacional Argentina, 5th Edn, Buenos Aires, Talleres Graficos del Ministerio de Asistencia Social y Salud Publica, 1966

Gelatina, pp. 412–13

acidity limit; arsenic; heavy metals; identification; solubility sulphite

Brazil: Farmacopéia Brasileira, 3rd Edn, Sao Paulo, Organizacao Andrei Editora S.A., 1977

Gelatinum, Gelatina, pp. 859–61

arsenic; bacterial content; gel strength; heavy metals; identification; solubility; sulphite

China: Pharmacopoeia of the People's Republic of China, Part 2, Peking, People's Hygiene Press Association, 1985

Mingjiao, Gelatinum, pp. 234–5

Europe: European Pharmacopoeia, 2nd Edn, Part II, 57160 Sainte-Ruffine, France, Maisonneuve S.A., 1984

Gelatina, Gelatin, Eighth Fascicule, pp. 330–330-6

appearance and pH of solution; arsenic; gel strength; heavy metals; identification; loss on drying; peroxides; phenolic preservatives; sulphated ash; sulphur dioxide

Countries that have adopted the standards of the European Pharmacopoeia include Austria, Belgium, Britain, Denmark, Eire, Finland, France, Germany (West), Greece, Iceland, Italy, Luxembourg, Netherlands, Norway, Spain, Sweden, Switzerland.

India: Pharmacopoeia of India, 3rd Edn, Delhi, Controller of Publications, 1985

Gelatin, Vol. 2, pp. 229–30

arsenic; ash; copper; heavy metals; identification; loss on drying; microbial limits; odour; solubility; water-insoluble matter; zinc

Japan: Pharmacopoeia of Japan, 10th Edn, Tokyo, Ministry of Health and Welfare, 1981

Gelatinum, Gelatin, pp. 1045–6 (English Edn)
Gelatinum Purificatum, Purified Gelatin, p. 1047 (English Edn)

arsenic; heavy metals; identity; loss on drying; mercury; odour; residue on ignition; sulphite; water-insoluble substances

Jugoslavia: Pharmacopoea Jugoslavica, 4th Edn, Belgrade, Izdanje Saveznog zavoda za zdravstvenu zaštitu, 1984

Gelatina Medicinalis, Ljekovite Galerte, Vol. 1, p. 241
Gelatina Alba, Gelatina Animalis, Bijela Zelatina, Bela Zwotinjska gelatina, Vol. 2, pp. 437–8

acidity; arsenic; bacterial content; gel strength; heavy metals; identification; moisture content; residue on ignition; sulphur dioxide

Roumania: Farmacopeea Română, 9th Edn, Bucharest, Editura Medicală, 1976

Gelatinum, Gelatină, pp. 330–1

acidity; albumen; arsenic; gel strength; heavy metals; identification; loss on drying; microbial test; residue on ignition; sulphur dioxide

Turkey: Türk Farmakopesi, Istanbul, Millî Eğitim Basimevi, 1974

Gelatinum, Jelatin, pp. 261–2

acidity, alkalinity; identification; purity; residue on ignition; solubility; sulphur dioxide

USA: The United States Pharmacopeia, 21st Revision, The National Formulary, 16th Edn, Rockville, United States Pharmacopeial Convention Inc., 1985

Gelatin, pp. 1563–4

arsenic; heavy metals; identification; microbial limits; odour; residue on ignition; sulphur dioxide; water-insoluble substances

USSR: State Pharmacopoeia of the Union of Soviet Socialist Republics, 10th Edn, Moscow, Ministry of Health, 1971

Gelatina Medicinalis, Medical Grade Gelatin, pp. 297–9

acidity; arsenic; clarity; gelling properties; identification; microbiological content; moisture content; colour; purity; residue on ignition; sulphur dioxide

2.2 Gelatin Testing

Castello, R.A. and Goyan, J.E., *J. pharm. Sci.*, 1964, *53*, 777–82

Rheology of gelatin films

capsules, soft gelatin: films, tensile relaxation modulus, effect of different gelatins

Veis, A., *The Macromolecular Chemistry of Gelatin*, New York, Academic Press, 1964

applications, manufacture, properties, testing

Smith, H. L. and Goyan, J. E., *J. pharm. Sci.*, 1965, *54*, 545–8

Method of studying rheology of gelatin melts

capsules, soft gelatin: films, tensile relaxation modulus, effect of formulation, plasticisers

Schott, H., *J. pharm. Educ.*, 1972, *36*, 104–7

Swelling of gelatin as a function of pH

gelatin, capsule, chemical properties

Robinson, J.A.J., Kellaway, I.W. and Marriott, C., *J. Pharm. Pharmac.*, 1975, *27*, 653–8

The effect of ageing on the rheological properties of gelatin gels

gelatin, hard capsule, manufacture; gelatin properties, gel rigidity, effect of storage

Robinson, J.A.J., Kellaway, I.W. and Marriott, C., *J. Pharm. Pharmac.*, 1975, *27*, 818–24

The effect of blending on the rheological properties of gelatin solutions and gels

gelatin, hard capsule, manufacture; gelatin properties, gel rigidity, effect of blending

Chesworth, K.A.C., Sinclair, A., Stretton, R.J. and Hayes, W.P., *J. Pharm. Pharmac.*, 1977, *29*, 60–1

An enzymic technique for the microbiological examination of pharmaceutical gelatin

gelatin, microbiological content

Kellaway, I.W., Marriott, C. and Robinson, J.A.J., *Can. J. pharm. Sci.*, 1978, *13*, 83–90

The mechanical properties of gelatin films. 1. The influence of water content and preparative conditions

gelatin, hard capsule, acid and alkaline ossein; gelatin, physical properties, film strength, Young's modulus, effect of moisture content

Ludwig, A., Van Ooteghem, M. and Delva, A., *Pharm. Ind., Berl.*, 1979, *41*, 796–8

Disintegration of hard gelatin capsules. Part 1: Composition and structure of the capsule wall

gelatin, hard capsule, analysis of type, isoelectric focusing; gelatin films, hard capsule, structure, microscopy, optical, scanning electron; 3.2.1

Melia, C.D., Kellaway, I.W. and Hadgraft, J., *J. Pharm. Pharmac.*, 1981, *33*, Suppl., 20P

Varietal differences in capsule grade gelatins: mechanical properties

gelatin, hard capsules, manufacture; gelatin properties, mechanical effect of moisture content

Thomas, M., Kellaway, I.W. and Jones, B.E., *J. Pharm. Pharmac.*, 1983, *55*, Suppl., 6P

A technique for studying gelatin gelation

gelatin, hard capsule, alkaline ossein; gelatin, physical properties, gelation process, measurement by photo correlation spectrometry

Tomka, I., Chapter III in *The Capsule, Basics, Technology and Biopharmacy, a Modern Dosage Form* [in German], Fahrig, W. and Hofer, U., (Eds.), Stuttgart, Wissenschaftliche Verlagsgesellschaft mbH, 1983, pp. 33–57

Gelatin: chemistry; manufacture; properties, testing (in German)

Hüttenrauch, R. and Fricke, S., *Naturwissenschaften*, 1984, *71*, 426–7

Importance of water structure to helical conformation and ageing of gelatin in aqueous solutions

gelatin, hard capsule, physical properties, molecular configuration, effect of water structure

2.3 Gelatin Manufacture and Applications

Smith, P.I., *Pharm. J.*, 1929, *122*, 617–18

The uses of gelatin in pharmacy

capsules, soft gelatin, pastes, pastilles and suppositories: formulation, capsule shells; gelatin testing

Charles B. Knox Gelatine Company, Inc., *British Patent* 1 836 082, 1960

Method of modifying type A gelatin and product thereof

capsules, hard gelatin: gelatin films, brittleness, drying rate; gelatin modification, polycarboxylic acids

Jones, R.T., *Process Biochem.*, 1970, *5*(12), 2–8

Pharmaceutical gelatin. Manufacture

review

Jones, R.T., *Process Biochem.*, 1971, *6*(7), 19–22

Pharmaceutical gelatin. Applications

capsules, hard and soft gelatin, emulsions, lozenges, pastes, pastilles, suppositories and tablets: review

Jones, R.T., *Mfg Chem.*, 1977, *48*(7), 23–4

The role of gelatin in pharmaceuticals

pharmaceutical applications, review

The Science and Technology of Gelatin, Ward, A. G. and Courts, A., (Eds.), London, Academic Press, 1977 applications, manufacture, properties, testing

Callahan, J.C., Cleavy, G.W., Elefant, M., Japlan, G., Kensler, T. and Nash, R.A., *Drug Dev. ind. Pharm.*, 1982, *8*, 355–69

Equilibrium moisture content of pharmaceutical excipients

gelatin, equilibrium moisture content, effect of relative humidity

Grouber, B., *Labo-Pharma Probl. Tech.*, 1983, *31*, 909–16

Gelatins, properties, standards, principal applications (in French)

applications, manufacture, properties, testing

2.4 Gelatin Substitutes

Murphy, H. W., assigned to Eli Lilly & Co., *U.S. Patent* 2 526 683, 1950

Methylcellulose capsules and process of manufacture

capsules, two-piece: capsule shell composition, methylcellulose; manufacturing method, dipping

Greminger, G.K. and Weaver, M.A., assigned to Dow Chemical Company, *U.S. Patent* 2 810 659, 1957

Thermoplastic compositions of water-soluble cellulose ethers

capsule, one-piece: capsule shell composition, cellulose ethers; formulation, plasticisers; manufacturing method, rotary die

Tanabe Seiyaku Co. Ltd, *Japanese Patent Application No. 70 01277*, 1970, through *Derwent Accession No.* 06531R, 1967

Polyvinyl alcohol-based soft capsules

capsules, one-piece: capsule shell composition, polyvinyl alcohol; manufacturing method, plate, rotary die; stability, bacteria, heat, light, moisture

Dow Chemical Company, *British Patent* 1 144 225, 1969

Preparation of medicinal capsule shells from hydroxyalkyl-alkylcellulose ethers

capsules, two-piece: capsule shell composition, hydroxyalkyl-alkylcellulose ethers; manufacturing method, dipping

Greminger, G.K. and Davis, L.E., assigned to Dow Chemical Company, *U.S. Patent* 3 493 407, 1970

Preparation of medicinal capsules from hydroxyalkylcellulose ethers

capsules, two-piece: capsule shell composition, hydroxyalkylcellulose ethers; aqueous and non-aqueous systems; manufacturing method, dipping

Centre de Recherches Marcel Midy and Rene Claude, *French Patent* 2 073 288, 1971, through *Derwent Accession No.* 00580T-B, 1969

Thermoplastic capsules for pharmaceutical use, administered orally, rectally or vaginally

capsules, one-piece: capsule shell composition, hydroxypropyl-cellulose, polyacrylic acid, polymethacrylates, polyoxyethylene, polyvinyl alcohol, vinylpyrrolidone/vinyl acetate copolymer; capsule type, oral, rectal, vaginal; manufacturing method, injection moulding, thermoforming

Langman, C.A.J., assigned to Dow Chemical Co., *U.S. Patent* 3 617 588, 1971

Dip coating for preparing cellulose ether capsules using induction heating

capsules, two-piece: capsule shell composition, hydroxyalkyl-cellulose ethers; manufacturing method, dipping, thermal gelation, means of heating moulds by induction

Tanabe Seiyaku Co. Ltd, *Japanese Patent Application No. 71 10199*, 1971 through *Derwent Accession No.* 19844S-B, 1967

Gelatin alkyl sulphate capsule base

capsules, one- or two-piece: capsule shell composition, gelatin alkyl sulphate or salt of; manufacturing method, standard; properties, physical strength, solubility

Röhm GmbH, *Belgian Patent* 785 702, 1972, through *Derwent Accession No.* 02444U-AB, 1971

Dissolvable pharmaceutical capsule

capsules, two-piece: capsule shell composition, polymer of vinylic monomer; capsule solubility, pH dependent; formulation of shell, aqueous dispersion; manufacturing method, dipping

Dow Chemical Co., *British Patent* 1 310 697, 1973

Dip coating process for preparing cellulose ether film products

capsules, two-piece: capsule shell composition, hydroxyalkyl-cellulose ethers; manufacturing method, dipping

Szymanski, C.D. and Helmstetter, G.J., assigned to National Starch and Chemical Corp., *U.S. Patent* 3 758 323, 1973

Dextrin-extended gelatin compositions

capsules, two-piece: capsule shell composition, gelatin and modified starch; method of manufacture, use; starch, liquid or thermal modification

National Starch and Chemical Corp., *Dutch Patent* 7 309 843, 1974, through *Derwent Accession No.* 08679V/05, 1972

Gelatin composition diluted with modified starch for capsule production

capsules, hard gelatin: capsule shell composition, gelatin and modified starch; manufacturing method, dipping; starch, liquid or thermal modification

Hoechst A.G., *German (BRD) Patent (Offen.)* 2 363 853, 1975, through *Derwent Accession No.* 4636W/28, 1976

Self carrying packages or capsules for medicaments

capsules, two piece: capsule shell composition, copolymer polyethylene oxides, vinyl acetate, vinyl alcohol; formulation of coating; manufacturing method, dipping

Christen, J.D. and Cheng, W.-J., assigned to Dow Chemical Company, *U.S. Patent* 4 026 986, 1977

Capsule shell

capsules, two-piece: capsule shell composition, hydroxyalkyl starches; capsule shell properties, formulation; manufacturing method, dipping

3 Capsule Practice and Manufacture

3.1 Capsule Practice

Bourjau, C., *Dt. ApothZtg*, 1963, *103*, 1093–5

Gelatin capsules in dispensing pharmacy (in German)

applications; capsule products, Germany (BRD); dispensing

Kuhn, T., *Pharm. Ztg, Berl.*, 1963, *108*, 130–5, 195–8

The testing of gelatin capsules (in German)

gelatin; manufacture; pharmacopoeial standards; properties; 3.7.1

Köchel, F., *Dt. ApothZtg*, 1967, *107*, 603–7

Incompatibilities with various medicinal dosage forms (in German)

pharmaceuticals: formulation, incompatibilities

Vestfal, N.I., *Sb. Nauch. Trud., Tsent. Aptech. Nauch.-Issled. Inst.*, 1971, *11*, 158–68

Analysis of medicinal substances contained in capsules. Preliminary report (in Russian)

capsules, hard and soft gelatin: products, USSR; review

Anon., *Drugs Germ.*, 1972, *15*, 64–72

Drugs in Scherer capsules

capsules, hard and soft gelatin: applications; filling; manufacture

Thoma, K., Siemer, E. and Pfaff, G., *4th International Pharmaceutical Study Week of the German Pharmaceutical Society*, Davos, 1974, pp. 42

Manufacture and review of capsule preparations

capsules, hard and soft gelatin: applications; filling; manufacture; testing

Anon., *Mfg Chem.*, 1977, *48*(7), 19–20

The techniques of drug encapsulation

capsules, hard and soft gelatin: applications; manufacture; properties

Nerlo, H., *Pharm. Ind., Berl.*, 1977, *39*, 488–91

Effects of excipients on properties of solid oral dosage forms

capsules, hard and soft gelatin and tablets: formulation

Stephan, D., *Packung Transport*, 1978, No. 9, 416, 418, 421

Hard or soft – liquid or powder. Gelatin capsule filling (in German)

applications; capsule performance, comparison of hard and soft; capsule shells, dimensions, volume; manufacture, capsules, soft gelatin, rotary die

Jones, T.M., *Drug Cosmet. Ind.*, 1979, *124*(3), 40, 42, 44, 46, 48, 50, 53–4, 56, 103–4

The influence of excipients on the design and manufacture of tablets and capsules

formulation, contents, general; review

Anon., *Pharm. J.*, 1981, *227*, 700–1

Capsule technology

capsules, hard and soft gelatin: drug release, hard and soft capsules; filling, hard gelatin capsules, machines and mechanisms; formulation of contents; meeting report

Anon., *Mfg Chem.*, 1983, *54*(10), 45, 47

Encapsulating technology

capsule products, cleaning and inspection; filling machines, hard gelatin capsules; manufacturing methods, soft gelatin capsules

Bauer, K.H., Chapter IV in *The Capsule, Basics, Technology and Biopharmacy, a Modern Dosage Form* [in German], Fahrig, W. and Hofer, U. (Eds), Stuttgart, Wissenschaftliche Verlagsgesellschaft mbH, 1983, pp. 58–82

The manufacture of hard and soft gelatin capsules (in German)

capsules, hard and soft gelatin: manufacturing methods, industrial

Fahrig, W., Chapter I in *The Capsule, Basics, Technology and Biopharmacy, a Modern Dosage Form* [in German], Fahrig, W. and Hofer, U. (Eds), Stuttgart, Wissenschaftliche Verlagsgesellschaft mbH, 1983, pp. 12–20

Introduction to capsules (in German)

Anon, *Drug Cosmet. Ind.*, 1986, *138*(3), 34–5, 76–7

OTC capsules threatened by new Tylenol crisis

capsules, hard gelatin: product tampering, case study, USA position

Anon, *Mfg. Chem.*, 1986, 57(6), 27, 30

Capsules – is their fate sealed?

capsules, hard and soft gelatin: product tampering. comparison of methods to prevent, review

Dickinson, J., *Pharm. Technol.*, 1986, *10*(5), 18–19

Washington report. The future of hard capsules

capsules, hard gelatin: history; product tampering, case study, USA position

Eith, L., Stepto, R.T.F., Tomka, I. and Wittwer, F., *Fourth International Conference on Pharmaceutical*

Technology, (Paris, APGI, June 3–5, 1986), 1986, *V*, 70–79

The injection-moulded capsule

capsules, two piece: manufacturing method, injection moulding, process conditions; material, starch, comparison with gelatin

Stetler, C.J., *Pharm. Technol.*, 1986, *10*(5), 14–15

An eye to the issues. Will outlawing capsules eliminate tampering?

capsules, hard gelatin: product tampering, USA position.

3.2 Capsules, Hard Gelatin
3.2.1 General References

Müller, G., *Dt. ApothZtg*, 1962, *102*, 1138–40

Hard gelatin capsules (in German)

capsules, enteric, formaldehyde treatment; filling small scale, equipment; manufacture, industrial scale; storage conditions

Childs, R.F., *Am. J. pharm. Educ.*, 1965, *29*, 119–24

Solid dosage forms: capsules

filling, small scale; identification; properties of capsules, capsule shells and products

Smith, Kline and French Laboratories, Selected Pharmaceutical Research References, Philadelphia, 1966

Manufacture of hard capsules: An annotated bibliography

capsule sealing; enteric capsules; gelatin; gelatin substitutes; manufacture

Hoffmann, A., Hoffmann, M.-A. and Meunier, A., *Bull. Soc. Pharm. Nancy*, 1968, *78*, 7–18

Hard gelatin capsules (in French)

applications; drug availability, *in vitro*, *in vivo*; enteric coating; filling, small scale, separation-resistant capsules; formulation, contents; history; manufacture; storage

Pochet, G., *Prod. Probl. Pharm.*, 1968, *23*, 313–16

Hard gelatin capsules (in French)

filling, small scale, industrial scale; manufacture; storage

Jones, B.E., *Mfg Chem.*, 1969, *40*(2), 25–8 (French translation in *Labo-Pharma Probl. Tech.*, 1969, *17*(179), 34–41)

Hard gelatin capsules: a literature review

drug availability, *in vitro*, *in vivo*; enteric coating; filling; formulation; history; manufacture; review; storage

Samková, M., *Čslká Farm.*, 1969, *18*, 262–6

The filling of drugs into gelatin capsules in pharmacies (in Czech)

capsule shells, volumes; filling, industrial, small scale; filling, capsule size determination; powder properties, bulk density

Van Herle, L., *Farmaco, Edn Prat.*, 1969, *24*, 745–58

Empty gelatin capsules (gélules). Manufacture and importance (in French)

colour; drug availability; filling machines; formulation; gelatin; manufacture; storage

Besenzon, C., *Boll. Soc. Ital. Farm. Osp.*, 1970, *16*, 433–5

The possibilities offered by hand gelatin capsules as against other pharmaceutical forms in modern hospital pharmacy (in Italian)

applications; enteric coating; filling, small scale

Bitallon, P., Capsules et Gélules Symposium (Paris Faculty of Pharmacy, University of Paris) 1970, *II*, 1–10

The hard gelatin capsule (in French)

filling; manufacture; requirements

Ceschel, G.C. and Fontani, F., *Boll. chim.-farm.*, 1970, *109*, 157–79

Hard gelatin capsules (in Italian)

applications; filling; testing

Miet, J., *Labo-Pharma Probl. Tech.*, 1970, *18*(194), 39–41

A "Capsugel" factory, affiliate of Parke, Davis implanted in France (in French)

applications; capsule shells, dimensions, colour; gelatin standards; history; manufacturing method; separation-resistant capsules

Schmitt, J.-P. and Mathis, C., *Prod. Probl. Pharm.*, 1970, *25*, 752–61

Problems arising in the industrial production of hard gelatin capsules (in French)

capsule shells, colorants, dimensions, separation resistant; drug availability, *in vitro*, disintegration; filling, industrial scale; formulation, contents; powder properties, angle of repose, bulk density; product, weight uniformity; storage, product stability, effect of carbon dioxide, light, moisture, oxygen

Bovis, A., *Bull. Soc. Pharm. Marseille*, 1971, *20*, 7–18

The hard gelatin capsule (in French)

filling, small scale; history; manufacture

Van Herle, L., *Pharmacy Int.*, 1971, *1*, 12–18

Gelatin capsules (gélules) – manufacture and importance

colour; drug availability; filling, industrial scale; formulation; gelatin; manufacture; storage

Sugihara, M., *Nippon Yakuzaishi kai Zasshi*, 1972, *24*(8), 21–8

Hard capsuled medicines (in Japanese)

filling, small scale, industrial scale; manufacture; storage, products

Forbes, D.R. and Jones, B.E., *J. Hosp. Pharm.*, 1974, *32*, 209–17

Hard gelatin capsules in hospital pharmacy

enteric capsules; filling, small scale; formulation, contents

Temperli, M., *Pharm. Acta Helv.*, 1974, *49*, 121–39

The filling and dispensing of hard gelatin capsules (in German)

capsule shells; drug availability, *in vitro*, disintegration testing, *Swiss P.* VI method; extemporaneous dispensing, equipment, official products; filling, capsule size determination; formulation, contents, official products; lubricants, Aerosil, calcium stearate, magnesium stearate; powder properties, bulk density, flow properties; product weight uniformity, comparison of filling equipment, official products; storage, stability at room temperature, official products

Newton, D.W. and Becker, C.H., *Pharmacy Times*, 1977, *43*(1), 66–70, 76–7

What's the impact of capsule and tablet formulation on product selection?

capsules, hard gelatin and tablets: dissolution; formulation of contents

Stamm, A., *Bull. Soc. Pharm. Strasb.*, 1978, *21*, 15–41

Problems posed by the choice of excipients for hard gelatin capsules, cachets and tablets (in French)

formulation, contents, general; review

Strittmatter, T., *Pharm. Ztg, Berl.*, 1978, *123*, 2238–41

The hard gelatin capsule in the dispensary

capsule shells, separation-resistant, volume and weight; filling, small scale; formulation of contents; product weight uniformity, pharmacopoeial standards; products, content weight by capsule size

Ludwig, A., Van Ooteghem, M. and Delva, A., *Pharm. Ind., Berl.*, 1979, *41*, 796–8

Disintegration of hard gelatin capsules. Part I: Composition and structure of the capsule wall

capsule shells, wall structure and thickness; 2.2

von Wattenwyl, A., *Mfg Chem.*, 1981, *52*(3), 37–8

Hard gelatin capsules – a drug form for better patient compliance

capsule colour; capsule filling, separation-resistant capsules; capsule printing, radial; market survey; patient compliance, effect of capsule

Fuhrer, C., Chapter II, in *The Capsule, Basics, Technology and Biopharmacy, a Modern Dosage Form* (in German), Fahrig, W. and Hofer, U. (Eds), Stuttgart, Wissenschaftliche Verlagsgesellschaft mbH, 1983, pp. 21–32

The capsule as a modern medical form in the pharmacy and industry (in German)

Jones, B.E., *Pharm. Technol.*, 1985, *9*, 106–8, 110, 112

Hard gelatin capsules and the pharmaceutical formulator

applications, capsule manufacture; filling machines, dosing mechanisms; formulation of contents

3.2.2 Manufacture of Hard Capsules

3.2.2.1 Capsule Shells

Colton, A., assigned to Parke, Davis & Co., *U.S. Patent* 1 787 777, 1931

Capsule machine

machine, fully automatic; manufacturing method

Dehn, F.B., *British Patent* 360 427, 1931

An improved machine for making medicinal capsules and the like

machine, fully automatic; manufacturing method

Norris, W.G., *Mfg Chem.*, 1959, *30*, 233–6

Hard gelatin capsules – how Eli Lilly make 500 million a year

filling, industrial scale; gelatin standards; manufacturing, machines, method

Norris, W.G., *Mfg Chem.*, 1961, *32*, 249–52, 258

P.D.'s new capsule plant

filling, industrial scale; gelatin standards; manufacturing, machines, method

Anon., *Pharm. J.*, 1965, *194*, 475–6

Capsule-making at Basingstoke

manufacturing, machines, method

Girombelli, A. and Michel, L., Capsules et Gélules, Symposium (Paris, Faculty of Pharmacy, University of Paris), 1970, *III*, 1–9

The production and control of the manufacture of hard gelatin capsules (in French)

manufacturing, method, quality control systems; printing; raw materials

Oglevee, H.G. and Clement, B.R., assigned to Parke, Davis & Co., *U.S. Patent* 3 632 700, 1972

Monitoring viscosity of gelatin to insure uniform walls

capsule wall thickness, automatic control by viscometry; gelatin solution, viscosity determination

Parke, Davis & Co., *British Patent* 1 297 739, 1972

Capsule production apparatus and method

capsule wall thickness, automatic control by viscometry

Parke, Davis & Co., *British Patent* 1 328 423, 1973

Apparatus suitable for use in the dip-moulding of capsules

capsule wall thickness, control by viscosity

Martyn, G.W., *Drug Devel. Comm.*, 1974–5, *1*, 39–49

The people computer interface in a capsule molding operation

manufacturing methods, computer control

Höfliger, O., *German (BRD) Patent (Offen.)* 2 557 601, 1977

Hard gelatin capsules and procedure for their manufacture

capsules, two-layer; coating internal surface, hydrophobic polyelectrolyte polymer

Kupferberg-Odle, M., *German (BRD) Patent* 2 259 387, 1981

Method for making hard gelatin capsules

capsule shells, protective coatings, application by dipping; manufacturing method

Jones, B.E., *Chem. Engr, Lond.*, 1982, No. 380, 174–7

The manufacture of hard gelatin capsules

gelatin; history; manufacturing, machines, method, quality control systems; packaging; printing; storage

3.2.2.2 Ancillary Manufacturing Processes

Jones, B.E., *Annls méd. Nancy*, 1974, *13*, 191–200

The manufacture and printing of hard gelatin capsules

printing, design of logo, dimensions of print; printing equipment, industrial scale; printing ink, formulation

Su, K.S.E., Snyder, R.R. and Scott, R.R., assigned to Eli Lilly & Co., *U.S. Patent* 3 992 215, 1976

Pharmaceutical suspension for opaquing empty gelatin capsules

colorants, opacifying agents; formulation of suspension; titanium dioxide

François, D., Berneis, D.H., Cole, E.T., Pracht, I. and Schatz, B., *Mfg Chem.*, 1979, *50*(4), 48, 51, 76

Canthaxanthin to colour hard gelatin capsules

colour, stability to light; colorants, acceptability for use; colorants, natural, canthaxanthin; formulation, capsule shell; manufacture

Lykens, D. N., *Pharm. Technol.*, 1979, *3*, 57–60

Edible printing inks

printing faults, diagnosis; printing ink, formulation; printing, machines

3.2.3 Filling Hard Capsules

3.2.3.1 Small Scale Filling

Lee, J.W., *J. Am. pharm. Ass., scient. Edn.*, 1935, *24*, 469–76

Accuracy and speed factors in hand-filling capsules

capsule shells, physical specifications, weight uniformity; filling, manual methods; product weight uniformity

Matthews, D.R., *Pharm. J.*, 1948, *161*, 112

A capsule filling device

manual device, wood

Cooper, M.L., *J. Am. pharm. Ass., pract. Pharm. Edn*, 1954, *15*, 300

A capsule size selector

filling, capsule size determination

Tice, L.F. and Moore, A.W., *J. Am. pharm, Ass., pract. Pharm. Edn*, 1954, *15*, 296–7

A slide rule for selecting capsule size

filling, capsule size determination

van Nunen, J.W., *Pharm. Weekbl. Ned.*, 1962, *97*, 122–5

Capsules in the dispensary (in Dutch)

filling, capsule size determination; manual device, plastic; powder properties, bulk density; product weight uniformity

Artemev, A.I., *Aptech. Delo*, 1963, *12*(4), 58–9

An apparatus for filling gelatin capsules and starch wafers (in Russian)

cachets: manual device

Buchnev, B.P., *Aptech. Delo*, 1964, *13*(4), 80–1

Machine for filling hard gelatin capsules (in Russian)

manual device, plastic

Sandell, E., *Pharm. Ztg, Berl.*, 1964, *109*, 1099

Small scale apparatus for filling hard gelatin capsules in the dispensary (in German)

manual device, plastic

Jaspersen, H.P., *Schweiz. ApothZtg*, 1965, *103*, 747–52

A filling device for hard gelatin capsules (in German)

capsule shell, volumes, weight uniformity; filling, capsule size determination; formulation, contents; powder properties, bulk density; product weight uniformity

Ericsson, B. and Persson, H., *Svensk farm. Tidskr.*, 1966, *70*, 202–8

Hard gelatin capsules in place of pills in prescription work (in Swedish)

pills: dispensing, comparison capsules and pills

Van Ooteghem, M., *J. pharm. Belg.*, 1966, *21*, 73–85

The filling of powders in cachets and hard gelatin capsules (in French)

cachets: capsule shells, dimensions, volume; filling, capsule size determination; powder properties, bulk density, packing theory

Reuter, H., *Pharm. Prax., Berl.*, supplement to *Pharmazie*, 1968, *23*, *Suppl.* 10, 271–4

The filling of single dose medicines in the dispensary (in German)

pills, powders and tablets: extemporaneous dispensing, comparison of dosage forms; filling, dispensary equipment; product weight uniformity, comparison of dosage forms

Allart, H.H.J., *Pharm. Weekbl. Ned.*, 1971, *106*, 25–31

Capsule filling machines for use in the dispensary (in Dutch)

Thompson, G.R. and Cunningham, A., *J. pharm. Sci.*, 1975, *64*, 320–22

Versatile unit for filling gelatin capsules with drugs or chemicals capsule shells, physical specification; filling machine, liquid dosing; formulation of contents, liquid fill; storage, refrigerated conditions

3.2.3.2 Industrial Scale Filling of Hard Capsules

Anon., *Labo-Pharma Probl. Tech.*, 1966, *14*(145), 69–79

Why and how to fill capsules (in French)

filling machines, automatic, manual, and semi-automatic; 3.8.2.4

Pluripharm, *French Patent* 1 454 013, 1966, through *Derwent Accession No. 24 048, 1965*

Capsules

filling machine, insertion of capsules and capsule parts; incompatible medicines, separation by encapsulating; stability, incompatible medicines

Aspro-Nicholas Limited, *British Patent* 1 204 580, 1970

Encapsulated pharmaceutical dosage forms

filling machine, tablet insertion; incompatible medicines, separation by tabletting

Clement, H. and Marquardt, H.G., *Pharm. Ind., Berl.*, 1970, *32*, 169–76

Experiences with machines for filling hard gelatin capsules (in German)

filling machines, auger, dosing tube, tamping mechanisms; review

Robin, J., Capsules and Gélules, Symposium (Paris, Faculty of Pharmacy, University of Paris), 1970, *II*, 11–21

Machines for filling hard gelatin capsules (in French)

filling machines, auger, dosing tube, tamping mechanism; product sealing, banding, dot welding

Christian Brunnengräber Chemische Fabrik & Co. mbH, *German (BRD) Patent (Offen.)* 2 021 147, 1971 through *Derwent Accession No. 72732S-B, 1970*

Medicinal capsule containing separate units

filling machine, tablet insertion; incompatible medicines, separation by tabletting; stability, incompatible medicines

Gallet, M.M., *Farmaco, Ed. prat.*, 1971, *26*, 251–68

The hard gelatin capsule, filling and closing (in French)

filling machines, automatic and semi-automatic

Eli Lilly & Co., *British Patent* 1 267 304, 1972

Method for making filled capsules

filling machine, capsule body only, sealing open end with gelatin solution

Ridgway, K. and Callow, J.A.B., *Pharm. J.*, 1973, *211*, 281–5

Capsule-filling machinery

filling machines, small scale, industrial scale, semi-automatic, automatic; product weight uniformity

Perry Industries Inc., *U.S. Patent* 3 874 431, 1975, through *Derwent Accession No.* 25588 W/15, 1969

Loading medicinal powder into capsules

filling machine, air operated dosing tube mechanism

Faust, R.N., Vandervalk, W. and Warnick, R., *Chem. Engng. Prog.*, 1976, *72*(6), 84–7

Selecting a high-speed capsule machine

filling machine, comparison of automatic and semi-automatic, performance, yields; product weight uniformity, effect of filling machine

Zanasi Nigris SpA., *German (BRD) Patent (Offen.)* 2 612 472, 1976, through *Derwent Accession No.,* 81492X/44, 1975

Metering device for use in filling capsules

filling machine, dosing tube mechanism, semi-solid fill

Anon., *Mfg Chem.*, 1977, *48*(7), 26, 28, 30

Latest capsule machines on UK market

machines, automatic; machines, filled capsules, cleaning, sorting

Teague, P., *Mfg Chem.*, 1977, *48*(7), 30

Choosing your machine

machines, performance, requirements

Beckley, J.N., *Drug Cosmet. Ind.*, 1978, *123*(4), 70, 70, and 150–1

Dust control in tablet-making and capsule filling

air handling systems; cross contamination; good manufacturing practice

Manesty Machines Ltd, *German (BRD) Patent,* 2 443 466, 1978

Gelatin capsule filling machine

dosing mechanism, tablet punches and dies

Anon., *Khim.-farm. Zh.*, 1980, *14*, 100–3

mG2 filling machine for hard gelatin capsules (in Russian)

filling machine, dosing tube mechanism

Cole, G.C., *Chem. Eng, Lond.*, 1982, No. 380, 473–7

Capsule filling

capsule contents, solids and semi-solids; filling machines, instrumentation; filling machines, mechanisms; filling machines, powder plug formation, forces, effect of lubricants; formulation of contents (powders), diluents, lubricants; powder characteristics

von Doehren, P.J., Forbes, F.St. J. and Shively, C.D., *Pharm. Technol.*, 1982, *6*(9), 139–40, 143–5, 147–9, 153–4, and 156

An approach to the characterization and technology transfer of solid dosage from processes

formulation of contents, process design and optimisation; pharmaceutical processes, planning and scale-up

Di Costanzo, F., Grandvuillemin, L., van der Mander, J. and Réaux, M., *Labo-Pharma Probl. Tech.*, 1983, *31*(337), 917–25

Filling hard gelatin capsules (in French)

fill materials, types; machines, methods of dosing, review

Hofer, U., Chapter V, in *The Capsule, Basics, Technology and Biopharmacy, a Modern Dosage Form* [in German], Fahrig, W. and Hofer, U., (Eds), Stuttgart, Wissenschaftliche Verlagsgesellschaft mbH, 1983, pp. 83–111

Dry filling (in German)

Yelvigi, M. *Pharm. Technol.*, 1984, *8*(3), 47–50, 52, 55–6

Principles of process automation for liquid and solid dosage forms

production, flow chart for automation process

3.2.3.3 Instrumented Machines, Physical Analysis

Ito, K., Hitomi, M., Kaga, S.I. and Takeya, Y., *Chem. pharm. Bull., Tokyo*, 1969, *17*, 1138–45

Studies on hard gelatin capsules II. The capsule filling of powders and effects of glidant by ring filling method-machine

filling machine, auger mechanism; filling machine, settings, speed of filling; product weight uniformity, effects of, formulation, machine settings; 3.2.4.1

Irwin, G.M., Dodson, G.J. and Ravin, L.J., *J. pharm. Sci.*, 1970, *59*, 547–50

Encapsulation of clomacran phosphate {2-chloro-9-[3-(dimethylamino)propyl]acridan phosphate} I. Effect of flowability of powder blends, lot-to-lot variability, and concentration of active ingredient on weight variation of capsules filled on an automatic capsule-filling machine

filling machine, industrial, dosing tube mechanism; powder processing, granulation, formulations, effect on product weight uniformity; powder properties, flow measurements

Cole, G.C. and May, G., *J. Pharm. Pharmac.*, 1972, *24*, *Suppl.*, 122P–3P

Instrumentation of a hard shell encapsulation machine

filling machine, dosing tube mechanism; filling machine, powder plug formation, compaction and ejection forces; formulation, diluents, lubricants; instrumented filling machine, strain gauges

Miyake, Y., Shinoda, A., Nasu, T., Furukawa, M., Uesugi, K. and Hoshi, K., *Yakuzaigaku*, 1974, *34*, 32–7

Packing properties of pharmaceutical powders into hard gelatin capsules (in Japanese)

filling machine, dosing tube mechanism; powder properties, angle of repose, density, moisture content, particle size, effect on filling; product weight uniformity, effect of machine settings and powder properties

Cole, G.C. and May, G., *J. Pharm. Pharmac.*, 1975, *27*, 353–8

The instrumentation of a Zanasi LZ/64 capsule filling machine

filling machine, dosing tube mechanism; filling machine, powder plug formation, compaction and ejection forces; formulation of contents, diluents and lubricants; instrumented filling machine, strain gauges

Kent, J.S. and Yost, M.T., *J. pharm. Sci.*, 1977, *66*, 1507–8

Strain-gauged Wheatstone bridge design for automatic capsule-filling machine

instrumented filling machine, strain gauges, design

Mony, C., Sambeat, C. and Cousin, G., *First International Conference of Pharmaceutical Technology*, (Paris, APGI, May 31–June 2, 1977), 1977, *II*, 98–108

Applications of the measure of force in the formulation and filling of hard gelatin capsules (in French)

filling machine, dosing tube mechanism; filling machine, powder plug formation, compaction and ejection forces, effects of formulation of contents; instrumented filling machine, piezo-electric capacitor; 3.2.4.1

Small, L.E. and Augsburger, L.L., *J. pharm. Sci.*, 1977, *66*, 504–9

Instrumentation of an automatic capsule-filling machine

filling machine, dosing tube mechanism; filling machine, powder plug formation, compaction and ejection forces; formulation of contents, diluents and lubricants; instrumented filling machine, strain gauges

Small, L.E. and Augsburger, L.L., *J. pharm. Sci.*, 1977, *66*, 1508

Clarification of nomenclature

instrumented machine, strain gauges, design

Kurihara, K. and Ichikawa, I., *Chem. pharm. Bull., Tokyo*, 1978, *26*, 1250–6

Effect of powder flowability on capsule-filling-weight-variation

filling machines, oscillating plate, tamping, mechanisms; powder properties, flow, angle of repose, discharge through orifice, minimum orifice diameter; product weight uniformity, effects of, filling machine mechanism, formulation of contents, powder properties; 3.2.4.1

Small, L.E. and Augsburger, L.L., *Drug Dev. ind. Pharm.*, 1978, *4*, 345–72

Aspects of the lubrication requirements for an automatic capsule filling machine

filling machine, dosing tube mechanism; filling machine, powder plug formation, compaction and ejection forces, effect of, compression force, piston height, powder bed height; formulation, machine settings; filling machine settings; 3.2.4.1

Jolliffe, I.G., Newton, J.M. and Walters, J.K., *J. Pharm. Pharmac.*, 1979, *31*, *Suppl.*, 70P

A theoretical approach to optimising capsule filling by a dosator nozzle filling machine, dosing tube mechanism; powder properties, relationship to machine

Woodhead, P.J., Newton, J.M., Hardy, J.G. and Jackson, S.A., *J. Pharm. Pharmac.*, 1979, *31*, *Suppl.*, 72P

A gamma-ray attenuation technique for assessing the distribution of porosity in powder beds

filling machine, dosing tube mechanism; powder properties, bulk density measurement, non-disruptive technique with gamma source

Gioia, A., *Pharm. Technol. Int.*, 1980, *3*(2), 29–32

Intrinsic flowability: a new technology for powder-flowability classification

filling machine, dosing tube mechanism; powder properties, flow, measurement, flow meter; powder properties, flow, relationship to uniformity of fill weight

Jolliffe, I.G., Newton, J.M. and Walters, J.K., *Powder Technol.*, 1980, *27*, 189–95

Theoretical considerations of the filling of pharmaceutical hard gelatin capsules

filling machine, dosing tube mechanism; filling machine, powder plug formation, theoretical analysis; powder properties, arch formation, relationship angle of powder/wall friction and machine compressive force

Mehta, A.M. and Augsburger, L.L., *Int. J. Pharmaceut.*, 1980, *4*, 347–51

Simultaneous measurement of force and displacement in an automatic capsule filling machine

capsule-filling machine, dosing tube mechanism; filling machine, powder plug formation, effects of, compression force, lubricant; formulation of contents, diluent, microcrystalline cellulose, lubricant, magnesium stearate; instrumented machine, displacement transducer, strain gauges

Chowan, Z.T. and Young, I.-C., *J. pharm. Sci.*, 1981, *70*, 927–30

Powder flow studies III: Tensile strength, consolidation ratio, flow rate and capsule-fill-weight variation relationships

capsule, uniformity of fill-weight, effect of powder properties; diluents, lactose, starch; formulation of contents, drug and excipients; lubricant, magnesium stearate; powder properties, consolidation ratio, flow rate, tensile strength, effects of, consolidation pressure, formulation

Mehta, A.M. and Augsburger, L.L., *Int. J. Pharmaceut.*, 1981, *7*, 327–34

A preliminary study of the effect of slug hardness on drug dissolution from hard gelatin capsules filled on an automatic capsule-filling machine

capsule-filling machine, dosing tube mechanism; filling machine, powder plug formation, plug hardness, effect of formulation of contents; formulation of contents, diluents, lactose, microcrystalline cellulose, lubricant, magnesium stearate; powder plugs, hardness measurement, three-point bending test; 4.2.3.4

Newton, J.M. and Bader, F., *J. Pharm. Pharmac.*, 1981, *33*, 621–6

The prediction of the bulk densities of powder mixtures, and its relationship to the filling of hard gelatin capsules

capsule filling, prediction of fill-weight, effect of powder properties; powder properties, bulk densities, effect of composition of mixtures, practical and theoretical values; powder properties, measurements of, apparent density, maximum tapped bulk density

Woodhead, P.J. and Newton, J.M., *J. Pharm. Pharmac.*, 1981, *33*, *Suppl.*, 21P

The influence of nozzle/piston clearance on the efficiency of a capsule-filling dosator

capsule filling, uniformity of weight, effects of, entrapped air, powder properties; dosing tube mechanism, powder plug formation, effects of, nozzle/piston clearance, powder properties; filling machine simulator, intermittent motion, dosing tube mechanism; instrumented dosing tube, displacement transducer, strain gauges; powder properties, particle size

Augsburger, L.L., *Pharm. Technol.*, 1982, *6*(9), 111–19

Instrumented capsule-filling machines: development and application

filling machine, dosing tube mechanism; filling machine, powder plug formation, compaction and ejection forces; formulation of contents, diluents, lubricants; instrumented filling machines, strain gauges, review of methods

Jolliffe, I.G., Newton, J.M. and Cooper, D., *J. Pharm. Pharmac.*, 1982, *34*, 230–5

The design and use of an instrumented mG2 capsule filling machine simulator

filling machine simulator, continuous motion, dosing tube mechanism; filling machine, powder plug formation, compaction and ejection forces; instrumented dosing tube, displacement transducers, strain gauges

Jolliffe, I.G. and Newton, J.M., *J. Pharm. Pharmac.*, 1982, *34*, 293–8

Practical implications of theoretical consideration of capsule filling by the dosator nozzle system

capsule filling, dosing tube mechanism; dosing tube, static assembly, measurement of nozzle surface texture; dosing tube, powder plug formation, force for arch formation, effects of, compression force, nozzle surface texture, powder properties; powder properties, measurements by Jenike shear cell, angle of internal friction, angle of wall friction; powder properties, particle size, powder flow, powder bed density

Jolliffe, I.G. and Newton, J.M., *J. Pharm. Pharmac.*, 1982, *34*, 415–19

An investigation of the relationship between particle size and compression during capsule filling with an instrumented mG2 simulator

capsule filling, uniformity of weight, effect of compression ratio; dosing tube mechanism, powder plug formation, compression and ejection forces, effect of powder properties;

instrumented dosing tube mechanism, displacement trans-ducers, strain gauges; machine simulator, continuous motion, dosing tube mechanism; powder properties, particle size

Jolliffe, I.G. and Newton, J.M., *J. Pharm. Pharmac.*, 1983, *35*, 7–11

The effect of dosator nozzle wall texture on capsule fill-ing with the mG2 simulator

capsule filling, uniformity of weight, effects of, compression rates, nozzle surface texture, powder properties; dosing tube mechanism, powder plug formation, effect of powder proper-ties; dosing tube, measurement of surface texture; instru-mented dosing tube mechanism, displacement transducers, strain gauges; machine simulator, continuous motion, dosing tube mechanism; powder properties, angle of powder/wall fric-tion, particle size

Jolliffe, I.G. and Newton, J.M., *J. Pharm. Pharmac.*, 1983, *35*, 74–8

Capsule filling studies using an mG2 production machine

capsule filling, uniformity of weight, effects of, compression ratio, nozzle surface texture, powder properties; filling machine, dosing tube mechanism; instrumented filling machine, strain gauges, comparison with machine simulator; powder properties, particle size

Jollife, I.G. and Newton, J.M., *Powder Technol.*, 1983, *35*, 151–7

Extension of theoretical considerations of the filling of pharmaceutical hard gelatin capsules to the design of dosator nozzles

filling machine, dosing tube mechanism, filling machine, powder plug formation, theoretical analysis, effect of nozzle surface texture; powder properties, arch formation and angle of powder/wall friction, relationship to nozzle surface design

Shah, K., Augsburger, L.L., Small, L.E. and Polli, G.P., *Pharm. Technol.*, 1983, *7*(4), 42, 44, 46, 48, 52–4

Instrumentation of a dosing disc automatic capsule fill-ing machine

filling machine, tamping mechanism; filling machine, powder plug formation, compaction and ejection forces; formulation of contents, diluents and lubricants; instrumented filling machine, strain gauges

Botzolakis, J.E. and Augsburger, L.L., *J. Pharm. Phar-mac.*, 1984, *36*, 77–84

The role of disintegrants in hard-gelatin capsules

filling machine, dosing tube mechanism; filling machine, powder plug formation, compaction and ejection forces; instru-mented filling machine, strain gauges; powder plug hardness tester; powder plug properties, hardness, effects of, formula-tion of contents, machine forces; 3.2.4.1–4.2.4

Maury, M., Héraud, P., Etienne, A., Aumonier, P. and Casahoursat, L., *Fourth International Conference on Pharmaceutical Technology*, (Paris, APGI, June 3–5, 1986), 1986, *I*, 384–8

Pressure measurements during the filling of hard gelatin capsules (in French)

filling machine, dosing tube mechanism; filling machine, powder plug formation, compaction and ejection forces; instru-mented filling machine, piezo-electric capacitor

Shah, K.B., Augsburger, L.L. and Marshall, K., *J. pharm. Sci.*, 1986, *75*, 291–6

An investigation of some factors influencing plug forma-tion and fill weight in a dosing-disc type automatic cap-sule-filling machine

capsule-filling machine, tamping mechanism; filling machine, powder plug formation, plug hardness, effects of formulation of contents; fill weight, theoretical determination from powder properties, effects of formulation of contents, machine settings; formulation of contents, diluents, lubricant; instrumented fill-ing machine, strain gauges; powder plugs, hardness measure-ment, effects of, formulation of contents, machine settings

3.2.3.4 Filling Semi-solids into Hard Capsules

Anon., *Packung & Transp. chem. Ind.*, 1978, No. 9, 421

Liquids in hard gelatin capsules

dose measurement, dosing pump; machine, automatic

Hoechst UK Ltd, *British Patent* 1 572 226, 1980

Improvements in and relating to pharmaceutical prepa-rations in solid unit dosage forms

filling machines, detection of capsule parts, photoelectric con-trol; filling machines, dosage of liquids; product weight unifor-mity; 3.2.4.2–4.2.4

Walker, S.E., Ganley, J.A., Bedford, K. and Eaves, T., *J. Pharm. Pharmac.*, 1980, *32*, 389–93

The filling of molten and thixotropic formulations into hard gelatin capsules

filling machines, detection of capsule parts, photoelectric con-trol; filling machines, dosing of liquids; product weight unifor-mity, effect of liquid dosing; 3.2.4.2–4.2.3.4–4.2.3.6

François, D., *Labo-Pharma Probl. Tech.*, 1983, *31*, 944–9

Technology of pastes and oils in hard gelatin capsules (in French)

filling machines, review

François, D., Chapter VI, in *The Capsule, Basics, Tech-nology and Biopharmacy, a Modern Dosage Form* (in German), Fahrig, W. and Hofer, U. (Eds), Stuttgart, Wissenschaftliche Verlagsgesellschaft mbH, 1983, pp. 112–26

Liquid and paste filling into hard gelatin capsules (in German)

filling machines, industrial; 3.2.4.2

McTaggart, C., Wood, R., Bedford, K. and Walker, S.E., *J. Pharm. Pharmac.*, 1984, *36*, 119–21

The evaluation of an automatic system for filling liquids into hard gelatin capsules filling machine, detection of capsule parts, photoelectric control; filling machine, dosing of liquids; formulation of contents; liquid properties, viscosity; product weight uniformity, effect of process conditions

Bowtle, W.J., *Br. J. pharm. Pract.*, 1986, *8*, 307–8

Semi-solid matrix capsules

thermosoftening formulation, manufacturing method, bench and industrial scale; 3.8.3.4; 4.2.3.4

3.2.3.5 Self-locking Capsules

Eli Lilly & Co., *French Patent* 1 343 698, 1963

Capsule resisting separation

Eli Lilly & Co., *British Patent* 970 761, 1964

Separation-resistant capsule

Carnaghi, A.J. and Logsdon, I., assigned to Eli Lilly & Co., *U.S. Patent* 3 285 408, 1966

Capsule with integral locking band

Eli Lilly & Co., *British Patent* 1 040 859, 1966

Capsule with integral locking band

Oglevee, H.J. and Mottin, R.E., assigned to Parke, Davis & Co., *U.S. Patent* 3 399 803, 1968

Self-locking medicament capsule

Parke, Davis & Co., *British Patent* 1 108 629, 1968

Hard shell capsule

R.P. Scherer Corporation, *British Patent* 1 133 715, 1968

Two-piece capsule

Vierna, D.S.G. and Herrera, D.L.G., *Auxiliary products for oral solid dosage forms*, Symposium (Barcelona, Faculty of Pharmacy, University of Barcelona), 1969, 153–63

Safety measures for the use of gelatin capsules (in Spanish)

manufacture; separation-resistant capsules; 3.8.3.7

Parke, Davis & Co., *British Patent* 1 302 343, 1973

Hard-shell locking capsule

Koepff, H. and Leiberich, R., *Pharm. Ind., Berl.*, 1976, *38*, 1064–72

Separation behaviour of hard gelatin capsules

capsule-filling machine, dosing tube mechanism; capsule separation force, effects, capsule type, storage; capsule separation force, measurement, Instron tester; formulation of contents

Controulis, J., *Drug Dev. ind. Pharm.*, 1985, *11*, 585–90

Hard gelatin capsules–New developments from Capsugel

capsule, shape, elongated cap; capsule, tamper resistant

3.2.3.6 Sealing Hard Capsules

Okie Inc., *U.S. Patent* 3 159 546, 1964, through *Derwent Accession No.* 14 823, 1962

Gelatin capsule sealing composition

coating composition, acetone, ethyl acetate, water; sealing, by coating at cap–body junction

Centre de Recherches Marcel Midy., *French Patent* 1 587 915, 1970

Radiation welding of gelatin capsules for medicines

contents, powders; sealing spot heat welding

Sankyo Co. Ltd, *Japanese Patent Application No.* 7 250 367, 1972, through *Derwent Accession No.* 00985U-AB, 1969

Gelatin capsule sealing

band sealing, composition of solution; coating material, hydroxypropyl cellulose, polyvinyl acetal diethylaminoacetate

Wittwer, F., *Pharm. Technol.*, 1985, *9*(6), 24, 26, 28–29

New developments on hermetic sealing of hard gelatin capsules

capsule sealing, by immersion; sealing solution, gelatin solvent

Cadé, D., Cole, E.T., Mayer, J.P. and Wittwer, F., *Fourth International Conference on Pharmaceutical Technology*, (Paris, APGI, June 3–5, 1986), 1986, *I*, 389–97

Liquid filled and sealed hard gelatin capsules

capsule sealing, method using liquid immersion and drying; formulation of contents, liquids; sealed capsules, applications

3.2.3.7 Cleaning Hard Capsules

Parke, Davis & Co., *German (BRD) Patent* 2 152 778, 1974

Capsule cleaning rig

apparatus, vibratory bowl; cleaning material, sodium chloride; filled capsules, cleaning

Parke, Davis & Co., *German (BRD) Patent* 2 152 807, 1974

Pharmaceutical capsule machine

cleaning machine; dust removal by airflow; empty capsule removal by suction

Taisho Pharmaceutical Co., *Japanese Patent Application No.* 5 004 727, 1975, through *Derwent Accession No.* 20244W/12, 1970

Polishing washing agents for the production of hard capsules

cleaning machine, coating pan; dust removal by sugar coated with non-toxic surfactant

Perry Industries Inc., *U.S. Patent* 4 058 868, 1977, through *Derwent Accession No.* 86280Y/48, 1976

Cleaning and polishing of capsules; by impact against electrically charged screen followed by tumbling in a napped fabric lined drum

3.2.4 Formulation of Contents of Hard Capsules

3.2.4.1 Dry Solids

Husa, W.J. and Becker, C.H., *J. Am. pharm. Ass.*,

scient. Edn, 1940, *29*, 78–86

Incompatibilities in prescriptions III. The use of inert powders in capsules to prevent liquefaction due to formation of a eutectic mixture

camphor, salol; diluents, various; storage trials

Husa, W.J. and Becker, C.H., *J. Am. pharm. Ass., scient. Edn*, 1940, *29*, 136–41

Incompatibilities in prescriptions IV. The use of inert powders in capsules to prevent liquefaction due to deliquescence

deliquescent drug mixtures; diluents, various; storage trials

Husa, W.J. and Macek, T.J., *J. Am. pharm. Ass., scient. Edn*, 1942, *31*, 213–16

Incompatibilities in prescriptions V. The use of tribasic calcium phosphate and silica gel in capsules to prevent liquefaction

deliquescent drug mixtures; diluents, calcium phosphate, silica gel; storage trials

Bellafiore, I.J., *J. Am. pharm. Ass., pract. Pharm. Edn*, 1953, *14*, 580–2

Stabilization of capsules of eutectic mixtures against liquefaction

aspirin, caffeine citrate, camphor, phenazone; diluent, kaolin; eutectic mixtures; storage

Boger, W.P. and Gavin, J.J., *New Engl. J. Med.*, 1959, *261*, 827–32

An evaluation of tetracycline preparations

tetracyclines; diluents, citric acid, dicalcium phosphate, glucosamine and lactose; 4.4.6.1

Jacobs, P., *Pharm. Weekbl. Ned.*, 1964, *99*, 719–21

Filling of capsules with voluminous substances (in Dutch)

powder compression devices; powder properties, bulk density

Czetsch-Lindenwald, H.V. and Tawashi, R., *Pharm. Ind., Berl.*, 1965, *27*, 146–51

Tests with hard gelatin capsules (in German)

glidant, fumed silica; nomogram, fill-weight, capsule size determination; 3.8.2.4; 3.8.3.6

Czetsch-Lindenwald, H.V. and Asker, A.F., *Pharm. Ind., Berl.*, 1966, *28*, 614–16

Lubricants for filling hard gelatin capsules (in German)

lubricants, various; powder properties, flow measurements; product weight uniformity

Zoglio, M.A., Maulding, H.V., Haller, R.M. and Briggen, S., *J. pharm. Sci.*, 1968, *57*, 1877–80

Pharmaceutical heterogeneous systems III. Inhibition of stearate lubricant induced degradation of aspirin by the use of certain organic acids

acetylsalicylic acid; lubricant, magnesium stearate; stability, effect of formulation

Czetsch-Lindenwald, H.V., *Auxilary products for oral solid dosage forms*, Symposium (Barcelona, Faculty of Pharmacy, University of Barcelona), 1969, 143–9

Influence of lubricants on the accuracy of fill of capsules (in Spanish)

lubricants, aluminium stearate, magnesium stearate, polyethylene glycol, silicon dioxide, talc; powder properties, flow, effect of lubricants; product weight uniformity, effect of lubricants; storage, high humidity, effect of lubricant

Delonca, H., Puech, A., Segura, G. and Youakim, Y., *J. Pharm. Belg.*, 1969, *24*, 317–31

Influence of excipients and conditions of storage on the stability of medicines. II. Capsules of acetylsalicylic acid (in French)

aspirin; diluents, calcium phosphate, calcium sulphate, maize starch, polyvinylpyrrolidone, sodium alginate; lubricant, talc; 3.8.3.7

Ito, K., Hitomi, M., Kaga, S.-I. and Takeya, Y., *Chem. pharm. Bull., Tokyo*, 1969, *17*, 1138–45

Studies on hard gelatin capsules II. The capsule filling on powders and effects of glidant by ring filling method-machine

diluents, lactose, starch; glidants, colloidal silicon dioxide, product weight uniformity, effect of formulation; 3.2.3.2

Fonner, D.E., Buck, J.R. and Banker, G.S., *J. pharm. Sci.*, 1970, *59*, 1587–96

Mathematical optimization techniques in drug product design and process analysis

formulation, processing, mathematical optimisation technique, Lagrangian analysis

Prista, L.N., Morgado, R.R., Fonseca, A. and Pinho, A.A., *Anais Fac. Farm. Porto*, 1970, *30*, 19–34

Studies on hard gelatin capsules I. Ease of filling with powders (in Portuguese)

filling materials, powder types, calcium carbonate, lactose, quinine hydrochloride, sodium chloride; lubricants, polyethylene glycol 4000, silicon dioxide, stearates, aluminium, magnesium, zinc; powder properties, flow, angles of repose, effect of lubricants

Samyn, J.C. and Jung, W.Y., *J. pharm. Sci.*, 1970, *59*, 169–75.

In vitro dissolution from several experimental capsule formulations

diluents, dibasic calcium phosphate, lactose, disintegrants, starch; lubricants, magnesium stearate, talc; 4.2.4

Caldwell, H.C. and Westlake, W.J., *J. pharm. Sci.*, 1972, *61*, 984–5

Magnesium lauryl sulfate, soluble lubricant

lithium carbonate; diluent, spray-dried lactose; lubricants, magnesium lauryl sulphate, magnesium stearate

Khalil, S.A. and Ali, L.M.M., *Acta pharm. suec.*, 1972, *9*, 563–72

Some formulation factors affecting disintegration and dissolution of chloramphenicol capsules

chloramphenicol; diluents, calcium phosphate, lactose; lubricants, magnesium stearate, talc; 4.2.4

Caldwell, H.C. and Westlake, W.J., *Can. J. pharm. Sci.*, 1973, *8*, 50–3

Magnesium lauryl sulfate–soluble lubricant

lithium carbonate; diluent, lactose; lubricants, magnesium lauryl sulphate, magnesium stearate, sodium lauryl sulphate; powder properties, particle size determination, Coulter counter; 3.8.3.6; 4.2.4

Goodhart, F.W., McCoy, R.H. and Ninger, F.C., *J. pharm. Sci.*, 1973, *62*, 304–10

New *in vitro* disintegration and dissolution test method for tablets and capsules

diluents, microcrystalline cellulose, starch; lubricants, magnesium stearate, stearic acid; wetting agents, sodium lauryl sulphate; 4.2.4

Caldwell, H.C., *J. pharm. Sci.*, 1974, *63*, 770–3

Dissolution of lithium and magnesium from lithium carbonate capsules containing magnesium stearate

lithium carbonate; diluent, lactose; lubricants, magnesium lauryl sulphate, magnesium stearate, sodium stearate, stearic acid; product weight uniformity, comparison and effect of lubricants; wetting agent, sodium lauryl sulphate; 4.2.3.4

Newton, J.M. and Razzo, F.N., *J. Pharm. Pharmac.*, 1974, *26*, *Suppl.*, 30P–36P

The influence of additives on the *in vitro* release of drugs from hard gelatin capsules

nitrofurantoin, nitrofurazone, oxytetracycline dihydrate, tetracycline hydrochloride; diluents, lactose, sodium starch glycolate, starch; lubricant, magnesium stearate; wetting agent, sodium lauryl sulphate; 4.2.3.4

Varthalis, S. and Pilpel, N., *J. Pharm. Pharmac.*, 1976, *28*, 415–9

Anomalies in some properties of powder mixtures

paracetamol, oxytetracycline; diluent, lactose; powder properties, bulk density

Mony, C., Sambeat, C. and Cousin, G., *First International Conference of Pharmaceutical Technology*, (Paris, APGI, May 31–June 2, 1977), 1977, *II*, 98–108

Applications of the measure of force in the formulation and filling of hard gelatin capsules (in French)

diluents, celluloses, microcrystalline and granular, lactose, powder and microcrystalline, starches, maize, potato and rice, starch modified, sodium carboxymethyl starch; lubricants, magnesium stearate, talc; product weight uniformity, effect of diluents, lubricants; 3.2.3.3

Ryder, J. and Thomas, A., *J. Pharm. Pharmac.*, 1977, *29*, *Suppl.*, 63p

A comparison of the effectiveness of several disintegrants in capsules of 4-ethoxycarbonylphenoxy-2′-pyridylmethane (BRL 10614)

4-ethoxycarbonylphenoxy-2′-pyridylmethane; disintegrants, polyvinylpyrrolidone, cross-linked (Polyclar AT), sodium carboxymethylcellulose, low substituted (Nymcel ZSB16), sodium starch glycolate (Primojel), starch (maize); 4.2.3.4

Seager, H., *Mfg Chem.*, 1977, *48*(4), 25–35

Spray-coating bulk drugs aids dosage form production

drug availability, *in vivo*, human, serum levels, comparisons of dosage forms and formulations; powder properties, modification by spray-coating techniques

Kurihara, K. and Ichikawa, I., *Chem. pharm. Bull., Tokyo*, 1978, *26*, 1250–6

Effect of powder flowability on capsule-filling-weight-variation

diluents, microcrystalline cellulose, lactose, potato starch; lubricant, magnesium stearate; product weight uniformity, effect of formulation; 3.2.3.3

Liedtke, R., *German (BRD) Patent (offen.)* 2 719 156, 1978

Two compartment medical capsules

capsule, hard gelatin, two compartment; formulation, incompatible ingredients

Mendes, R.W., Masih, S.Z. and Kanumuri, R.R., *J. pharm. Sci.*, 1978, *67*, 1613–16

Effect of formulation and process variables on bioequivalency of nitrofurantoin I: Preliminary studies

nitrofurantoin; diluents, compressible sugar, lactose, mannitol; lubricant, magnesium stearate; 4.2.3.4

Small, L.E. and Augsburger, L.L., *Drug Dev. ind. Pharm.*, 1978, *4*, 345–72

Aspects of the lubrication requirements for an automatic capsule filling machine

diluents, microcrystalline cellulose, lactose, compressible starch; formulation of contents, effect on filling machine; lubricants, magnesium lauryl sulphate, magnesium stearate, stearic acid; 3.2.3.3

Beecham Group Limited, *French Patent* 2 320 731, 1979

Oral antibiotic–polyvinylpyrrolidone capsules, with short disintegration times and which are rapidly soluble

disintegrant, crospovidone

Kassem, A.A., Zaki, S.A., Mursi, N.M. and Tayel, S.A., *Pharmazie*, 1979, *34*, 86–91

Effect of certain additives on the dissolution rate of chloramphenicol

adsorbents, colloidal silicon dioxide, various grades; diluents, dextrose, lactose, sucrose; solid dispersions, method of manufacture, fusion; surface-active agents, natural, dehydrocholic acid, sodium deoxycholate; surface-active agents, synthetic, macrogol esters, macrogol ethers, sodium lauryl sulphate; 4.2.3.4

Merle, C., Artaud, M. and Guyot-Hermann, A.M., *Farmaco, Edn prat.*, 1979, *34*, 210–19

Influence of glidants on the dissolution rate of acetylsalicylic acid in hard gelatin capsules (in French)

lubricants, hydrophilic, colloidal silicon dioxide (Aerosil, Levilite), hydrophobic, talc, magnesium stearate; powder properties, porosity, effects of lubricants, mechanism of action; 4.2.3.4

Stewart, A.G., Grant, D.J.W. and Newton, J.M., *J. Pharm. Pharmac.*, 1979, *31*, 1–6

The release of a model low-dose drug (riboflavine) from hard gelatin capsule formulations

diluents, dicalcium phosphate, kaolin, lactose, microcrystalline cellulose, modified starch, sodium bicarbonate, sodium carboxymethyl starch, starch; lubricant, magnesium stearate; 4.5.5

Shek, E., Ghani, M. and Jones, R.E., *J. pharm. Sci.*, 1980, *69*, 1135–42

Simplex search in optimisation of capsule formulation

diluent, lactose; formulation, mathematical optimisation technique, simplex method, level of disintegrant; disintegrant, maize starch; lubricant, stearic acid; powder properties, tapped bulk density, rate of consolidation; 4.2.3.4

Botzolakis, J.E., Small, L.E., and Augsburger, L.L., *Int. J. Pharmaceut.*, 1982, *12*, 341–9

Effect of disintegrants on drug dissolution from capsules filled on a dosator-type automatic capsule-filling machine

hydrochlorothiazide, paracetamol; diluent, dicalcium phosphate dihydrate; disintegrants, maize starch, sodium carboxymethylcellulose, sodium carboxymethyl starch, crospovidone; glidant, sodium silicoaluminate; 4.2.4.

Botzolakis, J.E. and Augsburger, L.L., *J. Pharm. Pharmac.*, 1984, *36*, 77–84

The role of disintegrants in hard-gelatin capsules

hydrochlorothiazide; diluents, dicalcium phosphate, lactose; disintegrants, croscarmellose types A and B, sodium carboxymethyl starch; lubricant, magnesium stearate; 3.2.3.3; 4.2.4

Stamm, A., Boymond, C. and Mathis, C., *Drug Dev. ind. Pharm.*, 1984, *10*, 355–80

Some aspects of the formulation of hard gelatin capsules

diluents, granulating materials, glycerol palmitostearate, hydrogenated castor oil, hydroxypropylmethylcellulose, methacrylic acid polymers, polyethylene glycol, polyvinylpyrrolidone; diluents, powders, lactose, microcrystalline cellulose, pregelatinised starch; glidant, colloidal silicon dioxide; lubricant, magnesium stearate; 4.2.3.4

Chowhan, Z.T. and Chi, L.-H., *Pharm. Technol.*, 1985, *9*(3), 84, 86, 90, 92, 94–97

Drug-excipient interactions resulting from powder mixing, I: Possible mechanisms of interaction with starch and its effect on drug dissolution

ketorolac tromethamine; diluents, lactose, starch, maize and pregelatinised; disintegrants, starch, maize and pregelatinised;

drug, content uniformity, effect of lubricant mixing; lubricant, magnesium stearate; 4.2.2.1; 4.2.3.4

Chowhan, Z.T., and Chi, L.-H., *Pharm. Technol.*, 1985, *9*(4), 30, 32–33, 36, 38–41

Drug-excipient interactions resulting from powder mixing. II: Possible mechanisms of interactions with crospovidone and its effect on in vitro dissolution

ketorolac tromethamine; diluent, lactose; disintegrant, crospovidone; drug, content uniformity, effect of lubricant mixing; lubricant, magnesium searate; 4.2.2.1; 4.2.3.4

Mehta, A.M. and Jones, D.M., *Pharm. Technol.*, 1985, *9*(6), 52, 54–55, 58–60

Coated pellets under the microscope

coating machines, tablet pan, conventional and modified, fluidised bed; coating materials, ethyl cellulose, hydroxypropylmethyl cellulose; pellets, coated, method of manufacture; pellets, physical properties, surface characteristics by scanning electron microscopy, effects of, coating device, position of spray

O'Connor, R.E. and Schwartz, J.B., *Drug. Dev. ind. Pharm.*, 1985, *11*, 1837–57

Spheronisation II: Drug release from drug-diluent mixtures

chlorothiazide, chlorpheniramine maleate, quinidine sulphate, theophylline; diluents, microcrystalline cellulose, microcrystalline cellulose/carmellose sodium; drug availability, dissolution rate of pellets, effect of formulation; pellets, method of manufacture, wet granulation, extrusion, spheronisation; pellets, physical properties, density, friability, particle size

Anno, E. M. and Rees, J. E., *Fourth International Conference on Pharmaceutical Technology*, (Paris, APGI, June 3–5, 1986), 1986, *V*, 61–69

Release of phenytoin sodium from capsules containing two- and three-component mixes

phenytoin sodium; diluents, calcium sulphate dihydrate, lactose; lubricant, magnesium stearate; powder properties, state of mixture, scanning electron microscopy, X-ray microanalysis; 4.2.3.4

Ari-Ulubelen, A., Akbuğa, J., Bayraktar-Alpmen, G. and Gülhan, S., *Pharm. Ind., Berl.*, 1986, *48*, 393–395

Effect of formulation factors on the in vitro dissolution characteristics of phenytoin sodium capsules

phenytoin sodium; diluents, calcium sulphate dihydrate, lactose, maize starch, sodium sulphate; lubricants, colloidal silicon dioxide, magnesium stearate, talc; 4.2.3.4

Chowhan, Z.T. and Chi, L.-H., *J. pharm. Sci.*, 1986, *75*, 534–541

Drug-excipient interactions resulting from powder mixing, III: Solid state properties and their effect on drug dissolution

prednisone; diluents, calcium hydrogen phosphate, pregelatinised starch; disintegrants, pregelatinised starch, sodium starch glycolate; drug, content uniformity, effects of, formulation of contents, lubricant mixing; lubricant, magnesium stearate; 4.2.2.1; 4.2.3.4

Chowhan, Z.T. and Chi, L.-H., *J. pharm. Sci.*, 1986, 75, 542–545

Drug-excipient interactions resulting from powder mixing, IV: Role of lubricants and their effect on in vitro dissolution

ketorolac tromethamine; diluent, lactose; disintegrant, crospovidone; lubricants, magnesium stearate, sodium stearyl fumarate; 4.2.2.1.; 4.2.3.4

Kohri, N., Mori, K.-I., Miyazaki, K. and Arita, T., *J. pharm. Sci.*, 1986, 75, 57–61

Sustained release of nifedipine from granules

binders, ethylcellulose, hydroxypropylmethylcellulose, hydroxypropylmethylcellulose phthalate; diluents, maize starch, microcrystalline cellulose; formulation, pH-dependent and pH-independent granules; 4.5.6.2

3.2.4.2 Formulation of Semi-solids

Centre de Recherches Marcel Midy, *Swiss Patent* 510550, 1971, through *Derwent Accession No.* 648585-BJ, 1969

Encapsulation process

diluents, fatty substances, non oxidisable, melting point 30–40°; filling machine, volumetric dosing

Broer, J., *Verpack.-Rdsch., Frankf.*, 1978, 28, 706–7

The filling of liquids into hard gelatin capsules (in German)

capsules, comparison of hard and soft; filling, liquids and semi-solids, industrial scale; formulation, contents, liquid and semi-solid

Cuiné, A., Mathis, C., Stamm, A. and François, D., *Labo-Pharma Probl. Tech.*, 1978, 26(274), 222–7

Filling hard gelatin capsules with viscous solutions of active principles. I – Preliminary studies – Excipients (in French)

capsule, sealing; excipients, oils and thickening agents; formulation properties, melting point, surface tension, viscosity; stability, effect of temperature and time

Cuiné, A., Mathis, C., Stamm, A. and François, D., *Labo-Pharma Probl. Tech.*, 1978, 26(276), 421–30

Filling hard gelatin capsules with viscous solutions of active principles. II – Rheological study of fatty excipients (in French)

excipients, thixotropic mixtures; formulation properties, viscosity, thixotropic mixtures

Cuiné, A., Mathis, C., Stamm, A. and François, D., *Pharm. Ind., Berl.*, 1978, 40, 654–7

The filling of viscous solutions of active materials into hard gelatin capsules (in German)

clofibrate, vitamin A; applications; capsule, sealing; excipients, oils and thickening agents; formulation properties, viscosity

Cuiné, A., Mathis, C., Stamm, A. and François, D., *Labo-Pharma Probl. Tech.*, 1979, No. 292, 863–8

Filling of hard gelatin capsules with viscous solutions (or suspensions) of active ingredients III. Formulation of active ingredients (in French)

active ingredients, powders and semi-solid materials; excipients, oils; filling machine, cold and hot filling; formulation properties, viscosity, effect of formulation; stability testing; thickening agents, colloidal silicon dioxide, waxes

François, D. and Jones, B.E., *Mfg Chem.*, 1979, 50(3), 37, 38, and 41

Making the hard capsules with the soft centre

capsules, comparison of hard and soft; filling, liquids and semi-solids, small scale, industrial scale; formulation, contents, liquids and semi-solids, adjuvants and diluents; history; review

Boymond, C. and Mathis, C., *Second International Conference on Pharmaceutical Technology*, (Paris, APGI, June 3–5, 1980), 1980, IV, 93–103

A study of the influence of formulation on the release of ephedrine hydrochloride from hard gelatin capsules (in French)

excipients, hydrophobic, glycerides; formulation, delayed release; 4.2.3.4

Cuiné, A., Mathis, C. and Stamm, A., *Second International Conference on Pharmaceutical Technology*, (Paris, APGI, June 3–5, 1980), 1980, I, 66–76

Hard gelatin capsules with paste contents: study of the rheological properties and *in vitro* release of active principles (in French)

capsule, sealing; excipients, oils; formulation properties, viscosity, effect of formulation; thickening agents, colloidal silicon dioxide, waxes; 4.2.3.4

Hoechst UK Ltd, *British Patent* 1 572 226, 1980

Improvements in and relating to pharmaceutical preparations in solid unit dosage forms

diluents, polyethylene glycols, polyvinyl acetate; formulation of contents, prolonged release; thickeners, colloidol silicon dioxide, hydrogenated castor oil; 3.2.3.4; 4.2.4

Kreuter, J., Speiser, P.P. and Prasad, N.K., *Second International Conference on Pharmaceutical Technology*, (Paris, APGI, June 3–5, 1980), 1980, II, 103–8

In vitro release of different dosage forms of 8-methoxypsoralen

excipients, solvents, oleyl oleate, polysorbate 80; 4.2.3.2

Walker, S.E., Ganley, J.A., Bedford, K. and Eaves, T., *J. Pharm. Pharmac.*, 1980, 32, 389–93

The filling of molten and thixotropic formulations into hard gelatin capsules

content uniformity, comparison of liquid and powder formulations; filling machine performance, effect of formulation; formulation, effect on dissolution rate, controlled-release and standard products; formulation, thermosetting and thixotropic mixtures, method of manufacture; product weight uniformity, comparison of liquid and powder formulations; 3.2.3.4; 4.3.3.4; 4.2.3.6

Lilly Industries Ltd, *British Patent* 1 590 864, 1981

Thixotropic filling medium for hard gelatin capsules

diluents, review of; physical properties, of contents, surface tension, viscosity, effect of formulation

François, D., Denmat, A., Waugh, A. and Woodage, T., *Pharm. Ind., Berl.*, 1982, *44*, 86–9

The *in vitro* and *in vivo* availability of phenylpropanolamine from oil/paste formulations in hard gelatin capsules

phenylpropanolamine; diluents, powders, lactose; diluents, semi-solids, hydrophilic, Labrafil M 2130 BS, lipophilic, arachis oil/beeswax; formulation of contents, semi-solids, prolonged release; 4.5.6.2

Hunter, E., Fell, J.T., Sharma, H. and McNeilly, A. -M., *Pharm. Ind., Berl.*, 1982, *44*, 90–1

The "in vivo" behaviour of hard gelatin capsules filled with thixotropic liquids

diluent, polyethylene glycol 1000; physical properties, viscosity of contents, effect of thickener; thickener, colloidal silicon dioxide; 4.4.3

Mathis, C. and Cuiné, A., *Labo-Pharma Probl. Tech.*, 1983, *31*, 935–43

Formulation, stability and *in vitro* availability of active principles as solutions or viscous suspensions filled in hard gelatin capsules (in French)

capsule sealing; excipients, natural and synthetic, physical properties; formulation, physical properties, effect of formulation, addition of colloidal silicon dioxide; 4.2.3.4

François, D., Chapter VI, in *The Capsule, Basics, Technology and Biopharmacy*, a *Modern Dosage Form* (in German), Fahrig, W. and Hofer, U. (Eds), Stuttgart, Wissenschaftliche Verlagsgesellschaft mbH, 1983, pp. 112–26

Liquid and paste filling into hard gelatin capsules (in German)

clofibrate, phenylpropanolamine, vitamin E, examples; 3.2.3.4

Bauer, K.H. and Dortunc, B., *Drug Dev. ind. Pharm.*, 1984, *10*, 699–712

Non-aqueous emulsions as vehicles for capsule fillings

caffeine, chloramphenicol, salicylic acid, sodium salicylate; diluents, polyethylene glycol, propylene glycol, rape seed oil, semi-solid triglyceride/wax mixtures; formulation, non-aqueous emulsions; 4.5.5

Djimbo, M. and Moës, A.J., *J. Pharm. Belg.*, 1984, *39*, 36–42

Release of drugs formulated as hard pastes filled into hard gelatin capsules. Part 1. Physical properties and *in vitro* testing

acetylsalicylic acid, theophylline; diluents, pastes, polyethylene glycols, suppository bases; paste properties, rheology, effect of formulation; disintegrants, Ac-Di-Sol, polyplasdone, sodium carboxymethyl starch; 4.2.3.4

Bowtle, W.J., Lucas, R.A. and Barker, N.J., *Fourth International Conference on Pharmaceutical Technology*, (Paris, APGI, June 3–5, 1986), 1986, *V*, 80–89

Formulation and process studies in semi-solid matrix capsule technology

fenoprofen, vancomycin; excipients, polyethylene glycols; excipients, physical properties, heating/cooling characteristics, rheology; fill materials, physical properties; semi-solid filling, process characteristics; 3.8.3.7; 4.5.5

Chatham, S.M., Newton, J.M. and Walker, S.E., *Fourth International Conference on Pharmaceutical Technology*, (Paris, APGI, June 3–5, 1986). 1986, *II*, 213–20

The influence of thermal history on the morphology of PEG 4000

polyethylene glycol 4000, structure, measurement by differential scanning calorimetry and X-ray crystallography, effect of thermal history

Hagenlocher, M., Hannula, A.M., Wittwer, F., Soliva, M. and Speiser P., *Fourth International Conference on Pharmaceutical Technology*, (Paris, APGI, June 3–5, 1986), 1986, *I*, 398–405

Hard gelatin capsules for rectal drug delivery

paracetamol; diluents, Labrafil M2130 BS, M2735 BS, Miglyol 812, Witepsol H15; 3.5.2; 4.5.3.4

Mathis, C. and Heimendinger, J., *Fourth International Conference on Pharmaceutical Technology*, (Paris, APGI, June 3–5, 1986), 1986, *V*, 90–98

Test of programming the release of active principles from pasty excipients in hard gelatin capsules (in French)

aspirin; excipients, Gelucires, Labrafils, Precirol, Simulsols; 4.2.3.4

3.3 Capsules, Soft Gelatin

3.3.1 General References

Baum, E., *Chemikerzeitung*, 1952, *76*, 847–50

The gelatin capsule, an economic packaging form (in German)

applications; manufacture

Kipphan, K., *Chemie-Ingr.-Tech.*, 1952, *24*, 299–301

The gelatin capsule, its manufacture and its use (in German)

applications; manufacture

Brass, H., *Pharm. Ind., Berl.*, 1954, *16*, 421–4

The gelatin capsule, its manufacture and pharmaceutical significance (in German)

applications; manufacture

Kipphan, K., *Dt. ApothZtg*, 1955, *95*, 1032–6

Gelatin capsules (in German)

applications; manufacture

Clemow, J., *Mfg Chem.*, 1957, *28*, 170–2

Gelatin capsules – 50 million a week

applications; manufacturing method, rotary die

Müller, G., *Fette Seifen Anstr-Mittel*, 1960, *62*, 395–9

The manufacture of gelatin capsules (in German)

applications; capsule properties; formulation of shell; manufacture, seamed capsules, automatic and semi-automatic machines

Müller, G., *Mfg Chem.*, 1961, *32*, 63–6

Methods and machines for making gelatin capsules

formulation, shell; manufacture, seamed and seamless capsules

Widmann, A., *Pharm. Weekbl. Ned.*, 1961, *96*, 669–71

The manufacture of gelatin capsules (in Dutch)

applications; manufacture

Clemow, J., *Labo-Pharma.*, 1962, *10*(104), 63–7

Soft gelatin capsules (in French)

applications; history; manufacture

Müller, G., *Pharm. Ztg, Berl.*, 1962, *107*, 444–6

Soft gelatin capsule – machines (in German)

manufacture, industrial scale, seamed and seamless capsules

Genet, H., *Capsules et Gélules*, Symposium (Paris, Faculty of Pharmacy, University of Paris), 1970, *I*, 1–28

The soft gelatin capsule (in French)

capsules, enteric; filling; history; manufacture, seamed and seamless; pharmacopoeial standards; raw materials, standards; requirements

Torrado Valeiras, J.J., *Monitor Farm. Terap.*, 1970, *76*, 181–4

Soft gelatin capsules (in Spanish)

applications; manufacture

Widmann, A., *Pharma Int.*, 1970, No. 1, 5–10

Soft gelatin capsules

applications, oral, rectal, vaginal, veterinary; manufacturing method, rotary die; pharmacopoeial standards; properties; storage, packaging, stability

Stephan, D., *Packung Transp. chem. Ind.*, 1975, No. 12, 2–4

Soft gelatin capsules: Convenience and optimum form for bitter medicines (in German)

applications; manufacturing method, rotary die

Hellberg, N., *Farmaceutisk Revy*, 1977, *76*, 30–1

Soft capsules – not only easy to swallow . . . (in Swedish)

applications; drug availability; manufacture

Maconachie, S., *Mfg Chem.*, 1977, *48*(8), 33, 35–6, 39

Soft gelatin capsules in product development

drug availability, *in vivo*; formulation, contents; stability

Stephan, D., *Packung Transp. chem. Ind.*, 1979, No. 4, 188

Soft gelatin capsules not only for medicines (in German)

applications, chemical and cosmetic; manufacturing method, rotary die

Baes, E. A., *Mfg Chem.*, 1981, *52*(3), 33–4

Soft shell capsules

applications; drug availability; manufacture; market analysis

Berry, I.R., *Drug Cosmet. Ind.*, 1982, *131*, 40

One-piece, sealed soft gelatin capsules—why tamper resistant

applications; packaging

Seager, H. *Pharm. Technol.*, 1985, *9*, 84, 86, 88, 90, 92, 94, 96, 98, 100, 102, 104

Soft gelatin capsules: a solution to many tabletting problems

applications; drug availability, *in vivo*, comparison with other dosage forms; manufacturing method, rotary die; physical properties, comparison with drugs and tablets; stability, effects of storage

3.3.2 Manufacturing and Filling Soft Capsules
3.3.2.1 Seamed Capsules

Scherer, R.P., *British Patent* 395 546, 1933

Method of and apparatus for making capsules

manufacturing method, rotary die

Ravenscroft, E.A. and Young, F.H., assigned to Abbott Laboratories, *U.S. Patent* 2 205 837, 1940

Capsule making machine

capsule identification, by embossing; manufacturing method, rotary die

Scherer, R.P., *U.S. Patent* 2 199 210, 1940

Method and apparatus for making capsules by needle injection

capsule fill, liquid; capsule filling, needle injection; manufacturing method, rotary die

Waring, O.I., assigned in part to Rothberg, P., *U.S. Patent* 2 199 425, 1940

Method and means for making capsules

capsule fill, solid, semi-solid, liquid; manufacturing method, rotary die

Ravenscroft, E.A., assigned to Abbott Laboratories, *U.S. Patent* 2 279 505, 1942

Capsule making machine

capsule fill, liquids; manufacturing method, rotary die

Anon., *Mfg Chem.*, 1955, *26*, 56–8

Pharmaceutical processing of aureomycin

tetracyclines; capsule fill, powder; manufacturing method

Cooke, C.H., assigned to Upjohn Company, *U.S. Patent* 3 081 234, 1963

Elimination of entrapped air in elastic capsules

capsule fill, granules and powders; manufacturing method, rotary die; processing conditions

Anon., *Mfg Chem.*, 1965, *36*(9), 65

Encapsulating machine for soft shell products

manufacturing method, rotary die

Kath, A.W., assigned to R.P. Scherer Corp., *U.S. Patent* 3 269 088, 1966

Opposed gelatin sheets pressed together after filling

manufacturing method, rotary die; processing conditions

Berry, I.R., *Drug Cosmet. Ind.*, 1984, *134*(4), 26–8, 30, 84–5

Process validation for soft gelatin capsules

capsule properties, seam thickness, wall thickness, weight uniformity; manufacturing method, rotary die, process conditions; product weight uniformity

3.3.2.2 Seamless Capsules

Merrill, E.C., Reddie, J.W. and Anderson, J.M., assigned to United Drug Company, *U.S. Patent* 2 275 154, 1942

Method for making capsules

manufacturing method, extrusion

Plourde, N.N., assigned to Gunnell Capsulations, Inc., *U.S. Patent* 2 692 404, 1954

Seamless moulded capsule

capsule shell composition, gelatin and gelatin substitute; manufacturing method, injection moulding; processing conditions

Briess, P., *Mfg Chem.*, 1961, *32*, 275

The "drop" method of capsule manufacture

manufacturing method, drop

Moreland, S.T., *U.S. Patent* 4 028 024, 1977

Manufacture of filled capsules or the like

capsule shell composition, moisture content; machine; manufacturing method, extrusion, gelatin low moisture content

3.3.3 Formulation of Soft Capsules

3.3.3.1 Capsule Shells

Patterson, S.J. and Lerrigo, A.F., *Q. J. Pharm. Pharmac.*, 1947, *20*, 83–6

Betanaphthol in gelatin capsules – its use as a preservative, with a method for its determination

preservative, betanaphthol, effect of storage on concentration

Scherer, J.O., assigned to R.P. Scherer Corporation, *U.S. Patent* 2 628 916, 1953

Process of preparing molten gelatin solution

manufacture, preparation bubble-free gelatin solution; manufacture, process for applying vacuum

Weidenheimer, J.F. and Callahan, F.M., assigned to American Cyanamid Company, *U.S. Patent* 2 770 553, 1956

Soft gelatin encapsulation

plasticisers, acetamide, formamide

Stanley, J.P. and Bradley, C.W., assigned to R.P. Scherer Corporation, *U.S. Patent* 2 870 062, 1959

Acid treated high Bloom gelatin

gelatin, manufacture, acid-treated bone; gelatin, properties, high Bloom, low viscosity; plasticisers

American Cyanamid Company, *British Patent* 1 037 463, 1966

Surface dyeing and pigment marking of gelatin capsules

colour, surface dyeing; formulation, printing inks; identification, colour, imprinting

Mima, H., Noda, E. and Banba, H., assigned to Takeda Chemical Industries, Limited, Japan, *U.S. Patent* 3 456 051, 1969

Protection against humidity by addition of buffer

gelatin film composition, inclusion of buffer; stability, protection of contents

R.P. Scherer Corporation, *British Patent* 1 252 200, 1971

Improved gelatine capsules

capsule shell properties, mechanical strength, moisture resistance; gelatin film composition, additives, glycerol, silicone fluid; 3.4.2.2

Rolle, F.J., assigned to R.P. Scherer Corporation, *U.S. Patent* 3 653 934, 1972

Gastro-resistant capsules

gelatin film composition (non-enteric), additives, glycerol, silicone fluid; 3.4.2.2

Hom, F.S., Veresh, S.A. and Miskel, J.J., *J., pharm. Sci.*, 1973, *62*, 1001–6

Soft gelatin capsules I: factors affecting capsule shell dissolution rate

gelatin, Bloom strength, type; plasticisers, glycerol, hexaglycerol, sorbitol; solution enhancers, lysine hydrochloride, urea; 4.2.3.1

Tanabe Seiyaku Company Limited, *Japanese Patent* 7 310 522, 1973, through *Derwent Accession No.* 19506U-AB,1969

Soft capsules

capsule properties, mechanical strength, solubility, stability; drug release, enteric and non-enteric capsules; gelatin film, composition

Hom, F.S., Veresh, S.A. and Ebert, W.R., *J. pharm. Sci.*, 1975, *64*, 851–7

Soft gelatin capsules II: oxygen permeability study of capsule shells pigments, titanium dioxide; plasticisers, decaglycerol, glycerol, hexaglycerol, sorbitol; 3.8.2.3

Hom, F.S., *Drug Dev. ind. Pharm.*, 1984, *10*, 275–87

Soft gelatin capsules III: an accelerated method for evaluating the dissolution stability of various gel formulations

plasticisers, glycerol, sorbitol; solution enhancers, 1-histidine, semicarbazide; 4.2.3.1

Armstrong, N.A., James, K.C., Collet, D. and Thomas, M., *Drug Dev. ind. Pharm.*, 1985, *11*, 1859–68

Solute migration from oily solutions into glycerol-gelatin mixtures

gelatin film composition, additives, glycerol; solute migration, measurement into glycerogelatin column from oily solution; solute migration, effect of composition of glycerogelatin base, nature of solutes

3.3.3.2 Formulation of Contents of Soft Capsules

Kreuger, P., assigned to N.V. Moutsuikerindustrie and Extractiebedrijf Maltostase, *U.S. Patent* 2 580 683, 1951

Aqueous fills of sugar syrup

contents, syrup vehicles; gelatin film composition, additives, glycerol, sugar; stability, protection of contents

Kurtz, W.M., assigned to Upjohn Company, *U.S. Patent* 3 126 321, 1964

Soft gelatin capsules

oleaginous vehicle, formulation, oil and purified cellulose; stability, protection of contents

Hom, F.S. and Miskel, J.J., *J. pharm. Sci.*, 1970, *59*, 827–30

Oral dosage form design and its influence on dissolution rates for a series of drugs

diluents, polyethylene glycol 400, polyol-surfactants, nonionic; 4.2.3.2

Hom, F.S. and Miskel, J.J., *Lex & Sci.*, 1971, *8*(1), 18–26

Enhanced dissolution rates for a series of drugs as a function of dosage form design

diluents, polyethylene glycol 400, polyol-surfactant, non-ionic; 4.2.3.2

Cardini, C. and Stacchini, A., *Boll. chim.-farm.*, 1973, *112*, 104–9

Studies of availability of certain drugs in oral pharmaceutical dosage forms (in Italian)

diluents, beeswax, hydrogenated vegetable oils, polyethylene glycol 400 and 4000, polysorbate 81, soya lecithin, vegetable oils; 4.2.3.2

R.P. Scherer Corporation, *British Patent* 1 341 121, 1973

Soft gelatin capsule containing a fill of high water content

capsule fill, liquid, gel-lattice vehicles, high water content; manufacturing method, rotary die

R.P. Scherer Ltd, *German (BRD) Patent (Offen.)* 2 513 601, 1975, through *Derwent Accession No.* 67705W/41, 1974

Gelatin capsules containing cardiac glycosides

cardiotonic glycosides; contents, solutions in dimethylacetamide, dimethylformamide, polyethylene glycol

Wellcome Foundation Ltd, *German (BRD) Patent (Offen.)* 2 507 635, 1975, through *Derwent Accession No.* 59151W/36, 1974

Digoxin solutions in capsule forms

capsules: digoxin; drug availability *in vivo*, comparison of dosage forms; formulation of contents, organic solvent solution; formulation of shell, plasticisers; manufacturing method, rotary die

Bobbé, D., Mathis, C., Stamm, A., Metziger, P. and Gabler, W., *Labo-Pharma Probl. Tech.*, 1976, *24*(258), 879–85

Study of the stability of oily suspensions in soft gelatin capsules (in French)

capsule fill, physical properties, effect of formulation; diluents, vegetable oils and waxes; powder properties, particle size distribution, specific surface area; stability of suspensions, sedimentation rate, effect of formulation; suspension, dicalcium phosphate; 3.8.3.7

Bobbé, D., Mathis, C., Stamm, A., Metziger, P. and Widmann, A., *First International Conference on Pharmaceutical Technology*, (Paris, APGI, May 31–June 2, 1977), 1977, *V*, 109–19

Study of the influence of several excipients and adjuvants on the dissolution rate of amidopyrine from soft gelatin capsules (in French)

amidopyrine; diluents, arachis oil, beeswax, dimethicones, Labrafils, Miglyol, polyethylene glycols; formulation of shell; surfactants, soya lecithin, Tweens; 4.2.3.4

Eckert, T. and Kemper, F., assigned to Kali-Chemie Pharma GmbH, *German (BRD) Patent (Offen.)* 2 631 214, 1978

Increasing the solubility of poorly soluble pharmaceuticals for their application in gelatin capsules

diluents, glycerol mono-oleate, monoglycerides of C_{12-18} fatty acids

Springolo, V., *Boll. chim.-farm.*, 1978, *117*, 113–21

The bioavailability of formulations of erythromycin base and stearate in gastric-resistant soft gelatin capsules (in Italian)

erythromycin, base, stearate; diluents, beeswax, fractionated coconut oil, hydrogenated vegetable oil, liquid paraffin, vegetable oil; surfactants, sodium lauryl sulphate, soya lecithin; 3.4.2.2; 4.4.7.1

Stelle, V., Haslam, J., Yata, N., Okada, H., Lindenbaum, S. and Higuchi, T., *J. pharm. Sci.*, 1978, *67*, 1375–7

Enhancement of bioavailability of a hydrophobic amine antimalarial by formulation with oleic acid in a soft gelatin capsule

diluents, oleic acid; 4.4.4.1

D'Onofrio, G.P., Oppenheim, R.C., and Bateman, N.E., *Int. J. Pharmaceut.*, 1979, *2*, 91–9

Encapsulated microcapsules

diluents, ethyl acetate, light liquid paraffin; formulation, controlled-release granules; manufacture, microencapsulation with ethyl cellulose; 4.2.3.6

R.P. Scherer Corporation, *German (BRD) Patent* 2 135 801, 1979

Soft gelatin capsules with aqueous filling in moisture equilibrium with shell

capsule shell, composition; contents, water-soluble polypeptides, polysaccharides, edible synthetic polymers; formulation of contents, high moisture content; manufacturing method, rotary die

Laboratories Negma, *French Patent* 2 500 302, 1982

Novel pharmaceutical compositions of indomethacin (in French)

indomethacin; diluents, hydrophilic, polyethylene glycols, lipophilic arachis oil, beeswax, hydrogenated soya oil, partially hydrogenated vegetable oils; surfactants, Tween 80; 4.5.5

Richard, J. and Andermann, G., *Pharm. Acta Helv.*, 1982, *57*, 116–21

A study of the stability of cyclandelate in soft gelatin capsules (in French)

diluents, polyethylene glycol 400; 3.8.3.7

Aiache, J.-M., Roca, R., Bastide, J., Bastide, M. and Kantelip, J.-P., *J. Pharm. Belg.*, 1983, *38*, 5–21

Biopharmaceutical study of indomethacin new drug dosage forms (in French)

indomethacin; diluents, hydrophilic, polyethylene glycols, lipophilic, arachis oil, beeswax, partially hydrogenated vegetable oils, soya oil; 4.5.5

Bateman, N.E. and Uccellini, D.A., *J. Pharm. Pharmac.*, 1984, *36*, 461–4

Effect of formulation on the bioavailability of retinol, D-α-tocopherol and riboflavine

retinol, D-α-tocopherol, riboflavine, diluents, Aqua-Biosorb, soya oil; 4.4.4.1

Schmidt, P.C. and Stockebrand, B., *Pharm. Res.*, 1986, *3*, 230–34

Capsules with prolonged action, II. Capsule filling by a gelation process

codeine, theophylline; excipients, triethyl citrate, ethylcellulose, polyethylene glycol 400, sesame oil; formulation of contents, physical properties, phase diagram, rheology; formulation of contents, prolonged release, formation of matrix by gelatin; 4.2.3.6

Serujuddin, A.T.M., Sheen, P-C. and Augustine, M.A., *J. pharm. Sci.*, 1986, *75*, 62–4

Water migration from soft gelatin capsule shell to fill material and its effect on drug solubility

drug, water insoluble; diluents, polyethylene glycol 400, Gelucine 44/14; drug solubility, determination, effects of encapsulation, comparison of hard and soft gelatin capsules; encapsulation, method, rotary die; formulation, physical properties, melting point

3.3.3.3 Protective Coatings for Soft Capsules

Yen, E.C. and Stirn, F. E., assigned to American Cyanamid Co., *U.S. Patent* 2 727 833, 1955

Washing and coating composition

coating compositions, moisture resistant, non-tacky; coating formulation; coating method, dipping

Vance, J.J. and Yen, E.C., assigned to American Cyanamid Company, *U.S. Patent* 2 770 571, 1956

Barrier layer of beta pinene polymer

coating compositions, protection of contents; coating formulation, β-pinene polymer; coating method, inside surface gelatin film

A. Nattermann & Co., *French Patent* 1 559 913, 1969, through *Derwent Accession No.* 37 929, 1967

Gelatin capsules coated with methacrylic acid/methyl methacrylate copolymer

coating compositions, heat resistant, sticking prevention; coating formulation, copolymer methacrylic acid/methyl methacrylate, plasticiser; coating method, by spraying

Ciba S.A., *Belgian Patent* 757 715, 1971, through *Derwent Accession No.* 283865-AB, 1969

Hydroxypropylmethyl cellulose coated gelatin capsules

coating materials, ethyl cellulose, hydroxypropylmethylcellulose, polyalkalene glycol, shellac; coating method, spray application; storage, tropical conditions

Engelking, C., assigned to A. Nattermann & Cie, GmbH, *U.S. Patent* 3 592 945, 1971

Increasing heat resistance by coating with copolymer

coating compositions, heat and moisture resistant; coating formulation, anionic copolymer and plasticiser; coating method, spraying

Ciba-Geigy, A. G., *British Patent* 1 324 242, 1973

Coated gelatine capsules and a process for their manufacture

capsule properties, moisture resistance; coating, formulation; coating method, coating pan, fluidised-bed spray technique

3.4 Capsules, Enteric

3.4.1 Gastric Resistant Shells

Bogin, H.H., assigned to Parke, Davis & Co., *U.S. Patent* 2 575 789, 1951

Process and apparatus for manufacturing capsules

capsules, hard gelatin: capsule shell composition, gelatin, metal salt partial ester polycarboxylic acid and cellulose ester; manufacturing method, dipping

Parke, Davis & Co., *British Patent* 672 814, 1952

Process and apparatus for manufacturing of capsules

capsules, hard gelatin: capsule shell composition, cellulose acetate phthalate, gelatin; manufacturing method, dipping

Golovkin, V.A. and Skorik, V.M., *Farmatsiya, Mosk.*, 1972, *21*, 20–2

On the formulation of entero-soluble gelatin capsules (in Russian)

capsules, soft gelatin: chloramphenicol; capsule shell composition, ammonium cellulose acetate phthalate, gelatin; drug availability, *in vitro*, disintegration testing; manufacture, small scale, seamless capsules

Parke, Davis & Co., *Belgian Patent* 802 585, 1973, through *Derwent Accession No.* 03496V-AB, 1972

Keratinised pharmaceutical capsules

capsules, hard gelatin: capsule shell composition, gelatin, hydroxypropylmethylcellulose phthalates; formulation of capsule film; manufacturing method, dipping

Hirai, M. and Shimizu, T., assigned to Parke, Davis & Co., *U.S. Patent* 3 826 666, 1974

Enteric capsules

capsules, hard gelatin: capsule shell composition, gelatin, hydroxypropylmethylcellulose phthalate; manufacturing method, dipping

Lilly Industries Ltd, *Dutch Patent* 7 401 812, 1974, through *Derwent Accession No.* 62413V/35

Capsules insoluble at low pH

capsules, hard gelatin: applications, catalysts, pharmaceuticals, textiles, water softeners; capsule shells, two-layer; capsule shell composition, gelatin layer, enteric layer; manufacturing method, dipping

Susai, M., *Japanese Patent Application No.* 9 116 219, 1974, through *Derwent Accession No.* 15108W/09, 1973

Enteric capsule preparations

capsules, soft gelatin: capsule shell composition, casein, cellulose acetate phthalate, gelatin, hydroxypropylmethylcellulose phthalate, latex

Lilly Industries Ltd, *British Patent* 1 455 884, 1976

Improvements in the production of capsules

capsules, hard gelatin: capsule shells, two-layer; capsule shell composition, gelatin layer, enteric layer; manufacturing method, dipping

Okajima, Y., *German (BRD) Patent (Offen.)* 2 616 748, 1976

Capsules soluble in the intestinal fluids

capsules, two-piece: formulation of shell, gelatin or hydroxypropylmethylcellulose and cellulose acetate phthalate, hydroxypropylmethylcellulose phthalate, methacrylate polymers; manufacturing method

3.4.2 Coatings for Enteric Capsules
3.4.2.1 General References

Dumez, A.G., *J. Am. pharm. Ass.*, 1921, *10*, 372–6

A contribution to the history of the development of the enteric capsule

capsules, hard and soft gelatin and pills: enteric coating, materials, methods; history

Lesser, M.A., *Drug Cosmet. Ind.*, 1941, *49*, 151–5, 161

Enteric coatings

capsules and tablets: coating, methods and materials, review; disintegration testing, *in vitro*, *in vivo*, review

Keefer, C.S., *J. Am. pharm. Ass., pract. Pharm. Edn*, 1945, *6*, 210–15

Status of oral penicillin

capsules, hard gelatin: penicillin; enteric, materials and methods

Kanig, J.L., *Drug Stand.*, 1954, *22*, 113–21

Production and testing of enteric coatings

capsules and tablets: disintegration testing, *in vitro*, *in vivo*, critical review

Parrott, E.L., *J. Am. pharm. Ass.*, 1961, *NS1*, 158–9

An extemporaneous enteric coating

capsules, hard gelatin: acetylsalicylic acid, potassium iodide; coating materials, *n*-butyl stearate/carnauba wax/stearic acid and cellulose acetate phthalate; coating method, small scale, hand dipping; 4.5.6.1

Smith, G. and Cox, P.H., *Pharm. J.*, 1963, *190*, 245–6

Enteric-coated capsules of cobalt chloride

capsules, hard gelatin: cobalt chloride; coating materials, cellulose acetate phthalate, salol, shellac; coating method, hand dipping; disintegration testing, modified *B.P.* method; formulation, coating

Morgado, R.R., Pinho, A.A. and Prista, L.N., *Anais Fac. Farm. Porto*, 1970, *30*, 47–53

Studies on gelatin capsules III – The treatment of capsules to make them gastric resistant (in Portuguese)

capsules, hard gelatin: coating materials, cellulose acetate phthalate, formaldehyde; coating methods, dipping; disintegration method, *U.S.P.* XVII; disintegration testing, comparison of coating methods; formulation, coating, plasticisers, solvents

Gumma, A. and Mirimanoff, A., *Pharm. Acta Helv.*, 1971, *46*, 278–89

Study of several pharmaceutical procedures applied to therapeutics of substitution by *Lactobacillus acidophilus* (in French)

capsules, hard gelatin and tablets, film-coated: *Lactobacillus acidophilus*; coating materials, cellulose acetate phthalate, formaldehyde, methacrylic polymers; coating method; disintegration testing, oscillating tube apparatus, comparison of methods

Cognyl, G., *Labo-Pharma Probl. Tech.*, 1974, No. 230, 249–51

Hard gelatin capsules and gastric resistance (in French)

capsules, hard gelatin: coating, materials, methods, testing; formulation of contents, gastric resistance; review

3.4.2.2 Formaldehyde Treatment of Capsules

Weyland, J., *Apothekerzeitung, Berl.*, 1931, *46*, 470–3

Hardened gelatin capsules (in German)

capsules, hard and soft gelatin: drug availability, *in vitro*, disintegration; gelatin, reaction with formaldehyde; history; manufacturing methods

Glassman, J.A., *U.S. Patent* 3 186 910, 1965

Method for producing peroral capsules

capsules, hard gelatin: drug release, variable, enteric, non-enteric parts; filling machine, multiple joining of capsules; formaldehyde treatment by spraying

Glassman, J.A., *U.S. Patent* 3 228 789, 1966

Peroral capsules and tablets and the method for making same

capsules, hard gelatin: drug release, variable, enteric and non-enteric parts; formaldehyde solutions, alcoholic, aqueous; formaldehyde treatment by dipping

Biorex Laboratories Ltd, *British Patent* 1 093 286, 1967

Improvements in or relating to dosage unit forms for the administration of medicaments and diagnostic agents

capsules, hard gelatin: capsules, insoluble shells; coating method, immersion; drug release, by pressure from pyloric sphincter; formulation of contents

Boymond, P., Sfiris, J. and Amacker, P., *Pharm. Ind., Berl.*, 1966, *28*, 836–42 and *Drugs Germ.*, 1967, *10*, 7–19

The manufacture and testing of enterosoluble capsules (in German; English translation in *Drugs Germ.*)

capsules, hard gelatin: coating method, formaldehyde vapour, heat treatment, dipping in silicone resin and shellac; stability testing, effect of relative humidity; 4.2.2.2; 4.4.7.1

R.P. Scherer Corporation, *British Patent* 1 252 200, 1971

Improved gelatine capsules

capsules, hard and soft gelatin: formulation of shell; manufacturing method; 3.3.3.1

Rolle, F.J., assigned to R.P. Scherer Corporation, *U.S. Patent* 3 653 934, 1972

Gastro-resistant capsules

capsules, soft gelatin: coating method, coating pan; formulation, formaldehyde solution; 3.3.3.1

Springolo, V., *Boll. chim.-farm.*, 1978, *117*, 113–21

The bioavailability of formulations of erythromycin base and stearate in gastric-resistant soft gelatin capsules (in Italian)

capsules, soft gelatin: coating method, immersion; 3.3.3.2; 4.4.7.1

3.4.2.3 Natural Coatings for Enteric Capsules

Stoklosa, M.J. and Ohmart, L.M., *J. Am. pharm. Ass., pract. Pharm. Edn*, 1953, *14*, 507, 514–15

Enteric coatings in dispensing pharmacy. 2. A practical method of extemporaneous enteric coating

capsules, hard gelatin and pills: sodium salicylate; coating materials, *n*-butyl stearate-carnauba wax; coating method, hot dipping; enteric coat, stability on storage, effects of plasticisers, thickness of coat; formulation; coating, plasticisers; 4.4.7.1

Mercer, W.G., *Australas J. Pharm.*, 1955, *36*, 1169

Enteric coated capsules of cobalt chloride

capsules, hard gelatin: cobalt chloride; coating materials, beeswax, salol; coating method, hand dipping; disintegration testing

3.4.2.4 Synthetic Coatings for Enteric Capsules

Volwiler, E.H., assigned to Abbott Laboratories, *U.S. Patent* 1 690 760, 1928

Enteric coated capsules

capsules, hard gelatin: coating materials, cellulose ester, nitrocellulose; coating method, dip coating

Caldwell, H.C. and Rosen, E., *J. pharm. Sci.*, 1964, *53*, 1387–91

New air suspension apparatus for coating discrete solids

capsules, hard gelatin, granules and tablets: coating material, cellulose acetate phthalate; coating method, fluidised-bed spray technique, capsule presealing with coat applied in coating pan

Cook, C.H. and Webber, M.G., *Am. J. Hosp. Pharm.*, 1965, *22*, 95–9

An extemporaneous method of preparing enteric-coated capsules

capsules, hard gelatin: coating materials, cellulose acetate phthalate, polyvinyl acetate resins; coating method, immersion; formulation, coating, plasticisers, solvents; 4.5.6.1

Rothgang, G., *Pharm. Ind., Berl.*, 1967, *29*, 869–70

The coating of hard gelatin capsules with Eudragit L and S for preparations resistant to gastric juice (in German)

capsules, hard gelatin: coating materials, methylacrylic polymers; coating method, coating pan, spray application; disintegration testing, *Ger. P.* (DAB 7); formulation, coating, plasticisers, solvents; product sealing, banding

Wolkoff, H.N., Pinchuk, G. and Shapiro, P.H., *J. pharm. Sci.*, 1968, *57*, 317–21

Design and evaluation of a miniature air-suspension coating apparatus

capsules, hard gelatin and tablets: coating material, cellulose acetate phthalate; coating method, fluidised-bed spray technique

Jones, B.E., *Mfg Chem.*, 1970, *41*(5), 53–4, 57

Production of enteric coated capsules

capsules, hard gelatin: coating materials, cellulose acetate phthalate, methacrylic polymers; coating method, fluidised-bed spray technique; manufacturing methods, review; pharmacopoeial standards; physical stability testing

Sanol-Arzneimittel Dr. Schwarz GmbH, *Belgian Patent* 750 379, 1970, through *Derwent Accession No.* 84509R-AB, 1969

Gelatin capsules resistant to gastric juice which dissolve when in small intestine

capsules, hard gelatin: coating materials, carboxyvinyl polymer, hydroxymethylpropylcellulose, polyvinylpyrrolidone; coating method, coating pan

Eckert, T., Cordes, G. and Seidel, R., *Arzneimittel-Forsch.*, 1971, *21*, 1403–6

Release of active substances from enteric-coated gelatin capsules *in vivo* and *in vitro*. Part 4. Study with the pH radiotransmitter in man (in German)

capsules, hard gelatin: coating film, measurement of thickness; coating material, cellulose acetate phthalate; coating method, fluidised-bed spray technique; formulation, coating; 4.5.2

Dedukh, N.G., Khanina, G.I., Pospelova, V.V., Kryazher, V.N., Shniger, N.U., Marko, O.P. and Bronshtein, A.S., *Farmatsiva, Mosk.*, 1972, *21*, 16–19

Characteristics of acid-proof gelatin capsules (in Russian)

capsules, hard gelatin: coating materials, cellulose acetate phthalate; enteric coating, comparison coating materials, storage

Ekberg, L. and Källstrand, G., *Svensk farm. Tidskr.*, 1972, *76*, 375–8

The enteric coating of hard gelatin capsules on a dispensary scale (in Swedish)

capsules, hard gelatin: coating materials, cellulose acetate phthalate; coating method, modified air-suspension technique; formulation, coating, plasticisers, solvents; 4.5.6.1

Festa, B., *French Patent* 2 137 170, 1972, through *Derwent Accession No.* 14835U-B, 1971

Coating process with gastric juice-resistant solution for gelatin capsules

capsules, hard gelatin: coating materials, cellulose acetate phthalate; coating method, coating pan under reduced pressure

Green Cross Corporation, *French Patent* 2 118 883, 1972, through *Derwent Accession No.* 74600T-B, 1970

Enteric coating of hard capsules – after pre-sealing with aqueous organic solvent mixtures

capsules, hard gelatin: capsule sealing, spraying with volatile organic solvent/water; coating materials, cellulose acetate phthalate; coating method, spraying

Aiache, J.-M., Vidal, J.L., Aiache, S., Jeanneret, A. and Cornat, F., *Labo-Pharma Probl. Tech.*, 1974, *22*(232), 457–63

Methods for the biopharmaceutical testing of enteric capsules: Test with "enterocaps" capsules (in French)

capsules, hard gelatin: coating material, cellulose acetate phthalate; coating method, coating pan, airless spray; enteric coating, materials, methods, review; 4.4.7.1; 4.5.6.1

Aiache, J.-M., Aiache, S., Jeanneret, A., Cornat, F. and Vidal, J.L., *Boll. chim.-farm.*, 1975, *114*, 636–50

Methods for the biopharmaceutical testing of enteric capsules: Tests with "enterocaps" capsules (in French)

capsules, hard gelatin: coating material, cellulose acetate phthalate; coating method, coating pan, airless spray; enteric coating, materials, methods, review; 4.4.7.1; 4.5.6.1

Tanabe Seiyaku Company Ltd, *Japanese Patent Application No.* J4 9030524, through *Derwent Accession No.* 68644V/39, 1975

Gelatin capsules soluble in small intestines

capsules, hard and soft gelatin: coating materials, acrylic acid; methyl acrylate, methacrylic acid; methyl acrylate copolymers

Eckert, T., Cordes, G. and Ollenschläger, G., *Pharm. Ind., Berl.*, 1976, *38*, 836–41

Release of active substances from enteric-coated gelatin capsules *in vitro* and *in vivo*. Part 5. Study with films of cellulose acetate phthalate (CAP) and hydroxypropylmethylcellulose phthalate (HP-50) (in German)

capsules, hard gelatin: coating materials, cellulose acetate phthalate, hydroxypropylmethylcellulose phthalate; coating method, fluidised-bed spray technique; coating quantities and thickness; formulations, coating, plasticisers, solvents; 4.5.2

Evans, B.K., Fenton-May, V.G. and Lee, M.G., *J. clin. Pharm.*, 1979, *4*, 173–7

Enteric-coated capsules: an oral preparation for sodium diethyldithiocarbamate

capsules, hard gelatin: coating material, cellulose acetate phthalate; coating method, coating tower; formulation, coating

Remon, J.P., Gyselinck, P., van Severen, R. and Braeckman, P., *Acta Pharm. Tech.*, 1983, *29*, 25–7

New small scale apparatus for enteric coating of hard gelatin capsules

capsules, hard gelatin: coating materials, cellulose acetate phthalate, methyl acrylic polymers; coating method, dipping, mechanical device, bench-scale; formulation, coating, plasticiser, triacetin, solvents, acetone, ethyl acetate/isopropyl alcohol; 4.2.2.2

Rhodes, J. and Evans, B.K., *International Patent* WO 83/00435, 1983

Orally administrable pharmaceutical compositions

capsules, hard gelatin: coating materials, methacrylic acid polymers; coating method, modified air-suspension technique; formulation, coating, plasticisers, solvents; 4.4.3; 4.4.7.2

Werchan, D., *Pharmazie*, 1984, *39*, 275–6

Film coating of gelatin capsules in the dispensary (in German) capsules, hard gelatin: coating materials, cellulose acetate phthalate, polyvinyl acetate phthalate; coating method, coating pan, bench-scale; formulation, coating, plasticiser, propylene glycol, solvents, acetone, dichloromethane; 4.2.2.2

3.5 Capsules, Non-oral

3.5.1 Inhalation Capsules

Fisons Pharmaceuticals Ltd, *British Patent* 1 182 779, 1970

Inhaler for finely powdered medicaments

capsules, hard gelatin: inhalation device

Fisons Pharmaceuticals Limited, *U.S. Patent* 3 507 277, 1970

Oral inhalation powdered medicament device for pierceable capsule

capsules, hard gelatin: inhalation device

Bell, J.H., Hartley, P.S. and Cox, J.S.G., *J. pharm. Sci.*, 1971, *60*, 1559–64

Dry powder aerosols 1: a new powder inhalation device

capsules, hard gelatin: aerosol powder, generating system; powder properties, particle size

ISF S.P.A., *Belgian Patent* 821 152, 1975, through *Derwent Accession No.* 29075W/18, 1974

Portable inhaler for powdered medicaments

capsules, hard gelatin: inhalation device

Chowhan, Z.T. and Amaro, A.A., *J. pharm. Sci.*, 1977, *66*, 1254–8

Powder inhalation aerosol studies I: selection of a suitable drug entity for bronchial delivery of new drugs

capsules, hard gelatin: 7-methylsulphinyl-2-xanthone carboxylic acid and sodium salt; drug availability, *in vitro*, air sampling device; drug availability, *in vitro*, effects of, formulation, moisture content, particle size; powder properties, cohesiveness, particle size; 3.8.3.4

Hallworth, G.W., *Br. J. clin. Pharmac.*, 1977, *4*, 689–90

An improved design of powder inhaler

capsules, hard gelatin and inhaler, aerosol: salbutamol sulphate; drug availability, *in vitro*, multi-stage liquid impinger, comparison of devices

Chowhan, Z.T. and Linn, E.E., *Int. J. Pharmaceut.*, 1979, *3*, 117–26

Powder inhalation aerosol studies II. *In vitro* rat lung model and its comparisons with the air sampler

capsules, hard gelatin: 7-methylsulphinyl-2-xanthone carboxylic acid, labelled, unlabelled; drug availability, *in vitro*, comparison of methods, air sampling device, rat lung model; drug availability, *in vitro*, effects of, dose, formulation, inhalation pattern; formulation of contents

Crompton, G.K., *Eur. J. respir. Dis.*, 1982, *63*, 96–9

Clinical use of dry powder systems

capsules, hard gelatin: inhalation device; comparison of products

Pover, G.M., Browning, A.K., Mullinger, B.M., Butler, A.G. and Dash, C.H., *Practitioner*, 1982, *226*, 565–7

A new dry powder inhaler

capsules, hard gelatin: inhalation device, patient preference study

3.5.2 Rectal and Vaginal Capsules

Widmann, A., *Pharm. Ind., Berl.*, 1960, *22*, 348–52

Rectal gelatin capsules (in German)

capsules, soft gelatin: paracetamol; formulation of contents, excipients; rectal use; 4.4.4.4

Fichsel, H., *Kinderärztl. Prax.*, 1963, *31*, 245–50

Experiences with a new antipyretic and analgesic in a new rectal capsule form (in German).

capsules, soft gelatin: phenacetin; salicylamide; rectal use; 4.4.4.4

Widmann, A. and Bauer, K.H., assigned to R.P. Scherer GmbH, Germany, *U.S. Patent* 3 197 369, 1965

Rectal capsule-coating from homogeneous melt of emulsifying agent and lubricating substance

capsules, soft gelatin: coating compositions, lubrication for rectal insertion; coating formulation, emulsifying agent and lubricant; coating method, coating pan; rectal use

Bauer, K., assigned to Ciba Corp., *U.S. Patent* 3 432 594, 1969

Rectal capsule-coating of 1:1 methylcellulose and acrylic acid polymer

capsules, soft gelatin: coating compositions, hydrophilic, nontacky; coating formulations, gel forming; coating method, pill coating machine; rectal and vaginal use

Widmann, A., assigned to R.P. Scherer GmbH, Germany, *U.S. Patent* 3 467 748, 1969

Rectal capsule-coating of polyethylene glycol and polyvinyl acetate

capsules, soft gelatin: coating compositions, lubrication for rectal insertion; coating formulation, polyethylene glycol or emulsifiable substance and polyvinyl acetate; coating method, coating pan, revolving drum; rectal use

Akzo, N.V., *Dutch Patent* 7 302 521, 1974, through *Derwent Accession No.* 65689V/37

Foaming effervescent capsules

capsules, hard gelatin: capsule shell composition, gelatin, polyethylene oxides, carbohydrate; formulation, contents, effervescent mixture, foaming agent; rectal and vaginal use

Hunger, G., assigned to E.R. Squibb & Sons, Inc., *U.S. Patent* 3 886 940, 1975

Capsule

capsules, hard gelatin: capsule, open-ended assembly, thimble form; vaginal use

Teijin, K.K., *Japanese Patent Application No. 2156–919, 1976, through Derwent Accession No. 11571A/06, 1977*

Gelatin capsules especially for rectal administration–coated with proteolytic enzymes have improved moisture and heat resistance and decomposing properties

capsules: capsule properties, disintegration, stability; coating materials, proteolytic enzymes and method; rectal use

Vibelli, C., Chierichetti, S., Sala, P., Ferrari, P. and Pasotti, C., *Clin. Trials J.*, 1977, *14*, 83–8

Feprazone. Bioavailability in a new suppository preparation

capsules, soft gelatin: rectal use; 4.4.4.4

Carp, G.B., Chemtob, C. and Chaumeil, J.C., *Second International Conference on Pharmaceutical Technology*, (Paris, APGI, June 3–5, 1980), 1980, V, 68–80

Availability from rectally administered solid dosage forms: use of rectal soft gelatin capsules (in French)

capsules, soft gelatin: capsule shape; formulation, contents, shell; rectal use; 4.2.4

Moës, A.J., *Pharm. Acta Helv.*, 1981, *56*, 21–5

Formulation of highly available theophylline rectal suppositories

capsules, soft gelatin: theophylline, anhydrous, monohydrate; rectal use; 4.5.3.4

Akbar, M.R. Ahmadi, S.M., Heydate, A.H. and Khami, M.A., *Drug Dev. Res.*, 1982, *2*, 87–90

A three-day study with miconazole gelatin capsules in vaginal candidosis

capsules, soft gelatin: miconazole; drug, clinical effects; vaginal use

Möller, H., *Pharm. Ind., Berl.*, 1984, *46*, 514–20

In vitro and in vivo dissolution of rectal indomethacin dosage forms (in German)

capsules, soft gelatin: formulation, contents; rectal use; 4.5.3.4

Hagenlocher, M., Hannula, A.M., Wittwer, F., Soliva, M. and Speiser, P., *Fourth International Conference on Pharmaceutical Technology,* (Paris, APGI, June 3–5, 1986), 1986, *I*, 398–405

Hard gelatin capsules for rectal drug delivery

capsules, hard gelatin; coating compositions, lubrication for rectal insertion; coating formulation, sealing coat, Eudragit, gliding coat, macrogols; coating method; fluidised bed spray coater; rectal use; 3.2.4.2; 4.5.3.4

3.6 Packaging of Capsules
3.6.1 Unit-dose Packaging

Samuels, T.M. and Guthrie, D.L., *Am. J. Hosp. Pharm.*, 1966, *23*, 5–11

Unit dose packaging. A new machine for strip packaging tablets and capsules

capsules and tablets: packaging materials, moisture permeability; strip packaging machine, swell scale

Angele, M.M., *Chem. Rdsch.*, 1972, *25*, 125–6, 128

The blister packing and strip packing of Parke-Davis pure gelatin capsules (in German)

capsules, hard gelatin: blister packaging machines; packaging materials, permeability, moisture and gases; strip packaging machines

Anon., *Drug & Ther. Bull.*, 1972, *10*, 101–3

The presentation of dispensed tablets and capsules

capsules, hard and soft gelatin and tablets: dispensing containers; safety

Dean, D.A., *Pharm. J.*, 1972, *209*, 238–41

Unit packaging of tablets and capsules

capsules, hard and soft gelatin and tablets: blister packaging, machines, materials; strip packaging, machines, materials

Auslander, D.E., *Package Development and Systems*, 1978, *8*(5), 20–2

Part II. Hermetic packaging of drugs: optimized sealing of foil pouches

capsules, hard gelatin: blister packaging machine operating conditions; packaging materials, foil laminate specifications; strip packaging, sealing efficiency, effect of sealing temparature

Reamer, J.T. and Grady, L.T., *Am. J. Hosp. Pharm.*, 1978, *35*, 787–93

Moisture permeation of newer unit dose repackaging materials

capsules and tablets: unit-dose systems, comparison of products, American market; storage testing, moisture permeation rate determinations

Gupta, V.D., Stewart, K.R. and Gupta, A., *Am. J. Hosp. Pharm.*, 1980, *37*, 165, 169

Stability of oral solid drugs after repackaging in single-unit containers

capsules and tablets: packaging materials; strip packaging machine, small scale; 3.8.3.7

3.6.2 Bulk Packaging

List, H, *Drugs Germ.*, 1963, *6*, 164, 166, 168

A new high in packaging efficiency. A striking improvement in the automatic packaging of tablets, coated tablets, and gelatin capsules

capsules, gelatin and tablets, plain and sugar-coated: packaging equipment, automatic machinery

Beal, H.M., Dicenzo, R.J., Jannke, P.J., Palmer, H.A., Pinsky, J., Salame, M. and Speaker, T.J., *J. pharm. Sci.*, 1967, *56*, 1310–22

Pharmaceuticals stored in plastic containers

pharmaceutical products: containers, high density polyethylene; official products, United States; seals, metal screw caps; 3.8.3.4; 3.8.3.7

Henry, K.W., *S. Afr. pharm. J.*, 1972, *39*, 85–8

Automation in pharmaceutical packaging with reference to tablets, sugar coated tablets and capsules

capsules and tablets: packaging materials, review

Li Wan Po, A., Morland, I. and Robins, L., *J. clin. Pharm.*, 1977, *2*, 131–5

Chemical cross-contamination in the pharmacy

capsules, hard gelatin: cross-contamination, identification and quantification, thin-layer chromatography; dispensing, automatic counting machines, cross-contamination; tablet friability, effect on cross-contamination

3.7 Capsule Standards
3.7.1 General References
Kern, W., *Pharm. Ind., Berl.*, 1956, *18*, 474–93

The importance of the gelatin capsule as a dosage form in different countries. The appropriate pharmacopoeia or codex for the manufacturing of these medicines (in German)

capsules, hard and soft gelatin: manufacture, industrial scale; pharmacopoeial products; pharmacopoeial standards

Kuhn, T., *Pharm. Ztg, Berl.*, 1963, *108*, 130–5, 195–8

The testing of gelatin capsules (in German)

capsules, hard and soft gelatin: gelatin; manufacture; pharmacopoeial standards; 3.1

Jones, B.E. and Törnblom, J.-F.V., *Pharm. Acta Helv.*, 1975, *50*, 33–45

Gelatin capsules in the pharmacopoeiae

capsules, hard and soft gelatin: review, official compendia, worldwide

3.7.2 Official Standards
Europe: European Pharmacopoeia, 2nd Edn, Part II, 57160 Sainte-Ruffine, France, Maisonneuve S.A., 1984

Capsulae, Capsules, First Fascicule pp. 16–16-3

disintegration; uniformity of mass

Countries that have adopted the standards of the European Pharmacopoeia include Austria, Belgium, Britain, Denmark, Eire, Finland, France, Germany (West), Greece, Iceland, Italy, Luxembourg, Netherlands, Norway, Spain, Sweden, Switzerland

India: Pharmacopoeia of India, 3rd Edn, Delhi, Controller of Publications, 1985

Capsules, Vol. 2, pp. 91–2

content of active ingredient; disintegration; uniformity of weight

Japan: Pharmacopoeia of Japan, 10th Edn, Tokyo, Ministry of Health and Welfare, 1981

Capsulae, Capsules, p. 9 (English Edn)

disintegration test; weight variation

Capsulae Operculatae, Capsules, p. 985 (English Edn)

odour; solubility; acidity or alkalinity

Jugoslavia: Pharmacopoea Jugoslavica, 4th Edn, Belgrade, Izdanje Saveznog zavoda za zdravstvenu zaštitu, 1984

Capsulae Medicinales, Ljekovite Kapsule, Vol. 1, pp. 234–5

content uniformity; disintegration; weight uniformity

Roumania. Farmacopeea Română, 9th Edn, Bucharest, Editura Medicală, 1976

Capsulae, Capsule, pp. 161–2

content uniformity; disintegration; enteric capsules; heavy metals; solubility; weight uniformity

Turkey: Türk Farmacopesi, Istanbul, Millî Eğitim Basimevi, 1974

Capsulae, Kapsüller, pp. 121–2

disintegration; weight uniformity

USA: The United States Pharmacopeia, 21st Revision, The National Formulary, 16th Edn, Rockville, United States Pharmacopeial Convention Inc., 1985

Capsules, p. 1335

acid neutralising capacity (pp. 1192–3); disintegration (pp. 1242–3); dissolution (pp. 1243–4); packaging (pp. 1240–1); uniformity of dosage units (*Suppl. 1*, pp. 1909–1910)

USSR: State Pharmacopoeia of the Union of Soviet Socialist Republics, 10th Edn, Moscow, Ministry of Health, 1971

Capsulae, Capsules, pp. 137–8

dimensions; disintegration; solubility; solution, clarity; weight uniformity

3.8 Properties of Capsules
3.8.1 General References
U.S. Government Printing Office, Federal Specification, U-C-115b. Capsule, Gelatin, 1958

capsules, hard gelatin: definition; inspection, procedures; packaging, requirements; tests, acid solubility, appearance, colour, water resistance

Anon., *Fr.-Pharm.*, 1967, *20*, 27–31

Capsules of pure gelatin. Tests on hard gelatin capsules (in French)

capsules, hard gelatin: capsule shell permeability, gases, moisture; capsule volumes

Marquardt, H.-G., *Fr.-Pharm.*, 1970, *23*, 13–15

Influence of chemical components, light, temperature and moisture on Parke, Davis hard gelatin capsules (in French)

capsules, hard gelatin: capsule product storage, effects of, light, moisture, temperature

LeBelle, M., Lauriault, G. and Wilson, W.L., *Can. J. pharm. Sci.*, 1978, *13*, 7–8

The determination of ampicillin and penicillin G as contaminants in tetracycline and erythromycin solid dosage forms

capsules and tablets: erythromycin, estolate, ethylsuccinate, stearate, tetracycline hydrochloride (capsules); identification, contamination by ampicillin, penicillin G

Kammerl, E., Chapter X in *The Capsule, Basics, Technology and Biopharmacy, a Modern Dosage Form* (in German), Fahrig, W. and Hofer, U. (Eds), Stuttgart, Wissenschaftliche Verlagsgesellschaft mbH, 1983, pp. 181–95.

Quality control in the manufacture of capsule preparations (in German)

capsules: industrial methods and systems

Bolton, S., *Drug Cosmet. Ind.*, 1984, *135*(2), 42–4, 46–7, 85–7

Process validation for hard gelatin capsules

capsules, hard gelatin: industrial scale filling, process control methods, validation

3.8.2 Properties of Capsule Shells

3.8.2.1 Colouring Agents

Pellerin, F., Gautier, J.-A. and Conrard, A.-M., *Annls pharm. fr.*, 1964, *22*, 621–7

Identification in pharmaceutical preparations of authorised synthetic organic colorants (in French)

capsules, hard gelatin, ointments, solutions, suppositories, syrups, and tablets, plain and sugar-coated: dyes, extraction, adsorption on fibres; dyes, identification, chromatography, paper

Balatre, P. and Traisnel, M., *Bull. Soc. Pharm. Lille*, 1965, *1*, 41–7

Identification of permitted dyes by thin-layer chromatography of their quaternary ammonium complex (in French)

capsules, hard gelatin, granules and syrups: dyes, extraction, predigestion with trypsin, formation quaternary ammonium complexes; dyes, identification, chromatography, thin-layer

Alary, J., Luu Duc, C. and Coeur, A., *Bull. Trav. Soc. Pharm. Lyon*, 1966, *10*, 78–86

Identification of synthetic colouring materials in several pharmaceutical preparations (in French)

capsules, hard and soft gelatin and tablets, film- and sugar-coated: dyes, extraction, solvent; dyes, identification, chromatography, paper, thin-layer; products, France

Brustier, V., Bourbon, P., Amselem, A., Achor, G., Casabonne, M. and Ferrand, J.C., *Annls pharm. Fr.*, 1966, *24*, 51–6

Contribution to the study of the identification of synthetic colorants in pharmaceutical preparations (in French)

capsules, hard and soft gelatin, granules, ointments, solutions, suppositories, syrups and tablets, coated and plain: dyes, extraction, formation quaternary ammonium complexes; dyes, identification, chromatography, thin-layer, silica gel

Berret, R., Gavaudan, A. and Hirtz, J., *Annls pharm. fr.*, 1967, *25*, 365–9

Rapid isolation of synthetic colorants for their identification from gelatin capsules. Applications to other pharmaceutical forms (in French)

capsules, hard gelatin, granules, powders and tablets, sugar-coated: dyes, extraction, ion-exchange paper; dyes, identification, chromatography, thin-layer, cellulose

Lehmann, G. and Collet, P., *Arch. Pharm., Berl.*, 1970, *303*, 855–60

The study of synthetic dyestuffs in pharmaceuticals. Part VIII. Identification of synthetic dyes in drugs (in German)

capsules, hard gelatin, granules and tablets: dye extraction, absorption polyamide powder; dye identification, chromatography, thin-layer, cellulose

Pharmacopée Française, 8th Edn. (Sainte-Ruffine: Maisonneuve S.A., 1965)

Substances used for the coloration of medicines; Synthetic organic dyes, pp. 1835–56

dyes, identification, chromatography and spectrophotometry; dyes, standards

Pharmacopoea Helvetica, 6th Edn. (Berne, Office Centrale Federale d'Imprimes,·1971)

Colouring materials for medical preparations, Vol. I, pp. 29–38

colorants, inorganic and organic

Sitzius, F. and Rentsch, H., *Pharm. Ind., Berl.*, 1973, *35*, 148–50

Identification of dyes in capsules and sugar-coated tablets (in German)

capsules, hard and soft gelatin and tablets, sugar-coated: dyes, extraction, powder adsorption; dyes, identification, chromatography, thin-layer; products, Germany (BRD)

Smith, H.L., *J. pharm. Sci.*, 1974, *63*, 639–41

Sorption rates of water-soluble dyes on soft gelatin capsules

capsules, soft gelatin: capsules, surface dyeing process; dyes, water-soluble, sorption rates on capsules; formulation of shell

Turi, P., *Pharm. Ind., Berl.*, 1977, *39*, 476–82

Benefits and risks of the use of colouring agents in pharmaceutical dosage forms

pharmaceuticals: colorant properties, review

Akade, Y., Kawano, S. and Tanase, Y., *J. pharm. Soc. Japan*, 1978, *98*, 1300–04

High-pressure liquid chromatographic determination of colouring matter in capsules (in Japanese)

capules: dye extraction, adsorption on activated charcoal; dyes, identification, chromatography, high pressure liquid

Anon., *Drug Cosmet. Ind.*, 1983, *133*(2), 44, 46, 48, 106–7

Colorants for drug tablets and capsules

capsules and tablets: colorant acceptability legislation, U.S.A.; colorant properties, review

3.8.2.2 Moisture Content of Shells

Notton, H.E.E., *Pharm. J.*, 1948, *161*, 250–1

Humidity in flexible gelatin capsules

capsules, soft gelatin: capsule deformation test, apparatus; capsule pliability, relationship to moisture content, effect of storage

Strickland, W.A. and Moss, M., *J. pharm. Sci.*, 1962, *51*, 1002–5

Water vapour sorption and diffusion through hard gelatin capsules

capsules, hard gelatin: pentobarbitone sodium; moisture content, shells and contents, effect of relative humidity; moisture transfer, effect of coating with stearic acid

List, P.H. and Schenk, G.D., *Arch. Pharm., Berl.*, 1974, *307*, 719–26

Investigation of hard gelatin capsules, part I: Measurement of the moisture content with thermistors (in German)

capsules, hard gelatin: capsule shells, dimensions, effect of relative humidity on; moisture content, effect of relative humidity on; storage conditions

List, P.H. and Schenk, G.D., *Pharm. Ind., Berl.*, 1975, *37*, 91–6

Investigation of hard gelatin capsules, part II: Measurement of the moisture content by continuous increase of the humidity (in German)

capsules, hard gelatin: capsule shells, formulation, colorants, titanium dioxide; gelatin properties, sol/gel transformation, effect of humidity; moisture content, effect of relative humidity on, relationship to capsule shell formulation

3.8.2.3 Physical Properties of Shells

Polderman, J., Simons, L.M. and Laundy, T. *Pharm. Weekbl. Ned.*, 1965, *100*, 813–21

An apparatus for determination of breaking strength of packaging materials

ampoules, capsules, hard and soft gelatin: impact tester; hard gelatin capsules, breaking force; soft gelatin capsules, pliability, effect of plasticiser concentration

Czetsch-Lindenwald, H.V., *Pharm. Ind., Berl.*, 1967, *29*, 145–9

Meaning and limits of "in vitro" tests. Part I (in German)

capsules, hard gelatin: gas permeability measurements, carbon dioxide, effects of concentration, storage

Prista, L.N., Morgado, R.R. and Pinho, A.A., *Anais Fac. Farm. Porto*, 1970, *30*, 35–46

Studies on gelatin capsules II – The effects of ultraviolet radiation (in Portuguese).

capsules, hard gelatin: menadione, chemical stability, UV light exposure, comparision of protection of different colours of capsules; disintegration testing, Erweka and *U.S.P.*, effects of, storage, heat, UV light exposure

Hom, F.S., Veresh, S.A. and Ebert, W.R., *J. pharm. Sci.*, 1975, *64*, 851–7

Soft gelatin capsules II: Oxygen permeability study of capsule shells

capsules, soft gelatin: formulation of shell, pigments, plasticisers; gas permeability, effects of shells, formulation, moisture content, thickness; 3.3.3.1

Hüttenrauch, R., Taubert, H. and Jacob, J., *Pharmazie*, 1984, *39*, 356

Gas permeability of hard gelatin capsules (in German)

capsules, hard gelatin: gas permeability measurements, carbon dioxide, ethylene oxide, effects of, capsule coating, pressure, temperature; capsule coating, methacrylic acid polymer; sterilisation, gaseous, ethylene oxide/carbon dioxide mixture; 3.8.3.3

3.8.2.4 Physical Specifications of Shells

Peck, G.E., Christian, J.E. and Banker, G.S., *J. pharm. Sci.*, 1964, *53*, 607–11

Determination of thickness of walls of hard gelatin capsules by radioisotopic means

capsules, hard gelatin: capsule shells, wall thickness; manufacture, industrial scale; thickness measurements, radioactive tracers

Czetsch-Lindenwald, H.V. and Tawashi, R., *Pharm. Ind., Berl.*, 1965, *27*, 146–51

Tests with hard gelatin capsules (in German)

capules, hard gelatin: capsule volumes, weights; 3.2.4.1; 3.8.3.6

Anon., *Labo-Pharma Probl. Tech.*, 1966, *14*(145), 69–79

Why and how to fill capsules (in French)

capsules, hard gelatin: capacity, dimensions, weight; 3.2.3.2

Stone, J.C., *J. pharm. Sci.*, 1970, *59*, 1364

Objective visual evaluation of the relative content of major and minor defects in tablets and capsules

capsules and tablets: product appearance defects; visual assessment, sampling methods, viewing procedure

Edmatsu, K. and Nitta, Y., *Pattern Recog.*, 1981, *14*, 365–74

Automated capsule inspection method

capsules, hard gelatin: visual faults, classification; visual faults, inspection, automatic by light projection, T.V. cameras

3.8.3 Properties of Capsule Products

3.8.3.1 Uniformity of Content

Garrett, E.R., *J. pharm. Sci.*, 1962, *51*, 672–5

Selection, evaluation, and control of the assay of the pharmaceutical product I. Reproducibilities of assay and drug recovery from dosage forms

capsules, hard and soft gelatin and tablets, uncoated: comparison of dosage forms

Ahuja, S., Spitzer, C. and Brofazi, F. R., *J. pharm. Sci.*, 1968, *57*, 1979–82

Study on dosage variations of individual capsules and tablets of desipramine and imipramine hydrochloride

capsules, hard gelatin and tablets: desipramine and imipramine hydrochloride, active ingredient weight and variability

Flann, B., *J. pharm. Sci.*, 1974, *63*, 183–99

Comparison of criteria for content uniformity

capsules, hard and soft gelatin and tablets: comparison of criteria, statistical evaluation, computer simulation

Fusari, S.A., Dittmar, D. and Perizzo, C.H., *Drug Dev. Communs*, 1974–5, *1*, 517–37

A generalized approach to content uniformity assays

capsules, hard gelatin and tablets: drug extraction by dialysis; intact capsule and tablet assays

Hersey, J.A. and Cook, P.C., *J. Pharm. Pharmac.*, 1974, *26*, 126–33

Homogeneity of pharmaceutical dispersed systems

capsules and tablets: homogeneity of content

Setnikar, I., *Pharm. Acta Helv.*, 1974, *49*, 302–8

The USP content uniformity test. Analysis and proposals

capsules, hard and soft gelatin, sterile solids and tablets: evaluation of U.S.P. XVIII test, statistical analysis

Pharmaceuticals Manufacturers' Association of Tokyo, *Iyakuhin kenkyu*, 1978, *9*, 581–8

Studies of content uniformity test method for tablets and capsules (in Japanese)

capsules and tablets: evaluation of Jpn P. and U.S.P. XVIII methods, statistical analysis; content uniformity, comparison of products

Warren, J.W., Shah, K.A., Benmaman, J.D., Freeman, D.B., Lewkowicz, R.T. and Friend, C.G., *Curr. ther. Res.*, 1979, *25*, 172–9

Variations among ten chlordiazepoxide hydrochloride 10 mg capsule products

capsules, hard gelatin: chlordiazepoxide hydrochloride, comparison of products; 3.8.3.6; 4.2.3.3

Aitenschmidt, W., Eggert, W., Liske, T., Lutz, G., Schepky, G., Sell, R. and Weskamp, R., *Pharm. Ind., Berl.*, 1980, *42*, 725–32

The consequences of content-uniformity requirements for production (in German)

capsules: pharmacopoeial content uniformity standards; quality assurance testing

Bolton, S., *J. pharm. Sci.*, 1985, *74*, 572–4

Some properties of the U.S.P. content-uniformity test as related to control charts and validation of solid dosage forms

capsules, hard and soft gelatin: U.S.P. XX content-uniformity test, assay variation, control charts, validation

3.8.3.2 Identification of Products

Fahrig, W., *Pharm. Ind., Berl.*, 1959, *21*, 460–6

Identification of solid dosage forms (in German)

capsules, hard and soft gelatin and tablets: physical characteristics, systematic identification scheme; product imprinting

Müller, R.K., *Pharm. Prax., Berl.*, supplement to *Pharmazie*, 1963, *18, Suppl.* 10, 215–19

Identification of sugar-coated tablets and capsules permitted in DDR (Germany) by external characteristics (in German)

capsules, hard and soft gelatin and tablets, sugar-coated: capsule products, Germany (DDR); physical characteristics, colour, size, taste, weight

Caldwell, J.G., Shoman A.F., Hurst, C.B. and Robertson, W.O., *J. Am. med. Ass.*, 1964, *187*, 951–3

Identification of drugs. Use of the *JAMA* drug identification guide

capsules, hard and soft gelatin and tablets: physical characteristics, colour, shape, size

McCaw, R.L., *Hosp. Pharmst*, 1965, *18*, 169–73

Identification of tablets and capsules

capsules and tablets: identification methods, review

Eisenberg, W.V. and Tillson, A.H., *J. forens. Sci.*, 1966, *11*, 529–51

Identification of counterfeit drugs particularly barbiturates and amphetamines by microscopic, chemical and instrumental techniques

capsules, hard and soft gelatin: ingredients, examination techniques, instrumental testing; physical characteristics, examination techniques

Reynolds, L.M., Kessler, W.V., Christian, J.E. and Ziemer, P.L., *J. pharm. Sci.*, 1967, *56*, 437–43

Use of activation analysis in problems of drug control

capsules, hard gelatin and tablets: dexamphetamine sulphate; drugs, illicit manufacture; drugs, official controls; identification, manufacture; identification trace elements, activation analysis

Bertrand, J.M. and Lorentz, J.F., *Bull. Soc. Pharm. Nancy*, 1969, *82*, 40–5

Preliminary note on the settlement of a rapid identification system for tablets, capsules hard and soft (in French)

capsules, hard and soft gelatin and tablets: confirmatory tests; information retrieval, punched cards; physical characteristics, colour, size, weight

Faurby, V., *Farmaceutisk Tid.*, 1971, *81*, 1013–7

Visual identification of solid oral dosage forms (in Danish)

capsules, hard and soft gelatin and tablets: physical characteristics, colour, size, weight

Larcan, A., Bertrand, J.-M., Lorentz, J.-F., Valantin, P. and Mauray, G., *Presse méd.*, 1971, *79*, 1853–6

A card which permits the identification of different solid pharmaceutical forms (tablets, cachets, pills, hard gelatin capsules and soft gelatin capsules) (in French)

cachets, capsules, hard and soft gelatin and tablets: confirmatory tests; information retrieval, punched cards; physical characteristics, colour, size, weight

Masayoshi, H., *Nippon Yakuzaishi kai Zasshi*, 1972, *24*(9), 14–16

Identification code for tablets and capsules (in Japanese)

capsules, hard gelatin and tablets: identification by code, Japanese national drug code system; product, marking and printing

Fischer, A., *Pharm. Ind., Berl.*, 1973, *35*, 435–7

Evaluation of identification tests for solid dosage forms (in German)

capsules, hard and soft gelatin and tablets: computer information retrieval, products, Germany (BRD); physical characteristics, definitions

Bertrand, J.M., Lorentz, J.F. and Larcan, A., *Annls méd. Nancy*, 1974, *12*, 23–8

Utilisation of a system of punched cards for the identification of tablets, soft gelatin capsules and hard gelatin capsules (in French)

capsules, hard and soft gelatin and tablets: information retrieval, punched card system; physical characteristics, dimensions and sensory features

Hauck, G., *Annls méd. Nancy*, 1974, *12*, 29–39

Our experiences with a punched card system for identifying solid dosage forms (in German)

capsules and tablets: confirmatory tests; information retrieval, punched card system; physical characteristics

McArdle, C. and Skew, E.A., *Annls méd. Nancy*, 1974, *12*, 15–21

Tablets and capsules, an aid to their identification

capsules, hard and soft gelatin and tablets: confirmatory tests, chemical; information retrieval, punched card system; physical characteristics, colour, diameter, shape, surface markings

Monterro, J.I., *Annls méd. Nancy*, 1974, *12*, 85–6

Guide to the identification of capsules (in French)

capsules, hard gelatin: products, Portugal

Pedersen, E.H., *Annls méd. Nancy*, 1974, *12*, 47–9

Identification of solid dosage forms

capsules, hard and soft gelatin and tablets, coated and uncoated: information retrieval, punched card system; physical characteristics

Robertson, K.A. and Robertson, W.O., *Clin. Toxicol.*, 1974, *7*, 83–9

Drug identification by imprint

capsules and tablets: identification by product code, practical trial

van Rossen-Iburg, J.C., *Pharm. Weekbl. Ned.*, 1974, *109*, 929–35

Identification of solid dosage forms of medicines registered in the Netherlands (in Dutch)

capsules, pills and tablets: physical characteristics, colour, imprints, shape, size

Allsup, V., Parker, J. and Walker, J., *Pharm. J.*, 1977, *219*, 529–30

An optical coincidence feature card system

capsules and tablets: information retrieval, optical coincidence system

Collier, W.A.L., *Drug Intell. & clin. Pharm.*, 1977, *11*, 170–5

Indexable imprinting of solid dosage forms

capsules and tablets: imprint catalogue; imprint classification system

Scharf, H., *Pharm. Ztg, Berl.*, 1977, *122*, 114–20

Identification system for oral dosage forms (in German)

capsules, hard and soft gelatin and tablets: imprint catalogue; physical characteristics, colour, size; products, Germany (BRD)

Chemist and Druggist Directory and Tablet and Capsule Identification Guide, 1986, Tonbridge, Kent, Benn Business Information Services Ltd, 1986, pp. 1–96

capsules, hard and soft gelatin and tablets, coated and uncoated: identification by colour, dimensions, shape, surface markings; products, Great Britain

3.8.3.3 Microbiology of Capsule Products

Wanandi, B. and Speiser, P., *Pharm. Acta Helv.*, 1970, *45*, 501–12

The microbiological contamination of dosage forms and raw materials (in German)

pharmaceuticals: microbiological levels, excipients, products; microbiological standards

Bruch, C.W., *Drug Cosmet. Ind.*, 1972, *110*(6), 32–7, 116–21

Possible modification of U.S.P. microbial limits and tests

pharmaceuticals: proposed limits and tests, sterile and non-sterile products

Waterman, R.F., Sumner, E.D., Baldwin, J.N. and Warren, F.W., *J. pharm. Sci.*, 1973, *62*, 1317–20

Survival of *Staphylococcus aureus* on pharmaceutical oral solid dosage forms capsules, hard gelatin and tablets: microbiological levels, effect of storage, humidity, temperature; microbiological levels, survey of products

Wallhäusser, K.H., *Pharm. Ind., Berl.*, 1977, *39*, 491–7

Microbiological aspects on the subject of oral solid dosage forms

capsules and tablets: microbiological levels, review

Schneller, G.H., *Drug Cosmet. Ind.*, 1978, *122*(2), 48, 52, 54, 58, 146–53

Microbial testing of oral dosage forms

capsules and tablets: microbiological levels, pathogens, salmonella; microbiological standards

Hüttenrauch, R., Taubert, H. and Jacob, J., *Pharmazie*, 1984, *39*, 356

Gas permeability of hard gelatin capsules

capsules, hard gelatin: gas permeability, ethylene oxide/carbon dioxide mixture, effect on bacteria; 3.8.2.3

3.8.3.4 Moisture Content of Capsule Products

Frauch, P. and Lang, E., *Pharm. Acta Helv.*, 1963, *38*, 676–89

Dielectric determination of moisture in solid forms of drugs with the "Super Beha" measurement device (in German)

capsules, hard and soft gelatin, granules and tablets: moisture content, dielectric measurement

Leupin, K., *Pharm. Ind., Berl.*, 1964, *26*, 524–7

Storage experiments with hard gelatin capsules (in German)

capsules, hard gelatin: moisture content, capsules, contents, shells, effects of, humidity, storage; stability testing

Beal, H.M., Dicenzo, R.J., Jannke, P.J., Palmer, H.A., Pinsky, J., Salame, M. and Speaker, T.J., *J. pharm. Sci.*, 1967, *56*, 1310–22

Pharmaceuticals stored in plastic containers

pharmaceutical products: official products, United States; stability, products, chemical and physical; storage trials, various simulated environments; 3.6.2; 3.8.3.7

Ito, K., Kaga, S.-I. and Takeya, Y., *Chem. pharm. Bull., Tokyo*, 1969, *17*, 1134–7

Studies on hard gelatin capsules I. Water vapor transfer between capsules and powders

capsules, hard gelatin: capsule shells, colourless and opaque; formulation of contents, diluents, lactose, starch, maize and potato; moisture content, capsules, contents, shells, effects of, humidity, storage; stability testing

Bond, C.M., Lees, K.A. and Packington, J.L., *Pharm. J.*, 1970, *205*, 210–14

Cephalexin: A new oral broad-spectrum antibiotic

capsules, hard gelatin and granules: cephalexin; moisture content, capsules, contents, shells, effects of, humidity, storage; stability testing

Smith, G., *Pharm. J.*, 1974, *213*, 176–78

The stability of dispensed medicines

pharmaceuticals: moisture content, capsules, hard gelatin, contents; review

Chowhan, Z.T. and Amaro, A.A., *J. pharm. Sci.*, 1977, *66*, 1254–8

Powder inhalation aerosol studies I: Selection of a suitable drug entity for bronchial delivery of new drugs

capsules, hard gelatin: 7-methylsulphinyl-2-xanthone carboxylic acid and sodium salt; formulation of contents; moisture content, sorption desorption isotherms, capsules, contents, shells; 3.5.1

York, P., *Drug Dev. ind. Pharm.*, 1980, *6*, 605–27

Studies of the effect of powder moisture content on drug release from hard gelatin capsules

capsules, hard gelatin: capsule, contents and shells, moisture content, effect of relative humidity; formulation of contents, diluents, lactose, maize starch, drug, barbitone, barbitone sodium; moisture content, measurement of sorption desorption isotherms; 4.2.3.4

York, P., *J. Pharm. Pharmac.*, 1981, *33*, 269–73

Analysis of moisture sorption hysteresis in hard gelatin capsules, maize starch, and maize starch: drug powder mixtures

capsules, hard gelatin: capsule, contents and shells, moisture content, effect of relative humidity; formulation of contents, diluents, lactose, maize starch, drug, barbitone, barbitone sodium; moisture content, theoretical analysis; measurement of sorption desorption isotherms; moisture distribution, location in components

Bowtle, W.J., *Br. J.pharm. Pract.*, 1986, *8*, 307–8

Semi-solid matrix capsules

capsules, hard gelatin: vancomycin hydrochloride; moisture content, effect of formulation, storage; formation of contents, semi-solid; 3.2.3.4; 4.2.3.4

3.8.3.5 Physical Properties of Capsule Products

Colombo, B.M, *Boll. chim.-farm.*, 1969, *108*, 810–13

Malacymeter, an apparatus for the determination of the softness on soft gelatin dosage forms

capsules, soft gelatin: malacymeter; softness units

Vemuri, S., *Drug Dev. ind. Pharm.*, 1984, *10*, 409–23

Measurement of soft elastic gelatin capsule firmness with a universal testing machine

capsules, soft gelatin: capsule property, firmness, effect of storage, temperature and humidity; Instron tester, firmness measurements; packaging, glass, polystyrene bottles

3.8.3.6 Uniformity of Weight

Anon., *Schweiz. ApothZtg*, 1928, *66*, 489–91

The reliability of dosage of specialities (in German)

capsules and tablets: products, Switzerland

Goldstein, S.W., *J. Am. pharm. Ass., scient. Edn.*, 1950, *39*, 505–6

Standard tolerances for pharmaceutical compounding. A basis for their establishment. III. Capsules

capsules, hard gelatin: filling small scale

Neuhaus, H.-J. and Richter, J., *Pharmazie*, 1960, *15*, 537–8 and *Pharm. Zentralhalle Dtl.*, 1961, *100*, 12–14

Proposals for the DAB 7, Part 14: Permitted weight variation for tablets, sugar-coated tablets, powders, capsules and pills as well as other dosage forms (in German)

capsules, hard and soft gelatin, pills, powders, suppositories and tablets, uncoated and sugar-coated: pharmacopoeial monograph, Germany (DDR)

Anon., *Med. Lett. Drug. Ther.*, 1961, *3*(2), 5–7

Tests of secobarbital

capsules, hard gelatin: quinalbarbitone; capsule products, comparison of price; product weight uniformity, *U.S.P.* XVI test, comparison of products

Suñé, J.M. and Peris, J., *Galenica acta.*, 1961, *14*, 293–301

A contribution to the study of the test for weight uniformity of gelatin capsules and its possible inclusion in the Spanish Pharmacopoeia (in Spanish)

capsules, hard gelatin: comparison of pharmacopoeial tests; products, Spain

Stock, F.G., *Pharm. J.*, 1962, *188*, 453–4

Uniformity of weight of contents of capsules

capsules, hard gelatin: product weight uniformity, *B.P.* 1958 addendum 1960 test; products, Great Britain

Anon., *Med. Lett. Drug. Ther.*, 1963, *5*(24), 94–5

Tests of chloral hydrate

capsules, hard gelatin: chloral hydrate; capsule products, comparison of price; product weight uniformity, *U.S.P.* XVI test, comparison of products; 4.2.2.1

Czetsch-Lindenwald, H.V. and Tawashi, R., *Pharm. Ind., Berl.*, 1965, *27*, 146–51

Tests with hard gelatin capsules (in German)

capsules, hard gelatin: nomogram, fill-weight, capsule size determination; product weight uniformity, effects of, formulation, method of filling; product weight uniformity, pharmacopoeial standards, method of determination; 3.2.4.1; 3.8.2.4

Roberts, C., *Technometrics*, 1969, *11*, 161–75

Fill weight variation release and control of capsules, tablets and sterile solids

capsules, hard and soft gelatin, sterile powders and tablets: evaluation of *U.S.P.* test, statistical analysis

Pietra, V. and Setnikar, I., *J. pharm. Sci.*, 1970, *59*, 530–5

Testing for uniformity: sampling plans in pharmacopoeias for weight, volume, and content uniformity

cachets, capsules, hard and soft gelatin, injections, pills, sterile solids, and tablets: comparison of pharmacopoeial standards, statistical analysis

Anon., *Pharm. J.*, 1971, *206*, 148

Automated computer-linked check weighing

capsules, hard gelatin: ampicillin; automatic weighing

Caldwell, H.C. and Westlake, W.J., *Can. J. pharm. Sci.*, 1973, *8*, 50–3

Magnesium lauryl sulfate; soluble lubricant

capsules, hard gelatin and tablets: lithium carbonate; filling machine, dosing tube mechanism; product weight uniformity, effect of formulation, comparison of lubricants; 3.2.4.1; 4.2.4.

Setnikar, I. and Fontani, F., *Boll. chim.-farm.*, 1975, *114*, 509–20

Control charts for capsule weights (in Italian)

capsules, hard gelatin: filling, industrial scale, production control charts; product weight uniformity, statistical parameters

Mehta, G.N., Bavitz, J.F. and Bohidar, N.R., *Drug Dev. ind. Pharm.*, 1979, *5*, 335–48

A comparative evaluation of four automatic weighing systems

capsules, hard gelatin and tablets, film-coated: automatic weighing, comparison of systems

Warren, J.W., Shah, K.A., Benmaman, J.D., Freeman, D.B., Lewkowicz, R.T. and Friend, C.G., *Curr. ther. Res.*, 1979, *25*, 172–9

Variations among ten chlordiazepoxide hydrochloride 10-mg capsule products

capsules, hard gelatin: chlordiazepoxide hydrochloride, comparison of products; 3.8.3.1; 4.2.3.3

Demorest, R.L., *Pharm. Technol.*, 1980, *4*(12), 41–4

Rapid weighing and sorting of filled capsules

capsules, hard gelatin: automatic weighing, capacitance measurements

Pfeifer, W. and Marquardt, G., *Pharm. Ind., Berl.*, 1984, *46*, 407–11

Possibilities of weight control when filling hard gelatin capsules (in German)

capsules, hard gelatin: automatic weighing, comparison of systems

Lacey, M.E., Davis, P.J., Johnson, E.S. and Koester, A.P., *Pharm. Technol.*, 1985, *9*(3), 98, 102–3, 106

Comparison of tablet and capsule weight-variation criteria by Monte Carlo simulation

capsules, hard gelatin and tablets: U.S.P. XX, content uniformity test, comparison with product weight variation, statistical analysis

Pfeifer, W. and Marquardt, G., *Pharm. Ind., Berl.*, 1985, *47*, 423–5

Investigations of the frequency and causes of dosage deviations during filling of hard gelatin capsules. Part 2. Dosage deviations during the filling of pellets in hard gelatin capsules (in German)

capsules, hard gelatin: capsule-filling machines for pellets, continuous and intermittent motion; product weight uniformity, comparisons of, filling machines, products

3.8.3.7 Storage of Capsules

Nilou, K., Lindholm, H. and Terp, P., *Arch. Pharm. Chemi*, 1950, *57*, 332–43

The stability of vitamins A and D in gelatin capsules (in Danish)

capsules, soft gelatin: vitamins A, D; stability, effect of storage

Siegel, S., Reiner, R.H., Zelinskie, J.A. and Hanus, E.J., *J. pharm. Sci.*, 1962, *51*, 1068–71

Tablets of pyrilamine resin adsorbate with aspirin and vitamin C

capsules, hard gelatin and tablets: aspirin, mepyramine, maleate and resin adsorbate, sodium ascorbate; stability, effect of chemical form, resins, and storage at high temperatures (45°)

Czetsch-Lindenwald, H.V., *Pharm. Ind., Berl.*, 1964, *26*, 454–6

Capsules and climate (in German)

capsules, hard and soft gelatin: disintegration testing, effect of storage, various relative humidities and temperatures; testing, packaging, containers and materials

Tingstad, J.E., *J. pharm. Sci.*, 1964, *53*, 955–62

Physical stability testing of pharmaceuticals

capsules, hard and soft gelatin, emulsions, ointments, solutions, suspensions and tablets: product stability, formulation requirements

Beal, H.M., Dicenzo, R. J., Jannke, P.J., Palmer, H.A., Pinsky, J., Salame, M and Speaker, T.J., *J. pharm. Sci.*, 1967, *56*, 1310–22

Pharmaceuticals stored in plastic containers

pharmaceutical products: containers, plastic, stability testing; official products, *U.S.P.*, stability, chemical and physical; storage trials, various simulated environments; 3.6.2; 3.8.3.4

Gore, D.N. and Ashwin, J., *J. mond. Pharm.*, 1967, No. 4, 365–75

Significance of relative humidity and moisture pick-up data in relation to pharmaceutical formulation

capsules, hard gelatin: penicillins, semi-synthetic; moisture content, capsules, penicillins, starches, sugars, effects of, relative humidity, storage

Delonca, H., Puech, A., Segura, G. and Youakim, Y., *J. Pharm. Belg.*, 1969, *24*, 317–31

Influence of excipients and conditions of storage on the stability of medicines. II. Capsules of acetylsalicylic acid (in French)

capsules, hard gelatin: aspirin; storage testing, effects of, container, diluent, light, relative humidity, temperature; 3.2.4.1

Vierna, D.S.G. and Herrera, D.L.G., *Auxiliary products for oral solid dosage forms*, Symposium (Barcelona, Faculty of Pharmacy, University of Barcelona), 1969, 165–63

Safety measures for the use of gelatin capsules (in Spanish)

capsules, hard gelatin: storage, empty capsules; 3.2.3.5

van Oudtshoorn, M.C.B., Koeleman, H.A., Kapp, C.J. and Potgieter, F.J., *S. Afr. pharm. J.*, 1970, *37*(3), 4–6

The correct storage of medicines: the task of the pharmacist (in Afrikaans)

capsules, hard gelatin, gels and tablets: chloramphenicol; disintegration testing, effect of storage; pharmacopoeial storage requirements; storage, effects of, conditions, containers

Rizescu, C., Tiutiu, F. and Popescu, V., *Revue Chim., Buc.*, 1973, *24*, 652–4

Analytical studies in the stability of medicines packed in gelatin capsules (in Roumanian)

capsules, soft gelatin: clofibrate, phenylethyl carbinol, vitamin F; content uniformity; disintegration testing, effect of storage; product weight uniformity; storage conditions, 35°, high humidity

Bobbé, D., Mathis, C., Stamm, A., Metziger, P. and Gabler, W., *Labo-Pharma Probl. Tech.*, 1976, *24*(258), 879–85

Study of the stability of oily suspensions in soft gelatin capsules (in French)

capsules, soft gelatin: suspensions, physical properties, sedimentation, viscosity, effect of storage; 3.3.3.2

Goldberg, R. and Nightingale, C.H., *Am. J. Hosp. Pharm.*, 1977, *34*, 267–9

Stability of aspirin in propoxyphene compound dosage forms

capsules, hard gelatin: aspirin, caffeine, dextropropoxyphene hydrochloride, phenacetin; stability, aspirin, measured by release of salicylic acid; storage, effects of, humidity, low and high, temperatures, 25°, 50°

York, P., *Pharmazie*, 1977, *32*, 101–4

The shelf life of some antibiotic preparations stored under tropical conditions

capsules, hard gelatin and tablets: chloramphenicol, sulphathiazole, tetracycline hydrochloride; stability testing, accelerated storage trials, prediction of shelf-life; storage trials, temperate and tropical conditions; 4.2.3.2

Conine, J.W., Johnson, D.W. and Coleman, D.L., *Curr. ther. Res.*, 1978, *24*, 967–79

A comparison of the stability of commercial cephradine and cephalexin capsules

capsules, hard gelatin: cephalexin, cephradine; identification, decomposition products; stability, effect of packing; stability, measurement of potency; storage conditions, humidity, ambient, 75%, temperature, 5°, 25°, 40°

Saito, T., Suzuki, S. Nambu, N. and Nagai, T., *Yakuzaigaku*, 1978, *38*, 29–34

Test of the physical stability regarding dissolution property of solid preparations (in Japanese)

capsules, hard gelatin and tablets: dissolution testing, effect of storage; storage conditions, 52% RH at 5°, 92% RH at 30°; 4.2.4

Gupta, V.D. and Gupta, A., *Am. J. Hosp. Pharm.*, 1979, *36*, 1539–41

Stability of some oral solid drug products when stored in a counting machine

capsules, hard gelatin: disintegration testing, *U.S.P.* XIX, comparison of products after storage; dissolution testing, *U.S.P.* XIX, comparison of products after storage; moisture content, comparison of products after storage; packaging, electronic counting machine, product storage in

Cutie, M.R. *Drug Cosmet. Ind.*, 1980, *126*(1), 40–3, 86

Effects of cold and freezing temperatures on pharmaceutical dosage forms

pharmaceutical dosage forms: stability, products, low temperatures; storage conditions, pharmacopoeial definitions

Gupta, V.D., Stewart, K.R. and Gupta, A., *Am. J. Hosp. Pharm.*, 1980, *37*, 165, 169

Stability of oral drugs after repackaging in single-unit containers

capsules and tablets: disintegration testing, *U.S.P.* XIX, effect of storage; product moisture content, effect of storage; stability, comparison of unit pack and original containers; storage conditions, ambient; 3.6.1

Matsuda, Y., Itooka, T. and Mitsuhashi, Y., *Chem. pharm. Bull., Tokyo*, 1980, *28*, 2665–71

Photostability of indomethacin in model gelatin capsules: Effects of film thickness and concentration of titanium dioxide on the coloration and photolytic degradation

capsules, hard gelatin: indomethacin, photostability, effect of capsule, opacity, thickness; capsule shell, formulation, concentration of opacifier, titanium dioxide

Binda, M.L. and Dondi, G., *Boll. chim.-farm.*, 1981, *120*, 544–9

Study on the influence of light and colorants on the stability of nifedipine capsules (in Italian)

capsules, soft gelatin: nifedipine; drug stability, effect of light exposure, protection by shell formulation; formulation of capsule shell, colorants; formulation of contents

Ikekawa, A., *Yakuzaigaku*, 1982, *42*, 79–83

Stabilisation of photosensitive medicines by colouring soft gelatin capsules (in Japanese)

capsules, soft gelatin: clofibrate, 1α-hydroxycholecalciferol, DL-α-tocopherol; drug stability, effects of, capsule colour, time of exposure, wavelength of light

Richard, J. and Andermann, G., *Pharm. Acta Helv.*, 1982, *57*, 116–21

A study of the stability of cyclandelate in soft gelatin capsules (in French)

cyclandelate; comparison of batches, effects of storage; 3.3.3.2

Gouda, H.W., Moustafa, M.A. and Al-Shora, H.I., *Int. J. Pharmaceut.*, 1984, *18*, 213

Effect of storage on nitrofurantoin solid dosage forms

capsules, hard gelatin and tablets: nitrofurantoin; product packaging, blister packs, plastic bags, glass vials; stability, testing, effects of, humidity, temperature, packaging; 4.5.4

Bowtle, W. J., Lucas, R. A. and Barker, N. J., *Fourth International Conference on Pharmaceutical Technology*, (Paris, APGI, June 3–5, 1986), 1986, *V*, 80–89

Formulation and process studies in semi-solid matrix capsule technology

capsules, hard gelatin: vancomycin; moisture content, effects of storage, comparison of drug and product; 3.2.4.2; 4.5.5

4 Drug Availability from Capsules

4.1 Reviews

Nelson, E., *Clin. Pharmac. Ther.*, 1962, *3*, 673–81

Physicochemical and pharmaceutic properties of drugs that influence the results of clinical trials

Kaplan, S.A., *Drug Metab. Rev.*, 1972, *1*, 15–33

Biopharmaceutical considerations in drug formulation design and evaluation

Lachman, L. and Roemer, W.C., *J. Am. pharm. Ass.*, 1972, *NS12*, 215–24

Pharmaceutical properties of drugs and dosage forms affecting physiological availability

Wurster, D.E., *J. mond. Pharm.*, 1972, *15*(1), 21–51

Some formulation factors influencing the efficacy of drug delivery systems

Withey, R.J., *Revue can. Biol.*, 1973, *32*, *Suppl.*, 21–30

Proceedings: bioavailability and therapeutic efficacy

Jones, B.E., *Labo-Pharma Probl. Tech.*, 1974, *22*(231), 349–53

Drug release from hard gelatin capsules (in French)

Thoma, K., Chapter VIII in *The Capsule, Basics, Technology and Biopharmacy, a Modern Dosage Form* (in German), Fahrig, W. and Hofer, U. (Eds), Stuttgart, Wissenschaftliche Verlagsgesellschaft mbH, 1983, pp. 138–71

The biopharmaceutics of the capsule (in German)

4.2 Drug Availability in vitro

4.2.1 Reviews

Carvalho, L.S., *Revta port. Farm.*, 1969, *19*, 37–48

Dissolution test of solid oral preparations (tablets and gelatin capsules) (in Portuguese)

Hersey, J.A., *Mfg Chem.*, 1969, *40*(2), 32–5

Methods available for the determination of in vitro dissolution rate

Blake, M.I., *J. Am. pharm. Ass.*, 1971, *NS11*, 603–11

Role of the compendia in controlling factors affecting bioavailability of drug products

Klie, H.-E., *Pharm. Ind., Berl.*, 1971, *33*, 454–9, 525–32 and *Drugs Germ.*, 1971, *14*, 147–65

The E 70 tablet testing apparatus. A contribution to friability, disintegration and dissolution time testing (in German; English translation in *Drugs Germ.*)

capsules and tablets: disintegration testing, apparatus; dissolution testing, apparatus

4.2.2 Disintegration

4.2.2.1 Standard Capsules

Borasi, M., Bellentani, L. and Picci, L., *Farmaco, Edn prat.*, 1955, *10*, 525–37

A study of the disintegration of pharmaceutical preparations for oral administration (in Italian)

cachets, capsules, hard and soft gelatin, pills and tablets: disintegration method, Erweka apparatus; disintegration testing, effects of, formulation of contents, test medium composition, enzymes, pH, salts

Richter, J. and Klein, H., *Pharmazie*, 1957, *12*, 190–4

Preliminary norms for the disintegration, solubility and other characteristics of solid dosage forms as well as the manufacturing of the official preparations (in German)

cachets, capsules, hard and soft gelatin, granules, pills and tablets, uncoated and sugar-coated: disintegration method, DAB 7; disintegration testing, pharmacopoeial standards, standard and enteric products

Czetsch-Lindenwald, H.V., *Pharm. Ind., Berl.*, 1962, *24*, 110–14

The disintegration of gelatin capsules (in German)

capsules, hard and soft gelatin: disintegration testing, effects of, apparatus, capsule contents, capsule type, test media, test temperature; disintegration testing, enteric-coated products; disintegration testing, pharmacopoeial standards

Anon., *Med. Lett. Drug. Ther.*, 1963, *5*(24) 94–5

Tests of chloral hydrate

capsules, hard gelatin: chloral hydrate; disintegration, method, modified *U.S.P.* XVI; disintegration testing, comparison of products; 3.8.3.6

Anon., *Annls pharm. belg.*, 1968, *19*(6), Fasc No. 77, 2–3

Questions and answers. 'I would like to know the precision with which capsules disintegrate' (in French)

capsules, hard and soft gelatin: disintegration testing, pharmacopoeial standards

Sandell, E., *Acta pharm. suec.*, 1970, *7*, 55–6

A disintegration test for evaluation of drug availability

capsules, hard gelatin and tablets: phenacetin; disintegration method, oscillating tube with sieves

Hüttenrauch, R., *Pharmazie*, 1971, *26*, 107–8

The importance of ionic strength for the disintegration time of gelatin capsules (in German)

capsules, hard and soft gelatin: disintegration method, Erweka apparatus; disintegration testing, effects of, contents, ionic strength of test media

Jones, B.E. and Cole, W.V.J., *J. Pharm. Pharmac.*, 1971, *23*, 438–43

The influence of test conditions on the disintegration time of gelatin capsules

capsules, hard and soft gelatin: disintegration method, *B.P.* 1968; disintegration method, capsule shells, steel ball emptying; disintegration testing, effects of, formulation, test conditions; capsule products, Great Britain

Jones, B.E., *Acta pharm. suec.*, 1972, *9*, 261–3

Disintegration of hard gelatin capsules

capsules, hard gelatin: disintegration testing, influence of formulation

Elliott, G.R. and Armstrong, M.F., *Clin. Pharmac. Ther.*, 1973, *13*, 459

Sodium bicarbonate and oral tetracycline

capsules, hard gelatin: tetracycline; disintegration method, manual; disintegration testing, effect of pH of test media

Juhl, R.P. and Blaug, S.M., *J. pharm. Sci.*, 1973, *62*, 170

Factors affecting release of medicaments from hard gelatin capsules

capsules, hard gelatin: chloramphenicol; disintegration method, beaker, stirring; disintegration testing, effects of, pH of test medium, temperature

Hagemann, R. and Leupin, K., *Pharm. Acta Helv.*, 1974, *49*, 75–6

Studies with hard gelatin capsules (in German)

capsules, hard gelatin: disintegration method, *Swiss P.* VI; disintegration testing, end-point, timing of powder release

Langenbucher, F., *Drug Dev. Communs*, 1974–5, *1*, 287–301

Improved standards for the disintegration test of solid products

capsules and tablets: disintegration method, oscillating tube with mesh; disintegration testing, specification for improved test

Ludwig, A. and Van Ooteghem, M., *Pharm. Ind., Berl.*, 1980, *42*, 405–6

Disintegration of hard gelatin capsules. Part 2: Disintegration mechanism of hard gelatin capsules investigated with a stereoscopic microscope

capsules, hard gelatin: disintegration method, stirred beaker; disintegration testing, capsule shell rupture, observation by microscope; disintegration testing, effect of contents, hydrophilic and hydrophobic; formulation of contents, aminophenazone, copper sulphate, phenacetin

Ludwig, A. and Van Ooteghem, M., *Pharm. Ind., Berl.*, 1980, *42*, 1040–3

Disintegration of hard gelatin capsules. Part 3: Penetration and diffusion of liquid through the capsule wall investigated by scanning electron microscopy

capsules, hard gelatin: disintegration method, solvent immersion; disintegration testing, capsule wall, measurement of solvent penetration, scanning electron microscopy

Ludwig, A. and Van Ooteghem, M., *Pharm. Ind., Berl.*, 1980, *42*, 1140–1

Disintegration of hard gelatin capsules. Part 4: Method for measuring the time of rupture of the capsule

capsules, hard gelatin: aminophenazone, phenacetin; disintegration method, oscillating tube with wire mesh, rotating paddle, stirred beaker; disintegration testing, comparison of methods, effect of drug, wetting, non-wetting

Polesuk, J., *J. pharm. Sci.*, 1980, *69*, 749

Disintegration test for hard gelatin capsules

capsules, hard gelatin: disintegration method, *U.S.P.* XX; disintegration testing, collaborative testing, effect of apparatus variables, disks, test volume, tube movement

Doelker, E., Doelker, C. and Mordier, D., *J. Pharm. Belg.*, 1981, *36*, 404–11

The role of wetting on the release of hydrophobic drugs from hard gelatin capsules, I. Liquid diffusion through the wall and capillary penetration into the powder bed (in French)

capsules, hard gelatin: disintegration method, falling ball bearing; disintegration testing, effect of test medium, surfactants; 4.2.3.4

Ludwig, A. and Van Ooteghem, M., *Pharm. Ind., Berl.*, 1981, *43*, 188–90

Disintegration of hard gelatin capsules. Part 5: The influence of the composition of the test solution on the disintegration of hard gelatin capsules

capsules, hard gelatin: aminophenazone; disintegration method, modified beaker; disintegration testing, effects of, test medium, pepsin, pH, polysorbate 80, sodium chloride; disintegration testing, time for shell rupture

Thoma, K. and Heckenmüller, H., *Pharm. Ind., Berl.*, 1982, *44*, 521–3

The development of additional instrumentation to improve the disintegration test (in German)

capsules and tablets: disintegration method, *Eur. P.*; disintegration testing, determination of end point, optical detection, automation

Chowhan, Z.T. and Ari, L.-H., *Pharm. Technol.*, 1985, *9*(3), 84, 86, 90, 92,94–97

Drug excipient interactions resulting from powder mixing, I: Possible mechanisms of interaction with starch and its effect on drug dissolution

capsules, hard gelatin: ketorolac tromethamine; disintegration method, USP; disintegration testing, effects of, formulation of contents, lubricant mixing; 3.2.4.1; 4.2.3.4

Chowhan, Z.T., and Chi, L.-H., *Pharm. Technol.*, 1985, *9*(4), 30, 32–33, 36, 38–41

Drug-excipient interactions resulting from powder mixing, II: Possible mechanisms of interaction with crospovidone and its effect on in vitro dissolution

capsules, hard gelatin: ketorolac tromethamine; disintegration method, USP; disintegration testing, effects of, drug particle size, lubricant mixing; 3.2.4.1; 4.2.3.4

Hüttenrauch, R., Zielke, P. and Moller, U., *Pharmazie*, 1985, *39*, 123

Gelatin structure and capsule disintegration

capsules, hard gelatin: disintegration testing, effects of, composition test media, contents; gelatin, solution properties, effects of, structure breakers and builders

Chowhan, Z.T. and Chi, L.-H., *J. pharm. Sci.*, 1986, *75*, 534–541

Drug-excipient interactions resulting from powder mixing, III: Solid state properties and their effect on drug dissolution

capsules, hard gelatin: prednisone; disintegration method, USP; disintegration testing, comparison of disintegrants, effect of lubricant mixing; 3.2.4.1; 4.2.3.4

Chowhan, Z.T. and Chi, L.H., *J. pharm. Sci.*, 1986, *75*, 542–545

Drug-excipient interactions resulting from powder mixing, IV: Role of lubricants and their effect on in vitro dissolution

capsules, hard gelatin; ketorolac tromethamine; disintegration method, USP; disintegration testing, comparison of lubricants, effect of lubricant mixing; 3.2.4.1; 4.2.3.4

4.2.2.2 Disintegration of Enteric Capsules

Boymond, P., Sfiris, J. and Amacker, P., *Pharm. Ind., Berl.*, 1966, *28*, 836–42 and *Drugs Germ.*, 1967, *10*, 7–19

The manufacture and testing of enterosoluble capsules (in German; English translation in *Drugs Germ.*)

capsules, hard gelatin: disintegration method, rotating tube, *Swiss P.* VI; disintegration method, capsule shells, falling ball bearing; disintegration testing, effect of test media; 3.4.2.2; 4.4.7.1

Remon, J.P., Gyselinck, P., van Severen, R. and Braeckman, P., *Acta Pharm. Tech.*, 1983, *29*, 25–7

New small scale apparatus for enteric coating of hard gelatin capsules

capsules, hard gelatin: disintegration method, *Eur. P.* 2nd Edn; disintegration testing, effects of, coating materials, device operator, solvent systems; 3.4.2.4

Werchan, D., *Pharmazie*, 1984, *39*, 275–6

Film coating of gelatin capsules in the dispensary (in German)

capsules, hard gelatin: disintegration method, DDR AB; 3.4.2.4

4.2.3 Dissolution
4.2.3.1 General References

Schroeter, L.C. and Wagner, J.G., *J. pharm. Sci.*, 1962, *51*, 957–62

Automated dissolution rate studies of capsules and tablets

capsules and tablets: dissolution method, continuous flow

Schroeter, L.C. and Hamlin, W.E., *J. pharm. Sci.*, 1963, *52*, 811–12

Modified automated apparatus for determination of dissolution rates of capsules and tablets

capsules and tablets: dissolution method, modified *U.S.P.* XVI disintegration apparatus, automatic sampling

Paikoff, M. and Drumm, G., *J. pharm. Sci.*, 1965, *54*, 1693–4

Method for evaluating dissolution characteristics of capsules

capsules, hard gelatin: dissolution method, beaker, capsule holder

Pernarowski, M., Woo, W. and Searl, R.O., *J. pharm. Sci.*, 1968, *57*, 1419–21

Continuous flow apparatus for determination of the dissolution characteristics of tablets and capsules

capsules and tablets: dissolution method, continuous flow

Baun, D.C. and Walker, G.C., *J. pharm. Sci.*, 1969, *58*, 611–16

Apparatus for determining the rate of drug release from solid dosage forms

capsules, hard gelatin and tablets: dissolution method, beaker, continuous flow; dissolution testing, effect of test medium; literature review

Arnold, K., Gerber, N. and Levy, G., *Can. J. pharm. Sci.*, 1970, *5*, 89–92

Absorption and dissolution studies on sodium diphenylhydantoin capsules

capsules, hard gelatin: dissolution method, beaker; dissolution testing, effect of test media; 4.4.6.1

Lin, S.-L. Menig, J. and Swartz, C.J., *J. pharm. Sci.*, 1970, *59*, 989–94

Comparative evaluation of various dissolution apparatus for capsule dosage forms

capsules, hard gelatin: dissolution method, beaker, rotating basket, *U.S.P.*; dissolution testing, comparison of methods, effects of, type of capsule holder, variation of test conditions

Beyer, W.F. and Smith, E.W., *J. pharm. Sci.*, 1971, *60*, 1556–9

Automation of NF method I-USP dissolution-rate test

capsules, hard gelatin: tetracycline hydrochloride; dissolution method, *U.S.N.F.*XIII and *U.S.P.* XVIII, automatic analysis, multiple samples

Khalil, S.A.H., Ali, L.M.M. and Khalek, M.M.A., *J. Pharm. Pharmac.*, 1971, *23*, 125–30

Dissolution rate studies using B.P. disintegration apparatus

capsules, hard gelatin and tablets: chloramphenicol (capsules); dissolution method, modified *B.P.* 1968 disintegration apparatus; dissolution testing, effect of test conditions

Hom, F.S., Veresh, S.A. and Miskel, J.J., *J. pharm. Sci.*, 1973, *62*, 1001–6

Soft gelatin capsules I: Factors affecting capsule shell dissolution rate

capsules, soft gelatin: dissolution method, *U.S.P.* XVIII; dissolution testing, effects of, formulation of capsule shell, test conditions; 3.3.3.1

Khan, K.A., *J. Pharm. Pharmac.*, 1975, *27*, 48–9

The concept of dissolution efficiency

capsules and tablets: dissolution testing, expression of results

Turi, P., Dauvois, M. and Michaelis, A.F., *J. pharm. Sci.*, 1976, *65*, 806–10

Continuous dissolution rate determination as a function of the pH of the medium

capsules, hard gelatin: theophylline; dissolution method, continuous flow; dissolution testing, effect of pH of test medium

Brossard, D., Massoum, R. and Chaumeil, J.-C., *Sciences Tech. pharm.*, 1977, *6*, 41–8

Control of dissolution rate in vitro. I. Studies with a continuous flow apparatus (in French)

capsules, hard gelatin, granules, powders and tablets: nitrofurantoin; dissolution method, continuous flow; dissolution testing, effects of, cell dimensions, product form, speed of flow of test medium

Hom, F.S. and Ebert, W.R., *J. pharm. Sci.*, 1977, *66*, 710–13

Determination of meclizine hydrochloride by ion-pair extraction with methyl orange

capsules, soft gelatin and tablets: meclozine hydrochloride; dissolution method, rotating bottle; dissolution testing, effect of drug in shell

Brossard, D., Massoum, R., Poelman, M.-C. and Chaumeil, J.-C., *Sciences Tech. pharm.*, 1978, *7*, 109–15

Control of dissolution rate in vitro. II. Critical study of the method of Poole (in French)

capsules, hard gelatin, granules, powders and tablets: nitrofurantoin; dissolution method, beaker; dissolution testing, effects of, mode of holding capsule, product form, speed of agitation of test medium

Moore, W.E., *J. pharm. Sci.*, 1979, *68*(2), iv

Non disintegration of a capsule's contents

capsules, hard gelatin: dissolution testing, effect of formulation, test method; formulation of contents, disintegrants; letter

Caldwell, H.C., *J. pharm. Sci.*, 1979, *68*(5), iv

Capsule dissolution

capsules, hard gelatin: dissolution testing, effect of contents, wetting; formulation of contents; letter, reply to Moore, W.E., *ibid.*, 1979, *68*(2), iv

El-Yazigi, A., *Int. J. Pharmaceut.*, 1980, *5*, 79–84

Dissolution of hard gelatin capsules 1. Simple method for calculating the rate constant

capsules, hard gelatin and tablets: ampicillin trihydrate, aspirin, chloramphenicol, quinine sulphate, quinidine sulphate, tetracycline hydrochloride, tetracycline phosphate complex; dissolution method, *U.S.P.* XIX; dissolution testing, effect of stirrer speed; dissolution testing, calculation of rate constants

Hom, F. S., *Drug Dev. ind. Pharm.*, 1984, *10*, 275–87

Soft gelatin capsules III: an accelerated method for evaluating the dissolution stability of various gel formulations

capsules, soft gelatin: dissolution method, *U.S.P.* XX basket; dissolution testing, effects of, formulation of capsule shell, moisture content of shell, storage; storage conditions, low humidity, elevated temperatures; 3.3.3.1

4.2.3.2 Comparative Dissolution of Dosage Forms

Hom, F.S. and Miskel, J.J., *J. pharm. Sci.*, 1970, *59*, 827–30

Oral dosage form design and its influence on dissolution rates for a series of drugs

capsules, soft gelatin and tablets: dicoumarol; digitoxin; ethinyloestradiol; hydrocortisone; phenobarbitone; phenylbutazone; propylthiouracil; reserpine; stilboestrol; sulphadiazine; dissolution method, rotating bottle; 3.3.3.2

Weintraub, H. and Gibaldi, M., *J. pharm. Sci.*, 1970, *59*, 1792–6

Rotating-flask method for dissolution-rate determination of aspirin from various dosage forms

capsules, hard gelatin and tablets: acetysalicylic acid; dissolution method, rotating flask

Hom, F.S. and Miskel, J.J., *Lex Scientia*, 1971, *8*(1), 18–26

Enhanced dissolution rates for a series of drugs as a function of dosage form design

capsules, soft gelatin and tablets: chloramphenicol; chlorothiazide; chlorpropamide; dapsone; griseofulvin; hydrochlorothiazide; *p*-hydroxyphenylbutazone; nitrofurantoin; prednisolone; primidone; dissolution method, rotating bottle; 3.3.3.2

Shepherd, R.E., Price, J.C. and Luzzi, L.A., *J. pharm. Sci.*, 1972, *61*, 1152–6

Dissolution profiles for capsules and tablets using a magnet basket dissolution apparatus

capsules, hard gelatin and tablets: lithium carbonate; dissolution method, magnetic basket

Cardini, C. and Stacchini, A., *Boll. chim.-farm.*, 1973, *112*, 104–9

Studies of availability of certain drugs in oral pharmaceutical dosage forms (in Italian)

capsules, hard and soft gelatin and tablets: chlordiazepoxide, diazoxide, ethambutol, isoniazid, oxazepam; disintegration; dissolution method, beaker; 3.3.3.2

Bates, T.R., Young, J.M., Wu, C.M. and Rosenberg, H.A., *J. pharm. Sci.*, 1974, *63*, 643–5

pH-Dependent dissolution rate of nitrofurantoin from commercial suspensions, tablets and capsules

capsules, hard gelatin, suspensions and tablets: nitrofurantoin; dissolution method, stirred flask; drug solubility determination, effect of pH

Huynh-Ngoc, T. and Sirois, G., *Pharm. Acta Helv.*, 1975, *50*, 69–72

Dissolution rate of commercial dosage forms of quinidine sulfate

capsules, hard gelatin and tablets: quinidine sulphate; dissolution method, *U.S.P.* XVIII and *U.S.N.F.* XIII; dissolution testing, calculation of release constants; dissolution testing, comparison of manufacturers; dissolution testing, effects of test media

Boggiano, B.G. and Gleeson, M., *J. pharm. Sci.*, 1976, *65*, 497–502

Gastric acid inactivation of erythromycin stearate in solid dosage forms

capsules and tablets, enteric and film-coated: erythromycin stearate; dissolution method, rotating flask; drug, gastric acid inactivation

York, P., *Pharmazie*, 1977, *32*, 101–4

The shelf life of some antibiotic preparations stored under tropical conditions

capsules, hard gelatin and tablets: chloramphenicol, sulphathiazole, tetracycline hydrochloride; dissolution method, stirred flask; dissolution testing, effect of storage conditions; 3.8.3.7

Chow, D.-N. and Parrott, E.L., *Drug Dev. ind. Pharm.*, 1978, *4*, 441–5

A comparison of dissolution from commercial tablets and from capsules containing a powdered tablet

capsules, hard gelatin and tablets: dissolution method, *U.S.P.*; dissolution testing, effect of encapsulating powdered tablets

Kreuter, J., Speiser, P.P. and Prasad, N.K., *Second International Conference on Pharmaceutical Technology*, (Paris, APGI, June 3–5, 1980), 1980, *II*, 103–8

In vitro release of different dosage forms of 8-methoxy-psoralen

capsules, hard gelatin and tablets: 8-methoxypsoralen; dissolution method, stirred flask; dissolution testing, effect of formulation; formulation of contents, adsorbates, solid dispersions, solutions; 3.2.4.2

4.2.3.3 Comparative Dissolution of Products

Luzzi, L.A. and Needham, T.E., *J. pharm. Sci.*, 1973, *62*, 1907–8

Importance of considering variables when using magnetic basket dissolution apparatus

capsules, hard gelatin and tablets: butobarbitone sodium; dissolution method, magnetic basket

El-Yazigi, A. and Hikal, A.H., *Can. J. pharm. Sci.*, 1974, *9*, 19–23

In vitro studies of products containing levodopa using a continuous flow dissolution apparatus

capsules, hard gelatin and tablets: levodopa; capsule, products, content uniformity; dissolution method, continuous flow

Hardwidge, E.A., Sarapu, A.C. and Laughlin, W.C., *J. pharm. Sci.*, 1978, *67*, 1732–5

Comparison of operational characteristics of different dissolution testing systems

capsules, hard gelatin and tablets: tetracycline hydrochloride (capsules); dissolution method, rotating basket, rotating filter; dissolution testing, comparison of manufacturers

Cartwright, A.C., *J. Pharm. Pharmac.*, 1979, *31*, 434–40

Sources of variation during collaborative evaluation of in vitro dissolution tests for two solid preparations

capsules, hard gelatin and tablets: oxytetracycline (capsules); dissolution method, *B.P.* 1973 Addendum 1977; dissolution testing, effects of, apparatus inter-laboratory variations, vibration

Duru, C., Jacob, M., Puech, A., Slany, J. and Lasserre, Y., *Pharm. Acta Helv.*, 1979, *54*, 37–43

The preparation of different oral dosage forms of phenobarbitone base. In vitro control of the release rate of the active principle (in French)

capsules, hard gelatin, powders and tablets, sugar-coated: phenobarbitone: disintegration method, French Pharmacopoeia; dissolution method, beaker; dissolution, effects of, method of preparation of dosage forms, direct compression, wet granulation; dissolution testing, effect of test media; formulation of products, common

Warren, J.W., Shah, K.A., Benmaman, J.D., Freeman, D.B., Lewkowicz, R.T. and Friend, C.G., *Curr. ther. Res.*, 1979, *25*, 172–9

Variations among ten chlordiazepoxide hydrochloride 10-mg capsule products

capsules, hard gelatin: chlordiazepoxide hydrochloride; dissolution method, *U.S.P.* XIX; dissolution testing, results, cumulative release pattern, $T_{50\%}$; 3.8.3.1; 3.8.3.6

El-Yazigi, A., *Drug Dev. ind. Pharm.*, 1982, *8*, 911–21

Dissolution characteristics of capsule shells and drug release from commercial tetracycline-HCl capsules

capsules, hard gelatin: tetracycline hydrochloride; disintegration method, stirred flask; disintegration testing, measurement of shell rupture; dissolution method, *U.S.P.* XIX; dissolution testing, determination of dissolution rate constant, effects of, ionic strength and pH of dissolution medium, stirrer depth

4.2.3.4 Dissolution and Formulation

Aguiar, A.J., Zelmer, J.E. and Kinkel, A.W., *J. pharm. Sci.*, 1967, *56*, 1243–52

Deaggregation behavior of a relatively insoluble substituted benzoic acid and its sodium salt

capsules, hard gelatin, suspensions and tablets: benzoic acid, substituted derivative and sodium salt; deaggregation rate testing, effects of, capsule filling, test media, wetting agent; dissolution method, beaker; dissolution testing, effects of, capsule filling, test media, wetting agent; formulation of contents, wetting agent, surfactants

Withey, R.J. and Mainville, C.A., *J. pharm. Sci.*, 1969, *58*, 1120–6

A critical analysis of a capsule dissolution test

capsules, hard and soft gelatin: chloramphenicol; dissolution method, modified *U.S.P* disintegration apparatus; dissolution testing, comparison of products; formulation of contents, diluent, lactose; powder properties, drug particle size

Rowley, G. and Newton, J.M., *J. Pharm. Pharmac.*, 1970, *22*, 966–7

Limitations of liquid penetration in predicting the release of drugs from hard gelatin capsules

capsules, hard gelatin: ethinamate; dissolution method, beaker; powder properties, liquid penetration

Shah, P.T. and Moore, W.E., *J. pharm. Sci.*, 1970, *59*, 1034–6

Dissolution behaviour of commercial tablets extemporaneously converted to capsules

capsules, hard gelatin and tablets: acetylsalicylic acid, diphenhydramine, meprobamate; dissolution method, beaker; dissolution testing, effect of tablets packed in capsules

Newton, J.M., Rowley, G. and Törnblom, J.-F.V., *J. Pharm. Pharmac.*, 1971, *23*, 452–3

The effect of additives on the release of drug from hard gelatin capsules

capsules, hard gelatin: ethinamate; dissolution method, beaker; dissolution testing, capsule; dissolution testing, effects of, capsule filling, formulation, powder properties

Newton, J.M., Rowley, G. and Törnblom, J.-F.V., *J. Pharm. Pharmac.*, 1971, *23*, *Suppl.*, 156S-160S

Further studies on the effect of additives on the release of drug from hard gelatin capsules

capsules, hard gelatin: ethinamate; dissolution method, beaker; dissolution testing, effects of, capsule filling, formulation, powder properties; formulation of contents, diluent, lubricant, wetting agent; powder properties, capsule packing density

Hill, S.A., Seager, H. and Taskis, C.B., *J. Pharm. Pharmac.*, 1972, *24*, 152P-3P

Comparative dissolution rates of the anhydrous and trihydrate forms of ampicillin

capsules, hard gelatin: ampicillin; dissolution method, stirred flask; dissolution testing, effect of drug crystal form

Newton, J.M., *Pharm. Weekbl. Ned.*, 1972, *107*, 485–98

The release of drugs from hard gelatin capsules

capsules, hard gelatin: dissolution testing, effect of formulation of contents, review

Simmons, D.L., Frechette, M., Ranz, R.J., Chen, W.S. and Patel, N.K., *Can. J. pharm. Sci.*, 1972, *7*, 62–5

A rotating compartmentalized disk for dissolution rate determinations

capsules, hard gelatin and tablets: chlordiazepoxide; dissolution method, rotating disk, *U.S.N.F.* basket; dissolution testing, effect of formulation; formulation of contents, lubricant, magnesium stearate

Davies, J.E. and Fell, J.T., *J. Pharm. Pharmac.*, 1973, *25*, 431–2

The influence of starch and lactose on the release rates of drugs from hard gelatin capsules

capsules, hard gelatin: phenobarbitone, phenobarbitone sodium; dissolution method, beaker; formulation of contents, diluents, lactose, starch

Bell, S.P. and Fell, J.T., *Can. J. pharm. Sci.*, 1974, *9*, 119–20

The effect of starch concentration on the release of phenobarbitone from hard gelatin capsules

capsules, hard gelatin: phenobarbitone; dissolution method, beaker; dissolution testing, effect of formulation; formulation of contents, diluent, starch

Caldwell, H.C., *J. pharm. Sci.*, 1974, *63*, 770–3

Dissolution of lithium and magnesium from lithium carbonate capsules containing magnesium stearate

capsules, hard gelatin: lithium carbonate; dissolution method, *U.S.N.F.* XIII; dissolution testing, effects of, formulation, magnesium dissolution rate, surface tension of test media; product weight uniformity, comparison and effect of lubricants; 3.2.4.1

Newton, J.M. and Razzo, F.N., *J. Pharm. Pharmac.*, 1974, *26. Suppl.*, 30P–36P

The influence of additives on the *in vitro* release of drugs from hard gelatin capsules

capsules, hard gelatin: nitrofurantoin, nitrofurazone, oxytetracycline dihydrate, tetracycline hydrochloride; dissolution method, beaker; dissolution testing, effect of formulation; 3.2.4.1

Newton, J.M. and Rowley, G., assigned to Lilly Industries Ltd, *U.S. Patent* 3 859 431, 1975

Drug formulations

dissolution testing, effect of formulation; formulation of contents, diluent, sodium starch glycolate

Bobbé, D., Mathis, C., Stamm, A., Metziger, P. and Widmann, A., *First International Conference on Pharmaceutical Technology*, (Paris, APGI, May 31–June 2, 1977), 1977, *V*, 109–19

Study of the influence of several excipients and adjuvants on the dissolution rate of amidopyrine from soft gelatin capsules (in French)

capsules, soft gelatin: amidopyrine; dissolution method, Sartorius apparatus; dissolution testing, comparison of formulations; 3.3.3.2

Bobbé, D., Mathis, C., Stamm, A., Metziger, P. and Widmann, A., *Labo-Pharma Probl. Tech.*, 1977, *25*(268), 637–44

Study using the apparatus of Stricker on the influence of several excipients and adjuvants on the dissolution rate of iron salts from soft gelatin capsules (in French)

capsules, hard and soft gelatin and tablets, sugar-coated: ferrous fumarate, sulphate; dissolution method, Stricker; dissolution testing, comparison of dosage forms, effect of formulation

Cadórniga, R., Abad, M.C. and Camacho, M.A., *Cienc. ind. Farm.*, 1977, *9*, 178–82

The dissolution rate of medicines from gelatin capsules (in Spanish)

capsules, hard gelatin: acetylsalicylic acid, caffeine, phenacetin; dissolution method, beaker; dissolution testing, effects of, formulation, interaction between active ingredients

Dingwall, D. and Karanjah, D.S., *J. clin. Pharm.*, 1977, *2*, 5–11

Extemporaneous reduction of commercial capsule dosage – Macrodantin

capsules, hard gelatin: nitrofurantoin; dissolution method, modified *U.S.P.* rotating basket; dissolution testing, effects of, capsule fill, capsule shell, formulation, test media; formulation of contents, diluents, lactose, starch

Fell, J.T., Calvert, R.T. and Riley-Bentham, P., *First International Conference on Pharmaceutical Technology*, (Paris, APGI, May 31–June 2, 1977), 1977, *V*, 121–5

A study of the dissolution and bioavailability of a hydrophobic drug

capsules, hard gelatin: griseofulvin; dissolution method, beaker, modified; dissolution testing, effect of hydrophilic coating; formulation of contents, hydrophilic treatment, particle coating by granulation, hydroxypropylcellulose; powder properties, intrinsic dissolution rate, measurement by non-disintegrating disk

Murthy, K.S. and Samyn, J.C., *J. pharm. Sci.*, 1977, *66*, 1215–19

Effect of shear mixing on *in vitro* drug release of capsule formulations containing lubricants

capsules, hard gelatin: nitrofurantoin, procainamide hydrochloride; dissolution method, beaker; dissolution testing, effect of, processing conditions, mixer shear rates; formulation of contents, diluent, lactose, lubricants, magnesium lauryl sulphate, magnesium stearate

Newton, J.M. and Razzo, F.N., *J. Pharm. Pharmac.*, 1977, *29*, 205–8

The *in vitro* bioavailability of various drugs formulated as hard gelatin capsules

capsules, hard gelatin: imipramine, nitrofurantoin, nitrofurazone, oxytetracycline dihydrate, phenylbutazone, tetracycline hydrochloride; dissolution method, beaker; dissolution testing, effect of formulation; formulation of contents, diluents, lactose, sodium starch glycolate, starch, lubricant, magnesium stearate, wetting agent, sodium lauryl sulphate

Newton, J.M. and Razzo, F.N., *J. Pharm. Pharmac.*, 1977, *29*, 294–7

The influence of additives on the presentation of a drug in hard gelatin capsules

capsules, hard gelatin: nitrofurazone; dissolution method, modified beaker; dissolution testing, effect of formulation, statistical evaluation; formulation of contents, diluents, lactose, starch, lubricant, magnesium stearate, wetting agent, sodium lauryl sulphate

Ryder, J. and Thomas, A., *J. Pharm. Pharmac.*, 1977, *29*, *Suppl.*, 63P

A comparison of the effectiveness of several disintegrants in capsules of 4-ethoxycarbonylphenoxy-2′-pyridyl methane (BRL 10614)

capsules, hard gelatin: 4-ethoxycarbonylphenoxy-2′-pyridyl methane; dissolution method, stirred flask; dissolution testing, effects of, formulation, storage; filling machine, dosing tube mechanism; 3.2.4.1

Bastami, S.M. and Groves, M.J., *Int. J. Pharmaceut.*, 1978, *1*, 151–64

Some factors influencing the in vitro release of phenytoin from formulations

capsules, hard gelatin and tablets: phenytoin, phenytoin sodium; dissolution method, stirred flask; dissolution testing, effects of, drug particle size, formulation, pH test medium; formulation of contents, diluents, lactose, starch; powder properties, particle size

Geneidi, A.S., Ali, A.A. and Salama, R.B., *J. pharm, Sci.*, 1978, *67*, 114–16

Solid dispersions of nitrofurantoin, ethotoin, and coumarin with polyethylene glycol 6000 and their coprecipitates with povidone 25 000

capsules, hard gelatin: coumarin, ethotoin, nitrofurantoin; dissolution method, beaker; formulation of contents; solid dispersions, method of manufacture

Gurny, R., Boymond-Genoud, M. and Guitard, P., *J. Pharm. Belg.*, 1978, *33*, 6–10

Study of the influence of particle size and lactose on the dissolution of phenacetin and acetanilide capsules using a multiple regression method

capsules, hard gelatin: acetanilide, phenacetin; dissolution method, continuous flow; dissolution testing, effects of, drug particle size, formulation; formulation of contents, diluent, lactose; powder properties, particle size

Lerk, C.F., Lagas, M., Fell, J.T. and Nauta, P., *J. pharm. Sci.*, 1978, *67*, 935–9

Effect of hydrophilization of hydrophobic drugs on release rate from capsules

capsules, hard gelatin: hexobarbitone; coating materials, hydroxyethylcellulose, methycellulose; coating method, granulation; dissolution method, beaker; dissolution testing, effects of, hydrophilic coating of hydrophobic drug, surface tension of test medium; formulation of contents, hydrophilic coating; powder properties, contact angle, density, particle size

Mendes, R.W., Masih, S.Z. and Kanumuri, R.R., *J. pharm. Sci.*, 1978, *67*, 1613–16

Effect of formulation and process variables on bioequivalency of nitrofurantoin I: Preliminary studies

capsules, hard gelatin and tablets, chewable and standard: nitrofurantoin; dissolution method, beaker; dissolution testing, effects of, drug particle size, formulation of contents; 3.2.4.1

Kassem, A.A., Zaki, S.A., Mursi, N.M. and Tayel, S.A., *Pharmazie*, 1979, *34*, 86–91

Effect of certain additives on the dissolution rate of chloramphenicol

capsules, hard gelatin: chloramphenicol; dissolution method, beaker; dissolution testing, effect of formulation; formulation of contents, solid dispersions; 3.2.4.1

Kassem, A.A., Zaki, S.A., Mursi, N.M. and Tayel, S.A., *Pharm. Ind., Berl.*, 1979, *41*, 390–3

Chloramphenicol solid dispersion system I

capsules, hard gelatin: chloramphenicol; dissolution method, beaker; dissolution testing, effect of formulation; formulation of contents, solid dispersions, carbowaxes, polyvinylpyrrolidones; solid dispersions, method of manufacture

Merle, C., Artaud, M. and Guyot-Hermann, A.M., *Farmaco, Edn prat.*, 1979, *34*, 210–19

Influence of glidants on the dissolution rate of acetylsalicylic acid in hard gelatin capsules (in French)

capsules, hard gelatin: acetylsalicylic acid; dissolution method, continuous flow; dissolution testing, effects of formulation; 3.2.4.1

Ammar, H.O., Kassem, M.A., Salama, H.A. and El-Ridy, M.S., *Pharm. Ind., Berl.*, 1980, *42*, 757–60

On the dissolution of digoxin

capsules, hard gelatin, powders and tablets: digoxin; dissolution method, beaker, rotating basket; dissolution testing, capsule filled with solid dispersion, powders, effect of particle size, solid dispersions, effect of formulation; dissolution testing, comparison of capsules and tablets; formulation of solid dispersions, polyethylene glycols, polyvinylpyrrolidones

Boymond, C. and Mathis, C., *Second International Conference on Pharmaceutical Technology*, (Paris, APGI, June 3–5, 1980), 1980, *IV*, 93–103

A study of the influence of the formulation on the release of ephedrine hydrochloride from hard gelatin capsules (in French)

capsules, hard gelatin: ephedrine hydrochloride; dissolution method, stirred flask; dissolution testing, effects of, capsule preparation, size, formulation, powder properties; stability, effect of formulation; 3.2.4.2

Cuine, A., Mathis, C. and Stamm, A., *Second International Conference on Pharmaceutical Technology*, (Paris, APGI, June 3–5, 1980), 1980, *I*, 66–76

Hard gelatin capsules with paste contents: study of the rheological properties and *in vitro* release of active principles (in French)

capsules, hard gelatin: acetylsalicylic acid, clofibrate, sodium salicylate; dissolution method, Sartorius apparatus, *U.S.P.* XVII modified; dissolution testing, effect of formulation; 3.2.4.2

Shek, E., Ghani, M., and Jones, R.E., *J. pharm. Sci.*, 1980, *69*, 1135–42

Simplex search on optimisation of capsule formulation

capsules, hard gelatin: dissolution method, stirred flask; dissolution testing, T_8 and T_{30} effects of formulation of contents; formulation, mathematical optimisation technique, simplex method, dissolution rate; 3.2.4.1

Walker, S.E., Ganley, J.A., Bedford, K. and Eaves, T., *J. Pharm. Pharmac.*, 1980, *32*, 389–93

The filling of molten and thixotropic formulations into hard gelatin capsules

capsules, hard gelatin: triamterene; dissolution method, *U.S.P.*; dissolution testing, comparison of liquid and powder formulations; formulation of contents, solid dispersion and solid solution; 3.2.3.4; 3.2.4.2; 4.2.3.6

York, P., *Drug Dev. ind. Pharm.*, 1980, *6*, 605–27

Studies of the effect of powder moisture content on drug release from hard gelatin capsules

capsules, hard gelatin: barbitone, sodium salt; dissolution method, modified beaker; dissolution testing, effect of powder properties; formulation of contents, diluents, lactose, maize starch; powder properties, contact angle, powder bed, liquid penetration and permeability; 3.8.3.4

Bremecker, K.-D. and List, P.H., *Pharm. Ind., Berl.*, 1981, *43*, 1026–8

The influence of relative humidity on drug release from hard gelatin capsules in vitro (in German)

capsules, hard gelatin: chlordiazepoxide, nortriptyline hydrochloride, pericyazine, procaine hydrochloride; capsule, contents and shells, moisture content, effect of relative humidity of storage; capsule shells, diffusion of contents, effects of hydrophilic/hydrophobic materials, moisture content; dissolution method, flow through cell; dissolution testing, effect of moisture content of capsule contents and shells

Doelker, E., Doelker, C. and Mordier, D., *J. Pharm. Belg.*, 1981, *36*, 404–11

The role of wetting on the release of hydrophobic drugs from hard gelatin capsules. I. Liquid diffusion through the wall and capillary penetration into the powder bed (in French)

capsules, hard gelatin: phenacetin; dissolution testing, effects of, powder wetting, test medium; formulation of contents; powder properties, particle size, wetting characteristics; 4.2.2.1

Mehta, A.M. and Augsburger, L.L., *Int. J. Pharmaceut.*, 1981, *7*, 327–34

A preliminary study of the effect of slug hardness on drug dissolution from hard gelatin capsules filled on an automatic capsule-filling machine

capsules, hard gelatin: hydrochlorothiazide; dissolution method, stirred flask; dissolution testing, effects of, formulation of contents, powder slug hardness; formulation of contents, diluents, lactose, microcrystalline cellulose, lubricant, magnesium stearate; 3.2.3.3

Miyazaki, S., Inoue, H. and Nadai, T., *Pharmazie*, 1981, *36*, 482–4

Effects of antacids on the dissolution of minocycline and demethylchlortetracycline from capsules

capsules, hard gelatin: demeclocycline, minocycline, antacids, adsorption and elution properties; antacids, aluminium silicate, magnesium aluminosilicate, magnesium trisilicate; dissolution method, rotating basket; dissolution testing, effect of antacids

Shah, K.A., Warren, J.W., Onwuelezi, G., Benmaman, J.D. and Monk, C.M., *Drug Dev. ind. Pharm.*, 1981, *7*, 683–91

In vitro release of hydrochlorothiazide from capsule formulations

capsules, hard gelatin: hydrochlorothiazide; dissolution method, rotating basket; dissolution testing, effect of formulation; formulation of contents, diluents, calcium hydrogen phosphate, lactose, maize starch, microcrystalline cellulose; product, content and weight uniformity

Akbuǧa, J., Gülhan, S. and Bayraktar-Alpmen, G., *Pharmazie*, 1983, *38*, 478–80

Studies on flufenamic acid capsules and tablets

capsules, hard gelatin and tablets: flufenamic acid; disintegration testing, comparison of products (capsules); dissolution method, rotating basket; dissolution testing, comparisons of, dosage forms, products (capsules); formulation of contents, diluents, lactose, maize starch, lubricant, magnesium stearate, surfactant, sodium lauryl sulphate

Mathis, C. and Cuiné, A., *Labo-Pharma Probl. Tech.*, 1983, *31*(337) 935–43

Formulation, stability and *in vitro* availability of active principles as solutions or viscous suspensions filled in hard gelatin capsules (in French)

capsules, hard gelatin: acetylsalicylic acid, ferrous sulphate, sodium salicylate; dissolution method, modified disintegration apparatus; dissolution testing, effects of formulation, comparison of excipients; 3.2.4.2

Muhammad, N.A.H. and Newton, J.M., *J. Pharm. Pharmac.*, 1983, *35*, 345–9

The influence of pH of dissolution fluid and particle size of drug on the in-vitro release of drug from hard gelatin capsules

capsules, hard gelatin: acetysalicylic acid; dissolution method, modified beaker; dissolution testing, effects of pH test media, powder properties; powder properties, particle size

Armstrong, N.A., James, K.C. and Pugh, W.K.L., *J. Pharm. Pharmac.*, 1984, *36*, 357–60

An in-vitro investigation of drug availability from lipophilic solutions

capsules, soft gelatin: 4-hydroxybenzoic acid; dissolution method, partition/permeation apparatus; dissolution testing, comparison of encapsulated and free solutions, effects of, capsule shell, formulation of contents; formulation of contents, solvents, isopropyl myristate, 1-octanol

Armstrong, N.A., James, K.C. and Pugh, W.K.L., *J. Pharm. Pharmac.*, 1984, *36*, 361–5

Drug migration into soft gelatin capsule shells and its effect on in-vitro availability

capsules, soft gelatin: acetomenaphthone, ephedrine, 4-hydroxybenzoic acid, phenobarbitone; dissolution method, partition/permeation apparatus; dissolution testing, effects of, capsule shell, drug, partition coefficient and solubility, formulation of contents; drug migration in capsule shell, effect of manufacturing process; formulation of contents, solvents, isopropyl myristate, 1-octanol

Djimbo, M. and Möes, A.J., *J. Pharm. Belg.*, 1984, *39*, 36–42

Release of drugs formulated as hard pastes filled into hard gelatin capsules. Part 1. Physical properties and *in vitro* testing

capsules, hard gelatin and tablets: acetylsalicylic acid, theophylline; dissolution method, paddle; dissolution method, intrinsic value, theophylline products, rotating disk; dissolution testing, comparison of dosage forms, effect of formulation; formulation of contents, semi-solids; 3.2.4.2

Elbary, A.A., Fadel, H.M. and Nour, S.A., *Pharmazie*, 1984, *39*, 110–12

Dissolution rate of chloramphenicol from hard gelatin capsules as a function of type of adjuvants and methods of granulation

capsules, hard gelatin: chloramphenicol; dissolution method, rotating basket; dissolution testing, comparison of excipients, effects of, content type, formulation; formulation of contents, granules, by dry and wet granulation

Newton, J.M. and Muhammad, N.A.H., *J. Pharm. Pharmac.*, 1984, *36*, 42–4

The influence of agitation intensity, particle size and pH of dissolution fluid on the in-vitro release of drug from hard gelatin capsules

capsules, hard gelatin: acetylsalicylic acid; dissolution method, modified beaker; dissolution testing, effects of, agitation intensity, pH test media, powder properties; powder properties, particle size

Stamm, A., Boymond, C. and Mathis, C., *Drug Dev. ind. Pharm.*, 1984, *10*, 355–80

Some aspects of the formulation of hard gelatin capsules

capsules, hard gelatin and tablets: griseofulvin, tetracycline hydrochloride; dissolution method, paddle; dissolution testing, comparison of dosage forms; effects of, formulation of contents, porosity of fill; 3.2.4.1

Chowhan, Z.T. and Chi, L.-H., *Pharm. Technol.*, 1985, *9*(3), 84, 86, 90, 92, 94–97

Drug-excipient interactions resulting from powder mixing, I; Possible mechanisms of interaction with starch and its effect on drug dissolution

capsules, hard gelatin: ketorolac tromethamine; dissolution method, paddle; dissolution testing, effects of, formulation of contents, lubricant mixing; powder properties, particle interactions, scanning electron microscopy; 3.2.4.1; 4.2.2.1

Chowhan, Z.T. and Chi, L.-H., *Pharm. Technol.* 1985, *9*(4), 30, 32–33, 36, 38–41

Drug-excipient interactions resulting from powder mixing, II: Possible mechanisms of interaction with crospovidone and its effect on in vitro dissolution

capsules, hard gelatin: ketorolac tromethamine; dissolution method, paddle; dissolution testing, effects of, drug particle size, lubricant mixing; powder properties, particle interactions, scanning electron microscopy; 3.2.4.1; 4.2.2.1

Combes, A., Bonnet, L. and Rouffiac, R., *Pharm. Acta Helv.*, 1985, *60*, 203–8

The influence of excipients on the rate of release of two non-steroidal anti-inflammatory drugs from capsules (in French)

capsules, hard gelatin: acetylsalicylic acid, indomethacin; dissolution method, continuous flow; dissolution testing, effects of formulation of contents, excipient salt type; formulation of contents, diluents, calcium and sodium salts of glucuronic, lactic and sulphuric acid, lactose; results, factorial analysis

De Beukelaer, P. and Van Ooteghem, M., *s.t.p. Pharma*, 1985, *1*, 956–61

Influence of powder bed porosity and wettability on liquid penetration and on drug release of powder mixtures filled into hard gelatin capsules

capsules, hard gelatin: dissolution method, beaker; drug availability, effects of, capsule content properties, liquid penetration, porosity, wettability, formulation of contents; formulation of contents, diluent, lactose; powder properties, liquid penetration, application of Washburn equation

Anno, E.M. and Rees, J.E., *Fourth International Conference on Pharmaceutical Technology*, (Paris, APGI, June 3–5, 1986), 1986, *V*, 61–69

Release of phenytoin sodium from capsules containing two- and three-component mixes capsules, hard gelatin: phenytoin sodium; dissolution method, paddle; dissolution testing, effect of, formulation of contents, method of mixing of contents; drug, solubility and swelling; 3.2.4.1

Ari-Ulubelen, A., Akbuğa, J., Bayraktar-Alpmen, G. and Gülhan, *Pharm. Ind., Berl.*, 1986, *48*, 393–395

Effect of formulation factors on the in vitro dissolution characteristics of phenytoin sodium capsules

capsules, hard gelatin: phenytoin sodium; dissolution method, rotating basket; dissolution testing, effects of, formulation of contents, method of preparation, powder mixing, slugging; formulation of contents, comparison of excipients and lubricants; 3.2.4.1

Bowtle, W.J., *Br. J. pharm. Pract.*, 1986, *8*, 307–8

Semi-solid matrix capsules

capsules, hard gelatin: indomethacin; dissolution testing, effect of formulation; formulation of contents, semi-solid, excipients differing HLB values; 3.2.3.4; 3.8.3.4

Chowhan, Z.T. and Chi, L.-H., *J. pharm. Sci.*, 1986, *75*, 534–541

Drug-excipient interactions resulting from powder mixing. III: Solid state properties and their effect on drug dissolution

capsules, hard gelatin: prednisone; dissolution method, paddle; dissolution testing, effects of, formulation of contents, lubricant mixing; powder properties, particle interactions, scanning electron microscopy; 3.2.4.1; 4.2.2.1

Chowhan, Z.T. and Chi, L.-H., *J. pharm. Sci.*, 1986, *75*, 542–545

Drug-excipient interactions resulting from powder mixing, IV: Role of lubricants and their effect on in vitro dissolution

capsules, hard gelatin: ketorolac tromethamine; dissolution method, paddle; dissolution testing, comparison of lubricants, effect of lubricant mixing; powder properties, particle interactions, scanning electron microscopy; 3.2.4.1; 4.2.2.1

Mathis, C. and Heimendinger, J., *Fourth International Conference on Pharmaceuticl Technology*, (Paris, APGI, June 3–5, 1986), 1986, *V*, 90–98

Test of programming the release of active principles from pasty excipients in hard gelatin capsules (in French)

capsules, hard gelatin: aspirin; dissolution method, paddle; dissolution testing, effects of formulation; 3.2.4.2

Matthieu, A.M., van Ooteghem, M. and Ludwig, A., *Fourth International Conference on Pharmaceutical Technology*, (Paris, APGI, June 3–5, 1986), 1986, *V*, 55–60

The influence of the solubility of adjuvants on the release of hydrophobic medicaments in hard gelatin capsules (in French)

capsules, hard gelatin: phenacetin; disintegration and dissolution method, beaker: disintegration and dissolution testing,

effects of, composition, pH and viscosity of test medium, formulation of contents; diluent and drug solubility, effect of pH; formulation of contents, diluents, dicalcium phosphate, lactose, saccharose, sodium chloride

4.2.3.5 Dissolution of Enteric Capsules

Jacob, M., Duru, C. and Puech, A., *Sciences Tech. pharm.*, 1979, *8*, 93–7

Preparation of fluoride dosage forms. In vitro control of the release of the active principle (in French)

capsules, hard gelatin and tablets, sugar-coated: sodium fluoride; capsule enteric coating, cellulose acetate phthalate; capsule, fill-weight and uniformity of fill; disintegration testing; dissolution method, Erweka; dissolution testing, comparison of dosage form, effect of enteric coating

4.2.3.6 Dissolution of Slow-release Capsules

Souder, J.C. and Ellenbogen, W.C., *Drug Stand.*, 1958, *26*, 77–83

Laboratory control of dextro amphetamine sulfate sustained release capsules

capsules, hard gelatin: dexamphetamine sulphate; dissolution method, rotating bottle

Royal, J., *Drug Stand.*, 1959, *27*, 1–6

A comparison of *in vitro* rates of release of several brands of dextro amphetamine sulfate sustained release capsules

capsules, hard gelatin: dexamphetamine sulphate; dissolution method, modified *U.S.P.* XV disintegration apparatus

Vliet, E.B., *Drug Stand.*, 1959, *27*, 97–9

A suggested *in vitro* procedure for measuring the rate of drug release from timed release tablets and capsules

capsules, hard gelatin and tablets: dissolution method, modified *U.S.P.* disintegration apparatus

Krueger, E.O. and Vliet, E.B., *J. pharm. Sci.*, 1962, *51*, 181–4

In vitro testing of timed release tablets and capsules

capsules, hard gelatin and tablets: dissolution method, rotating bottle; dissolution testing, collaborative study, sustained-release preparations

Chiaramonti, D., Giana, C., Innocenti, F. and Segre, A.D., *Farmaco, Edn prat.*, 1970, *25*, 257–62

Proposed method for the analysis of prolonged release medicines (in Italian)

capsules, hard gelatin: dissolution method, rotating flask; dissolution testing, effect of change in pH test medium; product, sustained-release granules

Goldman, R., *Drug Cosmet. Ind.*, 1970, *107*(3), 52–64, 151–6

Sustained release capsules

capsules, hard gelatin: review

Widmann, A., Eiden, F. and Tenczer, J., *Arzneimittel-Forsch.*, 1970, *20*, 283–9

Release of drugs from Depot soft gel capsules (in German)

capsules, soft gelatin: chlorpheniramine maleate, codeine; capsules shell, non-disintegrating; dissolution method, beaker; dissolution testing, effect of change in pH test medium, prolonged-release preparations; 4.4.3

Berkowitz, R.D., *Hosp. Pharm.*, 1971, *6*, 8–16

A study of in vitro release rates of sustained-release dextro amphetamine sulfate capsules

capsules, hard gelatin: dexamphetamine sulphate; dissolution method, *U.S.N.F.* XII; formulation of contents, sustained-release preparation

Schwarz, R., *ZentBl. Pharm.*, 1971, *110*, 1127–36

On the testing of sustained-release preparations (in German)

capsules, hard and soft gelatin: dissolution method, continuous flow, rotating bottle; dissolution testing, comparison of methods

Baichwal, M.R. and Yelvigi, M.S., *Indian J. Pharm.*, 1973, *35*, 146–50

Sustained release capsules using polyglycerol esters

capsules, hard gelatin: acetylsalicylic acid; dissolution method, modified disintegration apparatus; formulation of contents, polyethylene glycol esters

Bloch, R., Loebel, E. and Loschever, M., *German (BRD) Patent (Offen.)* 2 627 113, 1977

Capsule for controlled release of drugs

capsules, hard gelatin: capsule shell solubility, reduction with cross-linking agent; capsule sealing, epoxy resins

Steinbach, D. and Möller, H., *Int. J. Pharmaceut.*, 1978, *1*, 197–204

Investigations into the accuracy of dosage and release of active drug from sustained release preparations of isosorbide dinitrate

capsules, hard gelatin and tablets, coated and plain: isosorbide dinitrate; content uniformity, DAB 7, *U.S.P.* XIX; dissolution method, Diffutest and *U.S.N.F.* XIV; dissolution testing, prolonged-release preparations; product weight uniformity, DAB 7, *U.S.P.* XIX

Matheson, L.E., *Drug Dev. ind. Pharm.*, 1979, *5*, 459–71

Comparison of in vitro release rates of multisource sustained-release papaverine hydrochloride products

capsules, hard gelatin: papaverine hydrochloride; dissolution method, rotating bottle; dissolution testing, comparison between lots and manufacturers

D'Onofrio, G.P., Oppenheim, R.C. and Bateman, N.E., *Int. J. Pharmaceut.*, 1979, *2*, 91–9

Encapsulated microcapsules

capsules, soft gelatin: acetylsalicylic acid; dissolution method, continuous flow; dissolution testing, effects of, coating, drug dose; 3.3.3.2

Baggesen, S. and Bechgaard, H., *Pharm. Acta Helv.*, 1980, *55*, 312–15

In vitro evaluation of two controlled release propoxyphene hydrochloride formulations. Influence of the composition of dissolution media on drug release.

capsules, hard gelatin: dextropropoxyphene hydrochloride; dissolution method, modified rotating bottle; dissolution testing, effects of dissolution medium, buffer composition, ionic strength, pH, surface tension; experimental procedure, factorial experiment, statistical analysis; formulation of contents, pellets

Walker, S.E., Ganley, J.A., Bedford, K. and Eaves, T., *J. Pharm. Pharmac.*, 1980, *32*, 389–93

The filling of molten and thixotropic formulations into hard gelatin capsules

capsules, hard gelatin: nomifensine hydrogen maleate; dissolution method, *U.S.P.*; dissolution testing, effect of formulation; 3.2.3.4; 3.2.4.2; 4.2.3.4

Yalabik-Kaş, H.S., *Drug Dev. ind. Pharm.*, 1983, *9*, 1047–60

Microencapsulation and in vitro dissolution of oxazepam from ethyl cellulose microcapsules

capsules, hard gelatin: oxazepam; dissolution method, stirred flask; dissolution testing, effects of, formulation, test media, kinetic analysis; formulation of contents, controlled release, microencapsulation, ethylcellulose

Simons, K.J., Plett, K.D. and Simons, F.E.R., *Pharm. Acta Helv.*, 1984, *59*, 145–8

Dissolution studies of some regular and sustained-release dyphylline dosage forms

capsules, hard gelatin and tablets, standard and sustained-release: diprophylline; dissolution method, rotating basket; dissolution testing, effect of test media, simulated gastric and intestinal fluids

Paris, L. and Stamm, A., *s.t.p. Pharma*, 1985, *1*, 412–18

Study of the influence of pH on the in vitro dissolution of prolonged-release theophylline preparations (in French)

capsules, hard gelatin and tablets: theophylline; dissolution method, paddle; dissolution testing, comparison of dosage forms, effect pH test media; test media, pH change with time

Schmidt, P.C. and Stockebrand, B., *Pharm. Res.*, 1986, *3*, 230–34

Capsules with prolonged action, II. Capsule filling by a gelation process

capsules, soft gelatin: codeine, theophylline; dissolution method, paddle; dissolution testing, comparison of drugs, effects of; formulation; nature of matrix; 3.3.3.2

Schmidt, P.C. and Stockebrand, B., *Pharm. Res.*, 1986, *3*, 235–39

Capsules with prolonged action, III. Release of active ingredients from cast films capsules, soft gelatin: indomethacin, nifedipine, theophylline; dissolution method, paddle; dissolution testing, comparison with model systems; drug release, model systems, cast films, partition and permeation studies; drug release from membranes, effects of, film thickness, formulation, test conditions; formulation of membranes

4.2.3.7 Dissolution Methodology

Needham, T.E. and Luzzi, L.A., *J. pharm. Sci.*, 1974, *63*, 925–8

Comparison of dissolution profiles of tablets and capsules from the U.S.P., Levy, and magnetic basket methods

capsules, hard gelatin and tablets: butobarbitone sodium; dissolution methods, beaker, magnetic basket, *U.S.P.* XVIII

Cakiryildiz, C., Mehta, P.J., Rahmen, W. and Schoenleber, D., *J. pharm. Sci.*, 1975, *64*, 1692–7

Dissolution studies with a multichannel continuous-flow apparatus

capsules, hard gelatin: powders and tablets: tetracycline hydrochloride; dissolution methods, continuous flow, rotating basket

Brossard, D., Massoum, R., Poelman, M.C. and Chaumeil, J.C., *First International Conference on Pharmaceutical Technology*, (Paris, APGI, May 31–June 2, 1977). 1977, *V*, 182–93

Dissolution of solid oral dosage forms: critical study of two apparatus (in French)

capsules, hard gelatin, granules, powders and tablets: nitrofurantoin; dissolution methods, continuous flow, stirred flask; dissolution testing, comparison of dosage forms, effect of apparatus, speed of flow and stirring

Carstensen, J.T., Lai, T.Y.-F. and Prasad, V.K., *J. pharm. Sci.*, 1978, *67*, 1303–7

U.S.P. dissolution IV: Comparison of methods

capsules, hard gelatin and tablets: nitrofurantoin; dissolution methods, rotating filter, *U.S.P.*, rotating basket, disintegration apparatus, paddle; dissolution testing, comparison of dosage forms, effect of apparatus variables

Pharmaceutical Manufacturers' Association of Tokyo, *Iyakuhin kenkyu*, 1978, *9*, 573–80

Studies on dissolution method for tablets and capsules (in Japanese)

capsules, hard gelatin and tablets: indomethacin; dissolution methods, *U.S.P.* XIX methods I and II, modified disintegration apparatus (Jpn); dissolution testing, effect of inter-laboratory variations

Cartwright, A.C., *Drug Dev. ind. Pharm.*, 1979, *5*, 277–91

Practical aspects of dissolution testing

capsules and tablets: dissolution method, rotating basket; dissolution method, automatic sampling system, use of dissolution calibrators; dissolution testing, identification and review of test variables

Brossard, D., Massoum, R., Poelman, M.C. and Chaumeil, J.C., *Second International Conference on Pharmaceutical Technology*, (Paris, APGI, June 3–5, 1980), 1980, *II*, 119–33

Applications of the technique of continuous flux and of Poole's flask to different oral dosage forms: Study of hard gelatin capsules (in French)

capsules, hard gelatin: nitrofurantoin; dissolution methods, continuous flow, stirred flask; dissolution testing, effect of capsule holder, formulation of contents; dissolution testing, results, dissolution efficiency, reproducibility, sensitivity; formulation of contents, diluents, lubricants

Langenbucher, F. and Moeller, H., *Drugs Germ.*, 1981, *24*, 131–5

Possible improvements of the U.S.P. XX dissolution test standards

capsules and tablets: dissolution method, *U.S.P.* XX; dissolution testing, effects of, equipment variation, sampling techniques; dissolution testing, floating products, metal sinker (capsules)

Koch, H.P., Alcorn, G. and Ritschell, W.A., *Pharmazie*, 1983, *38*, 233–5

Comparison of two-dissolution apparatuses: Rotating basket versus rotating flask. Correlation of data from four commercial theophylline prolonged release dosage forms.

capsules, hard gelatin and tablets: theophylline; dissolution method, rotating basket, rotating flask; dissolution testing, comparisons of, method, products

Möller, H., *Pharm. Ind., Berl.*, 1983, *45*, 617–22

Dissolution testing of different dosage forms using the flow-through method

capsules, hard and soft gelatin, powders, suppositories and tablets: benzobromarone, isosorbide dinitrate, tetracycline; dissolution method, continuous flow, paddle; dissolution testing, comparison of methods, effects of formulation

Herzfeldt, C.D., *Pharm. Technol.*, 1984, *8*(9), 70–6

Automated dissolution testing of indomethacin capsules and tablets

capsules, hard gelatin and tablets: indomethacin; dissolution method, paddle, rotating basket, dissolution standards, *U.S.P.* XX, acceptance criteria; dissolution testing, automation, comparison of dosage forms, products, test methods

Baichwal, M.R., Deshpande, S.G. and Shetty, U.C., *Drug Dev. ind. Pharm.*, 1985, *11*, 1639–56

Comparative evaluation of four dissolution apparatus

capsules, hard gelatin: dissolution methods, basket and paddle, paddle, rotating basket, rotating basket with paddle; dissolution testing, comparison of methods, effect of agitation intensity; formulation of contents, pellets

Gander, B., Ventouras, K., Gurny, R. and Doelker, E., *Int. J. Pharmaceut.*, 1985, *27*, 117–24

In vitro dissolution medium with supramicellar surfactant concentration and its relevance for in vivo absorption

capsules, hard gelatin and tablets: palmitoylcatechin; disintegration method, *U.S.P.*; disintegration testing, comparison of dosage forms, effect of test media; dissolution method, paddle; dissolution testing, comparison of dosage forms, effect of test media

Pandit, N.K., Strykowski, J.M., McNally, E.J. and Waldbillig, A.M., *Drug Dev. ind. Pharm.*, 1985, *11*, 1797–1818

Surfactant solutions as media for dissolution testing of a poorly water-soluble drug

capsules, hard gelatin: 4-(4-biphenylyl-butanol); dissolution method, beaker; dissolution testing, effects of test media; drug solubility, effects of surfactants; surfactants, polyoxyethylene lauryl ether, sodium dodecyl sulphate; test media, addition of surfactants

Machida, Y., Tokumura, T., Komuro, S., Tsushima, Y., Tatsuishi, K., Kayano, M. and Nagai, T., *Chem. pharm. Bull., Tokyo*, 1986, *34*, 2637–41

A new method of dissolution testing for oily drug preparations using an improved apparatus

capsules, soft gelatin and tablets: d-α-tocopherol; dissolution method, modified paddle; dissolution testing, effects of, apparatus configuration, test media; dissolution testing, lipophilic materials

4.2.3.8 Dissolution and Storage

Akbufa, J., Ari-Ulubelen, A. and Bayraktar-Alpmen, G., *Pharmazie*, 1984, *39*, 695–6

Effect of relative humidity and ageing on drug release. Part 2: Experimental phenytoin sodium capsules

capsules, hard gelatin: phenytoin sodium; dissolution method, rotating basket; dissolution testing, effects of, formulation of contents, storage conditions; formulation of contents, lactose and magnesium stearate; storage conditions, humidity, RH 75% and 95%, time 2, 4 and 8 weeks

Martin, E.D., Frazer, R.J.L. and Camens, I., *Med. J. Aust.*, 1985, *143*, 634–5

Storage of phenytoin capsules

capsules, hard gelatin: phenytoin sodium; dissolution method, rotating basket; dissolution testing, effect of storage, comparison with standard capsules; drug clinical effect, effect of product storage; storage conditions, tropical

Rubino, J.T., Halterlein, L.M. and Blanchard, J., *Int. J. Pharmaceut.*, 1985, *26*, 165–74

The effects of ageing on the dissolution of phenytoin sodium capsule formulations

capsules, hard gelatin: phenytoin sodium; dissolution method, rotating basket; dissolution testing, effects of, formulation of contents, storage conditions; formulation of contents, excipients, diluents and diluent/drug ratio; pharmacokinetic analysis; storage conditions, humidity, RH, 11% and 67%, time 2 and 8 weeks

4.2.4 Disintegration/Dissolution Correlation

Sandell, E. and Eckemark, K.-E., *Acta pharm. suec.*, 1966, *3*, 235–9

Release of potassium chloride from hard gelatin capsules

capsules, hard gelatin: potassium bicarbonate, potassium chloride; disintegration testing, Paikoff and Drumm; dissolution method, beaker

Newton, J.M. and Rowley, G., *J. Pharm. Pharmac.*, 1970, *22*, *Suppl.*, 163S–8S

On the release of drug from hard gelatin capsules

capsules, hard gelatin: ethinamate; disintegration testing, effect of filling, particle size; dissolution method, beaker; powder properties, capsule powder bed permeability measurement

Samyn, J.C. and Jung, W.Y., *J. pharm. Sci.*, 1970, *59*, 169–75

In vitro dissolution from several experimental capsule formulations

capsules, hard gelatin: disintegration method, *U.S.P.* tablet test; disintegration testing, effect of formulation, diluents, disintegrants, lubricants; dissolution method, modified *U.S.P.* disintegration apparatus; dissolution testing, effects of, formulation, powder properties; powder properties, packing density, liquid penetration measurement, viscosity of powder blends, determination; 3.2.4.1

Sandell, E., Eriksson, K. and Mellström, G., *Acta pharm. suec.*, 1970, *7*, 559–66

A disintegration test for evaluation of drug availability from tablets and capsules

capsules, hard gelatin and tablets: chloramphenicol, indomethacin, tetracycline; disintegration method, oscillating tube with sieves; dissolution method, beaker

Siegfried, B., *Schweiz. ApothZtg*, 1970, *108*, 178–80

Comparative estimation of the oral dosage forms, capsule and pill, an example of a standard sedative capsule and pill (in German)

capsules, hard gelatin and pills: methylphenobarbitone; disintegration method, *Swiss P.* VI; dissolution method, beaker; dissolution testing, effect of storage; formulation, contents; product weight uniformity

Khalil, S.A. and Ali, L.M.M., *Acta pharm. suec.*, 1972, *9*, 563–72

Some formulation factors affecting disintegration and dissolution of chloramphenicol capsules

capsules, hard gelatin: chloramphenicol; disintegration method, *B.P.*; dissolution method, modified *B.P.* disintegration apparatus; powder properties, powder beds, liquid penetration measurements; 3.2.4.1

Caldwell, H.C. and Westlake, W.J., *Can. J. pharm. Sci.*, 1973, *8*, 50–3

Magnesium lauryl sulfate: soluble lubricant

capsules, hard gelatin and tablets: lithium carbonate; disintegration method, *U.S.N.F.* XIII Method II; disintegration testing, effect of formulation, comparison of lubricants; dissolution method, modified *U.S.N.F.* XIII disintegration; dissolution testing, effect of formulation, comparison of lubricants; 3.2.4.1; 3.8.3.6

Goodhart, F.W., McCoy, R.H. and Ninger, F.C., *J. pharm. Sci.*, 1973, *62*, 304–10

New *in vitro* disintegration and dissolution test method for tablets and capsules

capsules, hard gelatin and tablets: disintegration method, modified beaker, *U.S.P.*; dissolution method, modified beaker, *U.S.P.* XVIII disintegration apparatus; dissolution testing, effect of variation in test conditions; 3.2.4.1

Khalil, S.A.H. and Ali, L.M.M., *Indian J. Pharm.*, 1973, *35*, 59–62

Effect of dissolution medium and moisture content of the powder on the dissolution of chloramphenicol capsules

capsules, hard gelatin: chloramphenicol; disintegration method, *B.P.*; dissolution method, *B.P.* disintegration apparatus; dissolution testing, effects of, capsule contents, moisture content, test media

Cox, H.L.M., Breimer, D.D. and Freeke, G., *Pharm. Weekbl. Ned.*, 1974, *109*, 1018–26

In vitro testing of the release of chloral hydrate from soft gelatin capsules (in Dutch)

capsules, soft gelatin: chloral hydrate; disintegration testing, enteric-coated and untreated capsules; dissolution method, beaker; dissolution testing, comparison, enteric-coated and untreated capsules; dissolution testing, simulation of intestinal pH changes

Weyers, W. and Gebhart, U., *Pharm. Acta Helv.*, 1976, *51*, 233–7

Comparative examination of gastrointestinal absorption of tetracycline preparations (in German)

capsules, hard and soft gelatin and tablets, film- and sugar-coated: tetracycline hydrochloride; disintegration method, *Swiss P.* VI; dissolution method, Dibbern; dissolution testing, effect of pH on absorption

Merle, C., Mangin, C. and Guyot-Hermann, A.M., *Bull. Soc. Pharm. Lille*, 1977, *33*, 87–94

Trials with a continuous flow dissolution apparatus. Application to the study of the influence of powder packing in hard gelatin capsules (in French)

capsules, hard gelatin: acetylsalicylic acid, sodium salicylate; disintegration method, *U.S.P.* XVIII; disintegration testing, effect of capsule size/powder packing; dissolution method, continuous flow; dissolution testing, effects of, capsule size, powder packing

Grakovskaya, L.K., Nesterova, L.Y., Okhotnikova, V.F., Zak, A.F., Ermolova, O.B. and Batuashvili, T.A., *Antibiotiki*, 1978, *23*, 215–19 per *Chem. Abstr.*, 1978, *88*, 197546d

Effects of adjuvants on the bioavailability of tetracycline hydrochloride from capsules (*in vitro* studies) (in Russian)

capsules, hard gelatin: tetracycline hydrochloride; disintegration testing, effect of formulation; dissolution testing, effect of formulation; formulation of contents, diluents, magnesium carbonate, calcium phosphate, lactose, lubricant, calcium stearate

Saito, T., Suzuki, S., Nambu, N. and Nagai, T., *Yakuzaigaku*, 1978, *38*, 29–34

Test of the physical stability regarding dissolution property of solid preparations (in Japanese)

capsules, hard gelatin and tablets: indomethacin (capsules); disintegration method, oscillating tube; disintegration testing, effect of storage; dissolution method, rotating basket; dissolution testing, effect of storage; storage conditions, humidity (52%, 92%), temperature (5°, 30°); 3.8.3.7

Carp, G.B., Chemtob, C. and Chaumeil, J.C., *Second International Conference on Pharmaceutical Technology*, (Paris, APGI, June 3–5, 1980), 1980, *V*, 68–80

Availability from rectally administered solid dosage forms: use of rectal soft gelatin capsules (in French)

capsules, soft gelatin: phenobarbitone, free acid and sodium salt; disintegration method, *Fr.P.* 9th Edn, modified, *Pol.P.*, modified, *Swiss P.*, Widmann's (polythene bags); disintegration testing, comparison of methods; dissolution method, partitioning; dissolution testing, effect of formulation; 3.5.2

Hoechst UK Ltd, *British Patent* 1 572 226, 1980

Improvements in and relating to pharmaceutical preparations in solid unit dosage forms

capsules, hard gelatin: triamterene; disintegration method, *B.P.*; disintegration testing, effect of formulation of contents; dissolution method, *U.S.P.*; dissolution testing, effect of formulation of contents; formulation of contents, powder fill, semi-solid fill; 3.2.3.4; 3.2.4.2

Newton, J.M. and Bader, F., *J. Pharm. Pharmac.*, 1980, *32*, 167–71

The influence of drug and diluent particle size on the in vitro release of drug from hard gelatin capsules

capsules, hard gelatin: acetylsalicylic acid; disintegration method, *B.P.*; dissolution method, beaker; dissolution testing, effects of, formulation, powder properties; dissolution testing, results, analysis of variance of T50; formulation of contents, diluent, lactose; powder properties, particle size, porosity of powder bed

Grakovskaia, L.K., Garsheva, G.B., Dedukh, N.G., Khlystova, Z.I. and Koyal'chenko, N.D., *Antibiotiki*, 1981, *26*, 592–4

Effect of antibiotic granulation procedure on quality of capsules with semi-synthetic penicillins (with special reference to sodium dicloxacillin) (in Russian)

capsules, hard gelatin: sodium dicloxacillin; disintegration method, oscillating tube; disintegration testing, effect of powder properties; dissolution method, rotating basket; dissolution testing, effect of powder properties; formulation of contents; powder properties, method of preparation, dry compaction, wet granulation

Botzolakis, J.E., Small, L.E, and Augsburger, L.L., *Int. J. Pharmaceut.*, 1982, *12*, 341–9

Effect of disintegrants on drug dissolution from capsules filled on a dosator-type automatic capsule-filling machine

capsules, hard gelatin: hydrochlorothiazide, paracetamol; disintegration method, *U.S.P.*; disintegration testing, effects of, filling conditions, formulation of contents; dissolution method, stirred flask; dissolution testing, effects of, filling conditions, formulation of contents; disintegration/dissolution correlation, effect of drug type; 3.2.4.1

Botzolakis, J.E. and Augsburger, L.L., *J. Pharm. Pharmac.*, 1984, *36*, 77–84

The role of disintegrants in hard-gelatin capsules

capsules, hard gelatin: disintegration method, *U.S.P.* XX; disintegration testing, effects of, filling forces, formulation of contents; dissolution method, paddle; dissolution testing, effects of, filling forces, formulation of contents; 3.2.3.3; 3.2.4.1

Ritschel, W.P. and Parab, P., *Drug Dev. ind. Pharm.*, 1985, *11*(1), 147–67

Dissolution of some lithium dosage forms and correlation with Enslin number

capsules, hard gelatin and tablets: disintegration method, *U.S.P.*; disintegration testing, comparison of dosage forms; dissolution method, rotating basket; dissolution testing, comparison of dosage forms, correlation with powder properties; kinetic analysis, dissolution rate constants, correlation with powder properties; powder properties, water uptake measurement

4.3 Drug Availability in Animals

4.3.1 General References

Poole, J.W., *Revue can. Biol.*, 1973, *32, Suppl.*, 43–51

Penicillins: use of an animal model to predict bioavailability

capsules, hard gelatin and suspensions: ampicillin anhydrous, trihydrate, dicloxacillin, levels, serum (dog); drug availability, dog serum levels, correlation with human

Maeda, T., Takenaka, H., Yamahira, Y. and Noguchi, T., *J. pharm. Sci.*, 1977, *66*, 69–73

Use of rabbits for GI drug absorption studies

capsules, hard gelatin and tablets: griseofulvin, indomethacin, levels, plasma (rabbit); gastric emptying rate

4.3.2 Comparison of Dosage Forms

4.3.2.1 Comparison with Solid Preparations

Kagawa, C.M., Bouska, D.J. and Anderson, M.L., *J. pharm. Sci.*, 1964, *53*, 450–1

Oral absorption with various preparations of spironolactone in dogs

capsules, hard gelatin and tablets, uncoated and sugar-coated: spironolactone, levels, plasma (dogs); drug clinical effects, urine levels, sodium, potassium

Williams, J.F. and Trejos, A., *Res. vet. Sci.*, 1970, *11*, 392–4

The influence of gelatin capsules upon the activity of bunamidine hydrochloride against Echinococcus granulosus in dogs

capsules, hard gelatin and tablets: bunamidine hydrochloride, drug effects, parasite numbers (dogs); drug administration, tablet inside capsule; drug availability, effect of encapsulated tablet

Stella, V., Haslam, J., Yata, N., Okada, H., Lindenbaum, S. and Higuchi, T., *J. pharm. Sci.*, 1978, *67*, 1375–7

Enhancement of bioavailability of a hydrophobic amine antimalarial by formulation with oleic acid in a soft gelatin capsule

capsules, hard and soft gelatin: α-(dibutylaminomethyl)-6,8-dichloro-2-(3′,4′-dichlorophenyl)-4-quinolinemethanol, levels, serum (dogs); drug availability, effect of formulation; drug solubility, determination aqueous solubility; pharmacokinetic analysis, area under curve comparisons; 3.3.3.2

4.3.2.2 Comparison with Liquid Preparations

Andermann, G., Dietz, M. and Mergel, D., *Pharm. Acta Helv.*, 1979, *54*, 366–9

Bioavailability of medicines based on cyclandelate (in French)

capsules, hard and soft gelatin and suspensions: cyclandelate, levels, serum (rabbits); formulation of contents; pharmacokinetic analysis, relative bioavailability

4.3.2.3 Comparison with Injections

Helmi, R., Elian, A., Moustafa, M. and Sharaf, E., *J. Egypt. med. Ass.*, 1968, *51*, 70–7

A study of the serum concentrations of oxytetracycline after administration of different pharmaceutical preparations

capsules, hard gelatin and injections, intramuscular and intravenous: oxytetracycline hydrochloride, levels, serum (dogs)

Cabana, B.E., Willhite, L.E. and Bierwagen, M.E., *Antimicrob. Ag. Chemother.*, 1969, 35–41

Pharmacokinetic evaluation of the oral absorption of different ampicillin preparations in beagle dogs

capsules, soft gelatin and injections, intravenous: ampicillin, potassium, sodium and trihydrate, levels, serum, urine (dogs); pharmacokinetic analysis

Cotler, S., Holazo, A., Boxenbaum, H.G. and Kaplan, S.A., *J. pharm. Sci.*, 1976, *65*, 822–7

Influence of route of administration on physiological availability of levodopa in dogs boluses, intravenous and capsules, hard gelatin: levodopa, levels, plasma (dogs); pharmacokinetic analysis

4.3.2.4 Comparison with Rectal Preparations

Lambelin, G., Roncucci, R., Simon, M.-J., Orloff, S., Mortier, G., Veys, E. and Buu-Hoï, N.P., *Arzneimittel-Forsch.*, 1968, *18*, 56–60

Absorption and excretion of ^{14}C-p-butoxyphenylacet-hydroxamic acid in man and animals

capsules, hard gelatin, suppositories and tablets, enteric-coated: p-butoxyphenylacethydroxamic acid, levels, blood, serum, urine (rabbits, rats); radioactive isotope technique; 4.4.4.4

Anger-Braun, F., Sado, P.A., Le Verge, R. and Devis-saguet, J.P., *Second International Conference on Pharmaceutical Technology*, (Paris, APGI, June 3–5, 1980), 1980, *III*, 145–54

Bioavailability of quinidine in soft gelatin capsules after oral and rectal administration to rabbits (in French)

capsules, soft gelatin and solutions: quinidine sulphate and metabolites, levels, serum (rabbits); formulation of contents; pharmacokinetic analysis

4.3.2.5 Comparison with Multiple Dosage Forms

Walkenstein, S.S., Wiser, R., Gudmundsen, C.H., Kimmel, H.B. and Corradino, R.A., *J. pharm. Sci.*, 1964, *53*, 1181–6

Absorption, metabolism, and excretion of oxazepam and its succinate half-ester

capsules, hard gelatin, injections, intramuscular and suspensions: oxazepam, succinate half-ester, levels, faeces, plasma, urine (dogs); radioactive isotope technique; 4.4.4.3

Conklin, J.D., Sobers, R.J. and Wagner, D.L., *J. pharm. Sci.*, 1969, *58*, 1365–8

Urinary drug excretion in dogs during therapeutic doses of different nitrofurantoin dosage forms

capsules, hard gelatin, injections, intramuscular and tablets: nitrofurantoin, levels, serum, urine (dogs)

Mercer, H.D., Garg, R.C. Powers, J.D. and Powers, T.E., *Am. J. vet. Res.*, 1977, *38*, 1353–9

Bioavailability and pharmacokinetics of several dosage forms of ampicillin in the cat

capsules, hard gelatin, injections, intramuscular, intravenous and subcutaneous and suspensions: ampicillin, anhydrous, sodium, trihydrate, levels, serum (cats); pharmacokinetic analysis, dosage/route relationship

4.3.3 Comparison of Capsule Products

Agarwal, S.L., Tayal, J.N. and Deshmankar, B.S., *J. Indian med. Ass.*, 1966, *46*, 13–14

Studies on the oral absorption of antibiotics. Part 1. Chloramphenicol

capsules, hard gelatin: chloramphenicol, levels, serum (dogs)

Ogata, H., Aoyagi, N., Kaniwa, N., Ejima, A., Kitaura, T., Ohki, T. and Kitamura, K., *Int. J. Pharmaceut.*, 1986, *29*, 121–6

Evaluation of beagle dogs as an animal model for bioavailability testing of cinnarizine capsules

capsules, hard gelatin: cinnarizine, levels, plasma (dogs); drug availability, comparison with human data, effect of gastric pH; gastric pH measurement, comparison with human

4.3.4 Effect of Formulation on Absorption

Fincher, J.H., Adams, J.G. and Beal, H.M., *J. pharm. Sci.*, 1965, *54*, 704–8

Effect of particle size on gastrointestinal absorption of sulfisoxazole in dogs

capsules, hard gelatin: sulphafurazole, levels, blood (dogs); drug availability, effect of particle size

Paul, H.E., Hayes, K.J., Paul, M.F. and Borgmann, A.R., *J. pharm. Sci.*, 1967, *56*, 882–5

Laboratory studies with nitrofurantoin. Relationship between crystal size, urinary excretion in the rat and man, and emesis in dogs

capsules, hard gelatin: nitrofurantoin, levels, urine (rats); drug availability, effect of drug particle size; drug clinical effects, emesis (dogs); 4.4.4.1

Ljungberg, S. and Otto, G., *Acta pharm. suec.*, 1970, *7*, 449–56

Particle size and intestinal absorption of acetylsalicylic acid in dogs

capsules, hard gelatin: acetylsalicylic acid, levels, serum (dogs); drug availability, effect of particle size; powder properties, particle size, effect of granulation

Newmark, H.L. and Berger, J., *J. pharm. Sci.*, 1970, *59*, 1246–8

Coumermycin A_1 – Biopharmaceutical studies I

capsules, hard gelatin, injections, intravenous and solutions: coumermycin, soluble salts, sugar amines, complexing agents, levels, blood (dogs); drug availability, effect of formulation, drug chemical form; formulation of contents, N-methylglucamine gels

Hansford, D.T., Newton, J.M. and Wilson, C.G., *Pharm. Ind., Berl.*, 1980, *42*, 646–50

The influence of formulation on the absorption of orally administered griseofulvin preparations in rabbits

capsules, hard gelatin, solutions and suspensions: griseofulvin, levels, plasma (rabbits); drug availability, comparison of dosage forms, percentage of drug absorption

4.3.5 Availability from Enteric Capsules

Nash, J.F. and Crabtree, R.E., *J. pharm. Sci.*, 1961, *50*, 134–7

Absorption of tritiated d-desoxyephedrine in sustained-release dosage forms

capsules, hard gelatin: methylamphetamine hydrochloride, resinates, levels, blood, urine (dogs); enteric coating, cellulose acetate phthalate

4.4 Drug Availability in Humans

4.4.1 Reviews

Wagner, J. G., *J. pharm. Sci.*, 1961, *50*, 359–87

Biopharmaceutics: absorption aspects

Wagner, J.G., *Can. J. pharm. Sci.*, 1966, *1*, 55–68

Design and data analysis of biopharmaceutical studies in man

Riegelman, S., *The physiological equivalence of drug dosage forms*, Symposium (Food and Drug Directorate, Ottawa), 1969, 13–22

Pharmacokinetic analysis of drug dosage forms

capsules, hard gelatin and suspensions: griseofulvin, levels, plasma

Schneller, G.H., *J. Am. pharm. Ass.*, 1969, *NS9*, 455–9

Hazard of therapeutic nonequivalency of drug products

Wagner, J.G., *J. pharm. Sci.*, 1969, *58*, 1253–7

Interpretation of percent dissolved–time plots derived from *in vitro* testing of conventional tablets and capsules
capsules and tablets: presentation of results

Florence, A.T., *Pharm. J.*, 1972, *208*, 456–63

Generic equivalence: A look at the literature

Blanchard, J., *Am. J. Pharm.*, 1978, *150*, 132–51

Gastrointestinal absorption II. Formulation factors affecting drug availability

Ganderton, D., *Acta pharm. suec.*, 1978, *15*, 314–15

Effect of production variables on the properties of tablets and capsules related to bioavailability

Garcia, C.R., Siqueiros, A. and Benet, L.Z., *Pharm. Acta Helv.*, 1978, *53*, 99–109

Oral controlled release preparations

capsules and tablets: controlled-release products, capsules of coated granules

4.4.2 General References, Availability in Humans

Stelmach, H., Robinson, J.R. and Eriksen, S.P., *J. pharm. Sci.*, 1965, *54*, 1453–8

Release of a drug from a dosage form

capsules, hard gelatin, solutions and tablets: aspirin; drug availability, *in vivo*, computer (analog) simulation

Martin, C.M., *J. Am. med. Ass.*, 1968, *205*(9), 23–4, 30

Brand, generic drugs differ in man

capsules: chloramphenicol, phenytoin sodium, levels, serum; sulphafurazole, crushed tablets administered in capsules

Wheeler, L.M., *Drug Cosmet. Ind.*, 1972, *110*(2), 64, 66, 124–7

The standard dose form for pharmaceutical research

capsules, hard gelatin: clinical trials, double-blind; formulation of contents

Baars, R. E., Rapp, R.P., Young, B. and Canafax, D., *Drug Intell. & clin. Pharm.*, 1978, *12*, 584–8

Phenytoin 300 mg daily; not a dose for everyone. A comparison of a 300 mg capsule with three 100 mg capsules

capsules, hard gelatin: phenytoin, levels, serum; drug availability, effect of dosage levels

Cloyd, J.C., Gumnit, R.J. and Lesar, T.S., *Ann. Neurol.*, 1980, *7*, 191–3

Reduced seizure control due to spoiled phenytoin capsules

capsules, hard gelatin: phenytoin, levels, serum; drug availability, effect of capsule storage

Evens, R. P., Frazer, D. G., Ludden, T. M. and Sutherland, E.W., *Am. J. Hosp. Pharm.*, 1980, *37*, 232–5

Phenytoin toxicity and blood levels after a large oral dose

capsules, hard gelatin: phenytoin, levels, plasma; drug availability, effect of high dosage

Aiache, J.-M., Aiache, S., Renoux, R. and Mohamed, H., *Labo-Pharma Probl. Tech.*, 1983, *31*, 926–34

The place of the hard gelatin capsule: biopharmaceutical aspects (in French)

capsules, hard gelatin: disintegration; dissolution; drug availability, *in vivo*, effects of formulation, physiological factors; formulation of contents

Anon, *Med. Lett. Drug. Ther.*, 1983, *25*, 11–12

Digoxin solution in capsules (Lanoxicaps)
capsules, soft gelatin: digoxin, drug availability, review

Berry, I.R., *Mfg Chem.*, 1984, *55*(4), 54–5

Bioavailability and soft gelatin capsules

capsules, soft gelatin: drug availability, comparison with other dosage forms; review

4.4.3 Intestinal Performance

Oser, B.L., Melnick, D. and Hochberg, M., *Ind. Engng Chem. analyt. Edn*, 1945, *17*, 405–11

Physiological availability of the vitamins. Study of methods for determining availability of vitamins in pharmaceutical products

capsules, soft gelatin, solutions and tablets: thiamine, levels, urine; disintegration method, X-ray, radio-opaque contents; formulation of contents, adsorbents, acid clays and fuller's earth

Feinblatt, T.M. and Ferguson, E.A., *New Engl. J. Med.*, 1956, *254*, 940–3

Timed-disintegration capsules. An in vivo roentgenographic study

capsules, hard gelatin: barium sulphate; disintegration method, X-ray, radio-opaque contents; formulation of contents, granules, controlled release

Eckert, T., *Arzneimittel-Forsch.*, 1967, *17*, 645–6

The pH-endoradio probe: a method for determining the in vivo disintegration of oral dosage forms. Part I. The disintegration of hard gelatin capsules in vivo (in German)

capsules, hard gelatin: disintegration method, pH radiotransmitter; disintegration testing, capsule shell, release of contents

Widmann, A., Eiden, F. and Tenczer, J., *Arzneimittel-Forsch.*, 1970, *20*, 283–9

Release of drugs from Depot soft gel capsules (in German)

capsules, soft gelatin: chlorpheniramine maleate, codeine; capsule shell, non-disintegrating; disintegration method, X-ray, radio-opaque contents; drug availability, prolonged release; formulation of contents; 4.2.3.6

Casey, D.L., Beihn, R.M., Digenis, G.A. and Shambhu, M.B., *J. pharm. Sci.*, 1976, *65*, 1412–13

Method for monitoring hard gelatin capsule disintegration times in humans using external scintigraphy

capsules, hard gelatin: gastric behaviour, visualisation method, gamma scintigraphy, technetium–99 m; gastric behaviour, testing, effects of, formulation of contents, patient's fasting state

Evans, K.T. and Roberts, G.M., *Lancet*, 1976, *2*, 1237–9

Where do all the tablets go?

capsules, hard gelatin and tablets: gastric behaviour, clinical effects, disintegration in oesophagus, patient problems; visualisation method, X-ray, radio-opaque contents; disintegration testing, location of site

Carlborg, B., Kumlien, A. and Olsson, H., *Läkartidningen*, 1978, *75*, 4609–11

Oesophageal strictures caused by oral drug therapy (in Swedish)

capsules and tablets: oesophageal behaviour, effects of, physiological factors, products, review

Hunter, E., Fell, J.T., Calvert, R.T. and Sharma, H., *Int. J. Pharmaceut.*, 1980, *4*, 175–83

"In vivo" disintegration of hard gelatin capsules in fasting and non-fasting subjects

capsules, hard gelatin: disintegration method, *B.P.*; formulation of contents, ion-exchange resin, fast and slow disintegration; gastric behaviour, visualisation method, gamma scintigraphy, technetium-99 m; gastric behaviour, testing, dispersion of contents, gastric emptying, effect of patient's fasting state

Anon., *Drug & Ther. Bull.*, 1981, *19*(9), 33–4

Tablets and capsules that stick in the oesophagus

capsules and tablets: gastric and oesophageal behaviour, comparison of dosage forms, review

Evans, K.T. and Roberts, G.M., *J. clin. Hosp. Pharm.*, 1981, *6*, 207–8

The ability of patients to swallow capsules

capsules, hard and soft gelatin: barium sulphate; gastric and oesophageal behaviour, visualisation method, X-ray, radio-opaque contents; gastric and oesophageal behaviour, testing, comparison of dosage forms, effects of co-administration of water, condition of patient's oesophagus

Hunter, E., Fell, J.T. and Sharma, H., *J. Pharm. Pharmac.*, 1981, *33*, 617–18

A comparison of the behaviour of tablet and capsule formulations in vivo

capsules, hard gelatin and tablets: formulation of contents, ion-exchange resin; gastric behaviour, visualisation method, gamma scintigraphy, technetium-99 m; gastric behaviour, testing, comparison of, dosage form, effect of patient's fasting state

McCloy, E.C. and Kane, S., *Br. med. J.*, 1981, *282*, 1703

Drug-induced oesophageal ulceration

capsules, hard gelatin: oesophageal behaviour, adverse clinical effects, letter

Channer, K.S. and Virjee, J. *Br. med. J.*, 1982, *285*, 1702

Effect of posture and drink volume on the swallowing of capsules

capsules, hard gelatin: barium sulphate; gastric and oesophageal behaviour, visualisation method, X-ray, radio-opaque contents; oesophageal behaviour, effects of, co-administration of water, patient's posture, erect, supine

Dew, M.J., Hughes, P.J., Lee, M.G., Evans, B.K. and Rhodes, J., *Br. J. clin. Pharmac.*, 1982, *14*, 405–8

An oral preparation to release drugs in the human colon

capsules, hard gelatin: capsules, enteric-coated, methacrylic acid polymers; disintegration testing, estimation of site of disintegration, colon; gastric behaviour, visualisation method, X-ray, radio-opaque contents; 4.4.7.2

Hey, H., Jørgensen, F., Sørensen, K., Hasselbalch, H. and Wamberg, T., *Br. med. J.*, 1982, *285*, 1717–19

Oesophageal transit of six commonly used tablets and capsules

capsules, hard gelatin and tablets: barium sulphate; oesophageal behaviour, visualisation method, fluoroscopy; oesophageal behaviour, comparison of dosage form, effects of, co-administration of water, patient's posture, erect, supine, product, density, shape, size

Hunter, E., Fell, J.T. and Sharma, H., *Drug Dev. ind. Pharm.*, 1982, *8*, 751–7

The gastric emptying of pellets contained in hard gelatin capsules

capsules, hard gelatin: disintegration method, *B.P.*, formulation of contents, ion-exchange resin, fast and slow disintegration; gastric behaviour, visualisation method, gamma scintigraphy, technetium-99 m; gastric behaviour, testing, effects of patient's fasting state, product disintegration

Hunter, E., Fell, J.T., Sharma, H. and McNeilly, A.-M., *Pharm. Ind., Berl.*, 1982, *44*, 90–1

The "in vivo" behaviour of hard gelatin capsules filled with thixotropic liquids

capsules, hard gelatin: gastric behaviour, visualisation method, gamma scintigraphy, technetium-99 m; gastric behaviour, effects of, formulation, viscosity of contents; 3.2.4.2

Marvola, M., *Pharmacy Int.*, 1982, *3*, 294–6

Adherence of drug products to the oesophagus

capsules, hard gelatin and tablets: oesophageal transit, *in vitro* simulation, isolated pig oesophagus; oesophageal transit, measurement of oesophageal adherence force, comparison of products, product shape and size, effect of artificial saliva

Walker, R., *Br. J. pharm. Pract.*, 1982, *4*(9), 6, 8

A study of the fluid intake with tablets and capsules in geriatric patients

capsules and tablets: oesophageal behaviour, effect of co-administration of fluid, type and volume

Ardran, G.M., *Br. med. J.*, 1983, *286*, 304–5

Swallowing tablets and capsules

capsules and tablets: oesophageal transit, effect of administration of water, patient's ability to swallow particles

Channer, K.S., Wolinski, A., Kaye, B. and Virjee, J., *Br. J. clin. Pharmac.*, 1983, *15*, 560–3

The effect of hyoscine butylbromide on the swallowing of capsules

capsules, hard gelatin: gastric and oesophageal behaviour, visualisation method, X-ray, radio-opaque contents; gastric and oesophageal behaviour, testing, effects of, co-administration of hyoscine butylbromide and water, patient's posture, erect or supine, site of capsule disintegration

Deland, F.H., Beihn, R.M. and Digenis, G.A., *J. nucl. Med.*, 1983, *24*, P98

Novel techniques in the study of disintegration and dissolution of orally administered dosage forms in man

capsules and tablets: disintegration method, gamma scintigraphy, technetium-99 m; dissolution method, gamma scintigraphy, indium-111, technetium-99 m, labelled contents; dissolution testing, estimation from angular correlation measurements

Fell, J.T., *Am. J. Hosp. Pharm.*, 1983, *40*, 946, 948

Esophageal transit of tablets and capsules

capsules and tablets: oesophageal behaviour, critical review, letter, see Ponto, J.A., *Am. J. Hosp. Pharm.*, 1983, *40*, 38, 44

Hunter, E., Fell, J.T. and Sharma, H., *Int. J. Pharmaceut.*, 1983, *17*, 59–64

The gastric emptying of hard gelatin capsules

capsules, hard gelatin: disintegration method, *B.P.*; disintegration testing, correlation with *in vivo* behaviour; formulation of contents, Amberlite resin, particle size; gastric behaviour, visualisation method, gamma scintigraphy, indium-113 m, technetium-99 m; gastric behaviour, effects of, formulation of contents, patients' fasting state

Hunter, E., Fell, J.T., Sharma, H. and McNeilly, A.-M., *Pharm. Ind., Berl.*, 1983, *45*, 433–4

The in vivo behaviour of hard gelatin capsules filled with thixotropic liquids: Part 2: Quantitative aspects

capsules, hard gelatin: gastric behaviour, visualisation method, gamma scintigraphy, technetium-99 m; gastric behaviour, testing, mathematical model, lag time and emptying rate

Marvola, M., Rajaniemi, M., Marttila, E., Vahervuo, K. and Sothmann, A., *J. pharm. Sci.*, 1983, *72*, 1034–6

Effect of dosage form and formulation factors on the adherence of drugs to the esophagus

capsules, hard and soft gelatin and tablets: dosage forms coating, formulation; oesophageal transit, *in vitro* simulation, isolated pig oesophagus; oesophageal transit, measurement of oesophageal adherence, comparison of dosage forms, effect of surface coating

Ponto, J.A., *Am. Pharm.*, 1983, *NS23*, 6 and *Am. J. Hosp. Pharm.*, 1983, *40*, 38, 44

Esophageal retention of capsules

capsules and tablets: oesophageal behaviour, effects of physiological factors, letter

Rhodes, J. and Evans, B.K., *International Patent* WO 83/00435, 1983

Orally administerable pharmaceutical compositions

capsules, hard gelatin: capsules, enteric-coated; disintegration testing, estimation of site of disintegration, colon; gastric behaviour, visualisation method, X-ray, radio-opaque contents; 3.4.2.4; 4.4.7.2

Channer, K.S., Bell, J. and Virjee, J.P., *Br. Heart J.*, 1984, *52*, 223–7

Effect of left atrial size on the oesophageal transit of capsules

capsules, hard gelatin: barium sulphate; oesophageal behaviour, visualisation method, fluoroscopy; oesophageal behaviour, transit time, effects of, co-administration of water, 15, 60 ml, patient's cardiac and oesophageal state

Davis, S.S., Hardy, J.G., Taylor, M.J., Whalley, D.R. and Wilson, C.G., *Int. J. Pharmaceut.*, 1984, *21*, 167–77

A comparative study of the gastrointestinal transit of a pellet and tablet formulation

capsules, hard gelatin and tablet: capsule contents, pellets; gastric behaviour, visualisation method, gamma scintigraphy, indium-111 (tablet), technetium-99 m (capsule); gastric behaviour, gastric emptying, time to colon, comparison of dosage forms, effect of calorific value of meal

Djimbo, M., Fell, J.T., Kaus, L. and Moës, A.J., *J. Pharm. Belg.*, 1984, *39*, 43–9

Release of drugs formulated as hard pastes filled into hard gelatin capsules. Part 2. *In vivo* studies

capsules, hard gelatin and tablets: acetylsalicylic acid, levels, urine; drug availability, comparison of dosage forms, effect of capsule formulation; gastric behaviour, visualisation method, gamma scintigraphy, technetium-99 m; gastric behaviour, testing, gastric emptying, product disintegration; pharmacokinetic analysis, theophylline, predicted blood levels from dissolution data, effect of formulation

Kaus, L.C. and Fell, J.T., *J. clin. Hosp. Pharm.*, 1984, 9, 249–51

Effect of stress on the gastric emptying of capsules

capsules, hard gelatin: gastric behaviour, visualisation method, gamma scintigraphy, technetium-99 m; gastric behaviour, emptying rate, effect of patient's stress; patient stress, high noise levels

Kaus, L.C., Fell, J.T., Sharma, H. and Taylor, D.C., *Int. J. Pharmaceut.*, 1984, 20, 315–23

On the intestinal transit of a single non-disintegrating object

capsules, hard gelatin: capsule model, perspex; gastric behaviour, visualisation method, gamma scintigraphy, technetium-99 m, external markers, three-dimensional co-ordinates; gastric behaviour, distance travelled, effect of capsule density on rate of movement

Kaus, L., Sharma, H. and Fell, J.T., *J. Pharm. Pharmac.*, 1984, 36, 136–8

Simultaneous measurement of gastric emptying of the soluble and insoluble components of a formulation using a dual isotope, gamma scintigraphic technique

capsules, hard gelatin: disintegration method, *B.P.*; disintegration testing, correlation with *in vivo* behaviour; formulation of contents, Amberlite resin, sodium chloride; gastric behaviour, visualisation method, gamma scintigraphy, indium-113 m, technetium-99 m; gastric behaviour, effects of, formulation of contents, patient's fasting state

Channer, K.S. and Virjee, J.P., *J. Pharm. Pharmac.*, 1985, 37, 126–9

The effect of formulation on oesophageal transit

capsules, hard gelatin and tablets: barium sulphate; oesophageal behaviour, visualisation method, fluoroscopy; oesophageal behaviour, comparison of dosage forms, effects of, patient's posture, erect, supine, product, density, size, tablet form

Hardy, J.G., Wilson, C.G. and Wood, E., *J. Pharm. Pharmac.*, 1985, 37, 874–7

Drug delivery to the proximal colon

capsules and pellets: gastric behaviour, visualisation method, gamma scintigraphy, technetium-99 m; gastric behaviour, gastric emptying, transit times, small intestine, colon, comparison of non-disintegrating capsule and pellets

Hardy, J.G., Wood, E. and Wilson, C.G., *Dig. Dis. Sci.*, 1985, 30, 772

The intestinal transit of capsules and pellets

capsules and pellets: gastric behaviour, visualisation method, gamma scintigraphy, technetium-99 m; gastric behaviour, gastric emptying, transit times, small intestine, colon, comparison of non-disintegrating capsule and pellets

Tossounian, J.L., Mergens, W.J. and Sheth, P.R., *Drug Dev. ind. Pharm.*, 1985, 11, 1019–50

Bioefficient products. A novel delivery system

capsules, hard gelatin and tablets: riboflavine, thiamine, vitamin C and E; capsules, floating dosage form; gastric behaviour, visualisation method, gamma scintigraphy, technetium-99m; 4.5.5

Davis, S.S., Hardy, J.G. and Fara, J.W., *Gut*, 1986, 27, 886–92

Transit of pharmaceutical dosage forms through the small intestine

capsules, hard gelatin, solutions and tablets: intestinal behaviour, visualisation method, gamma scintigraphy, technetium-99m; intestinal behaviour, gastric emptying, small intestinal transit rate, comparison of dosage forms, effect of patient's fasting state

Spiller, R.C., *Gut*, 1986, 27, 879–85

Where do all the tablets go in 1986?

capsules, hard and soft gelatin and tablets: intestinal performance, review

4.4.4 Comparison of Dosage Forms in Humans

4.4.4.1 Comparison with Solid Preparations

Gantt, C.L., Gochman, N. and Dyniewicz, J.M., *Lancet*, 1962, 1, 1130–1

Gastrointestinal absorption of spironolactone

capsules, hard gelatin and tablets: spironolactone, spirolactone, levels, plasma; drug availability, effect of formulation; formulation of contents, surfactant, polysorbate 80; drug, clinical performance, urinary electrolytes, levels, sodium, potassium

Hollister, L.E., *New Engl. J. Med.*, 1962, 266, 281–3

Studies of delayed-action medication. 1. Meprobamate administered as compressed tablets and as two delayed-action capsules

capsules, hard gelatin and tablets: meprobamate, levels, plasma, urine; drug clinical effects

Lövgren, O. and Allander, E., *Br. med. J.*, 1965, 1, 996

Indomethacin and peptic ulcer

capsules, hard gelatin and tablets: indomethacin; drug side-effects, comparison of dosage forms

Wood, J.H., *J. pharm. Sci.*, 1965, 54, 1207–8

In vivo drug release rate from hard gelatin capsules

capsules, hard gelatin and tablets: acetylsalicylic acid, levels, serum

Rudhardt, M., Boymond, P. and Fabre, J., *Schweiz. med. Wschr.*, 1966, 96, 542–6

Micronisation, does it affect the efficacy of diuretics? Pharmaceutical and clinical study of micronised and non-micronised cyclothiazide (in French)

capsules, hard gelatin and tablets, sugar-coated: cyclothiazide, clinical effects, blood pressure reduction, serum levels, potassium and uric acid; drug availability, effect of drug particle size

Paul, H.E., Hayes, K.J., Paul, M.F. and Borgmann, A.R., *J. pharm. Sci.*, 1967, *56*, 882–5

Laboratory studies with nitrofurantoin. Relationship between crystal size, urinary excretion in the rat and man, and emesis in dogs

capsules, hard gelatin and tablets: nitrofurantoin, levels, urine; drug availability, effect of drug particle size; 4.3.4

Tannenbaum, P.J., Rosen, E., Flanagan, T. and Crosley, A.P., *Clin. Pharmac. Ther.*, 1968, *9*, 598–604

The influence of dosage form on the activity of a diuretic agent

capsules, hard gelatin and tablets: hydrochlorothiazide, triamterene, levels, urine; drug availability, comparison of dosage regimens; drug, clinical effects, urinary electrolytes, levels, sodium, potassium

Viala, A. and Cano, J.P., *Thérapie*, 1968, *23*, 775–8

Blood levels of diazepam ("Valium") following its administration in capsule form (in French)

capsules, hard gelatin and tablets: diazepam, levels, blood

Conklin, J.D. and Hailey, F.J., *Clin. Pharmac. Ther.*, 1969, *10*, 534–9

Urinary drug excretion in man during oral dosage of different nitrofurantoin formulations

capsules, hard gelatin and tablets: nitrofurantoin, levels, urine; drug availability, effect of drug particle size

Frisch, E.P. and Örtengren, B., *Acta psychiat. scand.*, 1969, *42*, 35–41

Plasma concentration of chlormethiazole following oral intake of tablets and capsules

capsules, soft gelatin and tablets: chlormethiazole, base and edisylate, metabolites, levels, plasma; drug, clinical effect, sleep onset

Raveux, R. and Gros, P., *Chim. Thér.*, 1969, *4*, 481–7

Study of the urinary excretion of dipotassium clorazepate and its metabolites. 3. Human experimentation with enteric-coated tablets and gelatin capsules (in French)

capsules, hard gelatin and tablets, enteric-coated: clorazepate, dipotassium, metabolites, levels, urine

Sidell, F.R., Groff, W.A. and Ellin, R.I., *J. pharm. Sci.*, 1969, *58*, 1093–8

Blood levels of oxime and symptoms in humans after single and multiple oral doses of 2-pyridine aldoxime methochloride

capsules, hard gelatin and tablets: pralidoxime chloride, levels, serum, urine; drug availability, comparison of dosage regimens, single and multiple dose; drug, side-effects; pharmacokinetic analysis

Lander, H., *Med. J. Aust.*, 1971, *2*, 984

L-Dopa – variation in response with different pharmaceutical preparations (Syndopa vs Larodopa)

capsules, hard gelatin and tablets: levodopa, clinical effect

Shaw, T.R.D., Howard, M.R. and Hamer, J., *Lancet*, 1972, *2*, 303–7

Variation in the biological availability of digoxin

capsules, hard gelatin and tablets: digoxin, levels, plasma; drug availability, effect of tablets packed in capsules

Beveridge, T., Schmidt, R., Kalberer, F. and Nüesch, E., *Lancet*, 1973, *2*, 499

Bioavailability of digoxin

capsules, hard gelatin and tablets: digoxin, levels, plasma, urine

Smyth, R.D., Lee, J.K., Polk, A., Chemburkar, P.B. and Savacool, A.M., *J. clin. Pharmac.*, 1973, *13*, 391–400

Bioavailability of methaqualone

capsules, hard gelatin and tablets: methaqualone hydrochloride, levels, plasma, urine

Williams, M.E., Kendall, M.J. and Mitchard, M., *Lancet*, 1973, *1*, 440

Variation in biological availability

capsules, hard gelatin and tablets: methaqualone, levels, plasma; drug availability, comparison of products

Albert, K.S., Sedman, A.J. and Wagner, J.G., *J. Pharmacokinet. Biopharm.*, 1974, *2*, 381–93

Pharmacokinetics of orally administered acetaminophen in man

capsules, soft gelatin and tablets: paracetamol, levels, plasma; pharmacokinetic analysis

Albert, K.S., Sedman, A.J., Wilkinson, P., Stoll, R.G., Murray, W.J. and Wagner, J.G., *J. clin. Pharmac.*, 1974, *14*, 264–70

Bioavailability studies of acetaminophen and nitrofurantoin

capsules, soft gelatin and tablets: nitrofurantoin, paracetamol, levels, plasma; drug availability, effect of formulation; formulation of contents, surfactant, poloxamers

Lund, L., *Eur. J. clin. Pharmac.*, 1974, *7*, 119–24

Clinical significance of generic inequivalence of three different pharmaceutical preparations of phenytoin

capsules, hard gelatin and tablets: phenytoin, free acid and sodium salt, levels, plasma; drug, clinical effects

Gundert-Remy, U., Bilzer, W., Kilgenstein, R. and Weber, E., *Pharm. Ind., Berl.*, 1975, *37*, 905–9

On the absorption of phenobarbitone from various dosage forms (in German)

capsules, soft gelatin and tablets: phenobarbitone, levels, plasma

Gundert-Remy, U., Bilzer, W. and Weber, E., *Drugs Germ.*, 1975, *18*, 99–104

Absorption of diphenhydramin-HCl of different dosage forms

capsules, hard and soft gelatin and tablets, sugar-coated: diphenhydramine hydrochloride, levels, plasma; formulation of contents, soft gelatin capsules, excipients

Manson, J.I., Beal, S.M., Magarey, A., Pollard, A.C., O'Reilly, W.J. and Sansom, L.N., *Med. J. Aust.*, 1975, *2*, 590–2

Bioavailability of phenytoin from various pharmaceutical preparations in children

capsules, hard gelatin and tablets: phenytoin, levels, blood; drug availability, comparison of 30- and 100-mg doses

Harvengt, C. and Desager, J.P., *Int. J. clin. Pharmac. Biopharm.*, 1976, *14*, 113–18

Pharmacokinetic study and bioavailability of three marketed compounds releasing *p*-chlorophenoxyisobutyric acid (CPIB) in volunteers

capsules, soft gelatin and tablets: clofibride and derivatives, levels, plasma, urine; drug availability, comparison of drug derivatives

Morris, J.G.L., Parsons, R.L., Trounce, J.R. and Groves, M.J., *Br. J. clin. Pharmac.*, 1976, *3*, 983–90

Plasma dopa concentrations after different preparations of levodopa in normal subjects

capsules, hard gelatin and tablets: levodopa, levels, plasma; drug availability, effect of co-administration of benserazide (combination capsule), comparison with tablet products

Smith, T.C. and Kinkel, A., *Clin. Pharmac. Ther.*, 1976, *20*, 738–42

Absorption and metabolism of phenytoin from tablets and capsules

capsules, hard gelatin and tablets: phenytoin, levels, plasma, urine

Frigo, G.M., Perucca, E., Teggia-Droghi, M., Gatti, G., Mussini, A. and Salerno, J., *Br. J. clin. Pharmac.*, 1977, *4*, 449–54

Comparison of quinidine plasma concentration curves following oral administration of some short-and long-acting formulations

capsules, hard gelatin and tablets: quinidine, salts, levels, plasma; drug availability, comparison of drug salts; pharmacokinetic analysis

Fuccella, L.M., Bolcioni, G., Tamassia, V., Ferrario, L. and Tognoni, G., *Eur. J. clin. Pharmac.*, 1977, *12*, 383–6

Human pharmacokinetics and bioavailability of temazepam administered in soft gelatin capsules

capsules, hard and soft gelatin: temazepam, levels, plasma; drug availability, effect of time of administration; pharmacokinetic analysis

Johnson, B.F., Smith, G. and French, J., *Br. J. clin. Pharmac.*, 1977, *4*, 209–11

The comparability of dosage regimens of Lanoxin tablets and Lanoxicaps

Capsules, soft gelatin and tablets: digoxin, levels, plasma

Longhini, G., Alvisi, V., Bagni, B., Portaluppi, F. and Fersini, C., *Curr. ther. Res.*, 1977, *21*, 909–12

Bioavailability of digoxin improved by pharmaceutical manufacturing process

capsules, soft gelatin and tablets: digoxin, levels, plasma, urine

Rodgers, E.M., Dobbs, S.M., Kenyon, W.I. and Poston, J.W., *Br. med. J.*, 1977, *2*, 234–5

Evaluation of digoxin capsules in outpatients

capsules, soft gelatin and tablets: digoxin, levels, serum; drug availability, comparison of dosage forms, relationship of dose

Padeletti, L. and Brat, A., *Int. J. clin. Pharmac. Biopharm.*, 1978, *16*, 320–2

Bioavailability of digoxin in capsules

capsules, soft gelatin and tablets: digoxin, levels, serum, urine; drug availability, comparison of single-dose and steady-state studies

Taylor, T., Chasseaud, L.F., Darragh, A. and O'Kelly, D.A., *Eur. J. clin. Pharmac.*, 1978, *13*, 49–53

Bioavailability of p-chlorophenoxyisobutyric acid (clofibrinic acid) after repeated doses of its calcium salt to humans

capsules, hard gelatin and tablets: clofibrinic acid and derivatives, levels, plasma

Wood, J.H., Flora, K.P. and Duma, R.J., *J. Am. med. Ass.*, 1978, *239*, 1874–6

Tetracycline, another example of generic bioinequivalence

capsules, gelatin and tablets: tetracycline hydrochloride, levels, plasma; pharmacokinetic analysis

Rameis, H., Hitzenberger, G. and Horwatitsch, H., *Dt. med. Wschr.*, 1979, *104*, 881–3

Bioavailability of spironolactone in two different pharmaceutical forms (in German)

capsules, hard gelatin and tablets: spironolactone, levels, serum, urine; drug availability, comparison of products

Rosenthal, J., Jaeger, H. and Specker, M., *Arzneimittel-Forsch.*, 1979, *29*, 1428–32

Comparative study of relative bioavailability of several spironolactone formulations in a steady-state test (in German)

capsules, hard gelatin and tablets: spironolactone, metabolites, levels, plasma; drug availability, comparison of products; drug availability, effect of product dose; pharmacokinetic analysis

Liedtke, R.K., Ebel, S., Missler, B., Haase, W. and Stein, L., *Arzneimittel-Forsch.*, 1980, *30*, 833–6

Single-dose pharmacokinetics of macrocrystalline nitrofurantoin formulations

capsules, hard gelatin and tablets: nitrofurantoin, levels, serum

d'Athis, P., Richard, M.-o., de Lauture, D., Rey, E., Bouvier d'Yvoire, M., Clement, E. and Olive, G., *Thérapie*, 1981, *36*, 443–9

Comparative bioavailability of two forms of spironolactone. Rationalisation applied to dosage (in French)

capsules, hard gelatin and tablets: spironolactone, levels, serum; drug availability, effect of particle size, comparison of micronised powder in capsule and standard powder in tablet; pharmacokinetic analysis

Gibberd, F.B., Spencer, K.M., Webley, M. and Berry, D., *Br. J. clin. Pharmac.*, 1982, *13*, 455–6

A comparison of the bioavailability of 2 brands of phenytoin

capsules, hard gelatin and tablets: phenytoin, levels, serum

Helfand, W.H. and Pejouan, B.L., *Annls pharm. fr.*, 1983, *41*, 401–8

New indomethacin formulations. Pharmacokinetic characteristics of an oral osmotic therapeutic system (in French)

capsules, hard gelatin and tablets, Oros system: indomethacin, levels, plasma; drug availability, comparison of dosage regimens

Jallad, N.S., Weidler, D.J., Dyal, C.G., McFarland, A., Kraml, M. and Fencik, M., *Clin. Res.*, 1983, *31*, A249

Comparison of the pharmacodynamics and bioavailability of two dosage forms of Inderal and placebo in man both with acute dosing and under steady state conditions

capsules, hard gelatin and tablets: propranolol, levels, serum; drug availability, comparison of controlled-release capsules and standard tablet; drug clinical effects, comparison of dosage forms, effects on, blood pressure, exercise tachycardia; pharmacokinetic analysis

Kirshner, H.S., *New Engl. J. Med.*, 1983, *308*, 1106

Phenytoin toxicity when tablets substituted for capsules

capsules, hard gelatin and tablets: phenytoin, levels, serum; drug side-effects, comparison of dosage forms, effect of product change

Lien, E. and Bakke, O.M., *Br. J. clin. Pharmac.*, 1983, *16*, 71–6

Sustained release disopyramide compared to plain capsules after change-over from intravenous infusion

capsules, hard gelatin, infusions, intravenous and tablets: disopyramide, levels, plasma; drug availability, comparison of standard capsule and sustained-release capsule; pharmacokinetic analysis

Malini, P.L., Strocchi, E., Negroni, S., Ambrosioni, E. and Magnani, B., *Curr. ther. Res.*, 1983, *33*, 646–50

Greater bioavailability of digoxin in a new capsule preparation

capsules, soft gelatin and tablets: digoxin, levels, plasma, urine; drug availability, comparison of dose, 100 µg in capsules and 125 µg in tablets; pharmacokinetic analysis

Rogers, J.D., Lee, R.B., Souder, P.R., Ferguson, R.K., Davies, R.O., Theeuwes, F. and Kwan, K.C., *Int. J. Pharmaceut.*, 1983, *16*, 191–201

Pharmacokinetic evaluation of osmotically controlled indomethacin delivery systems in man

capsules, hard gelatin and tablets: indomethacin, levels, plasma; drug availability, comparison of standard capsule and controlled-release (osmotic pump) tablet; pharmacokinetic analysis

Bateman, N.E. and Uccellini, D.A., *J. Pharm. Pharmac.*, 1984, *36*, 461–4

Effect of formulation on the bioavailability of retinol, D-α-tocopherol and riboflavine

capsules, hard and soft gelatin and tablets: vitamins A, B₂, E, levels, plasma; drug availability, comparison of formulations, capsules, soft gelatin; pharmacokinetic analysis; 3.3.3.2

Doherty, J.E., Marcus, F.I. and Binnion, P.F., *Curr. ther. Res.*, 1984, *35*, 301–6

A multicenter evaluation of the absolute bioavailability of digoxin dosage forms

capsules, soft gelatin, infusions, intravenous, solutions and tablets: digoxin, levels, serum; pharmacokinetic analysis

Nitsche, V., Mascher, H. and Schütz, H., *Int. J. clin. Pharmac. Ther. Toxic.*, 1984, *22*, 104–7

Comparative bioavailability of several phenytoin preparations marketed in Austria

capsules, hard gelatin and tablets: phenytoin, free acid, calcium and sodium salts, levels, plasma; drug availability, comparison of drug salts; pharmacokinetic analysis

Reynier, J.P., Bovis, A. and Bertocchio, M.-H., *Pharm. Acta Helv.*, 1984, *59*, 191–99

Bioavailability of clorazepate dipotassium from different oral dosage forms (in French)

capsules, hard gelatin, injections, intravenous and tablets: clorazepate dipotassium, metabolites, levels, serum; drug availability, comparison of standard release capsules and tablets with sustained release tablets; pharmacokinetic analysis

Stavchansky, S., Pearlman, R.S., Van Harken, D.R., Smyth, R.D., Hottendorf, G.H., Martin, A., Newburger, J. and Schneider, L.W., *J. pharm. Sci.*, 1984, *73*, 169–73

Evaluation of the bioavailability of sarpicillin, the methoxymethyl ester of hetacillin, in humans

capsules, hard and soft gelatin and tablets: sarpicillin, levels, plasma, saliva, urine; pharmacokinetic analysis

Kitzes, R., Ackerman, Z., Levy, M., Frumerman, I., Skved, A. and Garty, M., *Isr. J. med. Scis.*, 1985, *21*, 323–6

Bioavailability of phenytoin–comparison between 3 preparations

capsules, hard gelatin and tablets: phenytoin, levels, serum; pharmacokinetic analysis

Sertié, J.A.A., Zamini, A.C. and Oga, S., *Curr. ther. Res.*, 1985, *38*, 922–30

Serum levels of different formulations of oxytetracycline in adult healthy volunteers

capsules, hard gelatin and tablets, coated: oxytetracycline, levels, serum; drug availability, comparison of 2 × 250 mg capsules with 1 × 500 mg

Stolk, L.M.L., Siddiqui, A.H., Westerhof, W. and Cormane, R.H., *Br. J. Derm.*, 1985, *112*, 469–73

Comparison of bioavailability and phototoxicity of two oral preparations of 5-methoxypsoralen

capsules, hard gelatin and tablets: 5-methoxypsoralen, levels, serum; drug side effects, phototoxicity, comparison of dosage forms

Yakatan, G.J., Rasmussen, C.E., Feis, P.J. and Wallen, S., *J. clin. Pharmac.*, 1985, *25*, 36–42

Bioinequivalence of erythromycin ethylsuccinate and enteric-coated pellets following multiple oral doses

capsules, hard gelatin and tablets: erythromycin, base and ethylsuccinate, levels, plasma; capsule contents, erythromycin base, enteric coated pellets; pharmacokinetic analysis

4.4.4.2 Comparison with Liquid Preparations

Sjögren, J., Sölvell, L. and Karlsson, I., *Acta med. scand.*, 1965, *178*, 553–9

Studies on the absorption rate of barbiturates in man

capsules, hard gelatin, solutions, suspensions and tablets: amylobarbitone, butobarbitone, cyclobarbitone calcium, cyclopentobarbitone and sodium salt, hexobarbitone and sodium salt, pentobarbitone and sodium salt, quinalbarbitone and sodium salt, levels, plasma; formulation of contents, wetting agent, sodium lauryl sulphate

Wagner, J.G., Gerard, E.S. and Kaiser, D.G., *Clin. Pharmac. Ther.*, 1966, *7*, 610–19

The effect of the dosage form on serum levels of indoxole

capsules, hard and soft gelatin, emulsions and suspensions: indoxole, levels, serum; drug availability, comparison of dosage regimen, multiple and single dose

Bülow, K.B. and Larsson, H., *Pharmac. clinica*, 1969, *1*, 156–60

Absorption or orally administered tritium labelled theophylline preparations

capsules, hard gelatin and syrups: theophylline, levels, plasma, urine; radioactive isotope technique

Caldwell, H.C., Westlake, W.J., Connor, S.M. and Flanagan, T., *J. clin. Pharmac.*, 1971, *11*, 349–56

A pharmacokinetic analysis of lithium carbonate absorption from several formulations in man

capsules, hard gelatin, solutions and tablets: lithium carbonate, levels, serum; pharmacokinetic analysis

O'Callaghan, C.H., Tootill, J.P.R. and Robinson, W.D., *J. Pharm. Pharmac.*, 1971, *23*, 50–7

A new approach to the study of serum concentrations of orally administered cephalexin

capsules, hard gelatin, solutions and suspensions: cephalexin, levels, serum; drug availability, effects of, capsule filling, food; pharmacokinetic analysis

Welling, P.G., Lee, K.P., Patel, J.A., Walker, J.E. and Wagner, J.G., *J. pharm. Sci.*, 1971, *60*, 1629–34

Urinary excretion of ephedrine in man without pH control following oral administration of three commercial ephedrine sulfate preparations

capsules, hard gelatin and syrups: ephedrine sulphate, levels, urine; pharmacokinetic analysis

Ballard, D.L. and McQueen, E.G., *Proc. Univ. Otago med. Sch.*, 1972, *50*(N2), 23–4

Blood levels of rifampicin after its administration in capsules or in syrup

capsules, hard gelatin and syrups: rifampicin, levels, plasma

Friedman, H.L. and Wang, R.I.H., *J. pharm. Sci.*, 1972, *61*, 1663–5

Oral absorption of ^{14}C-labeled mepenzolate bromide in humans

capsules, hard gelatin and solutions: mepenzolate bromide, levels, faeces, urine; radioactive isotope technique

Wagner, J.G., Welling, P.G., Roth, S.B., Sakmar, E., Lee, K.P. and Walker, J.E., *Int. Z. klin. Pharmak. Ther. Toxik.*, 1972, *5*, 371–80

Plasma concentrations of propoxyphene in man 1. Following oral administration of the drug in solution and capsule forms

capsules, hard gelatin and solutions: dextropropoxyphene hydrochloride, metabolites, levels, plasma; pharmacokinetic analysis; solution, capsules dissolved in Coca Cola

Halpern, S., Alazraki, N., Littenberg, R., Hurwitz, S., Green, J., Kunsa, J. and Ashburn, W., *J. nucl. Med.*, 1973, *14*, 507–11

^{131}I Thyroid uptakes: capsule versus liquid

capsules, hard gelatin and solutions: Iodine-131, levels, thyroid; radioactive isotope technique

Robertson, J.S., Verhasselt, M. and Wahner, H.W., *J. nucl. Med.*, 1974, *15*, 770–4

Use of ^{123}I for thyroid uptake measurements and depression of ^{131}I thyroid uptakes by incomplete dissolution of capsule filler capsules, hard gelatin and solutions: iodine-123 and 131, levels, thyroid; radioactive isotope technique

Jepson, K., *J. int. med. Res.*, 1975, *3*, *Suppl.* (1), 27–35

A comparative study of clomipramine (Anafranil) capsules and tablets

capsules, hard gelatin, syrups and tablets: clomipramine, levels, plasma; drug, clinical effect, psychological assessment

Mallis, G.I., Schmidt, D.H. and Lindenbaum, J., *Clin. Pharmac. Ther.*, 1975, *18*, 761–8

Superior bioavailability of digoxin solution in capsules

capsules, soft gelatin, solutions and tablets: digoxin, levels, serum, urine

Sansom, L.N., O'Reilly, W.J., Wiseman, C.W., Stern, L.M. and Derham, J., *Med. J. Aust.*, 1975, *2*, 593–5

Plasma phenytoin levels produced by various phenytoin preparations

capsules, hard gelatin, suspensions and tablets: phenytoin, free acid, sodium salt, levels, plasma; drug availability, comparison of products; product, content uniformity

Dugal, R., Cooper, S.F. and Bertrand, M., *Can. J. pharm. Sci.*, 1976, *11*, 92–5

Plasma levels and relative systemic availability of erythromycin estolate capsule and liquid suspension formulations in man

capsules, hard gelatin and suspensions: erythromycin estolate, levels, plasma; pharmacokinetic analysis

Green, J.P., Wilcox, J.R., Marriott, J.D., Halpern, S.E. and Crews, Q.E., *J. nucl. Med.*, 1976, *17*, 310–12

Thyroid uptake of [131]I: Further comparisons of capsules and liquid preparations

capsules, hard gelatin and solutions: iodine-131, levels, thyroid; drug availability, comparison of capsule products

Miles, B.E., Attwood, E.C. and Seddon, R.M., *Lancet*, 1976, *1*, 255

Serum-phenytoin

capsules, hard gelatin, suspensions and tablets: phenytoin, levels, serum; drug availability, effect of multiple dosage

Colburn, W.A. and Gibaldi, M., *Can. J. pharm. Sci.*, 1977, *12*, 90–1

Pharmacokinetics of erythromycin absorption from capsules and suspensions

capsules, hard gelatin and suspensions: erythromycin estolate, levels, plasma; drug availability, comparison of products; pharmacokinetic analysis

Lindenbaum, J., *Clin. Pharmac. Ther.*, 1977, *21*, 278–82

Greater bioavailability of digoxin solution in capsules. Studies in the postprandial state

capsules, soft gelatin, solutions and tablets: digoxin, levels, serum, urine; pharmacokinetic analysis

Männistö, P., *Clin. Pharmac. Ther.*, 1977, *21*, 370–4

Absorption of rifampin from various preparations and pharmaceutic forms

capsules, hard gelatin, syrups and tablets: rifampicin, levels, serum, urine; drug availability, comparison of products; product, content uniformity

Mroszczak, E.J., Runkel, R., Strand, L.J., Tomlinson, R.V., Fratis, A. and Segre, E., *J. pharm. Sci.*, 1978, *67*, 920–3

Cloprednol bioavailability in humans

capsules, hard gelatin, solutions and tablets: cloprednol, levels, plasma; drug availability, effect of capsule formulation; pharmacokinetic analysis

Müller-Brand, J., Staub, J.J., Moeglen, C. and Peyer, P., *Nucl. Med.*, 1978, *17*, 70–3

The influence of the pharmaceutical form of ^{131}I on results in radio-iodine study. Comparison of ^{131}I-capsule and solution of [131]I (in German)

capsules, hard gelatin and solutions: iodine-131, levels, protein bound, thyroid

Vallner, J.J., Needham, T.E., Jun, H.W., Brown, W.J., Stewart, J.T., Kotzan, J.A. and Honigberg, I.L., *J. clin. Pharmac.*, 1978, *18*, 319–24

Plasma levels of clobazam after three oral dosage forms in healthy subjects

capsules, hard gelatin, solutions and tablets: clobazam, levels, plasma; drug clinical effects

Weintraub, H.S., Killinger, J.M. and Fuller, B.L., *Gastroenterology*, 1978, *74*, 1110

Human active pharmacokinetics and comparative bioavailability of loperamide hydrochloride from capsule and syrup formulations

capsules, hard gelatin and syrups: loperamide hydrochloride, levels, serum, urine

Kotzan, J.A., Needham, T.E., Honigberg, I.L., Vallner, J.J., Stewart, J.T., Brown, W.J. and Jun, H.W., *J. pharm. Sci.*, 1979, *68*, 1002–4

Examination of blood clobazam levels and several pupillary measures in humans

capsules, hard gelatin, solutions and tablets: clobazam, levels, blood; drug, clinical effects

Lesko, L.J., Canada, A.T., Eastwood, G., Walker, D. and Brousseau, D.R., *J. pharm. Sci.*, 1979, *68*, 1392–4

Pharmacokinetics and relative bioavailability of oral theophylline capsules

capsules, soft gelatin and solutions: theophylline, levels, serum

Arnold, J., Jacob, J.T. and Riley, B., *J. pharm. Sci.*, 1980, *69*, 1416–8

Bioavailability and pharmacokinetics of a new, slow-release potassium chloride capsule capsules, hard gelatin, elixirs and tablets, controlled-release: potassium chloride, levels, urine (potassium); drug side-effects, comparison of products

Ginsburg, C.M. and McCracken, G.H., *J. int. med. Res.*, 1980, *8*, Suppl. (1), 9–14

Bioavailability of cefadroxil capsules and suspension in pediatric patients

capsules, hard gelatin and suspensions: cefadroxil, levels, saliva, serum, urine; drug availability, effects of, patient's age (children) and fasting state; pharmacokinetic analysis

Aïache, J.M. and Aïache, S., *J. Pharm. Belg.*, 1981, *36*, 325–31

Comparative bioavailability of ampicillin after administration of two drug dosage forms (hard gelatin capsules and suspension) (in French)

capsules, hard gelatin and suspensions: ampicillin, levels, serum, urine; pharmacokinetic analysis

Aïache, J.M., Borel, J.P. and Kantelip, J.-P., *Biopharm. Drug Disp.*, 1982, *3*, 275–81

Comparative bioavailability of S-carboxymethylcysteine from two dosage forms: hard gelatin capsule and syrup

capsules, hard gelatin and syrups: S-carboxymethylcysteine, levels, plasma: pharmacokinetic analysis

Debbas, N.M.G., Mofs, R.M.J., Gordon, B.H., Richards, R.P., Jackson, S.H.D. and Turner, P., *Br. J. clin. Pharmac.*, 1985, *20*, 549

(+)-fenfluramine: relative and absolute bioavailability of a solution compared with capsule

capsules, hard gelatin, infusion, intravenous and solutions: fenfluramine, levels, plasma; pharmacokinetic analysis

Harcus, A.W., Ward, A.E., Ankier, S.I. and Kimber, G.R., *J. clin. Hosp. Pharm.*, 1983, *8*, 125–32

A comparative bioavailability study of Molipaxin capsules and a trazodone liquid formulation in normal volunteers

capsules, hard gelatin and syrups: trazodone, levels, plasma; drug clinical effect, comparison of dosage forms, double-blind trial; pharmacokinetic analysis

Randolph, W.C., Beg, M.M.A., Swagzdis, J.E. and Putterman, K., *Curr. ther. Res.*, 1985, *38*, 990–6

Bioavailability of a modified formulation capsule containing 25 mg hydrochlorothiazide and 50 mg triamterene

capsules, hard gelatin and solutions: hydrochlorothiazide, triamterene, levels, blood, urine; pharmacokinetic analysis

Noonan, P.K. and Benet, L.Z., *J. pharm. Sci.*, 1986, *75*, 241–3

The bioavailability of oral nitroglycerin

capsules, hard gelatin and solutions: nitroglycerin, dinitrate metabolites, levels, serum; drug availability, comparison of

results with sublingual administration; drug clinical effect, correlation with metabolites

4.4.4.3 Comparison with Injections

Walkenstein, S.S., Wiser, R., Gudmundsen, C.H., Kimmel, H.B. and Corradino, R.A., *J. pharm. Sci.*, 1964, *53*, 1181–6

Absorption, metabolism and excretion of oxazepam and its succinate half-ester

capsules, hard gelatin and injections, intramuscular: oxazepam, succinate half-ester, levels, faeces, plasma, urine; radioactive isotope technique; 4.3.2.5

Danhof, I.E., Schreiber, E.C., Wiggans, D.S. and Leyland, H.M., *Toxic. appl. Pharmac.*, 1968, *13*, 16–23

Metabolic dynamics of dicyclomine hydrochloride in man as influenced by various dose schedules and formulations

capsules, hard gelatin, injections, intravenous and tablets: dicyclomine hydrochloride, levels, faeces, plasma, urine; drug availability, comparison of dosage regimens, single, multiple, effect of prolonged-release product; radioactive isotope technique

Castegnaro, E., Iannotta, F. and Pollini, C., *Farmaco, Edn prat.*, 1974, *29*, 520–2

Preliminary studies on the pharmacokinetics of ketoprofen (in Italian)

capsules, hard gelatin and injections, intramuscular: ketoprofen, levels, plasma

Dubetz, D.K., Brown, N.N., Hooper, W.D., Eadie, M.J. and Tyrer, J.H., *Br. J. clin. Pharmac.*, 1978, *6*, 279–81

Disopyramide pharmacokinetics and bioavailability

capsules, hard gelatin and injections, intravenous: disopyramide, levels, plasma

Breuing, K.H., Gilfrich, H.J., Meinertz, T. and Jähnchen, E., *Arzneimittel-Forsch.*, 1979, *29*, 971–2

Pharmacokinetics of azapropazone following single oral and intravenous doses

capsules, hard gelatin and injections, intravenous: azapropazone, levels, plasma; pharmacokinetic analysis

Lintz, W., Barth, H., Osterloh, G. and Schmidt-Böthett, E., *Arzneimittel-Forsch.*, 1986, *36* (II), 1278–83

Bioavailability of enteral tramadol formulations. 1st Communication: Capsules

capsules, hard gelatin and injections, intravenous: tramadol hydrochloride, levels, serum; pharmacokinetic analysis

4.4.4.4 Comparison of Oral and Rectal Routes

Höbel, M. and Talebian, M., *Arzneimittel-Forsch.*, 1960, *10*, 653–6

The absorption of N-acetyl-p-aminophenol from gelatin suppositories (in German)

capsules, soft gelatin and suppositories: paracetamol, levels, urine; formulation of contents; rectal capsules

Widmann, A., *Pharm. Ind., Berl.*, 1960, *22*, 348–52

Rectal gelatin capsules (in German)

capsules, soft gelatin and suppositories: paracetamol, levels, urine; formulation of contents; rectal capsules; 3.5.2

Fichsel, H., *Kinderärztl. Prax.*, 1963, *31*, 245–50

Experiences with a new antipyretic and analgesic in a new rectal capsule form (in German)

capsules, soft gelatin and suppositories: phenacetin, salicylamide, levels, urine; drug, clinical effects, temperature reduction, sedation; rectal capsules; 3.5.2

Michotte, L.J., van Bogaert, P. and Wauters, M., *Acta rheum. scand.*, 1966, *12*, 146–52

The results of long-term treatment of coxarthrosis with indomethacin

capsules, hard gelatin and suppositories: indomethacin, clinical effects, side-effects

Lambelin, G., Roncucci, R., Simon, M.-J., Orloff, S., Mortier, G., Veys, E. and Buu-Hoï, N.P., *Arzneimittel-Forsch.*, 1968, *18*, 56–60

Absorption and excretion of ^{14}C-p-butoxyphenylacethydroxamic acid in man and animals

capsules, hard gelatin, suppositories and tablets, enteric-coated: *p*-butoxyphenylacethydroxamic acid, levels, blood, serum, urine; radioactive isotope technique; 4.3.2.4

Fuccella, L.M., Tosolini, G., Moro, E. and Tamassia, V., *Int. J. clin. Pharmac.*, 1972, *6*, 303–9

Study of physiological availability of temazepam in man

capsules, hard gelatin, solutions and suppositories: temazepam, metabolites, levels, serum, urine; pharmacokinetic analysis

Vibelli, C., Chierichetti, S., Sala, P., Ferrari, P. and Pasotti, C., *Clin. Trials J.*, 1977, *14*, 83–8

Feprazone. Bioavailability in a new suppository preparation

capsules, soft gelatin and suppositories: feprazone, levels, serum; drug availability, co-administration bromhexine; rectal capsules; 3.5.2

Doluisio, J.T., Smith, R.B., Chun, A.H.C. and Dittert, L.W., *J. pharm. Sci.*, 1978, *67*, 1586–8

Pentobarbital absorption from capsules and suppositories in humans

capsules, hard gelatin and suppositories: methylphenobarbitone, pentobarbitone sodium, levels, serum; drug availability, effect of dosage, two capsule strengths

Colombo, B., Carrabba, M. and Sarchi, C., *Boll. chim.-farm.*, 1979, *118*, 176–82

Bioavailability of Tolectin administered orally and rectally (in Italian)

capsules and suppositories: tolmetin, levels, plasma, urine; drug availability, comparison of dose, 200 mg sodium salt (capsules) and 400 mg free acid (suppositories); pharmacokinetic analysis

Fuccella, L.M., *Br. J. clin. Pharmac.*, 1979, *8*, *Suppl.* 1, 31S–35S

Bioavailability of temazepam in soft gelatin capsules

capsules, hard and soft gelatin, solutions and suppositories: temazepam, levels, plasma

Adams, K.R.H., Baber, B., Halliday, L.D.C., Littler, T.R., Orme, M.L.E. and Sibeon, R., *Br. J. clin. Pharmac.*, 1982, *14*, 612–3P

A clinical and pharmacokinetic study of indomethacin in standard and slow release formulations

capsules, hard gelatin, suppositories and tablets: indomethacin, levels, serum; drug, clinical effects, comparison of dosage forms; drug, side-effects, comparison of dosage forms

Battino, D., Biraghi, M., Cusi, C., Nespolo, A. and Avanzini, G., *Ital. J. neurol. Sci.*, 1982, *3*, 197–200

Comparison of the effectiveness of several formulations of sodium valproate : Tablets, enteric-coated capsules, solutions and rectal capsules

capsules, drops, syrups and tablets: valproate sodium, levels, plasma; drug availability, comparison of oral and rectal forms; drug side-effects, comparison of dosage forms, capsule, enteric-coated and standard oral forms; rectal capsules

Fredj, G., Farinotti, R., Hakkou, F., Astier, A. and Dauphin, A., *J. Pharm. Belg.*, 1983, *38*, 105–8

Oral and rectal comparative bioavailability of indomethacin (in French)

capsules, hard gelatin and suppositories: indomethacin, levels, serum; drug, side-effects, comparison of dosage forms; pharmacokinetic analysis

Reinicke, C., Hippius, M., Berles, R. and Grune, D., *Ztg Klin. Med.*, 1985, *40*, 125–9

Comparison of bioavailability of registered indomethacin preparations (in German)

capsules, hard gelatin, suppositories and tablets, sugar-coated: indomethacin, levels, serum; pharmacokinetic analysis

Äärynen, M. and Palho, J., *Arzneimittel-Forsch.*, 1986, *36*(1), 744–747

Piroxicam capsules versus suppositories: a pharmacokinetic and clinical trial

capsules, hard gelatin and suppositories: piroxicam, levels, serum; drug effect, pain relief; pharmacokinetic analysis

4.4.4.5 Comparison with Multiple Dosage Forms

Kleinsorge, H. and Gaida, P., *Arzneimittel-Forsch.*, 1961, *11*, 1100–2

The quantity and speed of excretion of the Rauwolfia alkaloid ajmalin following different forms of administration (in German)

capsules, soft gelatin, injections, intramuscular and intravenous, suppositories and tablets, enteric-coated: ajmaline, levels, urine

Hollister, L.E., Curry, S.H., Derr, J.E. and Kanter, S.L., *Clin. Pharmac. Ther.*, 1970, *11*, 49–59

Studies of delayed-action medication V. Plasma levels and urinary excretion of four different dosage forms of chlorpromazine

capsules, hard gelatin, injections, intramuscular, solutions and tablets: chlorpromazine, levels, plasma, urine; drug availability, comparison of dosage regimens

Hall, A.P., Czerwinski, A.W., Madonia, E.C. and Evensen, K.L., *Clin. Pharmac. Ther.*, 1973, *14*, 580–5

Human plasma and urine quinine levels following tablets, capsules and intravenous infusion

capsules, hard gelatin, infusions, intravenous and tablets: quinine sulphate, levels, plasma, urine

Binnion, P.F., *J. clin. Pharmac.*, 1976, *16*, 461–7

A comparison of the bioavailability of digoxin in capsule, tablet and solution taken orally with intravenous digoxin

capsules, soft gelatin, infusions, intravenous and tablets: digoxin, levels, serum, urine

Bolme, P., Dahlström, B., Diding, N.Å., Flink, O. and Paalzow, L., *Eur. J. clin. Pharmac.*, 1976, *10*, 237–43

Ampicillin: comparison of bioavailability and pharmacokinetics after oral and intravenous administration of three brands

capsules, hard gelatin, injections, intravenous and tablets: ampicillin, levels, serum; drug availability, comparison of products; pharmacokinetic analysis

Marcus, F.I., Dickerson, J., Pippin, S., Stafford, M. and Bressler, R., *Clin. Pharmac. Ther.*, 1976, *20*, 253–9

Digoxin bioavailability: Formulations and rates of infusion

capsules, soft gelatin, injections, intravenous, solutions and tablets: digoxin, levels, serum, urine; drug availability, comparison of dosage regimen, different dose levels; pharmacokinetic analysis

Mason, W.D., Covinsky, J.O., Valentine, J.L., Kelly, K.L., Weddle, O.H. and Martz, B.L., *J. pharm. Sci.*, 1976, *65*, 1325–9

Comparative plasma concentrations of quinidine following administration of one intramuscular and three oral formulations to 13 human subjects

capsules, hard gelatin, injections, intramuscular, solutions and tablets: quinidine sulphate, levels, plasma; pharmacokinetic analysis

Stafford, M.G., Marcus, F.I., Dickerson, J., Pippin, S. and Bressler, R., *Clin. Res.*, 1976, *24*, 94A

Comparative bioavailability of digoxin tablets, oral solution and capsules

capsules, soft gelatin, infusions, intravenous, solutions and tablets: digoxin, levels, serum, urine

Lloyd, B.L., Greenblatt, D.J., Allen, M.D., Harmatz, J.S. and Smith, T.W., *Am. J. Cardiol.*, 1978, *42*, 129–36

Pharmacokinetics and bioavailability of digoxin capsules, solution and tablets after single and multiple doses

capsules, hard gelatin, injections, intravenous and tablets: digoxin, levels, serum; drug availability, comparison of dosage regimen, single and multiple dose; pharmacokinetic analysis

Icasas-Cabral, E., Capa, H., Zarate, M.V. and Dayrit, C., *Phillipine J. intern. Med.*, 1979, *17*, 185–94

Evaluation of bioavailability of digoxin tablets and capsules

capsules, soft gelatin, injection, intravenous and tablets: digoxin, levels, serum, urine

Weidler, D.J., Garg, D.C., Vasquez, C.L., Allin, D. and Dragonetti, D.E., *Clin. Pharmac. Ther.*, 1980, *27*, 293

Absolute bioavailability of a new soft elastic gelatin (SEG) digoxin capsule in patients with functional class I, II and III cardiac failure

capsules, soft gelatin, injections, intravenous, and tablets: digoxin, levels, plasma; pharmacokinetic analysis

Rietbrock, N., Brecht, H.M., Rudorf, J.E. and Alken, R.G., *Münch. med. Wschr.*, 1982, *124*, 550–2

Absolute bioavailability of digoxin. Comparison of a soft gelatin capsule and a commercially available silicic acid–matrix preparation (in German)

capsules, soft gelatin, injection, intravenous and tablets: digoxin, levels, plasma, urine; pharmacokinetic analysis

Erb, R. and Stoltman, W., *J. Pharmacokinet. Biopharm.*, 1983, *11*, 611–21

Evaluation of 2 nitroglycerin dosage forms. A metered spray and a soft gelatin capsule

capsules, soft gelatin, inhalations, aerosol and tablets, sublingual: nitroglycerin, clinical effect, digital plethysmographic measurements; dosage form testing, blind trial with placebo

Kukovetz, W.R., Beubler, E., Kreuzig, F., Moritz, A.J., Nirnberger, G. and Werner-Breitenecker, L., *J. Rheumatol.*, 1983, *10*, 90–4

Bioavailability and pharmacokinetics of D-penicillamine

capsules, hard gelatin, injections, intravenous and tablets: D-penicillamine, levels, plasma; drug availability, comparison of oral forms of dimethylcysteine, effect of dose, 150 and 250 mg in capsules; pharmacokinetic analysis

Lücker, P.W., Tinhof, W., Wetzelsberger, N., Weyers, W. and Brodbeck, R., *Arzneimittel-Forsch.*, 1983, *33*, 453–8

Pharmacokinetics and absolute bioavailability of bromopride from various pharmaceutical formulations (in German)

capsules, hard gelatin, drops, injections and suppositories: bromopride, levels, serum; drug availability, comparison of dosage regimen, multiple and single dose, capsules and drops; pharmacokinetic analysis

Skoutakis, V.A., Acchiardo, S.R., Wojciechowski, N.J. and Carter, C.A., *Pharmacotherapy*, 1984, *4*, 392–7

Liquid and solid potassium chloride: bioavailability and safety

capsules, hard gelatin, solutions and tablets: potassium chloride, levels, potassium, serum and urine; drug, side-effects, comparison of products, standard and slow-release

Skoutakis, V.A., Acchiardo, S.R., Wojciechowski, N.J., Carter, C.A., Melikan, A.P. and Chremos, A.N., *J. clin. Pharmac.*, 1985, *25*, 619–21

The comparative bioavailability of liquid, wax-matrix and microencapsulated preparations of potassium chloride

capsules, hard gelatin, solutions and tablets: potassium chloride levels, potassium, urine

4.4.4.6 Comparison of Inhalation Capsules and Aerosols

Latimer, K.M., Roberts, R., Dolovich, J. and Hargreave, F.E., *Can. med. Ass. J.*, 1982, *127*, 857–9

Salbutamol: comparison of bronchodilating effect of inhaled powder and aerosol in asthmatic subjects

aerosols and capsules, hard gelatin: salbutamol; capsules, non-oral, inhalation; drug, clinical effects, forced expiratory volume, vital capacity

Sovijavv. A.R., Lahdensu, A. and Muittari, A., *Curr. ther. Res.*, 1982, *32*, 566–73

Bronchodilating effect of salbutamol inhalation powder and salbutamol aerosol after metacholine-induced bronchoconstriction

capsules, hard gelatin and inhalations, aerosol: salbutamol, clinical effects, flow-volume spirometry; patients' physiological state, induced bronchoconstriction with metacholine

4.4.5 Comparison of Capsule Products

Glazko, A.J., Kinkel, A.W., Alegnani, W.C. and Holmes, E.L., *Clin. Pharmac. Ther.*, 1968, *9*, 472–83

An evaluation of the absorption characteristics of different
chloramphenicol preparations in normal human subjects

capsules, hard gelatin: chloramphenicol, levels, plasma, urine

Sequeira, A.P., Saraiva Paiva, L.F.S. and Carvalho, L.S., *Revta port. Farm.*, 1969, *19*, 79–85

The availability and biological activity of several capsules of oxytetracycline hydrochloride (in Portuguese)

capsules, hard gelatin: oxytetracycline hydrochloride, levels, serum

Blair, D.C., Barnes, R.W., Wildner, E.L. and Murray, W.J., *J. Am. med. Ass.*, 1971, *215*, 251–4

Biological availability of oxytetracycline HCl capsules. A comparison of all manufacturing sources supplying the United States market

capsules: oxytetracycline, levels, serum

Mayersohn, M. and Endrenyi, L., *Can. med. Ass. J.*, 1973, *109*, 989–93

Relative bioavailability of commercial ampicillin formulations in man

capsules, hard gelatin: ampicillin, levels, plasma

Arcilla, J.D., Fiore, J.L., Resnick, O., Nadelmann, J.W., Huth, J.L. and Troetel, W.M., *Curr. ther. Res.*, 1974, *16*, 1126–36

Comparative bioavailability of doxycycline

capsules, hard gelatin: doxycycline hydrochloride, levels, plasma

Meyer, M.C., Dann, R.E., Whyatt, P.L. and Slywka, G.W.A., *J. Pharmacokinet. Biopharm.*, 1974, *2*, 287–97

The bioavailability of sixteen tetracycline products

capsules: tetracycline, hydrochloride, phosphate, levels, urine

Whyatt, P.L., Slywka, G.W.A., Melikian, A.P. and Meyer, M.C., *J. pharm. Sci.*, 1976, *65*, 652–6

Bioavailability of 17 ampicillin products

capsules, hard gelatin: ampicillin, anhydrous, trihydrate, levels, serum

Adir, J. and Barr, W.H., *J. pharm. Sci.*, 1977, *66*, 1000–4

Effect of sleep on bioavailability of tetracycline

capsules, hard gelatin: tetracycline hydrochloride, levels, urine; drug availability, effect of patient's condition, movement and sleep

DeSante, K.A., Stoll, R.G., Kaiser, D.G. and DiSanto, A.R., *J. pharm. Sci.*, 1977, *66*, 1713–6

Generic propoxyphene: Need for clinical bioavailability evaluation

capsules, hard gelatin: dextropropoxyphene hydrochloride, levels, plasma

Fedorcak, A., Mielenz, H., Bozler, G. and Mader, G., *Arzneimittel-Forsch.*, 1977, *27*, 659–65

Studies on the pharmacokinetic equivalence of pivampicillin base and hydrochloride in capsules and tablets (in German)

capsules, hard gelatin and tablets: pivampicillin base and hydrochloride, levels, plasma

Melikian, A.P., Straughn, A.B., Slywka, G.W.A., Whyatt, P.L. and Meyer, M.C., *J. Pharmacokinet. Biopharm.*, 1977, *5*, 133–46

Bioavailability of 11 phenytoin products

capsules, hard gelatin: phenytoin sodium, levels, plasma

Chonielewski, D.H., *J. pharm. Sci.*, 1978, *67*(9), iv

Propoxyphene bioavailability

comment on paper by DeSante, K.A., Stoll, R.G., Kaiser, D.G. and DiSanto, A.R., *J. pharm. Sci.*, 1977, *66*, 1713–6

Taylor, T., O'Kelly, D.A., Darragh, A. and Chasseaud, L.F., *Pharm. Ind., Berl.*, 1978, *40*, 155–6

Bioavailability of ampicillin measured after repeated oral doses

capsules, hard gelatin: ampicillin, levels, serum; drug availability, effect of dosage regimen, multiple doses

Chow, M., Quintiliani, R., Cunha, B.A., Thompson, M., Finkelstein, E. and Nightingale, C.H., *J. clin. Pharmac.*, 1979, *19*, 185–94

Pharmacokinetics of high-dose oral cephalosporins

capsules, hard gelatin: cephalexin, cephradine, levels, serum, urine; pharmacokinetic analysis

Erking, W., Lücker, P.W., Stöcker, K.-P. and Wetzelsberger, K., *Arzneimittel-Forsch.*, 1979, *29*, 1184–9

Relative bioavailability of a new spironolactone preparation (in German)

capsules, hard gelatin: spironolactone, metabolites, levels, serum, urine; pharmacokinetic analysis

Hamilton-Miller, J.M.T. and Brumfitt, W., *J. antimicrob. Chemother.*, 1979, *5*, 699–704

The bioavailability for four different commercially available brands of ampicillin compared with that of talampicillin

capsules, hard gelatin and tablets: ampicillin (capsules), levels, serum

Sorel, R.H.A. and Roseboom, H., *Int. J. Pharmaceut.*, 1979, *3*, 93–9

Rapid in vitro and in vivo conversion of hydroxymethylnitrofurantoin into nitrofurantoin as measured by HPLC

capsules, hard gelatin and tablets: nitrofurantoin, hydroxymethylnitrofurantoin, levels, urine

Welling, P.G., Elliott, R.L., Pitterle, M.E., Corrick-West, H.P. and Lyons, L.L., *J. pharm. Sci.*, 1979, *68*, 150–5

Plasma levels following single and repeated doses of erythromycin estolate and erythromycin stearate

capsules, hard gelatin, suspensions and tablets: erythromycin estolate and stearate, levels, plasma

Cid, E., Henriquez, A., Andrade, A., Olguin, R., Firmani, E. and Fuentes, B., *J. Pharm. Belg.*, 1980, *35*, 273–6

Relationship between bioavailability and clinical effect of chloramphenicol

capsules, hard gelatin: chloramphenicol, levels, urine; drug clinical effect, healthy volunteers and patients

Ali, H.M., *Int. J. Pharmaceut.*, 1981, *7*, 301–6

Comparative bioavailability of eight brands of ampicillin

capsules, hard gelatin: ampicillin, levels, urine; pharmacokinetic analysis

Ali, A.A. and Farouk, A., *Int. J. Pharmaceut.*, 1981, *9*, 239–43

Comparative studies on the bioavailability of ampicillin anhydrate and trihydrate

capsules, hard gelatin: ampicillin, anhydrous, trihydrate, levels, urine

Buniva, G., Pagani, V. and Carozzi, A., *Int. J. clin. Pharmac. Ther. Toxic.*, 1983, *21*, 404–9

Bioavailability of rifampicin capsules

capsules, hard gelatin: rifampicin, levels, serum; drug availability, comparison of experimental formulations with standard formulation, effect of manufacturing method; formulation of contents, excipients, particle size

Chaudhari, G.N., Tipnis, H.P., Doshi, B.S. and Kulkarni, R.D., *Eur. J. clin. Pharmac.*, 1984, *26*, 261–4

Bioequivalence studies in humans of indomethacin capsules marketed in India

capsules, hard gelatin: indomethacin, levels, plasma; pharmacokinetic analysis

Khalil, S. A., Mortada, L.M. and Ismail, F.A., *Drug Dev. ind. Pharm.*, 1984, *10*, 929–48

Bioavailability of eight brands of ampicillin capsules

capsules, hard gelatin: ampicillin, levels, urine; pharmacokinetic analysis

Dahmen, W., Pabst, G., Molz, K.-H., Lutz, D. and Jaeger, H., *Arzneimittel-Forsch.*, 1985, *35*, 1842–4

Bioavailability of new Nifedipine preparations in man. 2. Bio-equivalence of Nifedipine in form of soft gelatin capsules (in German)

capsules, soft gelatin: nifedipine levels, plasma; pharmacokinetic analysis

Del Arno, E., Cordoba, M. and Torrado, J.J., *Ann. Real Acad. Farm.*, 1985, *51*, 471–6

Bioavailability of rifampicin (in Spanish)

capsules, hard gelatin: rifampicin, levels, plasma; pharmacokinetic analysis

Ogunbona, F.A. and Akanni, A.O., *Pharmazie*, 1985, *40*, 479

Comparative bioavailability studies on some brands of ampicillin capsules

capsules, hard gelatin: ampicillin, levels, urine

Rossi, S.S., Clayton, L.M. and Hofmann, A.F., *J. pharm. Sci.*, 1986, *75*, 288–90

Determination of chenodiol bioequivalence using an unmobilized multi-enzyme bioluminescence technique

capsules: chenodiol, 7α-hydroxy bile acids, levels, serum; pharmacokinetic analysis

4.4.6 Effect of Formulation on Absorption
4.4.6.1 Solid Preparations
Boger, W.P. and Gavin, J.J., *New Engl. J. Med.*, 1959, *261*, 827–32

An evaluation of tetracycline preparations

capsules, hard gelatin and powders: tetracyclines, levels, serum, urine; drug availability, effect of formulation, diluents; 3.2.4.1

Kraml, M., Dubuc, J. and Gaudry, R., *Antibiotics Chemother.*, 1962, *12*, 239–42

Gastrointestinal absorption of griseofulvin: II. Influence of particle size in man

capsules, hard gelatin: griseofulvin, levels, serum; drug availability, effect of particle size; powder properties, particle size determination

Avery, G.S., Adams, E.F. and Samson, K.L., *N.Z. med. J.* 1968, *68*, 408–9

Phenytoin capsules

capsules, hard gelatin: phenytoin, adverse drug interactions, intoxications, review

McQueen, E.G., *N.Z. med. J.*, 1968, *68*, 332

Phenytoin capsules

capsules, hard gelatin: phenytoin; drug availability, effect of formulation; formulation of contents, diluent, identification method

Arnold, K., Gerber, N. and Levy, G., *Can. J. pharm. Sci.*, 1970, *5*, 89–92

Absorption and dissolution studies on sodium diphenyl-hydantoin capsules

capsules, hard gelatin: phenytoin sodium, levels, plasma; drug availability, comparison of dosage regimens, single and multiple doses, effect of co-administration of sodium bicarbonate solution; 4.2.3.1

Tyrer, J.H., Eadie, M.J., Sutherland, J.M. and Hooper, W.D., *Br. med. J.*, 1970, *4*, 271–3

Outbreak of anticonvulsant intoxication in an Australian city

capsules, hard gelatin: phenytoin, levels, blood, faeces; drug availability, effect of formulation, diluents; formulation of contents, diluents, calcium sulphate, lactose

Bochner, F., Hooper, W., Tyrer, J. and Eadie, M., *Proc. Aust. Ass. Neurol.*, 1973, *9*, 165–70

The explanation of the 1968 Australian outbreak of diphenylhydantoin intoxication

capsules, hard gelatin: phenytoin, levels, blood; formulation of contents, diluents, calcium sulphate, lactose

Taylor, T. and Chasseaud, L.F., *J. pharm. Sci.*, 1977, *66*, 1638–9

Plasma concentrations and bioavailability of clofibric acid from its calcium salt in humans

capsules, soft gelatin: clofibrate, calcium salt, clofibric acid, levels, plasma; drug effect, antilipaemic action calcium salts; formulation of contents, combination with calcium carbonate

O'Grady, J., Johnson, B.F., Bye, C. and French, J., *Eur. J. clin. Pharmac.*, 1978, *14*, 357–60

The comparative bioavailability of Lanoxin tablets and Lanoxicaps with and without sorbitol

capsules, soft gelatin and tablets: digoxin, levels, urine; drug availability, comparison of dosage forms; drug availability, effects of formulation; formulation of contents, diluent, sorbitol; pharmacokinetic analysis, comparative bioavailability

Neuvonen, P.J., *Clin. Pharmacokinet.*, 1979, *4*, 91–103

Bioavailability of phenytoin: clinical pharmacokinetic and therapeutic implications

capsules, hard gelatin: phenytoin, free acid, sodium salt; drug availability, comparison of products, effect of formulation, review; 4.5.1

Wolen, R.L., Carmichael, R.H., Ridolfo, A.S., Thompkins, L. and Ziege, E.A., *Biomed. mass Spectrom.*, 1979, *6*, 173–8

The effect of crystal size on the bioavailability of benoxaprofen: Studies utilizing deuterium labelled drug

capsules, hard gelatin and solutions: benoxaprofen, levels, plasma; drug availability, effect of drug particle size; radioactive isotope technique

4.4.6.2 Semi-solid Preparations

Calvert, R.T., Barker, M., Ganley, J.A. and McEwen, J., *J. Pharm. Pharmac.*, 1983, *35*, *Suppl.*, 58P

In-vivo evaluation of a rapidly dissolving glibenclamide formulation

capsules, hard gelatin: glibenclamide, levels, blood; drug availability, effect of formulation; drug levels, radioimmunoassay technique; formulation of contents, semi-solid fill, diluent, polyethylene glycols 400/3000; gastric behaviour, visualisation method, gamma scintigraphy, technetium-99m

Ganley, J.A., McEwen, J., Calvert, R.T. and Barker, M.C.J., *J. Pharm. Pharmac.*, 1984, *36*, 734–39

The effect of in-vivo dispersion and gastric emptying on glibenclamide absorption from a novel, rapidly dissolving capsule formulation

capsules, hard gelatin: glibenclamide, levels, plasma; formulation of contents, polyethylene glycol matrix; gastric behaviour, visualisation method, gamma scintigraphy, technetium-99 m; gastric behaviour, capsule disintegration, gastric emptying, correlation with plasma levels, effect of patient's fasting state; pharmacokinetic analysis

4.4.7 Availability from Controlled Release Products

4.4.7.1 Enteric Capsules

Bukey, F.S. and Rhodes, P., *J. Am. pharm. Ass.*, 1935, *24*, 567–70

A comparative study of enteric coatings

capsules, hard gelatin and tablets: coating materials, keratin, shellac; disintegration method, X-ray, radio-opaque contents

Goorley, J.T. and Lee, C.O., *J. Am. pharm. Ass.*, 1938, *27*, 379–84

A study of enteric coating

capsules, hard gelatin: coating material, shellac/castor oil; disintegration method, fluoroscopic examination, X-ray, radio-opaque contents

Lark-Horovitz, K. and Leng, H.R., *Nature*, 1941, *147*, 580–1

Radioactive indicators, enteric coatings and intestinal absorption

capsules, hard gelatin: coating material, castor oil/shellac; disintegration method, radioactive isotope technique

Hodge, H.C., Forsyth, H.H. and Ramsey, G.H., *J. Pharmac. exp. Ther.*, 1944, *80*, 241–9

Clinical trials of cellulose acetate phthalate as an enteric coating

capsules, soft gelatin and tablets: barium sulphate; coating material, cellulose acetate phthalate; disintegration method, fluoroscopic examination, X-ray, radio-opaque contents

Stoklosa, M.J. and Ohmart, L.M., *J. Am. pharm. Ass., pract. Pharm. Edn*, 1953, *14*, 507 and 514–5

Enteric coatings in dispensing pharmacy. 2. A practical method of extemporaneous enteric coating

capsules, hard gelatin and pills: sodium salicylate, levels, urine (human); disintegration method, fluoroscopic examination; 3.4.2.3

Boymond, P., Sfiris, J. and Amacker, P., *Pharm. Ind., Berl.*, 1966, *28*, 836–42 and *Drugs Germ.*, 1967, *10*, 7–19

The manufacture and testing of enterosoluble capsules (in German; English translation in *Drugs Germ.*)

capsules, hard gelatin: disintegration method, model system, stomach and urine marker; 3.4.2.2; 4.2.2.2

Mascoli, C.C., Leagus, M.B., Weibel, R.E., Stokes, J., Reinhart, H. and Hilleman, M.R., *Proc. Soc. exp. Biol. Med.*, 1966, *121*, 1264–8

Attempt at immunization by oral feeding live Rhinoviruses in enteric-coated capsules

capsules, hard gelatin: rhinoviruses; coating material, cellulose acetate phthalate; disintegration method, X-ray, radio-opaque contents

Eckert, T., Rothgang, G. and Seidel, R., *Arzneimittel-Forsch.*, 1968, *18*, 372–3

The pH-endoradio probe: a method for investigating the disintegration of medicinal preparations with gastric juice resistant coatings in the intestines. Part 2. The disintegration of gelatin capsules with gastric juice resistant coatings (in German)

capsules, hard gelatin: coating material, methacrylates; disintegration method, pH radiotransmitter

Lindup, W.E., Parke, D.V. and Colin-Jones, D., *Gut*, 1970, *11*, 555–8

The absorption of carbenoxolone administered orally as a positioned-release capsule

capsules, hard gelatin: carbenoxolone sodium, levels, serum; capsules, formaldehyde treatment, position release; disintegration method, X-ray, radio-opaque contents; disintegration testing, site of disintegration

Aiache, J.-M., Vidal, J.L., Aiache, S., Jeanneret, A. and Cornat, F., *Labo-Pharma Probl. Tech.*, 1974, *22*(232), 457–63

Methods for the biopharmaceutical testing of enteric capsules: Tests with "enterocaps" capsules (in French)

capsules, hard gelatin: disintegration method, X-ray, radio-opaque contents; 3.4.2.4; 4.5.6.1

Aiache, J.M., Aiache, S., Jeanneret, A., Cornat, F. and Vidal, J.L., *Boll. chim.-farm.*, 1975, *114*, 636–50

Methods for the biopharmaceutical testing of enteric capsules: Tests with "enterocaps" capsules (in French)

capsules, hard gelatin: disintegration method, X-ray, radio-opaque contents; 3.4.2.4; 4.5.6.1

Springolo, V., *Boll. chim.-farm.*, 1978, *177*, 113–21

The bioavailability of formulations of erythromycin base and stearate in gastric resistant soft gelatin capsules (in Italian)

capsules, soft gelatin: erythromycin, base and stearate, levels, plasma; enteric coating, formaldehyde treatment; 3.3.3.2; 3.4.2.2

Rees, W.D.W., Evans, B.K. and Rhodes, J., *Br. med. J.*, 1979, *2*, 835–6

Treating irritable bowel syndrome with peppermint oil

capsules, hard gelatin: peppermint oil; coating material, cellulose acetate phthalate; drug, clinical effect, comparison with placebo

Nassif, E.G., Younoszai, M.K., Weinberger, M.M. and Nassif, C.M., *J. Pediat.*, 1981, *98*, 320–3

Comparative effects of antacids, enteric coating and bile salts on the efficacy of oral pancreatic enzyme therapy in cystic fibrosis

capsules, hard gelatin: pancrelipase; drug, clinical effects, comparison of dosage forms, enteric-coated pellets in capsules, standard capsules, effects of co-administration of, antacids, bile salts; drug, clinical effects, fat absorption, nitrogen excretion; treatment costs, comparison of products

Dew, M.J., Hughes, P.J., Lee, M.G., Evans, B.K. and Rhodes, J., *Br. J. clin. Pharmac.*, 1982, *14*, 405–8

An oral preparation to release drugs in the human colon

capsules, hard gelatin: sulphapyridine, levels, plasma; coating material, methacrylic acid polymers; drug availability, correlation of plasma levels and site of disintegration; gastric behaviour, visualisation method, X-ray, radio-opaque contents; 4.4.3

Taylor, R.H., Mee, A.S., Misiewicz, J.J., Bernardo, D.E. and Polanska, N., *Br. med. J.*, 1982, *285*, 1392–3

Decrease in pancreatic steatorrhoea by positioned-release enzyme capsules

capsules, hard gelatin: pancreatin, drug, clinical effect, faecal fat levels; drug availability, comparison of standard and formaledehyde-treated capsule

Bell, G.D., Richmond, C.R. and Somerville, K.W., *Br. J. clin. Pharmac.*, 1983, *16*, 228-9P

Peppermint oil capsules (Colpermin) for the irritable bowel syndrome: a pharmacokinetic study

capsules, hard and soft gelatin: peppermint oil, menthol, levels, urine; drug availability, comparison of enteric-coated hard gelatin capsule and standard soft gelatin capsule; drug release, site of capsule disintegration

Boymond, C., Chanliau, J., Minck, R. and Stamm, A., *Pharm. Acta Helv.*, 1983, *58*, 266-9

The enteric coating of hard gelatin capsules with acrylic resins: coating technique and in vivo trial (in French)

ampoules and capsules, hard gelatin: bacteriophages; capsules, enteric-coated; drug, clinical effects, effect on urinary bacterial levels, comparison of dosage forms and effect of administration by fibroscope; 3.4.2.4

Thomas, P., Richards, D., Richards, A., Rogers, A., Evans, B.K., Dew, M.J. and Rhodes, J., *J. Pharm. Pharmac.*, 1985, *37*, 757-8

Absorption of delayed-release prednisolone in ulcerative colitis and Crohn's disease

capsules, hard gelatin; [^{3}H] prednisolone, levels, urine; coating material, methacrylates; drug availability, comparison of standard and coated capsules, effect of patient's disease state

Petroski, D., *Am. J. Gastroenterol.*, 1986, *81*, 26-8

A comparison of enteric-coated aspirin granules with plain and buffered aspirin; a report of two studies

capsules, hard gelatin and tablets: acetylsalicylic acid, levels, serum; drug availability, comparison of standard release tablets and enteric product in capsules; drug, side-effects, gastrointestinal damage measured by endoscopy, patient's subject record, comparison of dosage forms

4.4.7.2 Slow-release Capsules

Cass, L.J. and Frederik, W.S., *Curr. ther. Res.*, 1962, *4*, 263-9

Clinical evaluation of long-release and capsule forms of pentobarbital sodium

capsules, hard gelatin and tablets: pentobarbitone sodium; drug, clinical evaluation; drug availability, comparison of dosage regimens, single and multiple dose

Hollister, L.E., Kanter, S.L. and Clyde, D.J., *Clin. Pharmac. Ther.*, 1963, *4*, 612-8

Studies of prolonged-action medication. III. Pentobarbital sodium in prolonged-action form compared with conventional capsules: Serum levels of drug and clinical effects following acute doses

capsules, hard gelatin and tablets: pentobarbitone sodium, levels, serum; drug, clinical effect, Clyde mood scale

Beckett, A.H. and Tucker, G.T., *J. Pharm. Pharmac.*, 1966, *18*, Suppl., 72-5S

A method for the evaluation of some oral prolonged-release forms of dexamphetamine in man, using urinary excretion data

capsules, hard gelatin, granules and solutions: dexamphetamine sulphate, levels, urine, acid pH; drug availability, comparisons of, dosage forms, dosage regimens

Allen, E.S., *Curr. ther. Res.*, 1969, *11*, 745-9

Effect of timed release on the bioavailability of ascorbic acid: Ascorbicap vs. non-timed dosage forms

capsules, hard gelatin: ascorbic acid, levels, blood, urine; drug availability, comparison of dosage regimens; formulation of contents

Beckett, A.H. and Brookes, L.G., *J. Pharm. Pharmac.*, 1971, *23*, 837-41

Administration of two or more related drugs to investigate the effect of molecular modification and formulation on drug absorption, metabolism and excretion

capsules, hard gelatin and tablets: amphetamines, metabolites, levels, urine, acid pH; drug availability, comparison of dosage forms; formulation of contents, slow-release product

Testa, B. and Beckett, A.H., *Pharm. Acta Helv.*, 1974, *49*, 21-7

The metabolism of diethylpropion in man; influence of changes in drug formulation and urinary pH

capsules, hard gelatin: diethylpropion hydrochloride, metabolites, levels, urine, acid pH; formulation of contents, slow-release product

Maneksha, S., *Br. J. clin. Pract.*, 1975, *29*, 12-13

Prolonged action fenfluramine capsules versus fenfluramine tablets in general practice

capsules, hard gelatin and tablets: fenfluramine, clinical effect, mean weight loss; drug availability, comparison of dosage forms, slow-release forms

Soeterboek, A.M. and Van Thiel, M., *J. int. med. Res.*, 1976, *4*, 393-401

Serum quinidine levels after chronic administration of four different quinidine formulations

capsules, hard gelatin and tablets: quinidine bisulphate, levels, serum; drug availability, comparison of dosage forms, standard and controlled-release forms

Frigo, G.M., Perucca, E., Teggia-Droghi, M., Gatti, G., Mussini, A. and Salerno, J., *Br. J. clin. Pharmac.*, 1977, *4*, 449-54

Comparison of quinidine plasma concentration curves following oral administration of short- and long-acting formulations

capsules, hard gelatin and tablets, standard and soluble: quinidine, arabogalactane sulphate (capsules), bisulphate, polygalacturonate, sulphate, levels, plasma; drug availability, comparisons of, salt of drug, products, slow-release preparations; pharmacokinetic analysis

Jørgensen, A., *Eur. J. clin. Pharmac.*, 1977, *12*, 187-90

Comparative bioavailability of a sustained release preparation of amitriptyline and conventional tablets

capsules, hard gelatin and tablets: amitriptyline, levels, serum; drug availability, comparison of dosage forms, standard and controlled-release forms; formulation of contents (capsule), slow-release pellets; pharmacokinetic analysis

Manion, C.V., Lalka, D., Baer, D.T. and Meyer, M.B., *J. pharm. Sci.*, 1977, *66*, 981–4

Absorption kinetics of procainamide in humans

capsules, hard gelatin, infusions, intravenous and tablets, sustained-release: procainamide hydrochloride, levels, plasma, urine; drug availability, comparison of dosage forms, standard and slow-release forms; pharmacokinetic analysis

Bateman, N.E., Finnin, B.C., Jordan, G.J. and Reed, B.L., *Aust. J. pharm. Sci.*, 1978, *7*, 93–5

Bioavailability of theophylline from a prolonged-release soft gelatin capsule using HPLC assay of saliva samples

capsules, soft gelatin and elixirs: theophylline, levels, saliva; drug availability, comparison of dosage forms

Weinberger, M., Hendeles, L. and Bighley, L., *New Engl. J. Med.*, 1978, *299*, 852–7

The relation of product formulation to absorption of oral theophylline

capsules, hard gelatin, solutions and tablets: theophylline, levels, serum; drug availability, comparison of dosage forms

Campbell, D.B., Hopkins, V., Richards, R. and Taylor, D., *Curr. med. Res. Opinion*, 1979, *6*, Suppl. 1, 160–8

Fenfluramine plasma concentrations after administration of a sustained-release capsule formulation and rapid-release tablets

capsules, hard gelatin and tablets: fenfluramine, levels, plasma; drug availability, comparison of, dosage forms, dosage regimen; formulation of contents, slow release

Chubb, J.M., MacFarlane, M.D. and Woosley, R.L., *Fedn Proc.*, 1979, *38*, 585, No. 1887

Bioavailability of Theobid Duracap: sustained-release anhydrous theophylline

capsules, hard gelatin and elixirs: theophylline, levels, serum; drug availability, comparison of dosage forms

Douglas-Jones, A.P., *J. int. med. Res.*, 1979, *7*, 221–3

Comparison of a once daily long-acting formulation of propranolol with conventional propranolol given twice daily in patients with mild to moderate hypertension

capsules, hard gelatin: propranolol; drug availability, comparison of standard and slow-release products; drug, clinical effects

Falliers, C.J., *Int. J. clin. Pharmac. Biopharm.*, 1979, *17*, 125–30

Pharmacodynamic and spirometric responses to a sustained-release theophylline capsule

capsules, hard gelatin and elixirs: theophylline, levels, serum; drug, clinical effects; drug availability, comparison of dosage forms

Fleming, T.E., *Ann. Allergy*, 1979, *42*, 341

Re: Aerolate SR-JR-III capsules of theophylline

capsules, hard gelatin: theophylline; drug availability, controlled release, effect on side-effects; drug availability, serum levels for prophylaxis

Halkin, H., Almog, S. and Friedman, E., *Israel J. med. Scis*, 1979, *15*, 448–50

Serum concentrations of isosorbide dinitrate produced by a sustained-release capsule

capsules, hard gelatin and tablets: isosorbide dinitrate, levels, serum; drug availability, comparison slow-release capsules with standard tablets

Halkin, H., Vered, I., Saginer, A. and Rabinowitz, B., *Eur. J. clin. Pharmac.*, 1979, *16*, 387–91

Once daily administration of sustained release propranolol capsules in the treatment of angina pectoris

capsules, hard gelatin and tablets: propranolol, levels, serum; drug availability, comparison of slow-release capsule and standard tablet; drug, clinical effects

Meyer, M.C., Gollamudi, R. and Straughn, A.B., *J. clin. Pharmac.*, 1979, *19*, 435–44

The influence of dosage form on papaverine bioavailability

capsules, hard gelatin, elixirs and tablets: papaverine hydrochloride, levels, serum; drug availability, comparison of dosage forms, standard and slow-release; drug availability, comparison of products (capsules); pharmacokinetic analysis

Simmons, D.L., Legore, A.A., Picotte, P. and Cesari, F., *Can. J. pharm. Sci.*, 1980, *15*, 26–9

Peristaltic dissolution apparatus: Utility in new dosage form design

capsules, hard gelatin and tablets: ibuprofen, levels, plasma (human), serum (dog); dissolution method, peristaltic

Sinterhauf, K. and Bechtel, W.D., *Arzneimittel-Forsch.*, 1980, *30*, 1012–15

Plasma levels and renal excretion of [^{3}H]-codeine phosphate in humans receiving tablets or depot capsules (in German)

capsules, hard gelatin and tablets: codeine phosphate, levels, plasma; drug availability, comparison slow-release capsules and standard tablets; radioactive isotope technique

Green, E.R., Green, A.W., Lane, R., Slaughter, R. and Middleton, E., *J. Pediat.*, 1981, *98*, 832–4

Absorption characteristics of sustained release theophylline capsules administered in apple sauce

capsules, hard gelatin and syrups: theophylline, levels, plasma (children); drug availability, comparison of pellets and pellets filled in capsule, effect on free pellets of co-administration of apple sauce; pharmacokinetic analysis

Ryan, J.R. and Elliott, B.W., *Curr. ther. Res.*, 1981, *29*, 838–48

A multicenter trial of microencapsulated potassium chloride

capsules, hard gelatin: potassium chloride, levels, K^+ in serum, drug side-effects, comparison with previous treatments; formulation of contents, microencapsulated potassium chloride

Saletu, B., Grünberger, J., Amrein, R. and Skreta, M., *J. int. med. Res.*, 1981, *9*, 408–33

Assessment of pharmacodynamics of a new "controlled-release" form of diazepam (Valium CR Roche) by quantitative EEG and psychometric analysis in neurotic subjects

capsules, hard gelatin and tablets: diazepam; drug, clinical effects, comparison of slow-release capsule and standard tablets, measurement of quantitative EEG and psychometric analysis; drug, side-effects, comparison of dosage forms; formulation of contents, slow-release hydrodynamically-balanced capsule

Adams, K.R.H., Halliday, L.D.C., Sebeon, R.G., Baber, N., Littler, T. and Orme, M.L.E., *Br. J. clin. Pharmac.*, 1982, *14*, 286–9

A clinical and pharmacokinetic study of indomethacin in standard and slow release formulations

capsules, hard gelatin and suppositories: indomethacin, levels, plasma; drug availability, comparison of formulations, capsule, standard and slow release, routes, oral and rectal; pharmacokinetic analysis

Black, R., Levine, M.M., Young, C., Rooney, J., Levine, S., Clements, M.L., O'Donnell, S., Hughes, T., Germanier, R., Schuster, A., Rodriguez, H., Borgono, J.-M., Lobos, H., Vincent, P., Morales, A. and Pistori, C., *Dev. biol. Standard.*, 1982, *53*, 9–14

Immunogenicity of Ty21a attenuated 'Salmonella typhi' given with sodium bicarbonate or in enteric-coated capsules

capsules, hard gelatin: drug availability, comparison of dosage forms and dosage regimen; effect of co-administration of sodium bicarbonate

Bogentoft, C.B., *Pharmacy Int.*, 1982, *3*, 366–9

Oral controlled-release dosage forms in perspective

capsules, hard gelatin and tablets: drug availability, effect of physiological factors, review; formulation of capsule contents, slow release, enteric-coated capsules and microspheres, hydrodynamically-balanced capsules, review

Conard, G.J., Jernberg, M.J., Wong, F.N., Mildon, C.A. and French, I.W., *Int. J. Pharmaceut.*, 1982, *10*, 259–73

Clinical assessment of theophylline absorption from Theolair-SR and two other sustained-release formulations relative to a conventional formulation

capsules, hard gelatin and tablets: theophylline, levels, plasma; drug availability, comparison of slow-release capsules and tablets with standard tablets; pharmacokinetic analysis

Geigenberger, A., Degen, J. and Maier-Lenz, H., *Arzneimittel-Forsch.*, 1982, *32*, 1138–40

Comparative pharmacokinetics and bioavailability of isosorbide dinitrate and its metabolite 5-isosorbide mononitrate from two prolonged release formulations

capsules, hard gelatin and tablets: isosorbide dinitrate, metabolites, levels, serum; drug availability, comparison of slow-release capsule with standard tablet; pharmacokinetic analysis

Lückner, P.W., Kraus, M., Brenner, H., Kyrein, H.J. and Schnikker, J., *Arzneimittel-Forsch.*, 1982, *32*, 409–13

Investigations into gastric tolerance of a sustained release theophylline formulation

capsules, hard gelatin and solutions: theophylline; drug availability, gastric potential difference measurements; drug, clinical effect, comparison of dosage forms, effect on gastric irritation

Newth, C.J. and Isles, A.F., *J. Asthma*, 1982, *19*, 145–9

Comparison at steady state of sustained-release theophylline tablets and capsules

capsules, hard gelatin and tablets: theophylline, levels, serum; drug availability, comparison of controlled-release capsules and tablets; pharmacokinetic analysis

Wautrech, J.C., Vandenbossche, J.L., Englert, M., *Clin. Trials J.*, 1982, *19*, 239–47

A comparison of the physiological actions of propranolol tablets and capsules (Inderal and Inderal Retard)

capsules, hard gelatin and tablets: propranolol; drug availability, comparison of slow-release capsule with standard tablet; drug, clinical effect, ECG analysis of heart

Bottini, P.B., Caulfield, E.M., Devane, J.G., Geoghegan, E.J. and Panoz, D.E., *Drug Dev. ind. Pharm.*, 1983, *9*, 1475–93

Comparative oral bioavailability of conventional propranolol tablets and a new controlled-absorption propranolol capsule

capsules, hard gelatin and tablets: propranolol, levels, plasma; drug availability, comparison with standard tablets; pharmacokinetic analysis

Edwards, C., Cope, A.S., Jackson, A.H. and Purkiss, R., *J. clin. Hosp. Pharm.*, 1983, *8*, 63–7

The comparative bioavailability of slow release oral theophylline preparations

capsules, hard gelatin and tablets: theophylline, levels, plasma; drug availability, comparison of dosage forms; pharmacokinetic analysis

Gyselinck, Ph., Schacht, E., van Severen, R. and Braeckman, P., *Acta Pharm. Tech.*, 1983, *29*, 9–12

Preparation and characterisation of therapeutic hydrogels as dosage forms

capsules, hard gelatin, hydrogels and injections, intravenous: procainamide, levels, serum (rabbits); drug availability, comparison of drug in capsule with hydrogel; hydrogels, formulation, method of preparation; pharmacokinetic analysis, comparison of absolute availabilities of dosage forms

Laufen, H., Schmid, M. and Leitold, M., *J. pharm. Sci.*, 1983, *72*, 496–9

Use of isosorbide dinitrate saliva concentrations for bio-pharmaceutical investigations

capsules, hard gelatin: isosorbide dinitrate, levels, plasma, saliva; pharmacokinetic analysis, comparison of plasma and saliva data

Nauta, I.L.D., van de Calseyde, J. and Hertzberger, D.P., *Curr. med. Res. Opinion.*, 1983, *8*, 582–93

Plasma; levels of disopyramide after administration of conventional capsules and sustained-release tablets

capsules, hard gelatin and tablets: disopyramide, levels, plasma; drug availability, comparison of standard release capsules and slow-release tablets; drug, clinical effects, myocardial function

Osman, M.A., Patel, R.B., Irwin, D.S. and Welling, P.G., *Biopharm. Drug Disp.*, 1983, *4*, 63–72

Absorption of theophylline from enteric coated and sustained release formulations in fasted and non-fasted subjects

capsules, hard gelatin and tablets: theophylline, levels, plasma; drug availability, comparison of controlled-release pellets in capsule and slow-release tablet; drug availability, effect of patient's fasting state; pharmacokinetic analysis

Rhodes, J. and Evans, B.K., *International Patent* WO 83/00435, 1983

Orally administrable pharmaceutical compositions

capsules, hard gelatin: sulphapyridine, levels, plasma; capsules, enteric-coated; drug availability, correlation of plasma levels and site of disintegration; gastric behaviour, visualisation method, X-ray, radio-opaque contents; 3.4.2.4; 4.4.3

Wills, R.J. and Colburn, W.A., *Ther. Drug Monit.*, 1983, *5*, 423–4

Multiple-dose pharmacokinetics of diazepam following once-daily administration of a controlled-release capsule

capsules, hard gelatin: diazepam, metabolite, levels, plasma; drug availability, effect of time of dose; pharmacokinetic analysis

Fitzsimmons, E.J., Thomson, W. and Jacobs, A., *Br. J. clin. Pharmac.*, 1984, *17*, 111–3

Iron absorption from 'Feospan' capsules and ferrous sulphate tablets B.P.

capsules, hard gelatin and tablets: ferrous sulphate, levels, serum ferritin, haemoglobin; drug availability, comparison of slow-release capsule and standard release tablet

Green, L.D., Saccar, C.L., Helsel, C.L., Niehls, M.E., McGeady, J. and Mansmann, H.C., *J. Asthma*, 1984, *21*, 35–9

Forty-eight-hour absorption pharmacokinetic profiles of two sustained-release theophylline preparations

capsules, hard gelatin and tablets, standard and sustained-release: theophylline, levels, serum; drug availability, comparison of dosage forms; pharmacokinetic analysis

Houghton, G.W., Dennis, M.J., Templeton, R., Calvert, R.M. and Cresswell, D.G., *Int. J. clin. Pharmac. Ther. Toxic.*, 1984, *22*, 131–3

A pharmacokinetic study of repeated doses of a new controlled release form of ketoprofen

capsules, hard gelatin: ketoprofen, levels, plasma; pharmacokinetic analysis

Johnson, K.I., Hoppe, H.-J. and Schatton, W., *Arznei-mittel-Forsch.*, 1984, *34*, 1785–7

Relative bioavailability of Etofibrate. A comparison of an acute and a new sustained release formulation

capsules, soft gelatin: etofibrate, metabolite, levels, plasma; drug availability, comparison of standard and slow-release forms; pharmacokinetic analysis

Kolarou, G. and Staib, A.H., *Münch. med. Wschr.*, 1984, *126*, 353–6

Comparative test on 2 sustained-release preparations of theophylline; Bronchoretard and Euphylline retard (in German)

capsules, hard gelatin and tablets: theophylline, levels, serum; drug availability, comparison of dosage forms; pharmacokinetic analysis

Morley, K.D., Bernstein, R.M., Hughes, G.R.V., Black, C.M., Rajapakse, C.N.A. and Wilson, L., *Curr. med. Res. Opinion*, 1984, *9*, 28–34

A comparative trial of a controlled-release formulation of ketoprofen ('Oruvail') and a conventional capsule formulation of ketoprofen ('Orudis') in patients with osteoarthritis of the hip

capsules, hard gelatin: ketoprofen; drug availability, comparison of formulations, standard and slow-release; drug, clinical effect, hip disease

Pollack, G.M., Baswell, B., Szefler, S.J. and Shen, D.D., *Int. J. Pharmaceut.*, 1984, *21*, 3–16

Comparison of inter- and intra-subject variation in oral absorption of theophylline from sustained-release products

capsules, hard gelatin, solutions and tablets: theophylline, levels, serum; drug availability, comparison of dosage forms, effect of subject variation; pharmacokinetic analysis, comparison with solution

Soubeyra, J., Cornet, F., Gillet, A., Georges, D. and Brazier, J.L., *Eur. J. clin. Pharmac.*, 1984, *27*, 325–28

A 'once a day administration' sustained-release theophylline formulation: Disposition and pharmacokinetics

capsules, hard gelatin: theophylline, levels, plasma; drug availability, correlation of dose and serum levels

Levi, F. Le Louarn, C. and Reinberg, A., *Clin. Pharmac. Ther.*, 1985, *37*, 77–84

Timing optimizes sustained-release indomethacin treatment of osteoarthritis

capsules, hard gelatin: indomethacin; drug, clinical effects, slow-release form, pain relief, effect of time of administration, patient's selection for pain relief

Lutz, D., Gielsdorf, W., Rasper, J., Jaeger, H. and Loew, D., *Arzneimittel-Forsch*, 1985, *35*, 730–4

Comparative study of the bioavailability and pharmacokinetics of slow-release formulations of isosorbide dinitrate against standard drugs and determination of isosorbide-5-mononitrate

capsules, hard gelatin and tablets: isosorbide dinitrate, metabolite levels, plasma; drug availability, comparisons of, dosage forms and products; pharmacokinetic analysis

Sado, P.A., Gibassier, D., Le Verge, R., Acerbi, D. and Schiantarelli, P., *J. Pharm. Belg.*, 1985, *40*, 308–22

Relative bioavailability of vinburnine in man (microgranules/hard gelatin capsules) (in French)

capsules, hard gelatin: vinburnine, metabolite levels, plasma; drug availability, effect of formulation, standard and slow-release forms

Yeh, K.C., *Am. J. Med.*, 1985, *79*, Suppl. 4C, 3–12

Pharmakinetic overview of indomethacin and sustained-release indomethacin

capsule, hard gelatin: indomethacin, levels, plasma; drug availability, literature review, comparison of standard and slow-release products

4.4.8 Effect of Physiological Factors on Availability

Hansen, T., *Ugeskr. Laeg.*, 1967, *129*, 1506–11

Oxytetracycline (oxycyclin) serum concentration after oral administration (in Danish)

capsules, hard gelatin: oxytetracycline, levels, serum, urine; drug availability, comparison of dosage regimens

Wagner, J.G., Novak, E., Patel, N.C., Chidester, C.G. and Luminis, W.L., *Am. J. med. Sci.*, 1968, *256*, 25–37

Absorption, excretion and half-life of clinimycin in normal adult males

capsules, hard gelatin and tablets: clinimycin, levels, serum, urine; drug availability, comparison of dosage forms, effect of patient's fasting state

Barr, W.H., Adir, J. and Garrettson, L., *Clin. Pharmac. Ther.*, 1971, *12*, 779–84

Decrease of tetracycline absorption in man by sodium bicarbonate

capsules, hard gelatin and solutions: tetracycline hydrochloride, levels, urine; drug availability, effect of co-administration of sodium bicarbonate

Smith, R.B., Dittert, L.W., Griffen, W.O. and Doluisio, J.T., *J. Pharmacokinet. Biopharm.*, 1973, *1*, 5–16

Pharmacokinetics of pentobarbital after intravenous and oral administration

capsules, hard gelatin and injections, intravenous: pentobarbitone sodium, levels, serum; drug availability, effect of patient's fasting state; pharmacokinetic analysis

Greenblatt, D.J., Shader, R.I., Harmatz, J.S., Franke, K. and Koch-Weser, J., *Clin. Pharmac. Ther.*, 1976, *19*, 234–9

Influence of magnesium and aluminium hydroxide mixture on chlordiazepoxide absorption

capsules, hard gelatin: chlordiazepoxide hydrochloride, metabolites, levels, serum; drug availability, effect of co-administration of aluminium hydroxide and magnesium hydroxide; pharmacokinetic analysis

Musa, M.N. and Lyons, L.L., *Curr. ther. Res.*, 1976, *19*, 669–74

Effect of food and liquid on the pharmacokinetics of propoxyphene

capsules, hard gelatin and solutions: dextropropoxyphene hydrochloride, levels, plasma; drug availability, comparison of dosage forms, effects of, fluid intake, food type, carbohydrate, fat, protein, patient's fasting state; pharmacokinetic analysis

Rosenberg, H.A. and Bates, T.R., *Clin. Pharmac. Ther.*, 1976, *20*, 227–32

The influence of food on nitrofurantoin bioavailability

capsules, hard gelatin, suspensions and tablets: nitrofurantoin, levels, urine; drug availability, comparison of dosage forms, effects of, patient's fasting state, particle size of drug, microcrystalline in tablets, macrocrystalline in capsules

Welling, P.G., Lyons, L.L., Tse, F.L.S. and Craig, W.A., *Clin. Pharmac. Ther.*, 1976, *19*, 559–65

Propoxyphene and norpropoxyphene: Influence of diet and fluid on plasma level

capsules, hard gelatin: dextropropoxyphene, metabolites, levels, plasma; drug availability, effects of, co-administration of food, comparison of carbohydrate, fat, protein, of liquid, capsule dissolved in carbonated drink, of water; pharmacokinetic analysis

Galeazzi, R.L., *Eur. J. clin. Pharmac.*, 1977, *12*, 65–8

The effect of an antacid on the bioavailability of indomethacin

capsules, hard gelatin: indomethacin, levels, plasma, urine; drug availability, effect of co-administration of antacid; pharmacokinetic analysis

Jones, K.H., *Br. med. J.*, 1977, *2*, 232–3

Bioavailability of talampicillin

capsules, hard gelatin and tablets: ampicillin, talampicillin hydrochloride, levels, serum; drug availalbility, comparison of dosage forms, effect of patient's fasting state

Lindenbaum, J., *Clin. Pharmac. Ther.*, 1977, *21*, 278–82

Greater bioavailability of digoxin solution in capsules. Studies in the postprandial state

capsules, soft gelatin, solutions and tablets: digoxin, levels, serum, urine; drug availability, comparison of dosage forms, effect of food, high fat breakfast

Nation, R.L., Vine, J., Triggs, E.J. and Learoyd, B., *Eur. J. clin. Pharmac.*, 1977, *12*, 137–45

Plasma level of chlormethiazole and two metabolites after oral administration to young and aged human subjects

capsules, soft gelatin: chlormethiazole edisylate, levels, plasma; drug availability, effect of patient's age; pharmacokinetic analysis

Poust, R.I., Mallinger, A.G., Mallinger, J., Himmelhoch, J.M., Neil, J.F. and Hanin, I., *J. pharm. Sci.*, 1977, *66*, 609–10

Absolute availability of lithium

capsules, hard gelatin: lithium carbonate, levels, plasma; drug availability, effect of co-administration of chlorothiazide, improved renal clearance

Raghuram, T.C. and Krishnaswamy, K., *Eur. J. clin. Pharmac.*, 1977, *12*, 281–4

Influence of nutritional status on plasma levels and relative bioavailability of tetracycline

capsules: tetracycline hydrochloride, levels, plasma; drug availability, effects of, dosage regimen, single and multiple dose, patient's health, undernourished and well-nourished

Welling, P.G., Huang, H., Koch, P.A., Craig, W.A. and Madsen, P.O., *J. pharm. Sci.*, 1977, *66*, 549–52

Bioavailability of ampicillin and amoxicillin in fasted and nonfasted subjects

capsules, hard gelatin: ampicillin trihydrate, amoxycillin trihydrate, levels, serum; drug availability, effect of patient's fasting state; pharmacokinetic analysis

Welling, P.G., Koch, P.A., Lau, C.C. and Craig, W.A., *Antimicrob. Ag. Chemother.*, 1977, *11*, 462–9

Bioavailability of tetracycline and doxycycline in fasted and nonfasted subjects

capsules, hard gelatin: doxycycline, tetracycline hydrochloride, levels, serum; drug availability, patient's fasting state, pharmacokinetic analysis

Adir, J. and Barr, W.H., *J. Pharmacokinet. Biopharm.*, 1978, *6*, 99–110

Dose-dependent bioavailability of tetracycline in man

capsules: tetracycline hydrochloride, levels, urine; drug availability, comparison of products, effects of, dosage regimen, co-administration of water

Albert, K.S., Welch, R.D., DeSante, K.A. and DiSanto, A.R., *J. pharm. Sci.*, 1979, *68*, 586–8

Decreased tetracycline bioavailability caused by a bismuth subsalicylate antidiarrhoeal mixture

capsules, hard gelatin: tetracycline, levels, serum, urine; drug availability, effect of co-administration of bismuth salicylate

Allen, M.D., Greenblatt, D.J. and Smith, T.W., *Clin. Pharmac. Ther.*, 1979, *25*, 212

Effect of Maalox and Kaopectate on absorption of digoxin from tablets and capsules

capsules, soft gelatin and tablets: digoxin, levels, plasma, urine; drug availability, effect of co-administration of Kaopectate and Maalox

Chapron, D.J., Kramer, P.A., Mariano, S.L. and Hohnadel, D.C., *Archs Neurol., Chicago*, 1979, *36*, 436–8

Effect of calcium and antacids on phenytoin bioavailability

capsules, hard gelatin: phenytoin, levels, plasma; drug availability, effect of co-administration of antacids and calcium

Clementi, W.A., Ludden, T.M., Evens, R.P. and Bowden, C., *Clin. Pharmac. Ther.*, 1979, *25*, 217–8

The effect of sodium on the bioavailability of lithium

capsules, hard gelatin: lithium carbonate, levels, serum, urine; drug availability, effect of high and low sodium meals

Haginaka, J., Yamaoka, K., Nakagawa, T., Nishimura, Y. and Uno, T., *Chem. pharm. Bull., Tokyo*, 1979, *27*, 3156–9

Evaluation of effect of food ingestion on bioavailability of cephalexin by moment analysis

capsules, hard gelatin: cephalexin, levels, urine; drug availability, effect of patient's fasting state; pharmacokinetic analysis

Record, K.E., Rapp, R.P., Young, A.B. and Kostenbauder, H.B., *Ann. Neurol.*, 1979, *5*, 268–70

Oral phenytoin loading in adults: rapid achievement of therapeutic plasma levels

capsules, hard gelatin: phenytoin, levels, plasma; drug availability, effect of dosage regimen, patient's weight; pharmacokinetic analysis, therapeutic levels

Bustrack, J.A., Katz, J.D., Hull, J.H., Foster, J.R., Christenson, R.H. and Hammond, J.E., *Drug Intell. & clin. Pharm.*, 1981, *15*, 477

Effect of fluid volume on bioavailability of digoxin tablets and capsules

capsules, soft gelatin and tablets: digoxin, levels, serum, urine; drug availability, comparison of dosage forms, effect of co-administration of water; pharmacokinetic analysis

Clayton, D. and Leslie, A., *J. int. med. Res.*, 1981, *9*, 470–7

The bioavailability of erythromycin stearate versus enteric-coated erythromycin base when taken immediately before and after food

capsules, hard gelatin and tablets: erythromycin, base, stearate, levels, plasma; drug availability, comparison of dosage forms, effect of patient's fasting state; formulation of contents, enteric-coated pellets

Mather, L.E., Austin, K.L., Philpot, C.R. and McDonald, P.J., *Brit. J. clin. Pharmac.*, 1981, *12*, 131–40

Absorption and bioavailability of oral erythromycin

capsules, hard gelatin and tablets: erythromycin, base and stearate, levels, serum; drug availability, comparison of dosage forms, effect of patient's fasting state; pharmacokinetic analysis

Musatti, L., Maggi, E., Moro, E., Valzelli, G. and Tamassia, V., *J. int. med. Res.*, 1981, *9*, 381–6

Bioavailability and pharmacokinetics in man of acipimox, a new antilipolytic and hypolipemic agent

capsules, hard gelatin: acipimox, levels, plasma, urine; drug availability, effect of patient's fasting state; pharmacokinetic analysis

Shargel, L., Stevens, J.A., Fuchs, J.E. and Yu, A.B.C., *J. pharm. Sci.*, 1981, *70*, 599–602

Effect of antacid on bioavailability of theophylline from rapid and timed-release drug products

capsules, hard gelatin and tablets: theophylline, levels, serum; drug availability, comparison of slow-release pellets in capsules and standard tablets, effect of co-administration of magnesium aluminium hydroxide; pharmacokinetic analysis

Wills, R.J., Waller, E.S., Puri, S.K., Ho, I. and Yakatan, G.J., *Drug Dev. ind. Pharm.*, 1981, *7*, 385–96

Influence of food on the bioavailability of Trental (Pentoxifylline) in man

capsules, hard gelatin: oxpentifylline, metabolite, levels, plasma; drug availability, effect of patient's fasting state; pharmacokinetic analysis

Chan, K., Tse, J., Orme, M. and Sibeon, R.G., *J. clin. Hosp. Pharm.*, 1982, *7*, 155–60

The influence of urinary pH on the disposition of indomethacin in healthy volunteers

capsules, hard gelatin: indomethacin, levels, plasma, urine; drug availability, effect of control of urinary pH; pharmacokinetic analysis

Johnson, B.F., Bustrack, J.A., Urbach, D.R., Hull, J.H. and Marwaha, R., *Clin. Pharmac. Ther.*, 1984, *36*, 724–30

Effect of metoclopramide on digoxin absorption from tablets and capsules

capsules, soft gelatin and tablets: digoxin, levels, serum; drug availability, comparison of dosage forms, effect of coadministration of metoclopramide, gut motility, increased with metoclopramide; pharmacokinetic analysis

Khali, S.A.H., El-Khordagui, L.K. and El-Gholmy, Z.A., *Int. J. Pharmaceut.*, 1984, *20*, 99–106

Effect of antacids on oral absorption of rifampicin

capsules, hard gelatin: rifampicin, levels, urine; drug availability, effect of co-administration of antacids, comparison of aluminium hydroxide, magnesium trisilicate, sodium bicarbonate

Challenor, V.F., Renwick, A.G., Gruchy, B.S., Walker, D. and George, C.F., *Brit. J. clin. Pharmac.*, 1985, *20*, 550–1

The effects of food and posture on the pharmacokinetics of a novel formulation of nifedipine

capsules, soft gelatin and injection, intravenous: nifedipine, levels, plasma; drug availability, effects of patient's food intake and posture; pharmacokinetic analysis

Lesko, L.J., Hunter, J.R., Burgess, R.C. and Rodgers, G.P., *J. Pharm. Pharmac.*, 1986, *38*, 486–488

Accumulation of nifedipine after multiple doses

capsules, soft gelatin; nifedipine, levels, serum; drug availability, comparison of single and multiple doses; pharmacokinetic analysis

Ogata, H., Aoyagi, N., Kaniwa, N., Ejima, A., Sekme, N., Kitamura, M. and Inoue, Y., *Int. J. Pharmaceut.*, 1986, *29*, 113–120

Gastric acidity dependant bioavailability of cinnarizine from two commercial capsules in healthy volunteers

capsules, hard gelatin: cinnarizine, levels, serum; dissolution method, rotating basket; dissolution testing, comparison of products, effect of pH test medium; drug availability, comparison of products, effects of, patient's gastric pH, high and low, product dissolution rate; pharmacokinetic analysis

4.4.9 Effect of Psychological Factors on Availability

Weisker, J., *Pharm. Ind., Berl.*, 1963, *25*, 11–12

An interesting American consumption test (in German)

capsules, soft gelatin and tablets, plain and sugar-coated: patient preference, comparison of dosage forms, ease of swallowing

Cattaneo, A.D., Lucchelli, P.E. and Filippucci, G., *Eur. J. clin. Pharmac.*, 1970, *3*, 43–5

Sedative effects of placebo treatment

capsules, hard gelatin: placebo, clinical effects, sleep, onset and duration; clinical response, effects of, capsule colour, order of administration, patient's sex

Hussain, M.Z. and Ahad, A., *Br. med. J.*, 1970, *3*, 466

Tablet colour in anxiety states

capsules, hard gelatin and tablets: chlordiazepoxide, clinical effects; patient compliance, patient preference, comparison of dosage forms

Blackwell, B., Bloomfield, S.S. and Buncher, C.R., *Lancet*, 1972, *1*, 1279–82

Demonstration to medical students of placebo responses and non-drug factors

capsules, hard gelatin: placebo, clinical effects, sedative, stimulant; clinical effects, effects of, capsule colour, dose

Masheter, H.C., *Br. med. J.*, 1977, *1*, 973–4

Keep on taking the tablets

capsules, hard gelatin: flufenamic acid, phenylbutazone; patient compliance, effect of dosage form

Lucchelli, P.E., Cattaneo, A.D. and Zattoni, J., *Eur. J. clin. Pharmac.*, 1978, *13*, 153–5

Effect of capsule colour and order of administration of hypnotic treatments

capsules, hard gelatin: heptabarbitone; drug, clinical effects, sleep, onset and duration; drug, clinical response, effects of, capsule colour, order of administration, patient's sex, placebo

Hunter, R.H. and Kotzan, J.A., *J. pharm. Sci.*, 1979, 68, 272–4

Effect of obtrusive measures on antibiotic compliance

capsules, hard gelatin: ampicillin trihydrate, levels, urine; drug compliance, detection by urine levels

Radecki, B., *Am. J. Psychiat.*, 1980, 137, 259–60

Patient preference: Lithium pills versus capsules

capsules, hard gelatin and tablets: lithium carbonate; compliance, comparison of dosage forms

Bailie, G.R. and Kesson, C.M., *Drug Intell. & clin. Pharm.*, 1981, 15, 492–3

The effect of capsule color on hypnotic efficacy

capsules, soft gelatin: temazepam; drug, clinical effects, sleep, onset and duration; drug, clinical response, effects of, capsule colour, patient's sex; patient's preference for treatment

Buckalew, L.W. and Coffield, K.E., *J. clin. Psychopharmac.*, 1982, 2, 245–8

An investigation of drug expectancy as a function of capsule color and size and preparation form

capsules, hard gelatin and tablets: patient's perceptions, comparison of dosage forms, effects of, capsule colour and size; product colour, patient's association with disease states

Delaney, R., *Pharm. Exec.*, 1982, 2, 34–8

Surveying consumer preferences

capsules, hard and soft gelatin and tablets: consumer preference, comparison with industrial usage

Samo, I., *Pharm. Ind., Berl.*, 1983, 45, 386–90

Patient compliance: A literature review (in German)

capsules, hard gelatin: patient compliance, literature review

Webber, E., Fischer, B., Lehrl, S. and Gundert-Remy, U., Chapter VII in *The Capsule, Basics, Technology and Biopharmacy, a Modern Dosage Form* (in German), Fahrig, W. and Hofer, U. (ed.), Stuttgart, Wissenschaftliche Verlagsgesellschaft mbH, 1983, pp. 127–137

Better acceptance through colour (in German)

capsules: patient compliance, effect of colour

Blaustein, M., *Am. J. Psychiat.*, 1986, 143, 1066

Patients taking drug capsules may fear Tylenol-like poisoning

capsules, hard gelatin: patient compliance, effect of media reporting of tampering

4.5. Drug Availability, *in vitro*/*in vivo* Correlation

4.5.1 General References

Aguiar, A.J., Wheeler, L.M., Fusari, S. and Zelmer, J.E., *J. pharm. Sci.*, 1968, 57, 1844–50

Evaluation of physical and pharmaceutical factors involved in drug release and availability from chloramphenicol capsules

capsules, hard gelatin: chloramphenicol, levels, plasma; deaggregation rate testing; dissolution method, modified *U.S.P.* disintegration apparatus; drug availability, *in vitro*, drug permeation, rat intestine; powder properties, particle size

Mattila, M.J., Koskinen, R. and Takki, S., *Annls Med. intern. Fenn.*, 1968, 57, 75–9

Absorption of ethionamide and prothionamide *in vitro* and *in vivo*

capsules, hard gelatin and tablets, film- and sugar-coated: ethionamide, prothionamide, level, serum; drug availability, *in vitro*, rat intestinal perfusion studies; drug availability, *in vivo*, ethionamide, effect of co-administration of antacids

Poole, J.W., *Drug Inf. Bull.*, 1969, 3, 8–16

Some experiences in the evaluation of formulation variables on drug availability

capsules, hard gelatin and tablets: drug, levels, serum (dogs, human); dissolution method, beaker

Bell, H., Johansen, H., Lunde, P.K.M., Andersgaard, H.A., Finholt, P., Midtvedt, T., Holum, E., Martinussen, B. and Aarnes, E.D., *Pharmacology*, 1971, 5, 108–20

Absorption and dissolution characteristics of 14 different oral chloramphenicol preparations tested on healthy human male subjects

capsules, suspensions and tablets: chloramphenicol, palmitate, stearate, levels, serum; dissolution method, beaker, sink and non-sink conditions; drug availability, comparisons of, dosage forms, products

Kaplan, S.A. and Cotler, S., *J. pharm. Sci.*, 1972, 61, 1361–5

Use of cannulated everted intestinal sac for serial sampling as a drug absorbability (permeability) screen

capsules, injections, intravenous and solutions: drug levels, blood (dog); drug testing, *in vitro*, permeability through everted rat intestinal sac; drug availability, *in vitro-in vivo* correlation, comparison of dissolution, permeability data, effect of drug pK_a

Jusko, W.J. and Lewis, G.P., *J. pharm. Sci.*, 1973, 62, 69–76

Comparison of ampicillin and hetacillin pharmacokinetics in man

capsules, hard gelatin and injections, intravenous: ampicillin, hetacillin, levels, plasma, urine; dissolution method, beaker; pharmacokinetic analysis

Neuvonen, P.J., *Clin. Pharmacokinet.*, 1979, 4, 91–103

Bioavailability of phenytoin: clinical pharmacokinetic and therapeutic implications

capsules, hard gelatin and tablets: phenytoin, comparison of dosage forms and products; drug, chemical properties; drug, clinical effects, effects of, drugs, physiological factors; review; 4.4.2

Möller, H., Chapter IX, in *The Capsule, Basics, Technology and Biopharmacy, a Modern Dosage Form* (in German), Fahrig, W. and Hofer, U. (Ed.), Stuttgart, Wissenschaftliche Verlagsgesellschaft mbH, 1983, pp. 172–180

Tests and standards for capsule preparations with consideration to *in vivo* conditions (in German)

capsules, hard and soft gelatin and tablets: doxycycline, tetracycline, levels, plasma; dissolution methods, flow-through cell, paddle, rotating basket; dissolution testing, comparison of methods; drug availability, comparison of dosage forms; literature review

Möller, H., *Pharm. Ind., Berl.*, 1986, *48*, 514–9

Biopharmaceutical assessment of modified release oral dosage forms

capsules, hard gelatin and tablets: indomethacin, propranolol, theophylline, percentage release; dissolution method, flow through cell, paddle; dissolution testing, comparison of methods, pharmacopoeial requirements; drug availability, physiological factors, comparison of drugs; pharmacokinetic analysis

4.5.2 Disintegration and Performance

Eckert, T., Cordes, G. and Seidel, R., *Arzneimittel-Forsch.*, 1971, *21*, 1403–6

Release of active substances from enteric-coated gelatin capsules *in vivo* and *in vitro*. Part 4. Study with the pH radiotransmitter in man (in German)

capsules, hard gelatin: disintegration method, *in vitro*, *Ger. P.* (DAB 7); disintegration method, *in vivo*, pH radiotransmitter; disintegration testing, effect of coat thickness; 3.4.2.4

Eckert, T., Cordes, G. and Ollenschläger, G., *Pharm. Ind., Berl.*, 1976, *38*, 836–41

Release of active substances from enteric-coated gelatin capsules *in vitro* and *in vivo*. Part 5. Study with films of cellulose acetate phthalate (CAP) and hydroxypropylmethylcellulose phthalate (HP–50) (in German)

capsules, hard gelatin: capsule contents, glutamic acid hydrochloride; disintegration method, *in vitro*, *Ger. P.* (DAB 7) with pH electrode; disintegration method, *in vivo*, pH radiotransmitter; disintegration testing, comparison of polymers, effect of coating thickness; 3.4.2.4

Hey, H., Matzen, P., Andersen, J.T., Didriksen, E. and Nielsen, B., *Br. J. clin. Pharmac.*, 1979, *8*, 237–42

A gastroscopic and pharmacological study of the disintegration time and absorption of pivampicillin capsules and tablets

capsules, hard gelatin and tablets: pivampicillin, disintegration method, *U.S.P.* XIX; disintegration, *in vivo*, gastroscopy; dissolution method, *U.S.P.* XIX; drug availability, comparison of dosage forms, effect of gastroscopy

4.5.3 Comparison of Dosage Forms, *in vitro*/*in vivo*

4.5.3.1 Comparison with Solid Preparations

Graffner, C. and Sjögren, J., *Acta pharm. suec.*, 1971,

8, 19–26

Side-effects of potassium chloride in products with different dissolution rates

capsules, hard gelatin and tablets: potassium chloride; dissolution method, beaker; drug availability, side-effects, comparison of dosage forms; formulation of contents

Davis, C.M., Vandersarl, J.V. and Kraus, E.W., *Am. J. med. Sci.*, 1973, *265*, 69–74

Tetracycline inequivalence: the importance of 96-hour testing

capsules and tablets, film-coated: tetracycline hydrochloride, levels, serum, urine; dissolution method, rocking cylinder; drug availability, comparison of products

Davis, S.S., Poxon, R., Mitchard, M. and Williams, M.E., *Lancet*, 1973, *1*, 667–8

Biological availability of methaqualone

capsules, hard gelatin and tablets: methaqualone, levels, plasma; dissolution method, not stated; drug availability, comparison of products

Meyer, M.C., Slywka, G.W.A., Dann, R.E. and Whyatt, P.L., *J. pharm. Sci.*, 1974, *63*, 1693–8

Bioavailability of 14 nitrofurantoin products

capsules, hard gelatin and tablets: nitrofurantoin, levels, urine; content uniformity; disintegration method, *U.S.P.* XVIII; dissolution method, *U.S.P.* XVIII; drug availability, comparison of products

Okhotnikova, V.F., Geitman, I.Y., Yakhyaev, V.D., Grakovskaya, L.K. and Kivman, G.Y., *Antibiotiki*, 1974, *19*, 843–7

Correlation between disintegration and solubility of tablets and capsules of tetracycline and its blood level in humans (in Russian)

capsules, hard gelatin and tablets: tetracycline, levels, blood; disintegration testing; dissolution method, rotating basket

Williams, M.E., Kendall, M.J., Mitchard, M., Davis, S.S. and Poxon, R., *Br. J. clin. Pharmac.*, 1974, *1*, 99–105

Availability of methaqualone from commercial preparations: *in vitro* and *in vivo* studies in man

capsules, hard gelatin and tablets: methaqualone, levels, plasma; dissolution method, rotating basket; drug availability, comparison of products

Cartwright, A.C., Hatfield, H.L., Yeadon, A. and London, E., *J. antimicrob. Chemother.*, 1975, *1*, 317–22

A comparison of the bioavailability of minocycline capsules and film-coated tablets

capsules, hard gelatin and tablets, film-coated: minocycline, levels, serum; dissolution method, *U.S.P.* XVIII

Hart, A., Barber, H.E. and Calvey, T.N., *Br. J. clin. Pharmac.*, 1975, *2*, 277–80

Bioavailability and dissolution of different formulations of oxytetracycline preparations

capsules, hard gelatin and tablets, film-coated: oxytetracycline, dihydrate and hydrochloride, levels, plasma; dissolution method, *U.S.N.F.* XIII; drug availability, comparison of products

Angelucci, L., Petrangeli, B., Celletti, P. and Favilli, S., *J. pharm. Sci.*, 1976, *65*, 455–6

Bioavailability of flufenamic acid in hard and soft gelatin capsules

capsules, hard and soft gelatin: flufenamic acid, levels, plasma (dogs); dissolution method, *U.S.P.* XVIII; formulation of contents

Chemburkar, P.B., Smyth, R.D., Buehler, J.D., Shah, P.B., Joslin, R.S., Polk, A. and Reavey-Cantwell, N.H., *J. pharm. Sci.*, 1976, *65*, 529–33

Correlation between dissolution characteristics and absorption of methaqualone from solid dosage forms

capsules, hard gelatin and tablets: methaqualone hydrochloride, levels, serum; dissolution method, resin flask, rotating flask; drug availability, comparison of products

Morris, J.G.L., Parsons, R.L., Trounce, J.R. and Groves, M.J., *Br. J. clin. Pharmac.*, 1976, *3*, 983–90

Plasma dopa concentrations after different preparations of levodopa in normal subjects

capsules, hard gelatin and tablets, standard and slow-release: levodopa, levels, plasma; disintegration method, *B.P.*; disintegration testing, effect of pH test media; dissolution method, beaker; dissolution testing, effect of pH test media; drug availability, comparison of products, effects of, co-administration of carbidopa, metoclopramide, slow-release preparations; drug metabolism, effect of intestinal absorption site

Okhotnikova, V.F., Grakovskaya, L.K., Koroleva, V.G., Minasova, G.S. and Zak, I.R., *Antibiotiki*, 1976, *21*, 719–21

Rate of tetracycline dissolution from tablets and capsules and biological availability of the antibiotic (in Russian)

capsules, hard gelatin and tablets: tetracycline, levels, blood; dissolution method, rotating basket

Mendes, R.W., Masih, S. Z. and Kanumuri, R.R., *J. pharm. Sci.*, 1978, *67*, 1616–19

Effect of formulation and process variables on bioequivalency of nitrofurantoin II: *In vivo – in vitro* correlation

capsules, hard gelatin and tablets, chewable and standard: nitrofurantoin, levels, urine; disintegration; dissolution method, *U.S.P.*; drug availability, effects of, drug particle size, formulation

Needham, T.E., Shah, K., Kotzan, J. and Zia, H., *J. pharm. Sci.*, 1978, *67*, 1070–3

Correlation of aspirin excretion with parameters from different dissolution methods

capsules, hard gelatin and tablets: aspirin, levels, urine; dissolution method, basket, magnetic basket, modified beaker, *U.S.P.*; dissolution testing, comparison of methods; drug availability, comparison of products, controlled-release tablets and standard capsules

Papadimitriou, D.C. and Sheth, B.B., *Drug Dev. ind. Pharm.*, 1978, *4*, 373–87

Correlation of dissolution – dialysis rates with bioavailability of nitrofurantoin solid dosage forms

capsules, hard gelatin and tablets: nitrofurantoin, levels, urine; dissolution method, modified *U.S.P.* plus dialysis chamber; *in vivo–in vitro* correlation, correlation of apparent dialytic rate constant with biological parameters

Alvisi, V., Longhini, C., Bagni, B., Portaluppi, F., Ruina, M. and Fersini, C., *Arzneimittel-Forsch.*, 1979, *29*, 1047–50

An improvement in digoxin bioavailability. Studies with soft gelatin capsules containing a solution of digoxin

capsules, soft gelatin and tablets: digoxin, levels, plasma, urine; dissolution method, paddle; drug clinical effect, cardiac functions

Astorri, E., Bianchi, G., La Canna, G., Assanelli, D., Visioli, O. and Marzo, A., *J. pharm. Sci.*, 1979, *68*, 104–6

Bioavailability and related heart function index of digoxin capsules and tablets in cardiac patients

capsules, soft gelatin and tablets: digoxin, levels, serum; dissolution method, beaker; dissolution testing, effect of dissolution media; drug availability, chemical effects, heart function index; pharmacokinetic analysis, comparative bioavailability

Brandau, R. and Wehnert, H.-U., *Arzneimittel-Forsch.*, 1979, *29*, 552–5

Dissolution rates and bioavailability of phenytoin preparations (in German)

capsules, hard gelatin, suspensions and tablets: phenytoin, calcium, sodium salts, levels, plasma (human); dissolution method, *U.S.P.* XIX; drug availability, comparison of products; 4.5.3.2

Leonard, G.S., Tovey, G.D. and Lee, R.M., *Drug Dev. ind. Pharm.*, 1979, *5*, 217–26

The pharmaceutical development and bioavailability of cimetidine capsule and tablet formulations

capsules, hard gelatin and tablets: cimetidine, levels, blood; disintegration method, *B.P.* 1973; dissolution method, *U.S.P.* XIX

Needham, T.E., Javid, P. and Brown, W., *J. pharm. Sci.*, 1979, *68*, 952–4

Bioavailability and dissolution paramaters of seven lithium carbonate products

capsules, hard gelatin and tablets: lithium carbonate, levels, saliva, urine (human); dissolution method, modified beaker, *U.S.P.* XIX

Alam, A.S., Hagerman, L.M. and Imondi, A.R., *Int. J. Pharmacodyn.*, 1980, *247*, 180–9

Bioavailability of sulpiride tablet and capsule in dogs

capsules, hard gelatin and tablets: sulpiride, levels, urine, (dogs); dissolution method, rotating basket; dissolution testing, effect of test media; pharmacokinetic analysis; test media, simulated gastric and intestinal juice

Gröning, R., *Drug Dev. ind. Pharm.*, 1980, *6*, 475–91

Development and evaluation of dissolution tests using clinical data

capsules, hard gelatin and tablets: nitrofurantoin, levels, urine; dissolution methods, flow-through two-compartment cell, paddle, rotating basket; dissolution testing, comparison of, methods, products

Zak, A.F., Batuashvili, T.A. and Shchedrin, V.I., *Antibiotiki*, 1980, *25*, 24–8

Bioavailability of oral ampicillin (in Russian)

capsules, hard gelatin and tablets: ampicillin, anhydrous and trihydrate, levels, serum (human); dissolution method, basket

Cid, E., Morán, I., Monaris, M., Lasserre, C. and Vidal, V., *Biopharm. Drug Disp.*, 1981, *2*, 391–4

Bioavailability of four brands of phenytoin

capsules, hard gelatin and tablets: phenytoin sodium, levels, plasma; dissolution method, rotating basket; drug availability, comparison of products; pharmacokinetic analysis

El-Yazigi, A. and Sanchuk, R.J., *J. pharm. Sci.*, 1985, *74*, 161–4

In vitro – in vivo correlation and dissolution studies with oral theophylline dosage forms

capsule, hard gelatin and tablets: theophylline; dissolution methods, basket, rotating filter; dissolution testing, comparison of dosage forms, formulations, slow and standard release, effects of, pH test media, stirring rate; pharmacokinetic analysis, correlation with *in vivo*, blood levels (rabbit)

Neisingh, S.E., Sam, A.P. and de Nijs, H., *Drug Dev. ind. Pharm.*, 1986, *12*, 651–63

A dissolution method for hard and soft gelatin capsules containing testosterone undecanoate in oleic acid

capsules, hard and soft gelatin: testosterone undecanoate levels, plasma; dissolution method, flow-through cell; dissolution testing, comparison of dosage forms, effect of formulation; drug availability, comparison of dosage forms, effect of formulation

Sournac, M., Ducroux, P., Aiache, J. M., Renoux, R., Kantelip, J.P. and Ducros, M., *Fourth International Conference on Pharmaceutical Technology*, (Paris, APGI, June 3–5, 1986), 1986, II, 108–17

Studies in the comparative bioavailability of aspirin from four pharmaceutical forms. Application of statistical moments to the interpretation of the results and the establishment of *in vitro/in vivo* correlations (in French)

capsules, hard gelatin and tablets: acetylsalicylic acid, levels, plasma; dissolution method, rotating paddle; dissolution testing, comparison of dosage forms; drug availability, comparison of dosage forms; pharmacokinetic analysis

4.5.3.2 Comparison with Liquid Preparations

Baun, D.C., Bowen, B.M. and Wood, D.E., *Am. J. Hosp. Pharm.*, 1975, *32*, 1047–9

Comparison of the bioavailability of Cyanocobalamin from capsule and liquid dosage forms

capsules, hard gelatin and solutions: cyanocobalamin, levels, urine; dissolution method, continuous flow apparatus; radioactive isotope technique

Pandit, J.K., Jagadeesh, G., Nagabooshanam, M. and Tripathi, M.K., *Drug Dev. ind. Pharm.*, 1984, *10*, 85–99

Effect of some formulation additives on the oral absorption of indomethacin

capsules, hard gelatin and suspensions: indomethacin, levels, plasma (dog); dissolution method, modified beaker; dissolution testing, comparisons of, capsule products, dosage forms, effect of, drug treatment; drug availability, comparisons of, capsule products, dosage forms, effect of formulation; drug treatment, surface coating by co-precipitation with sodium taurocholate

4.5.3.3 Comparison with Injections

Flasch, H., Asmussen, B. and Heinz, N., *Arzneimittel-Forsch.*, 1978, *28*, 326–30

Enhanced bioavailability of digoxin from silica matrix formulations (in German)

capsules, hard gelatin, injections, intravenous and tablets, enteric, sugar-coated and uncoated: digoxin, levels, urine; disintegration method, DAB; dissolution method, continuous flow cell; drug availability, effect of formulation; formulation of contents, diluent, silicic acid; pharmacokinetic analysis

4.5.3.4. Comparison with Rectal Preparations

Wellauer, J., del Buono, M., Ory, A.M. and Steiger-Trippi, K., *Pharm. Acta Helv.*, 1960, *35*, 619–30

Gelatin-rectal-capsule, a new dosage form for rectal treatment

capsules, soft gelatin and suppositories: disintegration method, *in vitro*, Erweka apparatus; disintegration method, *in vivo*, X-ray, radio-opaque contents; rectal capsule

Parrott, E.L. and Matheson, L.E., *J. pharm. Sci.*, 1977, *66*, 955–8

Rectal absorption of nitrofurantoin

capsules, hard gelatin and suppositories: nitrofurantoin, levels, urine; dissolution method, *U.S.P.* disintegration apparatus

Moës, A.J., *Pharm. Acta Helv.*, 1981, *56*, 21–5

Formulation of highly available theophylline rectal suppositories

capsules, soft gelatin and suppositories: theophylline, anhydrous, monohydrate, levels, serum; dissolution method, suppositories, flow-through cell; drug properties, partition coefficient, solubility, measurements; intrinsic dissolution method, beaker; 3.5.2

Möller, H., *Pharm. Ind., Berl.*, 1984, *46*, 514–20

In vitro and *in vivo* dissolution of rectal indomethacin dosage forms (in German)

capsules, soft gelatin and suppositories: indomethacin; disintegration testing; dissolution method, flow-through cell; dissolution testing, effect of formulation; product properties, melting point, viscosity, effect of storage; 3.5.2

Hagenlocher, M., Hannula, A.M., Wittwer, F., Soliva, M. and Speiser, P., *Fourth International Conference on Pharmaceutical Technology*, (Paris, APGI, June 3–5, 1986), 1986, *I*, 398–405

Hard gelatin capsules for rectal drug delivery

capsules, hard gelatin, enema, solutions, oral and suppositories: paracetamol, levels, saliva; disintegration method DAB 8; disintegration testing, effect of capsule coating; dissolution testing, modified beaker; dissolution testing, comparisons of dosage forms, formulation of contents; pharmacokinetic analysis; 3.2.4.2; 3.5.2

4.5.3.5 Comparison with Multiple Dosage Forms

Calesnick, B., Katchen, B. and Black, J., *J. pharm. Sci.*, 1965, *54*, 1277–80

Importance of dissolution rates in producing effective diazoxide blood levels in man

capsules, hard gelatin, injections, intravenous, solutions and tablets: diazoxide, levels, blood; drug clinical effects, blood glucose levels, blood pressure; dissolution method, Stoll Gershberg

Flanagan, T.H., Broad, R.D., Rubinstein, M.H. and Longworth, A.R., *J. Pharm. Pharmac.*, 1969, *21, Suppl.*, 129S–34S

Dissolution and absorption of ICI 49,455

capsules, hard gelatin, solutions and tablets, film-coated and plain: ICI 49,455, levels, blood (dogs); dissolution method, beaker; drug availability, *in vitro*, goldfish death time

Chiou, W.L. and Riegelman, S., *J. pharm. Sci.*, 1970, *59*, 937–42

Oral absorption of griseofulvin in dogs: increased absorption via solid dispersion in polyethylene glycol 6000

capsules, hard gelatin, solutions and tablets: griseofulvin, levels, plasma, urine (dogs); dissolution method, modified *U.S.P.* disintegration apparatus; drug availability, effect of formulation; formulation of contents, solid dispersions in polyethylene glycol

Nash, J.F., Scholz, N.E. and Maxwell, S.B., *Toxic. appl. Pharmac.*, 1971, *19*, 537–45

A study of propoxyphene and salicylate concentrations in human plasma following the administration of propoxyphene napsylate and aspirin

capsules, hard gelatin, suspensions and tablets: aspirin, dextropropoxyphene hydrochloride and napsylate, caffeine, phenacetin, levels, plasma; disintegration method, *U.S.P.*; dissolution method, *U.S.P*; drug availability, effect of, capsule formulation, drug combination

Stricker, H., *Pharm. Ind., Berl.*, 1971, *33*, 446–54 and *Drugs Germ.*, 1971, *14*, 126–40

On the relationship between drug absorption and dissolution in the gastrointestinal tract (1) (in German, English translation in *Drugs Germ.*)

capsules, hard gelatin, solutions and tablets: aspirin, phenoxymethylpenicillin potassium, sulphapyrimidine, levels, plasma (human); dissolution method, Sartorius apparatus, *U.S.P.* XVIII; dissolution testing, comparison of methods

Fischler, M., Frisch, E.P. and Örtengren, B., *Acta pharm. suec.*, 1973, *10*, 483–92

Plasma concentrations after oral administration of different pharmaceutical preparations of clomethiazole

capsules, soft gelatin, solutions and tablets: clomethiazole, levels, plasma; disintegration method, *Nord.P.* apparatus

Wiseman, E.H., McIlhenny, H.M. and Bettis, J.W., *J. pharm. Sci.*, 1975, *64*, 1469–75

Flumizole, a new nonsteroidal anti-inflammatory agent

capsules, hard gelatin, infusions, intravenous, injections, intravenous and solutions: flumizole, levels, faeces, serum, urine (dogs, humans); dissolution method, *U.S.N.F.* XIII apparatus; pharmacokinetic analysis

Bergan, T., Berdal, B.P. and Holm, V., *Acta pharmac. tox.*, 1976, *38*, 308–20

Relative bioavailability of phenoxymethylpenicillin preparations in a cross-over study

capsules, hard gelatin, solutions, suspensions and tablets: phenoxymethylpenicillin, levels, serum; dissolution method, *U.S.P.*XVIII

Garrett, E.R., Roseboom, H., Green, J.R. and Schuermann, W., *Int. J. clin. Pharmac. Biopharm.*, 1978, *16*, 193–208

Pharmacokinetics of papaverine hydrochloride and the biopharmaceutics of its oral dosage forms

capsules, hard gelatin, injections, intravenous, solutions and tablets: papaverine hydrochloride, levels, serum; dissolution method, shaken flask; drug availability, comparison of dosage regimen, standard and slow-release preparation (capsule); pharmacokinetic analysis

Brandau, R. and Wehnert, H.-U., *Arzneimittel-Forsch.*, 1979, *29*, 552–5

Dissolution rates and bioavailability of phenytoin prepartions (in German)

capsules, hard gelatin, suspensions and tablets: phenytoin, calcium and sodium salts, levels, plasma; dissolution method, *U.S.P.* XIX; 4.5.3.1

Sved, S., Hossie, R.D., McGilveray, I.J., Beaudoin, N. and Brien, R., *Can.. J. pharm. Sci.*, 1979, *14*, 67–71

Bioavailability, absorption and dissolution kinetics of phenytoin formulations

capsules, hard gelatin, suspensions and tablets: phenytoin sodium, levels, plasma (human); dissolution method, modified beaker; drug availability, comparison of products; pharmacokinetic analysis

4.5.4 Comparison of Capsule Products

Bartelloni, P.J., Calia, F.M., Minchew, B.H., Beisel, W.R. and Ley, H.L., *Am. J. med. Sci.*, 1969, *258*, 203–8

Absorption and excretion of two chloramphenicol products in humans after oral administration

capsules, hard gelatin: chloramphenicol, levels, serum, urine; dissolution method, modified *U.S.P.* disintegration apparatus; drug availability, comparison of dosage regimens

Macdonald, H., Pisano, F., Burger, J., Dornbush, A. and Pelcak, E., *Clin. Med.*, 1969, *76*, 30–3

Physiologic availability of various tetracyclines

capsules: tetracyclines, levels, serum, urine; content uniformity; disintegration method, *U.S.P.*; dissolution method, rocking cylinder; drug availability, comparison of dosage regimens, single and multiple doses

Macdonald, H., Pisano, F., Burger, J., Dornbush, A. and Pelcak, E., *Drug Inf. Bull.*, 1969, *3*, 76–81

Physiological availability of various tetracyclines

capsules: tetracyclines, levels, serum, urine; content uniformity; disintegration method, *U.S.P.*; dissolution method, rocking cylinder; drug availability, comparison of dosage regimens, single and multiple doses

Ballin, J. C., *J. Am. med. Ass.*, 1971, *215*, 2095

Effectiveness of oxytetracyclines

capsules: oxytetracyclines; FDA certification

MacLeod, C., Rabin, H., Ruedy, J., Caron, M., Zarowny, D. and Davies, R.O., *Can. med. Ass. J.*, 1972, *107*, 203–9

Comparative bioavailability of three brands of ampicillin

capsules, hard gelatin: ampicillin trihydrate, levels, serum; dissolution method, *U.S.P.* XVIII; product, content uniformity

Butler, K., *Revue Can. Biol.*, 1973, *32, Suppl.*, 53–67

Biological availability of oxytetracycline HCl capsules

capsules, hard gelatin: oxytetracycline hydrochloride, levels, serum; dissolution method, Stoll-Gershberg apparatus; pharmacokinetic analysis

Andrade, L., Ortiz, S., Firmani, F. and Cid, E., *Annls pharm. fr.*, 1978, *36*, 639–44

Bioavailability of three brands of commercial ampicillin (in French)

capsules, hard gelatin: ampicillin, levels, urine (human); dissolution method, rotating basket

Berezovskaia, L.N., Koroleva, V.G., Granatova, E.K. and Grakovskais, L.K., *Antibiotiki*, 1979, *24*, 821–4

Bioavailability of doxycycline capsules (in Russian)

capsules, hard gelatin: doxycycline, levels, serum; dissolution testing, *U.S.P.* method; drug availability, comparison with American products

Bron, J., Vree, T.B., Damsma, J.E., Hekster, Y.A. and van der Kleijn, E., *Arzneimittel-Forsch.*, 1979, *29*, 1614–20

Dissolution, bioavailability and pharmacokinetics of three nitrofurantoin preparations in man

capsules, hard gelatin and tablets: nitrofurantoin, levels, plasma, urine; disintegration method, *U.S.P.* XIX; dissolution method, rotating basket; drug availability, formulation of contents, effect of particle size

Quay, J.F., Childers, R.F., Johnson, D.W., Nash, J.F. and Stucky, J.F., *J. pharm. Sci.*, 1979, *68*, 227–32

Cinoxacin in female mongrel dogs: effect of urine pH on urinary excretion and correlation of *in vitro* characteristics of oral dosage forms with bioavailability

capsules, hard gelatin, injections, intravenous and solutions: cinoxacin, levels, plasma, urine (dogs); dissolution method, modified basket; drug availability, formulation of contents, effect of powder properties, urinary pH; powder properties, particle size, surface area

Trivedi, B.M. and Patel, P.R., *Indian J. pharm. Sci.*, 1979, *41*, 66–8

Bioavailability of ampicillin in dogs

capsules, hard gelatin: ampicillin, levels, serum (dogs); dissolution method, rotating basket

Zak, A.F., Batuashvili, T.A. and Shchedrin, V.I., *Antibiotiki*, 1981, *26*, 728–31

Rifampicin drugs for oral use and their bioavailability (in Russian)

capsules, hard gelatin: rifampicin, levels, plasma; dissolution method, rotating basket; dissolution testing, comparison of products; drug availability, comparison of products

Kaniwa, N., Ogata, H., Aoyagi, N., Shibazaki, T., Ejima, A., Watanabe, Y., Motahashi, K., Sasahara, K., Nakajima, E., Morioka, T. and Nikanai, T., *Int. J. clin. Pharmac. Ther. Toxic.*, 1983, *21*, 56–63

The bioavailability of flufenamic acid and its dissolution rate from capsules

capsules, hard gelatin: flufenamic acid, levels, serum (dogs and humans); dissolution method, disintegration apparatus (*Jpn P.*), paddle, rotating basket, solubility simulator; dissolution testing, effects of, pH test medium, surfactant; pharmacokinetic analysis, comparison of dogs and humans

Shah, V.P., Prasad, V.K., Alston, T., Cabana, B.E., Gural, R.P. and Meyer, M.C., *J. pharm. Sci.*, 1983, *72*, 306–8

Phenytoin I: *In vitro – in vivo* correlation for 100-mg phenytoin sodium capsules

capsules, hard gelatin: phenytoin sodium, levels, plasma; dissolution method, paddle, rotating basket; dissolution testing, comparison of products; drug availability, comparison of products; pharmacokinetic analysis

Shah, V.P., Prasad, V.K., Freeman, C., Skelly, J.P. and Cabana, B.E., *J. pharm. Sci.*, 1983, *72*, 309–10

Phenytoin II: *In vitro – in vivo* bioequivalence standard for 100-mg phenytoin sodium capsules

capsules, hard gelatin: phenytoin sodium, levels, plasma; dissolution method, rotating basket; dissolution testing, comparison of products, fast and slow dissolving, proposed pharmacopoeial limit; drug availability, comparison of products; pharmacokinetic analysis

Shinozavva, S., Yoshimura, A. and Araki, Y., *Res. Commun. chem. Path. Pharmac.*, 1983, *42*, 161–4

The dissolution and bioavailability of Rifampicin products in healthy subjects and tubercular patients

capsules, hard gelatin: rifampicin, levels, plasma; dissolution method, rotating basket; dissolution testing, effect of test media; drug availability, effect of patient's disease state; pharmacokinetic analysis

Gouda, H.W., Moustafa, M.A. and Al-Shora, H.I., *Int. J. Pharmaceut.*, 1984, *18*, 213

Effect of storage on nitrofurantoin solid dosage forms

capsules, hard gelatin and tablets: nitrofurantoin, levels, urine; dissolution method, *U.S.P.*; dissolution testing, effects of, drug particle size in capsules, storage; 3.8.3.7

Aoyagi, N., Ogata, H., Kaniwa, N., Ejime, A., Nakata, H., Tsutsumi, J., Fujita, T. and Amada, I., *Int. J. clin. Pharmac. Ther. Toxic.*, 1985, *23*, 578–84

Bioavailability of indomethacin capsules in humans (III): correlation with bioavailability in beagle dogs

capsules, hard gelatin: indomethacin, levels, plasma (dogs); drug availability, effects of, formulation; gastric acidity; pharmacokinetic analysis, correlation with dissolution results

Kahr, R.K., Urumov, A. and Minkov, E., *Pharmazie*, 1985, *40*, 734–735

Comparative bioavailability studies of some oral amoxycillin products in rabbits

capsules, hard gelatin: amoxycillin, levels, serum (rabbit); dissolution methods, paddle, rotating basket, Sartorius; pharmacokinetic analysis

Mortada, L.M., Ismail, F.A. and Khalil, S.A., *Drug Dev. ind. Pharm.*, 1985, *11*(1), 101–30

Correlation of urinary excretion with *in vitro* dissolution using four dissolution methods for ampicillin capsules

capsules, hard gelatin: ampicillin, levels, urine; dissolution methods, disintegration apparatus modified, paddle, rotating basket, spiral stirrer method; dissolution testing, comparisons of, dissolution method, products, effect of stirrer speed

4.5.5 Effect of Formulation

Nelson, E. and Yuzuriha, Y., *J. Am. pharm. Ass., scient. Edn*, 1959, *48*, 96–103

Influence of dissolution rate and surface on tetracycline absorption

capsules, hard gelatin: tetracycline, hydrochloride phenolsulphonphthalein salt, sodium hexametaphosphate complex, levels, urine (human); dissolution method, solution rate of compressed disks; drug availability, effects of, diluent, sodium bicarbonate, particle size of active drug; formulation of contents, compressed disks, granules prepared by compression

Roland, M., *J. Pharm. Belg.*, 1967, *22*, 67–94

Formulation and availability of pharmaceutical tablets: applications to triamterene (in France)

capsules, hard gelatin and tablets: triamterene, levels, urine; disintegration method, Erweka apparatus; dissolution method, Souder and Ellenbogen; drug availability, comparison of dosage forms, effect of drug particle size

McGee, B.J., Kennedy, D.R. and Walker, G.C., *J. pharm. Sci.*, 1970, *59*, 1430–3

Some factors affecting release and availability of drugs from hard gelatin capsules

capsules, hard gelatin: acetylsalicylic acid, levels, plasma (rabbit); dissolution method, beaker; dissolution testing, effect of excipients

Koeleman, H.A. and van Oudtshoorn, M.C.B., *S. Afr. med. J.*, 1973, *47*, 94–9

An evaluation of the biological availability of chloramphenicol

capsules, hard gelatin: chloramphenicol, levels, urine; disintegration method, *B.P.*; dissolution method, beaker, modified *B.P.* disintegration apparatus; drug availability, effect of powder properties; powder properties, deaggregation rate determination, particle size determination; pharmacokinetic analysis

Dugal, R., Brodeur, J. and Caillé, G., *J. clin. Pharmac.*, 1974, *14*, 513–9

Ampicillin systemic bioavailability: the influence of dosage form

capsules, hard gelatin: ampicillin trihydrate, levels, serum; dissolution method, *U.S.P.* XVIII; formulation of contents, dry granulation, powder fill

Nash, J.F., Bechtel, L.D., Lowary, L.R., Rodda, B.E. and Rose, H.A., *Drug Devel. Comm.*, 1974–5, *1*, 443–57

The relationship between the particle size of dicumarol and its bioavailability in dogs. Part I. Capsules

capsules, hard gelatin: dicoumarol, levels, plasma, prothrombin time (dogs); dissolution method, *U.S.P.* XVIII; drug availability, effect of drug particle size

Nash, J.F., Childers, R.F., Lowary, L.R. and Rose, H.A., *Drug Devel. Comm.*, 1974–5, *1*, 459–70

The relationship between the particle size of dicumarol and its bioavailability in dogs. Part II. Drug substance

capsules, hard gelatin: dicoumarol, levels, plasma, prothrombin time (dogs); dissolution method, *U.S.P.* XVIII; drug availability, effect of drug particle size; powder properties, crystal structure

Allen, J.G. and Davies, C.A., *J. Pharm. Pharmac.*, 1975, *27*, 50–1

The effect of addition of lactose on the oral absorption of a highly lipid soluble drug capsules, hard gelatin and solutions: narcotic analgesic, levels, blood (dogs); dissolution method, modified beaker; drug availability, effect of drug particle size; formulation of contents, diluents, lactose, starch

Hill, S.A., Jones, K.H., Seager, H. and Taskis, C.B., *J. Pharm. Pharmac.*, 1975, *27*, 594–8

Dissolution and bioavailability of the anhydrate and trihydrate forms of ampicillin

capsules, hard gelatin: ampicillin anhydrous and trihydrate, levels, serum; dissolution method, flask apparatus

Johnson, B.F., Mcauley, P.V., Smith, P.M. and French, J.A.G., *J. Pharm. Pharmac.*, 1977, *29*, 576–8

The effects of storage upon *in vitro* and *in vivo* characteristics of soft gelatin capsules containing digoxin

capsules, soft gelatin: digoxin, levels, plasma; dissolution method, beaker; drug availability, effect of storage

Kassem, M.A., Salama, H.A., Ammar, H.O. and El-Ridy, M.S., *Pharm. Ind., Berl.*, 1977, *39*, 396–9

On the dissolution and bioavailability of phenindione. III. Dissolution and bioavailability of phenindione capsules

capsules, hard gelatin and powders: phenindione, levels, from blood clotting times (rabbit); dissolution method, beaker, *U.S.P.* XVIII; dissolution testing, effects of, capsule shell, drug particle size, formulation; formulation of contents, solid dispersions

Kent, J.S., Mroszczak, E. and Yost, M., *Drug Dev. ind. Pharm.*, 1977, *3*, 507–22

The use of radio-labelled drug in early dosage form development to provide a relation between physical dosage form characteristics and bioavailability

capsules, hard gelatin: dibenzthiepin, acetic acid derivative, ^{14}C-labelled, levels, serum, urine (monkey); dissolution method, *U.S.P.* type; formulation of contents; powder properties, particle shape, specific area; radioactive isotope technique

Kranz, O., Soliva, M. and Speiser, P.P., *Pharm. Ind., Berl.*, 1977, *39*, 712–5

The bioavailability of paracetamol from formulated hard gelatin capsules (in German)

capsules, hard gelatin and solutions: paracetamol, levels, saliva; dissolution method, column; drug availability, effect of formulation of capsule shells and contents; formulation of contents, lubricant, magnesium stearate

Kranz, O. and Speiser, P., *First International Conference on Pharmaceutical Technology*, Paris, APGI, 1977, IV, 209–13

The biopharmacy of capsules (in French)

capsules, hard gelatin: paracetamol, levels, saliva, urine ; dissolution method, flow-through cell; dissolution testing, effects of, formulation of capsule contents and shells; drug availability, effects of, formulation of capsule contents and shells; formulation of capsule shells, bone gelatin, skin gelatin, mixed gelatins; formulation of contents, hydrophilic, granules coated with

polyvinylpyrrolidone, hydrophobic, mixed with magnesium stearate

Fell, J.T., Calvert, R.T. and Riley-Bentham, P., *J. Pharm. Pharmac.*, 1978, *30*, 479–82

Bioavailability of griseofulvin from a novel capsule formulation

capsules, hard gelatin: griseofulvin, levels, urine; coating materials, hydroxypropylcellulose; coating method, granulation; dissolution method, beaker; dissolution testing, effect of hydrophilic coating of hydrophobic drug; formulation, hydrophilic coatings; pharmacokinetic analysis

Lerk, C.F., Lagas, M., Lie-A-Huen, L., Broersma, P. and Zuurman, K., *J. pharm. Sci.*, 1979, *68*, 634–8

In vitro and *in vivo* availability of hydrophilized phenytoin from capsules

capsules, hard gelatin: phenytoin, levels, plasma; disintegration method, *B.P.* 1973; dissolution method, beaker; formulation of contents, drug particle coating, methylcellulose

Nash, J.F., Bechtol, L.D., Bunde, C.A., Bopp, R.J., Farid, K.Z. and Spradlin, C.T., *J. pharm. Sci.*, 1979, *68*, 1087–90

Linear pharmacokinetics of orally administered fenoprofen calcium

capsules, hard gelatin: fenoprofen calcium, levels, plasma, urine; dissolution method, rotating basket

Ridolfo, A.S., Thompkins, L., Bechtol, L.D. and Carmichael, R.H., *J. pharm. Sci.*, 1979, *68*, 850–2

Benoxaprofen, a new anti-inflammatory agent: particle-size effect of dissolution rate and oral absorption in humans

capsules, hard gelatin: benoxaprofen, levels, plasma, urine; dissolution method, rotating basket; formulation of contents, particle size

Stewart, A.G., Grant, D.J.W. and Newton, J.M., *J. Pharm. Pharmac.*, 1979, *31*, 1–6

The release of a model low-dose drug (riboflavine) from hard gelatin capsule formulations

capsules, hard gelatin: riboflavine, levels, urine; dissolution method, beaker; 3.2.4.1

Wagner, J.G., Stoll, R.G., Weidler, D.J., Ayres, J.W., Hallmark, M.R., Sakmar, E. and Yacobi, A., *J. Pharmacokinet. Biopharm.*, 1979, *7*, 147–58

Comparison of the *in vitro* and *in vivo* release of digoxin from four different soft gelatin capsule formulations

capsules, soft gelatin: digoxin, levels, serum, urine; disintegration, capsule bursting time; dissolution method, *U.S.P.* XVIII; drug availability, effects of capsule disintegration

Bowtle, W., Woodage, T. and Waugh, A., *Int. J. Pharmaceut.*, 1981, *9*, 305–13

Bromhexine: *in vitro* and *in vivo* studies of release from mono- and bi-component preparations capsules, hard gelatin: bromhexine, base, hydrochloride, levels, plasma; cefaclor, levels, plasma; dissolution method, rotating basket; dissolution testing, effect of cefaclor presence; drug availability, effect of cefaclor presence; formulation of contents, bromhexine with or without cefaclor; pharmacokinetic analysis

Rosenberg, J.M., *N.Y. St. J. Med.*, 1981, *81*, 759

Please provide information concerning the differences between prompt phenytoin sodium capsules and extended phenytoin sodium capsules

capsules, hard gelatin: phenytoin; drug availability, comparison with *in vitro* dissolution standards, effect of fast and slow release forms

Boymond-Genoud, M., Eide-Jurgensen, G., Mordier, D., Doelker, E. and Buri, P., *J. Pharm. Belg.*, 1982, *37*, 135–40

The role of wetting in the release of hydrophobic drugs from hard gelatin capsules. II Deaggregation, dissolution and bioavailability in man (in French)

capsules, hard gelatin: phenacetin, levels, plasma; dissolution methods, continuous flow, paddle, rotating basket; dissolution testing, effects of, formulation of contents, powder properties, test media; powder properties, deaggregation, particle size; test media, inclusion of surfactants, polysorbate 80, dioctyl sodium sulphosuccinate

Laboratoires Negma, *French Patent* 2 500 302, 1982

Novel pharmaceutical compositions of indomethacin (in French)

capsules, soft gelatin: indomethacin, levels, plasma (rabbit); dissolution method, *U.S.P.*; dissolution testing, effect of formulation of contents; drug side-effects, gastric intolerance, effect of formulation of contents; 3.3.3.2

Aiache, J.-M., Roca, R., Bastide, J., Bastide, M. and Kantelip, J.-P., *J. Pharm. Belg.*, 1983, *38*, 5–21

Biopharmaceutical study of indomethacin new drug dosage forms (in French)

capsules, soft gelatin: indomethacin, levels, plasma (human); dissolution method, paddle; dissolution testing, effect of lipophilic contents; drug availability, animal, comparison of formulations and drug substance by LD50 in mice and rats; drug clinical effects (rat), anti-inflammatory activity on paw swelling, comparison of drug, excipients and products; drug side-effects (rat), effect on gastro-intestinal tract, comparison of drug, excipients and products; pharmacokinetic analysis; 3.3.3.2

Bauer, K.H. and Dortunc, B., *Drug Dev. ind. Pharm.*, 1984, *10*, 699–712

Non-aqueous emulsions as vehicles for capsule fillings

capsules, hard gelatin: riboflavine, salicylic acid, levels, urine; dissolution method, flow-through cell; 3.2.4.2

Shinkuma, D., Hamaguchi, T., Yamanaka, Y. and Mizuno, N., *Int. J. Pharmaceut.*, 1984, *21*, 187–200

Correlation between dissolution method and bioavailability of different commercial mefenamic acid capsules

capsules, hard gelatin: mefenamic acid, levels, plasma; disintegration method, *Jpn. P.* X; disintegration testing, comparison of products, effect of encapsulation; dissolution method, paddle; dissolution testing, comparison of products, fast and slow dissolving; drug availability, comparison of capsule contents, encapsulated, free; pharmacokinetic analysis

Aoyagi, N., Ogata, H., Kaniwa, N. and Ejima, A., *Int. J. clin. Pharmac. Ther. Toxic.*, 1985, *23*, 529–34

Bioavailability of indomethacin capsules in humans (II): correlation with dissolution rate

capsules, hard gelatin: indomethacin; disintegration method, *Jpn. P.* X; disintegration testing, effects of, formulation of contents, pH test media; dissolution methods, paddle, oscillating basket, rotating basket, solubility simulator; dissolution testing, effects of, pH of test media, stirrer speed; pharmacokinetic analysis, correlation with *in vivo* results

Aoyagi, N., Ogata, H., Kaniwa, N. and Ejima, A., *Int. J. clin. Pharmac. Ther. Toxic.*, 1985, *23*, 469–74

Bioavailability of indomethacin capsules in humans (1): bioavailability and effects of gastric acidity

capsules, hard gelatin: indomethacin, levels, serum; dissolution method, paddle; dissolution testing, effects of formulation of contents; drug availability, effects of, formulation of contents, patient's gastric acidity; pharmacokinetic analysis

Bowtle, W.J.., Lucas, R.A. and Barker, N.J., *Fourth International Conference on Pharmaceutical Technology*, (Paris, APGI, June 3–5, 1986), 1986, *V*, 80–89

Formulation and process studies in semi-solid matrix capsule technology

capsules, hard gelatin: fenoprofen, levels, serum; dissolution method, flow through cell; dissolution testing, effect of formulation; drug availability, effect of formulation; 3.2.4.2.; 3.8.3.7

Tossounian, J.L., Mergens, W.J. and Sheth, P.R., *Drug Dev. ind. Pharm.*, 1985, *11*, 1019–1050

Bioefficient products. A novel delivery system

capsules, hard gelatin and tablets: riboflavine, levels, urine; capsules, floating dosage form; dissolution method, beaker; dissolution testing, comparison of dosage forms and formulations; 4.4.3

Mohamad, H., Renoux, R., Aïache, S., Aïache, J.-M. and Kantelip, J.-P., *Sciences tech. pharm.*, 1986, *2*(18), 630–635

Study on the biopharmaceutical stability of medicines: application to tetracycline hydrochloride capsules: II *in vivo* study

capsules, hard gelatin: tetracycline hydrochloride, levels, plasma, urine; dissolution testing, comparison of batches, effect of storge; drug availability, comparison of batches, effect of storage; pharmacokinetic analysis; pharmacokinetic parameters, comparison of formulas, effect of storage

4.5.6 Controlled Release Products

4.5.6.1 Enteric Capsules

Bauer, C.W. and Geraughty, R.J., *J. Am. pharm. Ass., pract. Pharm. Edn*, 1953, *14*, 504–7 and 512

Enteric coatings in dispensing pharmacy. I. The preliminary investigation

capsules, hard gelatin and tablets: sodium salicylate, levels, urine; coating materials, carnauba wax, *n*-butyl stearate; coating method, hot dipping; disintegration method, *in vitro*, *U.S.P.*, disintegration method, *in vivo*, timed urine analysis; disintegration testing, *in vitro*, effect of solvents; formulation of coating, stability

Parrott, E.L., *J. Am. pharm. Ass.*, 1961, *NS1*, 158–9

An extemporaneous enteric coating

capsules, hard gelatin: acetylsalicylic acid, levels, urine; potassium iodide, levels, saliva; disintegration method, *in vitro*, *U.S.P.* apparatus; drug availability, *in vivo*, comparison of coating materials; 3.4.2.1

Cook, C.H. and Webber, M.G., *Am. J. Hosp. Pharm.*, 1965, *22*, 95–9

An extemporaneous method of preparing enteric-coated capsules

capsules, hard gelatin: disintegration method, *in vitro*, modified *U.S.P.* XVI; disintegration method, *in vivo* (dogs), X-ray, radio-opaque contents; 3.4.2.4

Cordes, G., *Pharm. Ind., Berl.*, 1969, *31*, 328–31 and *Drugs Germ.*, 1969, *12*, 111–7

Enteric-coated hard gelatin capsules as a dosage form for enzyme preparations (in German: English translation in *Drugs Germ.*)

capsules, hard gelatin and tablets: pancreatin; disintegration method, *in vitro*, Ger. P. (DAB 7); disintegration method, *in vivo*, radiotransmitter; disintegration testing, effects of, enteric film thickness, filling method; dissolution method, beaker; dissolution testing, measurement of lipase activity

Ekberg, L. and Källstrand, G., *Svensk farm. Tidskr.*, 1972, *76*, 375–8

The enteric coating of hard gelatin capsules on a dispensary scale (in Swedish)

capsules, hard gelatin: capsules, enteric coated; disintegration method, *in vitro*, Nord. P.; disintegration method, *in vivo*, gamma scintigraphy, technetium-99m; disintegration testing, *in vitro*, effect of film thickness; disintegration testing, *in vivo*, comparison of coated and uncoated capsules; 3.4.2.4

Aiache, J.-M., Vidal, J.L., Aiache, S., Jeanneret, A. and Cornat, F., *Labo-Pharma Probl. Tech.*, 1974, *22*(232), 457–63

Methods for the biopharmaceutical testing of enteric capsules: Tests with 'enterocaps' capsules (in French)

capsules, hard gelatin: doxapram base, levels, blood (human); 3.4.2.4; 4.4.7.1

Aiache, J.-M., Aiache, S., Jeanneret, A., Cornat, F. and Vidal, J.L., *Boll. chim.-farm.*, 1975, *114*, 636–50

Methods for the biopharmaceutical testing of enteric capsules: Tests with 'enterocaps' capsules (in French)

capsules, hard gelatin: doxapram base, methylenecycline, levels, blood; 3.4.2.4; 4.4.7.1

Jain, N.K. and Naik, S.U., *J. pharm. Sci.*, 1984, *73*, 1806–11

Design of a slow-release capsule using laser drilling

capsules, hard gelatin: tetracycline hydrochloride; capsule shells, perforated walls, laser drilling; capsules, enteric, formaldehyde treatment; disintegration method, rotating basket, gastric and intestinal fluids; disintegration testing, effect of formaldehyde; dissolution method, rotating basket; dissolution testing, effects of, formulation of contents, hole, size and number; gastric behaviour, visualisation method, X-ray, radio-opaque contents; formulation of contents, diluents, drug particle size, surfactants; gastric behaviour, transit times

4.5.6.2 Slow-release Capsules

Rosen, E. and Swintosky, J.V., *J. Pharm. Pharmac.*, 1960, *12*, *Suppl.*, 237–44T

Preparation of a ^{35}S labelled trimeprazine tartrate sustained action product for its evaluation in man

capsules, hard gelatin: trimeprazine tartrate, levels, blood, urine; dissolution method, Souder and Ellenbogen; formulation of contents; radioactive isotope technique

Heimlich, K.R., MacDonnell, D.R., Flanagan, T.L. and O'Brien, P.D., *J. pharm. Sci.*, 1961, *50*, 232–7

Evaluation of a sustained release form of phenylpropanolamine hydrochloride by urinary excretion studies

capsules, hard gelatin: phenylpropanolamine hydrochloride, levels, urine; dissolution method, Souder and Ellenbogen; formulation of contents

Rosen, E., *J. pharm. Sci.*, 1963, *52*, 98–100

Relationship of *in vitro* release to urinary recovery in man of a sustained-release preparation of ^{35}S prochlorperazine

capsules, hard gelatin: prochlorperazine maleate, levels, urine; dissolution method, Souder and Ellenbogen; drug availability, comparison of formulation, normal and slow-release; product form, sustained-release pellets; radioactive isotope technique

Rosen, E., Ellison, T., Tannenbaum, B., Free, S.M. and Crosley, A.P., *J. pharm. Sci.*, 1967, *56*, 365–9

Comparative study in man and dog of the absorption and excretion of dextroamphetamine-^{14}C sulphate in sustained-release and nonsustained-release dosage forms

capsules, hard gelatin: dexamphetamine sulphate, levels, urine (dogs, humans); dissolution method, Souder and Ellenbogen; dissolution testing, effect of formulations; radioactive isotope technique

Rosen, E., Polk, A., Free, S.M., Tannenbaum, P.J. and Crosley, A.P., *J. pharm. Sci.*, 1967, *56*, 1285–7

Comparative study in man of the absorption and excretion of amobarbital-^{14}C from sustained-release and non-sustained-release dosage forms

capsules, hard gelatin: amylobarbitone sodium, levels, plasma, urine; dissolution method, Souder and Ellenbogen

Beckett, A.H. and Tucker, G.T., *J. Pharm. Pharmac.*, 1968, *20*, 174–93

Application of the analogue computer to pharmacokinetic and biopharmaceutical studies with amphetamine-type compounds

capsules, hard gelatin, granules and solutions: amphetamines, levels, urine, acid pH; dissolution method, modified B.P. disintegration apparatus, rolling bottle, rotating bottle; drug availability, comparison of dosage forms, normal and slow-release forms; pharmacokinetic analysis, computer simulation

Simmons, D.L., Legore, A.A., Klapka, M. and Joshi, N.N., Can. J. pharm. Sci., 1973, 8, 139–41

An in vitro – in vivo evaluation of phenformin formulations

capsules, hard gelatin: phenformin, clinical effect, blood glucose level (guinea pig); dissolution method, rotating disk; drug administration by duodenal implantation; drug availability, comparison of normal and slow-release forms; formulation of contents, prolonged release

Bauguess, C.T., Fincher, J.H., Sadik, F. and Hartman, C.W., J. pharm. Sci., 1975, 64, 1489–92

Blood concentration profiles of acetaminophen following oral administration of fatty acid esters of acetaminophen with pancreatic lipase to dogs

capsules, hard gelatin: paracetamol, acetate and decanoate, levels, blood (dogs); drug availability, effect of co-administration of lipase; formulation of contents, slow release; pharmacokinetic analysis

Bauer, K.H., Otten, H. and Weuta, H., Pharm. Ind., Berl., 1976, 38, 823–7

Serum concentrations and urinary excretion quotient obtained from coated and uncoated oral ampicillin preparations (in German)

capsules, hard gelatin and tablets, film-coated: ampicillin, anhydrous, trihydrate, levels, serum, urine; dissolution method, beaker; drug availability, comparison of dosage forms, standard and slow-release forms; formulation of contents, controlled-release pellets

Schneider, H., Nightingale, C.H., Quintiliani, R. and Flanagan, D.R., J. pharm. Sci., 1978, 67, 1620–2

Evaluation of an oral prolonged-release antibiotic formulation

capsules, hard gelatin, injections, intravenous and tablets, prolonged-release: cephalexin, levels, serum, urine; dissolution method, U.S.P.; drug availability, comparison of commercial capsule product and slow-release tablet

Schoenwald, R.D., Garabedian, M.E. and Yakatan, G.J., Drug Dev. ind. Pharm., 1978, 4, 599–609

Decreased bioavailability of sustained release acetazolamide dosage forms

capsules, hard gelatin and tablets: acetazolamide, levels, plasma; dissolution method, paddle; drug availability, comparison of slow-release capsule and standard tablets

Gröning, R., Pharm. Ind., Berl., 1979, 41, 369–75

An in vitro and in vivo study of the release of nitrofurantoin from dosage forms (in German)

capsules, hard gelatin and tablets: nitrofurantoin, levels, urine; dissolution method, flow-through cell, paddle; drug availability, comparison of dosage forms; drug availability, slow-release capsule

Möller, H., Ali, S. L. and Steinbach, D., Int. J. Pharmaceut., 1980, 7, 157–67

Pharmaceutical and biological availability of sustained release preparations of potassium chloride

capsules, hard gelatin and tablets: potassium chloride, levels, K^+ in urine; dissolution method, rotating basket, paddle; dissolution testing, comparison of dosage forms; drug availability, comparison of slow-release pellets in capsules and coated tablets; patient's state, control of K^+ intake by diet

Chambliss, W.G., Cleary, R.W., Fischer, R., Jones, A.B., Skierkowski, P., Nicholes, W. and Kibbe, A.H., J. pharm. Sci., 1981, 70, 1248–51

Effect of docusate sodium on drug release from a controlled-release dosage form

capsules, hard gelatin: chlorpheniramine, levels, plasma; dissolution method, rotating basket; dissolution testing, effect of surfactant, docusate sodium; drug availability, effect of co-administration of 2×100 mg capsules of docusate sodium; drug availability, in vitro, measurement of micellar entrapment of chlorpheniramine in docusate sodium solutions; formulation of contents, controlled-release pellets; pharmacokinetic analysis

Laven, R. and Schäfer, E.-A., Arzneimittel-Forsch., 1981, 31, 353–6

Release of norfenefrine from sustained-release formulations by an in vitro dissolution model/simulation of 'drug levels' by calculation using pharmacokinetic constants and comparison with in vivo course of action

capsules, hard gelatin: norfenefrine hydrochloride; dissolution method, Stricker; dissolution testing, comparison of delayed-release and prolonged-release formulations; drug availability, in vitro simulation, calculation of blood levels; drug, clinical effects (cat), effect on blood pressure, comparison of formulations; pharmacokinetic analysis

Row, J.S. and Carless, J.E., J. Pharm. Pharmac., 1981, 33, 561–4

Comparison of the in vitro dissolution behaviour of various indomethacin formulations with their in vivo bioavailability

capsules, hard gelatin: indomethacin, levels, plasma; dissolution method, modified beaker; dissolution testing, comparison of standard and controlled-release products, effects of formulation of microcapsules; drug availability, comparisons of, standard and microencapsulated drug, controlled-release and microencapsulated drug; drug side-effects, comparison of formulations; formulation of contents, controlled-release pellets and powders; formulation of drug microcapsules, gelatin/acacia coacervates, various drug/colloid ratios; pharmacokinetic analysis

Schneider, G.F., Heese, G.U., Huber, H.J., Janzen, N., Jünger, H., Moser, C. and Stanislaus, F., Arzneimittel-Forsch., 1981, 31, 1489–97

Bioavailability of theophylline in a new oral sustained-release preparation (in German)

capsules, hard gelatin, solutions and tablets: theophylline, levels, plasma; dissolution method, paddle; dissolution testing, comparison of slow-release capsules and tablets; drug availability, comparison of dosage forms, effect of dose (capsules); formulation of contents, controlled-release pellets; pellet properties, density, friability, stability, uniformity of content; pharmacokinetic analysis

Yau, M.K.T. and Meyer, M.C., *J. pharm. Sci.*, 1981, *70*, 1017–24

In vivo – in vitro correlations with a commercial dissolution simulator I: Methenamine, nitrofurantoin and chlorothiazide

capsules, hard gelatin and tablets: nitrofurantoin, levels, urine, literature; dissolution method, rotating basket, Sartorius apparatus; dissolution testing, comparisons of, dosage forms, products; drug availability, correlation, in vitro simulator, Sartorius apparatus and in vivo data

Bechgaard, H., Brodie, R.R., Chasseaud, L.F., Houmoller, P., Hunter, J.O., Siklos, P. and Taylor, T., *Eur. J. clin. Pharmac.*, 1982, *21*, 511–5

Bioavailability of indomethacin from 2 multiple-units controlled-release formulations

capsule, hard gelatin: indomethacin, levels, plasma; dissolution method, rotating flask; dissolution testing, effects of, formulation, pH test media; drug availability, comparison of standards and slow-release formulations; formulation of contents, enteric-coated pellets; pharmacokinetic analysis

El-Egakey, M.A. and Speiser, P.P., *Acta pharm. Tech.*, 1982, *28*, 169–75

The in vitro and in vivo release studies of slow release phenylpropanolamine; polymethylcyanoacrylate entrapment products

capsules, hard gelatin: phenylpropanolamine, levels, urine; dissolution method, stirred flask; dissolution testing, contents, effect of formulation of pellets; drug availability, effect of formulation of pellets; formulation of contents, pellets, drug entrapment in methyl cyanoacrylate polymers; pellets, physical properties, particle size, effect of varying drug/monomer ratio

François, D., Denmat, A., Waugh, A. and Woodage, T., *Pharm. Ind., Berl.*, 1982, *44*, 86–9

The in vitro and in vivo availability of phenylpropanolamine from oil/paste formulations in hard gelatin capsules

capsules, hard gelatin: phenylpropanolamine hydrochloride, levels, plasma; dissolution method, Poole's apparatus; dissolution methodology, effect of lipophilic contents, correction for solvent evaporation; dissolution testing, comparison of formulations, powder and semi-solid fills; drug availability, comparison of formulations, powder and semi-solid fills; formulation of contents, semi-solid, hydrophilic, standard release, hydrophobic, slow release; pharmacokinetic analysis; 3.2.4.2

Yau, M.K.T. and Meyer, M.C., *J. pharm. Sci.*, 1983, *72*, 681–6

In vivo – in vitro correlations with a commercial dissolution simulator II: papaverine, phenytoin and sulfisoxazole

capsules, hard gelatin, elixirs and tablets: phenytoin sodium, papaverine hydrochloride, levels, plasma, literature; dissolution method, rotating basket, Sartorius apparatus; dissolution testing, comparison of dosage forms, papaverine hydrochloride, comparison of products, phenytoin sodium; drug availability correlation, in vitro simulator, Sartorius apparatus and in vivo data

Suryakusuma, H. and Jun, H.W., *J. Pharm. Pharmac.*, 1984, *36*, 497–501

Encapsulated hydrophilic polymer beads containing indomethacin as controlled release drug delivery systems

capsules, hard gelatin: indomethacin, levels, serum (dog); dissolution method, rotating basket; drug availability, comparison of formulations, standard powder and slow-release beads, effects of, bead coating polymers and thickness; formulation of bead coatings; production of hydrophilic polymer beads

Kohri, N., K.-I., Miyazaki, K. and Arita, T., *J. pharm. Sci.*, 1986, *75*, 57–61

Sustained release of nifedipine from granules

capsules, hard gelatin: nifedipine levels, serum (rabbits); dissolution method, rotating paddle; dissolution testing, comparison of formulations, effects of, binder type, drug content, pH of test media; drug availability, comparisons of, formulations, products; 3.2.4.1

Magbi, M., Beukaddour, N., Rodriguez, F., Michaud, P. and Rouffiac, R., *Fourth International Conference on Pharmaceutical Technology*, (Paris, APGI, June 3–5, 1986), 1986, *II*, 118–127

Comparison of controlled release formulations of theophylline, in vitro correlations (in French)

Capsules, hard gelatin, solutions and tablets: theophylline levels, saliva; dissolution method, rotating paddle; dissolution testing, comparisons of dosage forms, effect of pH test medium; drug availability, comparison of dosage forms; pharmacokinetic analysis

Morimoto, M., Yamashita, K., Koyama, H., Fujimoto, H., Toguchi, H. and Kitamori, N., *Chem. pharm. Bull., Tokyo*, 1986, *34*, 1257–63

Evaluation of sustained-release capsules of molsidomine (SIN-10) in dogs and monkeys

capsules, hard gelatin and tablets: molsidomine, levels, plasma (dog, monkey); dissolution method, rotating basket; dissolution testing, effects of, formulation of contents, pH of test medium; drug availability, comparison of dosage form, controlled release capsule, standard release tablet; formulation of contents, controlled release pellets; pharmacodynamic study; pharmacokinetic analysis

Steinijans, V.W., Schulz, H.-U., Beier, W. and Radtke, H.W., *Int. J. Clin. Pharmac. Ther. Toxic.*, 1986, *24*, 438–47

Once daily theophylline: multiple-dose comparison of an encapsulated micro-osmotic system (Euphylong) with a tablet (Uniphyllin)

capsules, hard gelatin and tablets: theophylline, levels, serum; dissolution method, paddle; drug availability, comparison of dosage forms; pharmacokinetic analysis

4.6 Investigational Drug Administration

4.6.1 Comparison of Drugs

White, W.F. and Gisvold, O., *J. Am. pharm. Ass., scient. Edn*, 1952, *41*, 42–6

Absorption rate studies of orally administered cardiac glycosides in cats

capsules, hard gelatin, solutions and tablets: acetyldigoxin (capsules), digitoxin, digoxin, lanatoside C; drug clinical effect, survival time (cats)

Weikel, J.H., *J. Am. pharm. Ass., scient. Edn*, 1958, *47*, 477–9

A comparison of human serum levels of acetylsalicylic acid, salicylamide and N-acetyl-*p*-aminophenol following oral administration

capsules, hard gelatin: aspirin, paracetamol, salicylamide, levels, serum

Steigbigel, N.H., Reed, C.W. and Finland, M., *Am. J. med. Sci.*, 1968, *255*, 296–312

Absorption and excretion of five tetracycline analogues in normal young men

capsules: tetracycline, demeclocycline, doxycycline, methacycline, minocycline, levels, serum, urine

Speirs, C.F., Stenhouse, D., Stephen, K.W. and Wallace, E.T., *Br. J. Pharmac.*, 1971, *43*, 242–7

Comparison of human serum, parotid and mixed saliva levels of phenoxymethylpenicillin, ampicillin, cloxacillin and cephalexin

capsules, hard gelatin and tablets: phenoxymethylpenicillin, levels, saliva (human); drug availability, effect of tablets in capsule

Nauta, E.H. and Mattie, H., *Br. J. clin. Pharmac.*, 1975, *2*, 111–21

Pharmacokinetics of flucloxacillin and cloxacillin in healthy subjects and patients on chronic intermittent haemodialysis

capsules, hard gelatin and infusions, intravenous: cloxacillin sodium, flucloxacillin sodium, levels, urine (human); drug availability, effect of patient's health, kidney performance; pharmacokinetic analysis

Harvengt, C. and Desager, J.-P., *Curr. ther. Res.*, 1976, *19*, 145–51

Pharmacokinetics and bioavailability of simfibrate, a clofibric acid derivative

capsules, soft gelatin: clofibric acid and derivatives, levels, plasma

Risberg, A.-M., Henricsson, S. and Ingvar, D.H., *Eur. J. clin. Pharmac.*, 1977, *12*, 105–9

Evaluation of the effect of fosazepam (a new benzodiazepine), nitrazepam and placebo on sleep patterns in normal subjects

capsules, hard gelatin: fosazepam, nitrazepam, clinical effects, sleep

Frithz, G. and Groppi, W., *J. int. med. Res.*, 1981, *9*, 338–42

Temazepam versus nitrazepam: A comparative trial in the treatment of sleep disturbances

capsules, soft gelatin and tablets: nitrazepam (tablets), temazepam (capsules); drug clinical effects, sleep, duration, onset, quality, comparison of drugs

4.6.2 Drug, Clinical Effects

Sandell, E., *Acta pharm. suec.*, 1967, *4*, 223–5

Tolerance to ammonium, potassium and sodium chloride in hard gelatin capsules

capsules, hard gelatin: ammonium chloride, potassium chloride, sodium chloride; formulation, effect on emesis (human)

Sterner, W., Voss, B. and Widmann, A., *Arzneimittel-Forsch.*, 1968, *18*, 1056–8

On the gastro-intestinal compatibility of orally applied drugs (in German)

capsules, soft gelatin and powders: capsicum oleoresin, podophyllin; drug, clinical effect, gastro-intestinal irritation (rats)

Husain, S.L., *Lancet*, 1969, *1*, 1069–71

Oral zinc sulphate in leg ulcers

capsules, hard gelatin: zinc sulphate, clinical effect, wound healing

Wilson, D.E., Quertermus, J., Raiser, M., Curran, J. and Robért, A., *Ann. intern. Med.*, 1976, *84*, 688–91

Inhibition of stimulated gastric secretion by an orally administered prostaglandin capsule

capsules, hard gelatin and solutions: 16,16-dimethylprostaglandin, clinical effect, gastric acid secretion

Baugh, R. and Calvert, R.T., *Eur. J. clin. Pharmac.*, 1977, *12*, 201–4

The effect of diphenhydramine alone and in combination with ethanol on histamine skin response and mental performance

capsules, hard gelatin: diphenhydramine hydrochloride, clinical effects, histamine skin response, serial seven subtraction, digit symbol substitution, tracking clinical effects, effect of co-administration of ethanol

Lithell, H., Boberg, J., Hedstrand, H., Hellsing, K., Ljunghall, S. and Vessby, B., *Eur. J. clin. Pharmac.*, 1977, *12*, 51–7

Effects of clofibrate on glucose tolerance, serum insulin, serum lipoproteins and plasma fibrinogen capsules, soft gelatin: clofibrate, biochemical effects, blood glucose, glucose intolerance, plasma fibrinogen, serum insulin; drug, clinical effects, body-weight, serum lipoprotein

Phillips, B.M. and Palermo, B.T., *J. pharm. Sci.*, 1977, *66*, 124–7

Physical form as a determinant of effect of buffered acetylsalicylate formulations on G.I. microbleeding

capsules, hard gelatin, powders, suspensions and tablets: aspirin, drug effects, gastro-intestinal bleeding (dogs); powder properties, particle size

Sutton, D.R. and Gosnold, J.K., *Br. med. J.*, 1977, *1*, 1598

Oesophageal ulceration due to clindamycin

capsules, hard gelatin: clindamycin, side-effects, oesophageal ulceration

Baars, R., Rapp, R., Young, B. and Canafax, D., *Ann. Neurol.*, 1978, *4*, 90

Phenytoin therapy – a comparison of one 300 mg capsule with three 100 mg capsules

capsules, hard gelatin: phenytoin; drug clinical effects, comparison of products, dosage regimen

Francis, M.E., Marshall, A.B. and Turner, W.T., *Vet. Rec.*, 1978, *102*, 377–80

Amoxycillin: clinical trial in dogs and cats

capsules, hard gelatin, injections and suspensions: amoxycillin, trihydrate; drug availability, comparison of dosage forms

Hennies, O.L., *J. int. med. Res.*, 1981, *9*, 62–8

A new skeletal muscle relaxant (DS 103–282) compared to diazepam in the treatment of muscle spasm of local origin

capsules, hard gelatin: diazepam, 5-chloro-4-(2-imidazolin-2-ylamino)-2,1,3-benzothiadiazole hydrochloride; drug, clinical effects, back pain reduction

Russell, A.S. and Le Morvan, P., *Curr. ther. Res.*, 1985, *38*, 599–605

Double-blind comparison between ketoprofen capsules four times daily and enteric-coated tablets twice daily in patients with osteoarthritis

capsules, hard gelatin and tablets, enteric coated: ketoprofen; drug, clinical effects, comparison of standard release capsule with delayed release tablets; drug, side-effects, comparisons of, dosage forms, dosage regimens

Wittig, R., Zorick, F., Roehrs, T., Paxton, C., Lamphere, J. and Roth, T., *Curr. ther. Res.*, 1985, *38*, 15–22

Effects of temazepam soft gelatin capsules on the sleep of subjects with insomnia

capsules, soft gelatin: temazepam; drug, clinical effects, polysomnographic measuring technique; drug, clinical trial, comparison with placebo

4.6.3 Drug, Formulation Effects

Aguiar, A.J. and Zelmer, J.E., *J. pharm. Sci.*, 1969, *58*, 983–7

Dissolution behaviour of polymorphs of chloramphenicol palmitate and mefenamic acid

capsules, hard gelatin: mefenamic acid, levels, blood; dissolution method, modified beaker; drug availability, effect of drug form, comparison of polymorphs

Khalafallah, N., Gouda, M.W. and Khalil, S.A., *J. pharm. Sci.*, 1975, *64*, 991–4

Effect of surfactants on absorption through membranes IV: effects of dioctyl sodium sulfosuccinate on absorption of a poorly absorbable drug, phenolsulfonphthalein, in humans

capsules and solutions: phenolsulphonphthalein (solution), levels, urine; drug availability, effect of co-administration of surfactant, dioctyl sodium sulphosuccinate (capsules or solution); drug trial, side-effects, effect of dosage form; surfactants, effect on biological membranes

Allen, P.V., Rahn, P.D., Sarapu, A.C. and Vanderwielen, A.J., *J. pharm. Sci.*, 1978, *67*, 1087–93

Physical characterization of erythromycin: anhydrate, monohydrate and dihydrate crystalline solids

capsules, hard gelatin: erythromycin, anhydrous, mono- and dihydrate; dissolution method, modified *U.S.P.*; dissolution testing, comparison of drug forms, effect of powder properties; powder properties, thermal analysis, surface area measurements

Kreuter, J. and Higuchi, T., *J. pharm. Sci.*, 1979, *68*, 451–4

Improved delivery of methoxsalen

capsules, hard gelatin and solutions: methoxsalen, levels, blood (dogs and rats); formulation of contents, liquid filling

Coronelli, M., Zuzolo, V., Tonti, M., Carosi, M. and Teggia, L., *Curr. ther. Res.*, 1983, *33*, 639–45

Antianginal activity of nifedipine in 5 mg capsules for acute administration

capsules, hard gelatin: nifedipine; drug, clinical effects, antianginal activity, measurements, cardiac performance

4.6.4 Drug Metabolism

Rubin, A., Rodda, B.E., Warrick, P., Ridolfo, A.S. and Gruber, C.M., *J. pharm. Sci.*, 1972, *61*, 739–45

Physiological disposition of fenoprofen in man II. Plasma and urine pharmacokinetics after oral and intravenous administration

capsules, hard gelatin and injections, intravenous: fenoprofen, calcium and sodium salts, metabolites, levels, plasma, urine; fenoprofen-^{14}C, calcium, metabolites, levels, faeces, plasma, urine; formulation of contents, radioactive isotope technique

Martin, L.E., Tanner, R.J.N., Clark, T.J.H. and Cochrane, G.M., *Clin. Pharmac. Ther.*, 1974, *15*, 267–75

Absorption and metabolism of orally administered beclomethasone dipropionate

capsules, hard gelatin and solutions: beclomethasone dipropionate, levels, faecal, plasma, urine; radioactive isotope technique

Verebely, K. and Inturrisi, C.E., *Clin. Pharmac. Ther.*, 1974, *15*, 302–9

Disposition of propoxyphene and norpropoxyphene in man after a single oral dose

capsules, hard gelatin: dextropropoxyphene hydrochloride, metabolite (norpropoxyphene), levels, plasma, urine

Cotler, S., Holazo, A., Boxenbaum, H.G. and Kaplan, S.A., *J. pharm. Sci.*, 1976, *65*, 822–7

Influence of route of administration on physiological availability of levodopa in dogs

capsules, hard gelatin, catheter, hepatoportal and injections, intravenous: levodopa, levels, serum, urine (dogs); drug metabolism, gastro-intestinal tract

Farid, N.A., Born, G.S., Kessler, W.V., Russell, H.T., Shaw, S.M. and Lange, W.E., *J. pharm. Sci.*, 1977, *66*, 536–8

Synthesis of ^{14}C-meglumine salicylate and its disposition in humans after oral administration

capsules, hard gelatin: meglumine salicylate, metabolites, levels, blood, faeces, urine; radioactive isotope technique

Sasahara, K., Nitanai, T., Habara, T., Kojima, T., Kawahara, Y., Morioka, T. and Nakajima, E., *J. pharm. Sci.*, 1981, *70*, 730–3

Dosage form design for improvement of bioavailability of levodopa IV: Possible causes of low bioavailability of oral levodopa in dogs

capsules, hard gelatin: levodopa, levels, serum (dogs); drug availability, comparison of route of administration; drug metabolism, effects of, gut position, intestinal flora; intestinal flora, effect of antibiotics; pharmacokinetic analysis

4.6.5 Pharmacokinetic Analysis

Nelson, E. and Schaldemose, I., *J. Am. pharm. Ass., scient. Edn*, 1959, *48*, 489–95

Urinary excretion kinetics for evaluation of drug absorption I. Solution rate limited and nonsolution rate limited absorption of aspirin and benzyl penicillin; absorption rate of sulfaethylthiadiazole

capsules, hard gelatin, suspensions and tablets: aspirin (tablets), benzylpenicillin, potassium and procaine, sulphaethidole (suspensions), levels, urine; drug form, compressed disks; drug availability, effect of formulation; formulation of contents, diluent, sodium bicarbonate

Nelson, E., *J. Am. pharm. Ass., scient. Edn*, 1960, *49*, 54–6

Urinary excretion kinetics for evaluation of drug absorption II. Constant, rate-limited release of tetracycline after ingestion by humans

capsules, hard gelatin and suspensions: tetracycline, disodium mucate and hydrochloride, levels, urine; drug availability, comparison of dosage forms, effect of formulation; drug form, compressed disks; formulation of contents, diluent, sodium bicarbonate

Nelson, E., *J. Am. pharm. Ass., scient. Edn*, 1960, *49*, 437–40

Urinary excretion kinetics for evaluation of drug absorption III. Method for calculation of absorption rate and application to tetracycline absorption in humans

capsules, hard gelatin: tetracycline, disodium mucate and hydrochloride, levels, urine; drug availability, effect of formulation; drug form, pellets; formulation of contents, diluents, sodium bicarbonate; pharmacokinetic analysis, absorption rate determination

Nelson, E., Long, S. and Wagner, J.G., *J. pharm. Sci.*, 1964, *53*, 1224–7

Correlation of amount of metabolite excreted and its excretion rate with available surface area of tolbutamide in dosage forms

capsules, hard gelatin: tolbutamide, metabolites, levels, urine; drug form, coated granules, compressed disks; drug availability, correlation surface area of drug form with urinary excretion; powder properties, surface area determination

Newmark, H.L., Berger, J. and Carstensen, J.T., *J. pharm. Sci.*, 1970, *59*, 1249–51

Coumermycin A_7 — Biopharmaceutical studies II

capsules, hard gelatin and injections, intravenous: coumermycin, and *N*-methylglucamine salt, levels, blood (dogs and humans)

Coutinho, C.B., Spiegel, H.E., Kaplan, S.A., Yu, M., Christian, R.P., Carbone, J.J., Symington, J., Cheripko, J.A., Lewis, M., Tonchen, A. and Crews, T., *J. pharm. Sci.*, 1971, *60*, 1014–19

Kinetics of absorption and excretion of levodopa in dogs

capsules, hard gelatin and injections, intravenous: levodopa, 2-^{14}C-levodopa, levels, serum, urine (dogs); drug availability, comparison acute and chronic dosage; radioactive isotope technique

Rubin, A., Rodda, B.E., Warrick, P., Ridolfo, A. and Gruber, C.M., *J. pharm. Sci.*, 1971, *60*, 1797–1801

Physiological disposition of fenoprofen in man I: pharmacokinetic comparison of calcium and sodium salts administered orally

capsules, hard gelatin: fenoprofen, calcium and sodium salts, levels, plasma

DiSanto, A.R. and Wagner, J.G., *J. pharm. Sci.*, 1972, *61*, 1086–90

Pharmacokinetics of highly ionised drugs II: Methylene blue – absorption, metabolism and excretion in man and dog after oral administration

capsules, hard gelatin: methylene blue, levels, urine (dogs, humans)

Macdonald, H., Kelly, R.G., Allen, E.S., Noble, J.F. and Kanegis, L.A., *Clin. Pharmac. Ther.*, 1973, *14*, 852–61

Pharmacokinetic studies on minocycline in man

capsules, hard gelatin and injections, intravenous: demeclocyc-line, doxycycline, methacycline, minocycline, levels, faeces, serum, urine; drug availability, comparison of dosage regimens, single and multiple dose; pharmacokinetic analysis, comparison of drugs; tissue distribution, minocycline

Kaplan, S.A., Alexander, K., Jack, M.L., Puglisi, J.C.V., de Silva, J.A.F., Lee, T.L. and Weinfeld, R.E., *J. pharm. Sci.*, 1974, *63*, 527–35

Pharmacokinetic profiles of clonazepam in dog and humans and of flunitrazepam in dogs

capsules, hard gelatin, injections, intravenous, solutions, and tablets: clonazepam, flunitrazepam, metabolites, levels, blood (dogs, humans); drug availability, effect of drug particle size

Loo, J.C.K., Foltz, E.L., Wallick, H. and Kwan, K.C., *Clin. Pharmac. Ther.*, 1974, *16*, 35–43

Pharmacokinetics of pivampicillin and ampicillin in man

capsules, hard gelatin, injections, intramuscular and intravenous and tablets: ampicillin, anhydrous, trihydrate, pivampicillin, levels, serum, urine; drug availability, comparison of dosage regimen, single and multiple dose

Lund, L., Alvan, G., Berlin, A. and Alexanderson, B., *Eur. J. clin. Pharmac.*, 1974, *7*, 81–6

Pharmacokinetics of single and multiple doses of phenytoin in man

capsules, hard gelatin and injections, intravenous: phenytoin, levels, plasma; drug availability, comparison of dosage regimens, single and multiple dose

Albert, K.S., Hallmark, M.R., Sakmar, E., Weidler, D.J. and Wagner, J.G., *J. Pharmacokinet. Biopharm.*, 1975, *3*, 159–70

Pharmacokinetics of diphenhydramine in man

capsules, hard gelatin, infusions, intravenous and solutions: diphenhydramine hydrochloride, levels, plasma, urine

Nauta, E.H. and Mattie, H., *Br. J. clin. Pharmac.*, 1975, *2*, 111–21

Pharmacokinetics of flucloxacillin and cloxacillin in healthy subjects and patients on chronic intermittent haemodialysis

capsules, hard gelatin, infusions, intravenous and suspensions: cloxacillin, flucloxacillin, levels, serum, urine; drug availability, comparison of dosage forms; pharmacokinetic analysis, comparison of parameters, absorption, elimination process, effect of patient's state of health

Greenblatt, D.J., Schillings, R.T., Kyriakopoulos, A.A., Shader, R.I., Sisenwine, S.F., Knowles, J.A. and Ruelius, H.W., *Clin. Pharmac. Ther.*, 1976, *20*, 329–41

Clinical pharmacokinetics of lorazepam 1. Absorption and disposition of oral ^{14}C-lorazepam

capsules, soft gelatin: lorazepam, metabolites, levels, faeces, plasma; radioactive isotope technique

Gugler, R., Manion, C.V. and Azarnoff, D.L., *Clin. Pharmac. Ther.*, 1976, *19*, 135–42

Phenytoin: pharmacokinetics and bioavailability

capsules, hard gelatin and infusions, intravenous: phenytoin, levels, plasma; drug availability, comparison of dosage regimens, single and multiple dose

Johnson, B.F., Bye, C.E., Jones, G.E. and Sabey, G.A., *Eur. J. clin. Pharmac.*, 1976, *10*, 231–6

The pharmacokinetics of beta-methyl digoxin compared with digoxin tablets and capsules

capsules, soft gelatin, injections, intravenous and tablets: digoxin, beta-methyl digoxin, levels, serum, urine; drug availability, comparison of dosage regimens, single and multiple dose

Jusko, W.J., Koup, J.R. and Alván, G., *J. Pharmacokinet. Biopharm.*, 1976, *4*, 327–36

Nonlinear assessment of phenytoin bioavailability

capsules, hard gelatin and injections, intravenous: phenytoin, levels, serum

Lesne, M., Sturbois, X. and Mercier, M., *Pharm. Acta Helv.*, 1976, *51*, 367–70

Comparative pharmacokinetic study of two pharmaceutical forms of nicotinic acid (in French)

capsules, hard gelatin: nicotinic acid, levels, plasma; drug availability, comparison, standard and slow-release forms

Altamura, A.C., Gomeni, R., Sacchetti, E. and Smeraldi, E., *Eur. J. clin. Pharmac.*, 1977, *12*, 59–63

Plasma and intracellular kinetics of lithium after oral administration of various lithium salts

capsules, hard gelatin: lithium, carbonate, chloride, sulphate, levels, plasma; drug availability, effect of salt type

Alván, G., Siwers, B. and Vessman, J., *Acta pharmac. tox.*, 1977, *40, Suppl.*, 1, 40–51

Pharmacokinetics of oxazepam in healthy volunteers

capsules, hard gelatin: oxazepam, metabolites, levels, faeces, plasma, urine; drug availability, comparison of dosage regimens, single and multiple doses

Boxenbaum, H.G., Geitner, K.A., Jack, M.L., Dixon, W.R., Spiegel, H.E., Symington, J., Christian, R., Moore, J.D., Weissman, L. and Kaplan, S.A., *J. Pharmacokinet. Biopharm.*, 1977, *5*, 3–23

Pharmacokinetic and biopharmaceutic profile of chlordiazepoxide hydrochloride in healthy subjects: single-dose studies by the intravenous, intramuscular and oral routes

capsules, hard gelatin and injections, intramuscular and intravenous: chlordiazepoxide hydrochloride, levels, plasma

Boxenbaum, H.G., Geitner, K.A., Jack, M.L., Dixon, W.R. and Kaplan, S.A., *J. Pharmacokinet. Biopharm.*, 1977, *5*, 25–39

Pharmacokinetic and biopharmaceutic profile of chlordiazepoxide hydrochloride in healthy subjects: multiple-dose oral administration

capsules, hard gelatin: chlordiazepoxide hydrochloride, metabolites, levels, plasma; drug availability, comparison of dosage regimens

Luders, R.C., Maggio-Cavaliere, M.B., Egger, H., Gum, O.B., Resnick, O., Bartlett, F., Gaito, M.J., Soo, A. and Li, C., *Clin. Pharmac. Ther.*, 1977, *21*, 721–30

Disposition of pirprofen, a new anti-inflammatory drug

capsules, hard gelatin: pirprofen, levels, plasma, urine; drug availability, comparison of dosage regimens, chronic dosing; drug metabolism; radioactive isotope technique

Stenbaek, Ø., Myhre, E., Rugstad, H.E., Arnold, E. and Hansen, T., *Eur. J. clin. Pharmac.*, 1977, *12*, 117–23

Pharmacokinetics of methyldopa in healthy man

capsules, hard gelatin: methyldopa, levels, serum, urine; radioactive isotope technique

Swaisland, A.J., Franklin, R.A., Southgate, P.J. and Coleman, A.J., *Br. J. clin. Pharmac.*, 1977, *4*, 61–5

The pharmacokinetics of ciclazindol (Wy 23409) in human volunteers

capsules, hard gelatin: ciclazindol, levels, plasma, urine; radioactive isotope technique

Finkelstein, E., Quintiliani, R., Lee, R., Bracci, A. and Nightingale, C.H., *J. pharm. Sci.*, 1978, *67*, 1447–50

Pharmacokinetics of oral cephalosporins: cephradine and cephalexin

capsules, hard gelatin and tablets: cephalexin, cephradine, levels, serum, urine; drug availability, comparisons of, dosage form, drug, effect of dosage regimen; pharmacokinetic parameters, serum, urine

Rodenstein, D., De Coster, A. and Gazzaniga, A., *Clin. Pharmacokinet.*, 1978, *3*, 247–54

Pharmacokinetics of oral acetylcysteine: absorption, binding and metabolism in patients with respiratory disorders

capsules, hard gelatin: ^{35}S-acetylcysteine, metabolites, levels, endobronchial mucus, lung tissue, serum, urine; radioactive isotope technique

Friis, M.L., Grøn, U., Larsen, N.-E., Pakkenberg, H. and Hvidberg, E.F., *Eur. J. clin. Pharmac.*, 1979, *15*, 275–80

Pharmacokinetics of bromocriptine during continuous oral treatment of Parkinson's disease

capsules: bromocriptine, levels, plasma

Palmieri, A., *Am. J. pharm. Educ.*, 1979, *43*, 21–3

An undergraduate experiment in biopharmaceutics: serum and urine bioavailability of ampicillin

capsules, hard gelatin: ampicillin, levels, urine; drug availability, effect of co-administration of probenecid; urine excretion data

Sasahara, K., Nitanai, T., Habara, T., Morioka, T. and Nakajima, E., *J. pharm. Sci.*, 1980, *69*, 1374–8

Dosage form design for improvement of bioavailability of levodopa III: influence of dose on pharmacokinetic behaviour of levodopa in dogs and parkinsonian patients

capsules, hard gelatin and injections, intravenous: levodopa, metabolites, blood, urine (dogs, humans); drug availability, effect of dose

Tanigawara, Y., Yamaoka, K., Nakagawa, T. and Uno, T., *J. pharm. Sci.*, 1982, *71*, 1129–33

Moment analysis for the separation of mean *in vivo* disintegration, dissolution, absorption, and disposition time of ampicillin products

capsules, hard gelatin, injections, intravenous and powders: ampicillin, anhydrous, trihydrate, levels, urine; drug availability, comparisons of, drug and product form; pharmacokinetic analysis, calculation of mean absorption, disintegration, dissolution, residence times and urinary recovery

Park, G.B., Kershner, R.P., Angellotti, J., Williams, R.L., Benet, L.Z. and Edelson, J., *J. pharm. Sci.*, 1983, *72*, 817–9

Oral bioavailability and intravenous pharmacokinetics of amrinone in humans

capsules, hard gelatin and injections, intravenous: amrinone, levels, plasma; drug availability, comparison of routes of administration

Groning, R., *Pharm. Ind., Berl.*, 1984, *46*, 88–96

Gastrointestinal passage and bioavailability of oral dosage forms. Application of statistics to description of limited absorption (in German)

capsules and tablets: drug availability, comparisons of, dosage forms and products; pharmacokinetic analysis, statistical evaluation; pharmacokinetic rate constant, absorption probability, relationship to gastrointestinal tract position

4.6.6 Methods of Administration to Animals

Jurgelsky, W. and Morison, R., *Am. J. vet. Res.*, 1964, *25*, 563–64

A method for administering capsules to rabbits

capsules, hard gelatin: dosage administration, rabbits; stomach tube

Brunk, R., *Berl. Münch. tierärztl. Wschr*, 1968, *81*, 203–4

The technique of administering capsules to dogs by means of an applicator (in German)

capsules, hard and soft gelatin: dosage administration, dogs; hand applicator

Conzelman, G.M., *Lab. Anim. Care*, 1970, *20*, 280–2

A stomach tube for the administration of gelatin capsules to nonhuman primates

capsules, hard gelatin: carcinogens; dosage administration, primates; stomach tube

Shani, J., Givant, Y. and Sulman, F.G., *Lab. Anim. Care*, 1970, *20*, 1154–5

A capsule-feeder for small laboratory animals

capsules, hard gelatin: dosage administration, mice, rats, capsule-feeder device

Fisk, S.K. and Soave, O.A., *Lab. Anim. Sci.*, 1971, *21*, 752–3

A device for the administration of capsules and tablets to cats

capsules, hard and soft gelatin and tablets: dosage administration, cats; stomach tube

Stanislaus, F., Schneider, G.F. and Hofrichter, G., *Arzneimittel-Forsch.*, 1979, *29*, 186–7

The technique of administration of medicines in solid forms to rats (in German)

capsules, hard gelatin: capsules, special small sizes; dosage administration, rats, anaesthetised; stomach tube

Lax, E.R., Militzer, K. and Trauschel, A., *Lab. Anim.*, 1983, *17*, 50–4

A simple method for oral administration of drugs in solid form to fully conscious rats

capsules, hard gelatin: capsules, special small sizes; dosage administration, rats; stomach tube

4.6.7 Diagnostic Tests

Beal, C.B. and Brown, J.W., *Am. J. dig. Dis.*, 1968, *13*, 113–22

A rapid screening test for gastric achlorhydria

capsules, hard gelatin: congo red, thread impregnated; gastric pH determination, *in vivo*

Kleeberg, J.J., *Israel J. med. Scis.*, 1968, *4*, 149–52

Estimation of gastric acidity by X-ray

capsules, hard gelatin: barium sulphate; disintegration, *in vivo*, X-ray testing; drug availability, *in vitro*, disintegration; gastric pH determination; protective coating, acid sensitive

Haas, S., *Ann. intern. Med.*, 1970, *72*, 549–52

Contamination of protein-bound iodine by pink gelatin capsules colored with erythrosine

capsules, hard gelatin: capsule colorants, erythrosine; dye levels, serum-bound iodine

Beal, C.B., *U.S. Patent* 3 683 890, 1972, through *Derwent Accession No.* 558437-B, 1970

Duodenum sample collecting device

capsules, hard gelatin: capsule, double unit, small capsule inside larger capsule; capsule solubility, outer one soluble, inner one insoluble; diagnostic sampling device, containing radio-opaque flexible yarn with sampling tube, weighted capsule

Farbwerke Hoechst A.G., *Dutch Patent* 7 210 728, 1973, through *Derwent Accession No.* 11868U-BK, 1971

Radioactive iodine capsules – for thyroid function tests

capsules, hard gelatin: capsule filling, low melting point solid; formulation of contents, diluent, suppository base

Babb, R.R. and Beal, C.B., *Gut*, 1974, *15*, 492–3

Use of a duodenal capsule for localisation of upper gastro-intestinal haemorrhage

capsules, hard gelatin: blood detection, upper gastro-intestinal tract; capsule, size 00, filled, silicone rubber bag, yarn

McDonald, J.W.D., Barr, R.M. and Barton, W.B., *Ann. intern. Med.*, 1975, *83*, 827–9

Spurious Schilling test result obtained with intrinsic factor enclosed in capsules

capsules, hard gelatin: cyanocobalamin; ^{57}Co, levels, urine; radioactive isotope technique

Hoffman, N.E., LaRusso, N.F. and Hofmann, A.F., *Mayo Clin. Proc.*, 1976, *51*, 171–5

Sampling intestinal content with a sequestering capsule. A noninvasive technique for determining bile acid kinetics in man

capsules, hard gelatin: capsule contents, dialysis tube, identification system, X-ray marker; *in vivo* sampling, radioactive labelled bile acids

Directory of Manufacturers

The names and addresses of the manufacturers (or agents) of products mentioned in the text are listed below in alphabetical order.

Anritsu Corporation, 5–10–27 Minamiazabu, Minato-ku, Tokyo 106, Japan.
U.K. agent: Skerman Group of companies, 162 Windmill Road West, Sunbury on Thames, Middx TW16 7HB, England

Bonapace/Zuma, Via Canova 6–72, P.O. Box 1840 Milano, Italy.
U.K. agents: Fred Rogers, 6 Knowle Park Ave, Staines, Middx TW18 1AN, England.

Chemical and Pharmaceutical Industries Co., Inc., 225 West Broadway, New York, NY 10007, U.S.A.

C.I. Electronics Ltd, Brunel Rd, Churchfields, Salisbury, Wilts, England.

Davcaps, P.O. Box 11, Monmouth, Gwent NP5 3NX, Wales.

Elanco Qualicaps (a division of Eli Lilly Company), Lilly Corporate Center, IN 46285–9400, U.S.A.
U.K. office: Elanco Qualicaps, Lilly Industries Ltd, Kingsclere Rd, Baskingstoke, Hants RG21 2XA, England

Farmatic s.r.l., Via Progresso 2/C, 40064 Ozzano Emilia, Bologna, Italy.
U.K. office: Imapak UK Ltd, Coworth Park, Ascot, Berks SL5 7SF, England.

Feton, 799 Chaussée de Louvain, Brussels 1140, Belgium.
U.K. agent: ACM Machinery, Old Kiln House, Silchester Rd, Tadley, Hants RG26 6RY, England.

Harro Höfliger, Helmholtzstrasse 4, 7151 Allmersback, Im Ta., W. Germany.
U.K. agent: Raupack Ltd, 131 High Street, Old Woking, Surrey GU22 9LD, England.

R.W. Hartnett Company, 1021–27 Cherry St, Philadelphia 7, U.S.A.

Höfliger & Karg, division of Robert Bosch GmbH, Stuttgarter Strasse, 130 D-7050, Waiblingen, W. Germany.
U.K. office: Robert Bosch Packaging Machinery (U.K.) Limited, Invincible Road, Farnborough, Hants GU17 7QU, England

IMA Group (agents for Farmatic s.r.l. and Nuova Zanasi s.p.a.), Via Emilia 281, 40064 Ozzano Emilia, Bologna, Italy.
U.K. office: Imapak UK Ltd, Coworth Park, Ascot, Berks SL5 7SF, England.

Kruger, Willi KG, Preussenstr. 56, 4030 Ratingen 6, W. Germany.

Leidsche Apparatenfabriek N.V. (LAF), OS-en Paardenlaan 41–43, Leiden, Holland.

Macofar s.a.s., Via Bellini 6, Sesto di Rastignano, Bologna, Italy.
U.K. agent: B.S.A.L. Agencies Ltd, 2 Portsmouth Rd, Kingston-on-Thames, KT1 2LU, England.

Manesty Machines Ltd, Evans Rd, Speke, Liverpool L24 9LQ, England.
Agents for: Osaka Automatic Machine Mfg Co. Ltd, 7–9–4 Nishigatanda, Shinagawa-Ku, Tokyo 141, Japan.

Markem Machines Ltd, Ladywell Trading Estate, Eccles New Rd, Salford, Lancs, England.

mG2 s.p.a., 18 Via del Savena, 40065 Pianoro, Bologna, Italy.
U.K. agent: Servital Ltd, 42 Bankside, Park Rd, High Barnet, Herts EN5 5RU, England.

MOCON/Modern Controls Inc., Elk River, Minnesota, U.S.A.

Nuova Zanasi s.p.a., Via 1 Maggio 14, 40064 Ozzano Emilia, Bologna, Italy.
U.K. agent: Imapak UK Ltd, Coworth Park, Ascot, Berks SL5 7SF, England.

Parke, Davis & Co. Ltd, Usk Rd, Pontypool, Gwent NP4 0YH, Wales.

Perry Industries Inc., 121 New South Rd, Hicksville, New York, NY 11802, U.S.A.

R.P. Scherer Ltd, Frankland Rd, Blagrove, Swindon, Wilts SN5 8YS, England.

Tevopharm-Schiedam N.V., 13 Rubenslaan, Schiedam, Netherlands.

Index

Page numbers for entries within the Bibliography (pp. 205–300) are distinguished by *italic* type.